NEUROSONOLOGY

NEUROSONOLOGY

Charles H. Tegeler, M.D.

Associate Professor of Neurology,
Head, Section on Stroke and Cerebrovascular Disease;
Director, Neurosonology Laboratory,
Bowman Gray School of Medicine,
Wake Forest University,
Winston-Salem, North Carolina

Viken L. Babikian, M.D.

Director, Neurovascular Intensive Care Unit,
Boston Veterans Administration Medical Center;
Associate Visiting Neurologist,
Boston University Medical Center;
Associate Professor of Neurology,
Boston University School of Medicine,
Boston, Massachusetts

Camilo R. Gomez, M.D.

Director, Comprehensive Stroke Center;
Associate Professor of Neurology,
University of Alabama at Birmingham,
Birmingham, Alabama

with 715 illustrations,
including 115 color plates

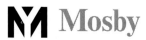 Mosby

St. Louis   Baltimore   Boston   Carlsbad   Chicago   Naples   New York   Philadelphia   Portland
London   Madrid   Mexico City   Singapore   Sydney   Tokyo   Toronto   Wiesbaden

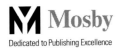

Mosby
Dedicated to Publishing Excellence

A Times Mirror Company

Vice President and Publisher, Medicine: Anne S. Patterson
Editor: Laura DeYoung
Developmental Editor: Carolyn A. Malik
Associate Developmental Editor: Jennifer J. Byington
Project Manager: Mark Spann
Senior Production Editor: Steve Hetager
Editing and Production: Graphic World Publishing Services
Designer: Dave Zielinski

Printed in the United States of America
Composition by Graphic World, Inc.
Printing/binding by Maple Vail Press

Mosby–Year Book, Inc.
11830 Westline Industrial Drive
St. Louis, Missouri 63146

Library of Congress Cataloging-in-Publication Data

Neurosonology / [edited by] Charles H. Tegeler, Viken L. Babikian,
  Camilo R. Gomez.
      p.   cm.
   Includes bibliographical references and index.
   ISBN 0-8151-8792-0
   1. Nervous system — Ultrasonic imaging.   I. Tegeler, Charles H.
II. Babikian, Viken L.   III. Gomez, Camilo R.
   [DNLM: 1. Nervous System Diseases — ultrasonography. 2. Nervous
System — ultrasonography. 3. Ultrasonography, Doppler — methods. WL
141 N4993 1995]
RC349.U47N48   1995
616.8′047543 — dc20
DNLM/DLC
for Library of Congress   95-32584
                                                                         CIP

96 97 98 99 00 / 9 8 7 6 5 4 3 2 1

Viken L. Babikian, M.D.
Director, Neurovascular Intensive Care Unit,
Boston Veterans Administration Medical Center;
Associate Visiting Neurologist,
Boston University Medical Center;
Associate Professor of Neurology,
Boston University School of Medicine,
Boston, Massachusetts

Eva Bartels, M.D.
Department of Neurology and Clinical Neurophysiology,
Städtisches Krankenhaus Bogenhausen,
Munich, Germany

Georg Becker, M.D.
Department of Neurology,
University of Würzburg,
Würzburg, Germany

Edward I. Bluth, M.D.
Associate Head, Section of Ultrasound
Ochsner Clinic,
New Orleans, Louisiana

Ulrich Bogdahn, M.D.
Professor of Neurology,
University of Würzburg,
Würzburg, Germany

Maura Bragoni, M.D.
Fellow in Cerebrovascular Disorders,
Department of Neurology,
Brown University School of Medicine,
Rhode Island Hospital,
Providence, Rhode Island

Rainer Brucher, Ph.D.
Professor of Biomedical Engineering,
Fachhochschule Ulm,
Ulm, Germany

Ramon Castello, M.D.
Assistant Professor of Medicine,
Department of Internal Medicine,
Saint Louis University Health Sciences Center,
St. Louis, Missouri

David P. Chason, M.D.
Assistant Professor of Radiology,
Neuroradiology Division,
Department of Radiology,
The University of Texas
Southern Medical Center at Dallas,
Dallas, Texas

George J. Dohrmann, M.D., Ph.D.
Associate Professor of Neurosurgery,
Section of Neurosurgery,
University of Chicago Medical Center,
Chicago, Illinois

B. Martin Eicke, M.D.
Department of Clinical Neurophysiology,
University of Göttingen,
Göttingen, Germany

Edward Feldmann, M.D.
Associate Professor of Neurology,
Department of Clinical Neurosciences,
Brown University School of Medicine,
Providence, Rhode Island

Asma Fischer, M.D.
President, International Institute of Neurosonology,
University Hospital;
Associate Clinical Professor,
Pediatrics, Medical College of Georgia,
Augusta, Georgia

Cole A. Giller, M.D., Ph.D.
Assistant Professor,
Department of Neurosurgery and Radiology,
University of Texas Southwestern Medical School,
Dallas, Texas

Camilo R. Gomez, M.D.
Director, Comprehensive Stroke Center,
Associate Professor of Neurology,
The University of Alabama at Birmingham,
Birmingham, Alabama

Daryl R. Gress, M.D.
Assistant Professor of Clinical Neurology,
Director of Neurovascular Service,
University of California at San Francisco Medical Center,
San Francisco, California

James H. Halsey, Jr., M.D.
Professor of Neurology,
Neurologic Institute,
Columbian Presbyterian Medical Center,
New York, New York

Anne M. Jones, R.N., B.S.N., R.V.T., R.D.M.S.
Department of Neurology,
Bowman Gray School of Medicine,
Wake Forest University,
Winston-Salem, North Carolina

Sandra L. Katanick, R.N., R.V.T.
Executive Director,
Intersocietal Commission for the
  Accreditation of Vascular Laboratories,
Rockville, Maryland

Roger E. Kelley, M.D.
Professor and Chairman of Neurology,
Louisiana State University School of Medicine,
Shreveport, Louisiana

Morton J. Kern, M.D.
Professor of Medicine,
Department of Internal Medicine,
Division of Cardiology;
Director,
The J. Gerard Mudd Cardiac Catheterization Laboratory,
Saint Louis University Medical Center,
St. Louis, Missouri

Jürgen Klingelhöfer, M.D.
Professor of Neurology,
Department of Neurology,
Technical University of Munich,
Munich, Germany

Volker A. Knappertz, M.D.
Department of Neurology,
Bowman Gray School of Medicine,
Wake Forest University,
Winston-Salem, North Carolina

Arthur J. Labovitz, M.D.
Professor of Medicine,
Department of Internal Medicine,
Saint Louis University Health Sciences Center,
St. Louis, Missouri

Paul Maertens, M.D.
Associate Professor in Child Neurology,
University of South Alabama,
Mobile, Alabama

Marc D. Malkoff, M.D.
Associate Professor of Neurology, Neurosurgery,
  and Anesthesiology,
Director, Neurocritical Care,
Indiana University Medical Center,
Indianapolis, Indiana

Hugh Markus, M.D.
Senior Lecturer in Neurology,
Kings College School of Medicine and Dentistry,
London, United Kingdom

David W. Newell, M.D.
Associate Professor,
Department of Neurological Surgery,
University of Washington Medical Center,
Harborview Medical Center,
Seattle, Washington

Stanton P. Newman, D.Phil., Dip.Psych., C.Psychol.
Professor of Health Psychology,
Chairman, Board of Psychiatry,
Head, Department of Psychiatry,
University College London Medical School,
London, United Kingdom

Shirley M. Otis, M.D.
Chair, Department of Medicine,
Medical Director of Primary Care,
Medical Director of Vascular Laboratory,
Scripps Clinic,
La Jolla, California

Jeffrey M. Perlman, M.D.
Associate Professor,
Pediatrics, Obstetrics and Gynecology,
Southwestern Medical Center at Dallas,
University of Texas;
Clinical Director,
Neonatal Intensive Care Nursery,
Parkland Memorial Hospital,
Dallas, Texas

Gary J. Peterson, M.D.
Associate Professor of Surgery,
Director, Division of Vascular Surgery,
Saint Louis University,
Health Services,
St. Louis, Missouri

Joseph F. Polak, M.D., MPH
Director, Non-Invasive Vascular Imaging,
Co-director, Vascular Diagnostic Laboratory,
Department of Radiology,
Cardiovascular and Interventional Radiology,
Brigham and Women's Hospital;
Associate Professor of Radiology,
Harvard Medical School,
Boston, Massachusetts

Fernand Ries, M.D.
Department of Neurology,
University Clinic Bonn,
Bonn, Germany

Ward A. Riley, B.A., M.S., Ph.D.
Associate Professor of Neurology,
Associate, Public Health Sciences,
Departments of Neurology and Public Health Sciences,
Bowman Gray School of Medicine,
Wake Forest University,
Winston-Salem, North Carolina

E. Bernd Ringelstein, M.D.
Professor and Chairman of Neurology,
Westfalian-Wilhelms University,
Münster, Germany

Jonathan M. Rubin, M.D., Ph.D.
Professor of Radiology,
Director, Division of Ultrasound,
University of Michigan Medical Center,
Ann Arbor, Michigan

David Russell, M.D., Ph.D.
Professor of Neurology,
Rikshospitalet,
The National Hospital,
University of Oslo,
Oslo, Norway

Dirk Sander, M.D.
Department of Neurology,
Technical University of Munich,
Munich, Germany

Jens J. Schwarze, M.D.
Department of Neurology,
Boston University School of Medicine,
Boston, Massachusetts

Michael A. Sloan, M.D.
Associate Professor of Neurology,
University of Maryland School of Medicine;
Director, Neurovascular Laboratory,
University of Maryland Medical Center,
Baltimore, Maryland

David A. Stump, Ph.D.
Associate Professor of Anesthesia and Neurology,
Director, Cerebral Blood Flow Laboratories,
Bowman Gray School of Medicine,
Wake Forest University,
Winston-Salem, North Carolina

Charles H. Tegeler, M.D.
Associate Professor of Neurology,
Head, Section on Stroke and Cerebrovascular Disease,
Director, Neurosonology Laboratory,
Bowman Gray School of Medicine,
Wake Forest University,
Winston-Salem, North Carolina

Edward J. Truemper, M.D., F.A.A.P., F.C.C.M.
Assistant Professor of Pediatrics,
Pediatric Critical Care Medicine,
Medical College of Georgia,
Augusta, Georgia

Francis O. Walker, M.D.
Associate Professor of Neurology,
Bowman Gray School of Medicine,
Wake Forest University,
Winston-Salem, North Carolina

Lawrence R. Wechsler, M.D.
Clinical Associate Professor of Neurology,
Department of Neurology,
University of Pittsburgh School of Medicine,
Pittsburgh, Pennsylvania

Jesse Weinberger, M.D.
Professor of Neurology,
The Mount Sinai School of Medicine;
Chief, Division of Neurology,
North General Hospital;
Director, Neurovascular Laboratory,
Mount Sinai School of Medicine,
New York, New York

Neurosonology has come of age. The book you are holding in your hands clearly proves that the application of ultrasound to the evaluation of the nervous system is now mature and relates to a significant body of knowledge. This body of knowledge is anything but static. Having had the pleasure of witnessing the work of many of the authors of this book over the past few years, I know that the field of neurosonology enjoys a dynamic present and a bright future.

At a time when cost-consciousness in medicine is everywhere, ultrasound provides a less expensive alternative for the imaging of the vascular tree that supplies the brain, and for pediatric neuroimaging. However, to view neurosonology as only a cheap replacement for magnetic resonance angiography would ignore many of the facts eloquently expressed in this book. In vascular work, ultrasound provides visualization of the vessel wall with a degree of detail unavailable to other modalities. Periodic vascular events, such as emboli, and changes in blood flow over time can be best monitored with ultrasound. Newer applications of ultrasound, such as intravascular work, are likely to increase the accuracy and applicability of this modality.

Mobility and flexibility are major assets of ultrasound. The capability of bringing the imaging study to the patient, wherever he or she may be, is particularly critical in the intensive care unit and in the emergency room. Perhaps less dramatic but just as useful is the ability to investigate the status of the vascular tree in an ambula-tory setting. The rapid integration of imaging with clinical findings allows for the best care to be provided to patients with neurological disorders.

It is no pure coincidence that many of the authors of this book are recognized as leading clinicians and researchers in the field of stroke. Ultrasound facilitates the diagnostic workup of patients with cerebrovascular disease by depicting not the damaged brain, about which little can be done, but the responsible cardiac and vascular structures. Prevention of stroke is not just the best way; it is still the only way. Modalities that can be used to stem the harm produced by the scourge of stroke and cerebrovascular disease have a major role to play in the practice of the neurological sciences.

The community of physicians who care for patients with neurological diseases, including specialists in radiology, is indebted to the editors and authors of *Neurosonology* for having contributed a tool that will greatly facilitate their work.

Joseph C. Masdeu, M.D.
President, American Society of Neuroimaging;
Professor and Chairman of Neurology,
New York Medical College;
Clinical Professor of Neurology,
New York University School of Medicine;
Visiting Professor of Neurology,
Albert Einstein College of Medicine

PREFACE AND ACKNOWLEDGMENTS

Neurosonology is the clinical science devoted to the use of various ultrasound techniques to study the nervous system and its supporting structures, particularly the cerebrovascular system, in both health and disease. It is a complex and dynamic subspecialty of the clinical neurosciences that provides a unique diagnostic perspective. As seen in this book, the scope of neurosonology encompasses the study of both children and adults, in outpatient, inpatient, and intraoperative settings. Neurosonology is also an evolving subspecialty, and the introduction of new technological developments is expected to increase its usefulness in clinical practice.

This book represents the culmination of an idea originally discussed during the 1987 meeting of the American Society of Neuroimaging. It then became apparent that there was no single and comprehensive source of neurosonological information for clinicians and researchers. Although ultrasound techniques had been used by physicians in several specialties for more than two decades, neurosonology had not been considered as a separate discipline. As a result, the relevant body of information was spread throughout numerous textbooks and thousands of research articles.

We hope that this book will fill this void and provide a practical source of information for anyone involved in neurosonology, particularly those just embarking on the journey to master this exciting field.

This book would not have been finished without the efforts of our publishers, particularly Laura DeYoung, Carolyn Malik, and Jennifer Byington. We owe them an enormous debt, one which we hope will be partially repaid by the success of the book. With their time spent editing and revising manuscripts, organizing meetings, arranging conference calls, and countless other activities requiring special skills, our respective secretaries and assistants also contributed significantly to the completion of the book. For their invaluable help, we wish to thank Judy Schulze, Mary Althage, Val Pochay, and Michelle Aaron. Mr. Andrew J. Hartley also made significant contributions with his editing of some manuscripts.

Finally, and above all, our wives and children were our true support. They tolerated and accepted our all-too-frequent absences required to prepare this book. To them we express not only our gratitude, but our deep love.

Charles H. Tegeler
Viken L. Babikian
Camilo R. Gomez

CONTENTS

Basic Principles

Physics and Principles of Ultrasound and Instrumentation

Ward A. Riley

A detailed discussion of the physics of diagnostic ultrasound and instrumentation has been provided by Kremkau[1] and an overview of the present status of ultrasonic imaging in medicine has been provided by Wells.[2] This chapter provides an introduction to the basic concepts needed for the study of ultrasonic energy, the important units of physical measurement required for its description, ultrasound transducers, the two fundamental principles from which medical ultrasound instruments derive their ability to provide diagnostic information (the pulse-echo and Doppler principles), image resolution and ultrasound instruments. The basic concepts and units of measurement discussed in this chapter are summarized in Tables 1-1 and 1-2. These tables should be referred to as needed to help clarify concepts and units as they are introduced in the text.

ULTRASOUND

Ultrasound is defined as the propagating acoustical energy that arises from mechanical vibrations exceeding a frequency of 20 kHz. The diagnostic applications of ultrasound use considerably higher frequencies between 1 MHz and 20 MHz. The upper frequency limit is due to a rapid loss of energy (attenuation) from ultrasonic

Table 1-1. Standard unit prefixes

Prefix	Definition	Abbreviation
mega	1,000,000	M
kilo	1000	k
centi	0.01	c
milli	0.001	m
micro	0.000001	μ

beams as they travel through soft tissue. Attenuation increases with the ultrasound frequency. This relationship acts as a practical limit on the depth to which ultrasound can penetrate. At lower frequencies, the ability to resolve detail is severely limited, and image resolution is not adequate to provide useful information.

The average propagation speed of ultrasonic energy in soft tissue is approximately 1540 m/s. In bone and solid media, propagation speeds are much higher (between 3000 and 5000 m/s) in contrast to that in air, where it is much lower (330 m/s). For comparison, the propagation speed of light, radio waves, and diagnostic x-rays is many orders of magnitude higher (above 100,000,000 m/s).

3

Table 1-2. Basic concepts and units

Concept	Unit	Abbreviation
distance, wavelength	meters	m
	centimeters	cm
	millimeters	mm
volume	cubic meters	m^3
time	seconds	s
	milliseconds	ms
	microseconds	μs
mass	kilogram	kg
mass density	kilograms/cubic meter	kg/m^3
speed	meters/second	m/s
frequency	(1/s) = Hertz	Hz
	kiloHertz	kHz
	megaHertz	MHz
acoustic impedance	(kg/m^{2}s) = rayl	rayl

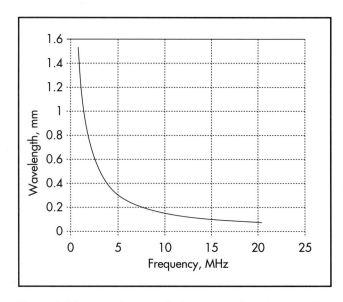

Fig. 1-1. The wavelength of ultrasound decreases as the transducer frequency increases. This graph shows the inverse relationship between wavelength and frequency in soft tissue, where the average propagation speed is assumed to be 1540 m/s.

As an ultrasonic disturbance propagates, a periodic spatial variation in pressure arises. The distance associated with this periodic variation is called the *wavelength* and is determined by the distance traveled by the disturbance during the cycle time (period) associated with one vibration.

The basic relationship between the three important wave parameters (frequency, propagation speed, and wavelength) can be expressed by

$$\text{wavelength} = \text{propagation speed/frequency}$$

or

$$\text{wavelength} = \text{propagation speed} \times \text{period}$$

For example, the wavelength of 5 MHz ultrasound in soft tissue is approximately 0.3 mm, and the corresponding wavelength of 10 MHz ultrasound is 0.15 mm. The general relationship between wavelength and frequency in soft tissue is illustrated in Figure 1-1.

ULTRASOUND TRANSDUCERS

Medical ultrasound is generated by applying a short-duration electrical pulse or high-frequency alternating electrical current to the larger, smooth conducting surfaces of a thin piezoelectric crystal, whose thickness determines the natural frequency of vibration of the crystal. In the 5 to 10 MHz frequency range, the required crystal thickness is only a few tenths of a millimeter. The dimensions of the conducting surfaces are normally 15 to 20 times the thickness.

The crystal expands or contracts in response to the electrical charge applied to the surfaces. When a short burst of electrical current is applied, the crystal vibrates for a short period of time, depending upon the degree of vibration damping applied to the crystal surfaces within the housing containing the crystal. For heavily damped

transducers excited by a short-duration electrical pulse such as those used for high-resolution imaging, the transducer vibrates only two or three times before ceasing transmission of ultrasound. The vibration creates a sound wave that travels away from the crystal.

When the same transducer is exposed to an incoming ultrasonic disturbance, the incident wave causes contraction and expansion of the crystal and induces an electrical signal across the crystal. The induced electrical signal closely resembles the time variation of the incident sound wave. As a consequence, ultrasonic echoes arising from that portion of the transmitted pulse that is reflected and returns to the transducer can be detected and the electrical signal processed in a variety of ways. Information related to the position and motion of the source of the echoes can be extracted using the pulse-echo and Doppler principles described later in this chapter.

Circular and rectangular surface geometries of single-element transducers are used in some applications, and the development of multiple-element arrays for real-time imaging applications includes both linear and annular arrays. Transducers can be focused by carefully shaping the large surfaces of the crystals or by electronic time-delay methods in multiple-element arrays.

PULSE-ECHO PRINCIPLE

When short pulses of ultrasound (two or three cycles in duration) are directed into tissue, echoes can be observed. These echoes are due to the reflection or scattering of the ultrasound waves as they encounter the bound-

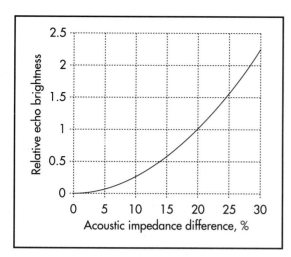

Fig. 1-2. The intensity (image brightness) of an echo from a boundary between two tissues increases as the acoustic impedance difference between the two tissues increases. This graph shows how the relative echo brightness from a boundary located at a fixed depth from the transducer would vary as the acoustic impedance difference increases.

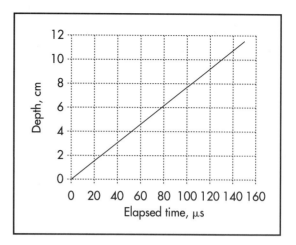

Fig. 1-3. The pulse-echo principle permits the depth (distance of a tissue boundary from the transducer) to be computed if the elapsed time from transmission to reception of the echo is measured. This graph shows the depth computed for different elapsed times, assuming a value for the average ultrasound propagation speed in soft tissue of 1540 m/s. For example, if the elapsed time for a boundary is approximately 80 μs, the depth is computed to be 6.2 cm and the boundary is assumed to be located 6.2 cm from the transducer.

aries or interfaces of tissues having significantly different values of acoustic impedance (mass density × propagation speed). The strength (intensity) of these echoes increases as the acoustic impedance difference increases and corresponds to the relative brightness of echoes on an ultrasound image. The relationship between relative echo brightness and acoustic impedance difference is shown in Figure 1-2.

At most soft tissue boundaries, the echoes are weak, and most of the incident energy continues into the tissue and yields additional echoes from deeper structures. These observations lead to an important principle, implemented in medical ultrasound systems, for locating structures within the body that are not visible from the surface. It is referred to as the *pulse-echo* principle.

Application of this principle requires a knowledge of the elapsed times between the transmission of the ultrasound pulse and the reception of the various echoes, as well as the propagation speed of the tissues through which the pulse is traveling. From this information, the distance from the source of ultrasound (transducer) to the location of the boundary can be calculated with the equation:

$$\text{distance} = (\text{propagation speed} \times \text{elapsed time})/2$$

For example, if an elapsed time of 20 μs was observed for one echo, the distance from the transducer of the tissue boundary associated with this reflection is approximately 1.54 cm, assuming a propagation speed in soft tissue of 1540 m/s. Very short elapsed time intervals can be accurately measured electronically, and propagation speeds vary only a few percent from the average value in soft tissues. Consequently, these calculated distances are

generally accurate to within a few percent of the true distances. Figure 1-3 illustrates the general relationship between depth and elapsed time to a depth of 12 cm.

Due to ultrasonic attenuation as described previously, the echo strength from the deeper structures may be too small to detect. A lower-frequency transducer for which the signal is less attenuated as it passes through the soft tissues would need to be used to detect any echoes at all. This limitation results in a degradation of image resolution as described later in this chapter.

Using the pulse-echo principle, it is possible to construct images or displays that record the relative locations of tissue boundaries within a volume of tissue. The position information contained in an ultrasonic B-mode image is derived from this basic principle. This important type of ultrasound image is discussed in greater detail in Chapter 3.

DOPPLER PRINCIPLE

In addition to measuring the elapsed time associated with each echo, it is possible to measure accurately the frequency of the scattered or reflected ultrasonic signal. If the echo arises from a stationary tissue boundary or interface, the echo frequency is identical to that of the transmitted pulse. If, however, the boundary is moving toward or away from the transducer, a small but measurable corresponding increase or decrease in frequency can be observed.

The change in frequency is proportional to the speed of the component of boundary motion parallel to the direction of propagation of the ultrasonic beam. The

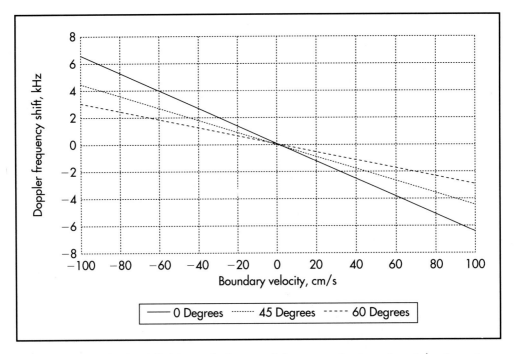

Fig. 1-4. The Doppler shift (change in frequency) from a moving boundary depends on the velocity of the boundary, the transmitted frequency, and the angle between the direction of propagation of the ultrasonic beam and the velocity of the boundary. This graph shows the Doppler frequency shift resulting from a range of boundary velocities for angles of 0°, 45°, and 60°. The frequency of the transmitted ultrasound is assumed to be 5 MHz. A large error in determination of the boundary velocity is possible if this angle is not accurately known.

frequency change associated with reflection or scattering from a moving boundary is referred to as the *Doppler effect.* Figure 1-4 illustrates the variation of the Doppler frequency shift, depending on the boundary velocity and angle between the direction of boundary motion and the ultrasound beam propagation direction angle of insonation for a 5-MHz transmitted signal. When this angle is 60°, the Doppler shift frequency from a boundary moving at a speed of 60 cm/s toward the ultrasound transducer is about +2 kHz. There is an inverse relationship between the angle of insonation and the frequency shifts due to the Doppler effect.

Information displays of Doppler frequency shifts can provide important information concerning tissue boundary motion, including that of blood, which acts as a moving scatterer. Doppler ultrasound is discussed in greater detail in Chapter 2. By combining Doppler information with that derived from the pulse-echo principle in the form of B-mode images, both the position and speed of tissue boundaries can be determined. Systems that simultaneously display both kinds of information are referred to as *duplex* systems.

IMAGE RESOLUTION

The term *resolution* refers to the degree of detail that can be revealed in an image. Two types of resolution are important in medical ultrasound imaging: axial and lateral.

Axial resolution refers to the smallest separation of tissue boundaries along the direction of propagation of the ultrasonic beam for which the corresponding echoes can be distinctly separated (resolved) and thus seen to have originated from two distinct boundaries. Although it depends in a complex manner on many characteristics of the ultrasound system and the tissues being imaged, it is primarily determined by the duration of the ultrasonic pulse generated by the transducer. In general, it is possible to generate shorter pulses with higher-frequency transducers. Consequently, axial resolution improves with increasing transducer frequency.

Axial resolution in ultrasound images can be very small compared to other medical imaging modalities and for high-resolution imaging systems can approach 0.1 mm to 0.2 mm. Because it is primarily determined by the pulse duration, axial resolution remains essentially constant with depth or distance from the transducer. The manner in which axial resolution typically varies with frequency in a high-resolution system is illustrated in Figure 1-5.

Lateral resolution refers to resolution in the plane perpendicular to the propagation direction of the ultrasonic beam. Lateral resolution is considerably greater than axial resolution because it is primarily

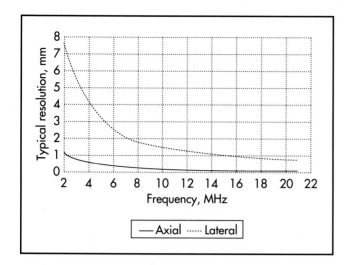

Fig. 1-5. Image resolution depends on many factors but is primarily determined by the frequency and dimensions of the ultrasound transducer. This graph shows the typical axial and lateral resolutions of an unfocused imaging system in the plane located at the depth where the beam diameter is smallest. The pulse duration is assumed to be three cycles long, giving a spatial pulse length of 3 wavelengths. The lateral resolution is assumed to be the diameter of the beam at the depth where it is minimum. Lateral resolution is larger outside this plane.

determined by the dimensions of the larger crystal surfaces, which vibrate. Lateral resolution typically ranges between 1 and 10 mm and can be reduced by focusing of the ultrasound beam. The manner in which lateral resolution typically varies with frequency is also shown in Figure 1-5 for comparison to axial resolution.

In general, lateral resolution is dependent on the distance from the transducer due to wave diffraction effects and beam focusing. At large distances from all transducers, lateral resolution becomes poor, whereas axial resolution remains essentially unchanged.

INSTRUMENTS

A wide variety of ultrasonic instruments that make use of the pulse-echo and Doppler principles are discussed in this volume. They include B-mode imaging systems, both continuous and pulsed-wave Doppler systems, duplex systems combining both B-mode and Doppler systems, and color flow Doppler. The details of presentation of images and displays are varied, as well as the transducer designs. Only two general comments on ultrasound instruments are given here.

Because echoes from deeper boundaries are generally weaker due to the attenuation of ultrasound with depth, all instruments have a method for adjusting image brightness for depth. Referred to as *time gain compensation* (TGC) or *depth gain compensation* (DGC), these methods amplify the returning echoes a greater amount in proportion to their arrival times after transmission of the pulse. This results in echoes from a tissue boundary associated with a given acoustic impedance difference being displayed in approximately the same brightness, independently of their depth. The visual appearance of the image is of nearly uniform brightness throughout, despite the progressively weaker signals from boundaries at greatest depth, due to attenuation.

In real-time B-mode imaging systems, very useful in studying dynamic behavior, an important limitation is placed on the number of image frames that can be obtained each second by the information given in Figure 1-3. When deeper structures are imaged, a longer time is required to acquire and process echoes and thus to form each line of the image. Consequently, the frame rate, number of image lines, and maximum depth of structures being imaged are interrelated. In general, in imaging shallow structures, a higher frame rate and image line density are possible. Typical image frame rates can range from 4 to 30 Hz.

REFERENCES

1. Kremkau FW: *Diagnostic ultrasound: principles, instruments and exercises,* ed 4, Philadelphia, 1993, WB Saunders.
2. Wells PNT: The present status of ultrasonic imaging in medicine, *Ultrasonics* 31:345-352, 1993.

2

Doppler Ultrasonography: Physics and Principles

B. Martin Eicke
Charles H. Tegeler

PRINCIPLES OF DOPPLER ULTRASOUND

The Doppler effect was first described by its namesake, Austrian physicist Christian Andreas Doppler (1803-1853) to explain color shifts in the visible light of double stars. This principle has proven valid for most other waveforms, including sound. As applied to ultrasound, the Doppler effect implies that a reflected or scattered sound wave will be shifted to a frequency higher or lower than the incident frequency if the reflector is moving relatively toward or away from the transducer. When the reflector is moving relatively toward the transducer, the sound waves are compressed, increasing the frequency, and just the opposite occurs when the reflector is moving relatively away from the transducer (Fig. 2-1). The term *frequency shift* describes the difference between transmitted and reflected or scattered frequencies.

Frequency shift = reflected − transmitted frequency

For vascular ultrasound applications, a positive frequency shift indicates flow toward the transducer, and negative frequency shift implies the opposite. The magnitude of the Doppler frequency shift (F) is directly related to the speed of the reflector (blood flow speed) and transmitted frequency and is inversely related to the angle of insonation. When the direction of the sound beam is parallel to the direction of flow (0° angle of insonation):

$$F \text{ (Hz)} = \frac{2 \times \text{reflector speed (m/s)} \times \text{incident frequency (Hz)}}{\text{propagation speed (m/s)}}$$

Depending on the operating frequency (usually 2 to 10 MHz in diagnostic ultrasound), the Doppler frequency shifts for physiologic blood flow are between 0.5 and 15 kHz, which also is in the audible frequency range.

The problem of angle correction

The previous equation assumes that the direction of the sound beam is identical to the flow direction. When the direction of the sound beam is not identical to the direction of the target, the sound beam may be reflected, scattered, or transmitted. At smooth interfaces, reflection will occur, and the reflection angle will be the same

8

as the incident angle (Fig. 2-2, *A*). Irregular interfaces cause scattering in different directions (Fig. 2-2, *B*). Another determinant of reflection or transmission is acoustic impedance, which is the product of the propagation speed and the density of each specific medium. Accurate estimation of the Doppler frequency shift from the reflector speed (flow speed), or vice versa, requires knowledge of the angle described between the sound beam and flow direction, the angle of insonation or Doppler angle. The cosine of the angle of insonation is used to correct for the apparent decrease in the Doppler frequency shift when the direction of the ultrasound path is not identical to the flow direction (Fig. 2-3).

$$\text{Reflector speed} = \frac{\text{Doppler shift} \times \text{propagation speed}}{2 \times \text{incident frequency} \times \cos{(\partial)}}$$

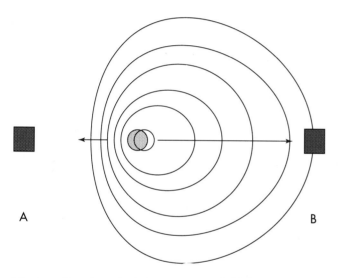

Fig. 2-1. Doppler principle. A spectator is hit by more waves per second if the sound source is moving toward the spectator.

When the propagation speed for soft tissue is inserted, this equation changes to:

$$\text{Reflector speed (cm/s)} = \frac{\text{Doppler shift (kHz)} \times 77}{\text{incident frequency} \times \cos{(\partial)}}$$

In the body the angle of insonation may change dramatically, depending on in situ anatomy. Accurate estimation of blood flow velocity with Doppler sonography requires accurate information regarding the angle of insonation. Accurate angle correction is possible only when B-mode imaging is combined with the Doppler function, as with virtually all duplex ultrasound instruments. To minimize this problem in extracranial carotid applications using nonduplex instruments, it is assumed that the vessel is positioned parallel to the skin surface. The operator positions the probe in a 60° angle as compared to the skin to produce standardized results. However, this assumption is not always accurate, and conversions from frequency shifts to velocity estimates (cm/s) without the ability to visualize the vessel and correct for the angle of insonation should be avoided. A common problem in extracranial Doppler sonography is the occurrence of so-called kinking or coiling. This vascular abnormality, which occurs mostly in the proximal common carotid or in the distal internal carotid, causes the vessel to bend directly away from or toward the skin surface and the transducer. In these cases the previously mentioned assumption does not apply. This bending causes a much higher frequency shift, which may be misinterpreted as flow acceleration due to a stenosis.

In current applications of transcranial Doppler (TCD) sonography, a 0° angle of insonation is assumed. Preliminary work with transcranial color flow duplex imaging suggests the angle of insonation for vessels studied via the transtemporal window may vary to a much greater degree than previously believed.[6] However, at present, this potential variability does not appear to affect appreciably the clinical importance and role of TCD.

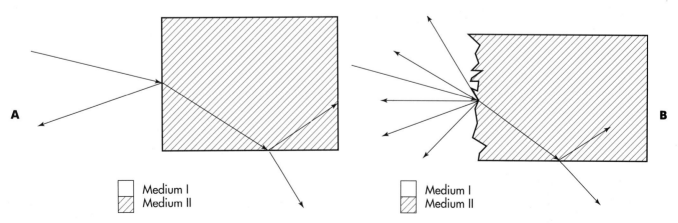

Fig. 2-2. Transmission, reflection, scattering. **A,** An ultrasound beam at a regular interface between two media will be partly transmitted and reflected at the same angle of incidence. **B,** At an irregular interface, the beam will be partly transmitted and scattered.

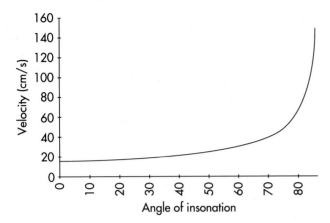

Fig. 2-3. Impact of the angle of insonation on the conversion from frequency shifts (Hz) to velocifier (mls). A specific frequency shift may represent very different flow velocifier depending on the angle of insonation. This example used a transmitted frequency of 5 mHz and a Doppler frequency shift of 1 KHz.

Continuous-wave and pulsed-wave Doppler

When Doppler sonography is the only modality used to evaluate the extracranial vessels, it is usually performed using continuous-wave Doppler instruments that constantly transmit, receive, and process ultrasound waves. All structures and targets causing a frequency shift along the beam are continuously displayed. This type of Doppler sonography does not have a timing element from which to calculate the depth of the moving scatterer, so it cannot localize the source of the Doppler shifted signal. This is acceptable as long as only one vessel of interest is insonated at a given time. Depending on the specific vascular application, information concerning the depth of the insonated vessel may be important. Particularly transcranial Doppler sonography requires depth information for accurate identification of specific vessels. Pulsed-wave Doppler helps to overcome this problem. The transducer can be activated to produce short pulses or packets of ultrasound. This pulse moves away from the transducer at a known propagation speed for soft tissue. If a signal is reflected or scattered back to the transducer, the range equation, which uses the propagation speed and the time for the round trip, can be used to determine the depth of the reflector.

$$\text{Depth (m)} = \frac{\substack{\text{Propagation speed (m/s)} \\ \times \text{ round trip travel time(s)}}}{2}$$

Conversely, the time interval during which any returning signals are processed can be manipulated to allow sampling only from a specific range of depths. This range gate, based on the timing of the returning signal from a specific sonic pulse, can be "opened" to allow sampling from a larger volume of tissue, "closed" to sample from a very discrete point, or shifted to sample from a different depth.

Pulsed Doppler, or pulsed-wave ultrasound devices emit a series of such short pulses of ultrasound. Pulse repetition period (PRP) describes the total duration from the beginning of one pulse to the start of the next; pulse duration describes the length of the pulse itself. Pulse repetition frequency (PRF) describes how many pulses per second are generated (1/PRP). One pulse usually includes between 5 and 30 cycles. The pulsed-wave Doppler device can evaluate a specific sample volume, but there must be adequate time between pulses for signals to return from the desired depths. This places limits on the maximum PRF and fundamentally limits the highest Doppler shift that can be accurately detected. A PW Doppler device cannot accurately determine Doppler frequency shifts that exceed PRF/2. When this limit is exceeded, "aliasing" may occur. This phenomenon results from inadequate Doppler sampling (fewer than two sampling pulses per cycle) and provides erroneous Doppler frequency shift information, suggesting Doppler shifts that are too low or even reversed. This is manifested on the spectral display as a cutoff of the signal and as wrapping around to the other side of the scale. An analogy from visible light is the illusion that the spokes of a wagon wheel appear to spin too slowly or reverse direction when watched with electrical light.

Spectral analysis

Blood flow in arteries does not produce a single Doppler frequency shift as from a single moving reflector or scatterer. The signal received is a mixture of different frequency shift components caused by reflectors moving at a variety of different velocities within the vessel. This "spectrum" of different frequency shifts (velocities) can be visually displayed by use of the fast Fourier transform (FFT) (Fig. 2-4). A variety of spectral parameters, criteria, and indices may then be used to evaluate the velocity and characteristics of flow (see Chapters 6, 7, and 9).

Instrumentation for Doppler sonography

Different applications of neurovascular Doppler ultrasound require different instrumentation. Now three major groups of instruments are commercially available for this purpose.

1. Continuous-wave Doppler instruments are used for extracranial carotid, vertebral, ophthalmic, and subclavian artery evaluations. In many ultrasound centers, these devices are used for screening of high-grade stenosis or to follow known stenoses. In such instruments, one transducer crystal is continuously producing an ultrasound wave, which usually has an incident frequency between 4 and 8 MHz. These devices are relatively inexpensive and easy to use and provide good sensitivity concerning the Doppler signal.

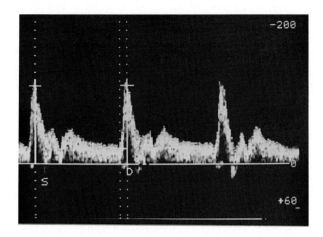

Fig. 2-4. Typical example of a spectral Doppler frequency display.

The major disadvantages are an inability to correct for the angle of insonation or to determine the depth of an insonated vessel.

2. Dedicated PW Doppler instruments are mainly used for transcranial Doppler (TCD) applications. They use a single crystal transducer to generate a pulsed wave form. For TCD an incident frequency of 2-2.5 MHz is used. These devices often have additional transducers with higher frequencies (4 to 8 MHz) for extracranial or neonatal transcranial use. These instruments can sample from a specific depth, an essential requirement of TCD, but still lack the capability to correct for the angle of insonation.

3. Duplex instruments have become the standard for vascular ultrasound. These instruments perform both B-mode gray scale real-time imaging and simultaneous pulsed-wave Doppler sonography. This capability allows visual guidance for placement of the Doppler sample gate in the desired location. Hemodynamics and morphology can be evaluated at the same time, and the B-mode image can help to define accurately the angle of insonation. Thus, frequency shifts can be converted to velocity estimates, providing that careful angle correction is performed. Color duplex instruments provide an even more sophisticated approach. These instruments have a multirange gated pw Doppler function and display color-coded velocity information superimposed on the B-mode image (see Chapter 9). Disadvantages of duplex scanning include a frequent inability to study the subclavian artery and the origin of the vertebral arteries, its greater expense, and the much greater operator training.

Most duplex scanners are equipped with a multicrystal transducer. These 64 to 256 elements are aligned either in a linear (linear array) or circular (annular array) fashion. The crystals gather information sequentially, with each crystal providing a part of the entire image. This is the case not only for B-mode imaging but also for color Doppler techniques. The image is created pixel by pixel and scan line by scan line. Multielement transducers also allow electronic steering and beam focusing. Electronic steering is an essential option in these instruments because these transducers cannot usually be angled adequately on the skin to achieve a sufficient Doppler angle. Without beam steering, the Doppler angle would often be between 70° and 90°, almost perpendicular to the vessel walls with a high risk for false and inaccurate Doppler readings. By precisely delaying the activation of specific transducer elements, the ultrasound beam can be steered to either side, achieving Doppler angles between 50° and 60°. This technology helps to minimize the problems of cosine-dependent Doppler errors by avoiding perpendicular angles of insonation. Even with beam steering, accurate angle correction remains an essential requirement.

SAFETY CONSIDERATIONS

The widespread acceptance of diagnostic ultrasound by both physicians and patients is based on the wide range of new diagnostic possibilities, the cost effectiveness, and a remarkable safety record. However, there are few epidemiologic studies regarding the safety of ultrasound. Those that have been published demonstrate no increased risk associated with the clinical use of diagnostic ultrasound. The most stringent epidemiologic work on ultrasound safety has been done with fetal ultrasound; it has shown no clinically apparent differences in newborns whose mothers had diagnostic ultrasound during pregnancy.[2] Nevertheless, therapeutic use of high-intensity ultrasound as used in lithotripsy emphasizes the important potential effects of ultrasound on tissue. Guidelines for diagnostic ultrasound should be followed to ensure the safety of this method; however, such guidelines may require periodic revision as new applications of diagnostic ultrasound are developed.

Bioeffects of ultrasound

The two potential physical effects of ultrasound most relevant to safety considerations are nonthermal and thermal effects.

Nonthermal effects. The most important potential nonthermal effect of ultrasound is the occurrence of cavitation. Ultrasound-induced cavitation includes both the production and motion of bubbles in a fluid. The term *stable cavitation* describes the oscillation of bubbles with the pressure variations induced by ultrasound. There is no known clinical risk associated with this physical phenomenon.

Potentially of more clinical importance is transient cavitation,[8] which occurs when the magnitude of bubble oscillations becomes large enough to cause sudden collapse of the bubbles, generating pressure discontinuities or so-called shock waves. Transient cavitation has the potential for tissue damage and is used therapeutically in lithotripsy. A secondary complication of transient cavitation is the formation of free radicals[3] and so-called sonochemicals,[2] which may cause further damage to the cell structure or even have a mutagenic effect.[4] These secondary potential complications of transient cavitation have never been demonstrated in vivo. The Bioeffects Committee of the American Institute of Ultrasound in Medicine (AIUM) suggests that transient cavitation may appear in soft tissue at an ultrasound pressure amplitude of more than 3300 W/cm^2.[1] Over the last decade, power and intensity outputs have continuously increased. Power outputs for pulsed Doppler instruments have risen from 10 W/cm^2 to 100 W/cm^2 SPPA.*[1,5] Some B-mode sector scanners now work with a SPPA of about 1000 W/cm^2,[5] which begins to raise concerns about possible transient cavitation. Transient cavitation is not a major concern for conventional pulsed-wave transcranial Doppler, but the growing interest in transcranial color duplex sonography will necessitate continued attention to this issue.

Thermal effects. Heating of the insonated medium due to the conversion of ultrasound energy is unavoidable. Heating becomes more pronounced with increased ultrasound intensities and depends on the transducer frequency. Due to greater attenuation, greater superficial heating occurs with higher frequency transducers, whereas more distant heating occurs with lower transducer frequency. Ultrasound attenuation in bone is much greater than the attenuation in typical soft tissues. Thus, the heating rate in bone can be up to 50 times faster than that in soft tissues. This is of potential clinical interest, particularly regarding both transcranial Doppler of the fetal skull and long-term TCD monitoring. Temperature elevation of 1°C during an ultrasound study is usually considered inconsequential.[1] However, scanning times should be considered carefully in patients who already have an elevated body temperature. Temperatures of 41°C have been cited as dangerous for a fetus.

There are no reports of adverse thermal ultrasound effects with a spatial average–temporal average (SATA; SPTA divided by the beam uniformity ratio) intensity of less than 200 mW/cm^2 (equals an SPTA of about 1000 mW/cm^2).[8] An SPTA intensity value of 100 mW/cm^2 (1

W/cm^2 for focused probes) is considered completely safe for all aspects of ultrasound transmission in both adult and fetal applications.[1] Current U.S. government regulations allow maximum SPTA intensities ranging from 17 mW/cm^2 for ophthalmic scanning to 720 mW/cm^2 for peripheral vessels. For neonatal cephalic and adult cephalic applications, 94 mW/cm^2 are considered to be upper limits. The problem of high attenuation due to bone becomes clinically relevant when the transtemporal approach is used in adult TCD. The greater attenuation requires higher power and intensity outputs to get adequate signal through the bony acoustic window. Ultrasound intensity is decreased by approximately 80% by the skull.[7] The SPTA intensity of a typical transcranial device (Eden Medical Electronics TC2-64B) in water at a maximum power output and maximum PRF (10.26 kHz) reaches up to 550 mW/cm^2. However, the estimated SPTA intensity through the skull, even at a maximum power output level, is well below 100 mW/s^2. Thus, thermal effects of TCD on brain tissue should not be a major concern. Although not reported clinically, the theoretical risk of periostial heating, especially with recent interest in long-term monitoring, remains a potential concern.

Likewise, use of the transorbital window evokes concern for adverse effects on the eye, specifically the risk of cataract formation. By limiting the length of exposure and reducing the maximum power output to 10-25%, no clinical cases of cataract formation due to ultrasound have been reported.

Thus, cerebrovascular Doppler sonography, including TCD, is a safe diagnostic method for which there have been no reported clinical adverse effects. No detrimental effects of ultrasound on adults or fetuses have been reported at SPTA intensity levels below 100 mW/cm^2. Power levels exceeding 100 mW/cm^2 should be avoided if possible, particularly for fetal applications. Transient cavitation has been observed at SPPA intensities exceeding 3300 W/cm^2. Conventional extracranial and transcranial Doppler instruments operate well below this limit, but this may become a concern in the future as color flow duplex instruments become more popular.

---

*SPPA (spatial peak-pulse average) intensity means the value of the pulse average intensity at the point in the acoustic field where the pulse average is a maximum or is a local maximum within a specified region. SPTA (spatial peak-temporal average) intensity means the value of the temporal average intensity at the point in the acoustic field where the temporal average intensity is a maximum or is a local maximum within a specified region.

REFERENCES

1. American Institute of Ultrasound in Medicine, Bioeffect Committee: Bioeffects considerations for the safety of diagnostic ultrasound, *Ultrasound Med Biol* 7:S1-S38, 1988.
2. Atchley AA, Crum LA: *Acoustic cavitation and bubble dynamics.* In Suslick KS, editor: *Ultrasound: its chemical, physical, and biological effects,* New York, 1988, VCH Publishers.
3. Carmichael AJ, Mossoba MM, Riesz P, Christman CL: Free radical production in aqueous solutions exposed to simulated ultrasonic diagnostic conditions, *IEEE Trans UFFC* 33:148-155, 1986.
4. Doida Y, Miller MW, Cox C, Church CC: Confirmation of an ultrasound-induced mutation in two in-vitro mammalian cell lines, *Ultrasound Med Biol* 16:699-705, 1990.

5. Duck FA: Output data from European studies, *Ultrasound Med Biol* 15(suppl 1):61-65, 1989.
6. Eicke BM, Tegeler CH, Dalley G, Myers LG: Angle correction in transcranial Doppler sonography, *J Neuroimaging* 4:29-33, 1994.
7. Grolimund P: *Transmission of ultrasound through the temporal bone.* In Aaslid R, editor: *Transcranial Doppler sonography,* New York, 1986, Springer-Verlag.
8. Kremkau FW: Biologic effects and safety. In Rumack CM, Wilson SR, Chorboneau JW, editors: *Diagnostic ultrasound,* vol 1, St Louis, 1991, Mosby–Year Book.

9. Stark Cr, Orleans M, Haverkamp Ad et al: Short- and long-term risks after exposure to diagnostic ultrasound in utero, *Obstet Gynecol* 63:194-200, 1984.

SUGGESTED READING

1. Bushong SC, Archer BR: *Diagnostic ultrasound: physics, biology, and instrumentation,* St Louis, 1991, Mosby–Year Book.
2. Kremkau FW: *Diagnostic ultrasound: principles, instruments, and exercises,* ed 4, Philadelphia, 1993, WB Saunders.

3

Ultrasonic B-mode Imaging Systems

Ward A. Riley

The major components of an ultrasonic B-mode (B = brightness) image system are shown in Figure 3-1. They include an ultrasound transducer, pulser, beam former, receiver, memory, and image display. The ultrasound transducer was discussed in Chapter 1. The function of the other major electronic components are discussed in this chapter to provide a basic understanding of how an ultrasonic B-mode image is formed.

THE PULSER

The pulser consists of a number of electronic circuits that generate very short electric voltage pulses at regular time intervals in order to excite the ultrasound transducer and to generate a burst of ultrasonic energy by means of the piezoelectric effect. Separate pulses, coinciding with these pulses, are also sent to the receiver, image display, and memory to initiate electronic sequences in the circuits of these components so that their functions can be accurately performed.

A typical timing sequence associated with the pulser is shown in Figure 3-2. Short (less than 1 µs) electric voltage pulses are produced with a pulse repetition period of 100 µs or greater. The pulse repetition period (PRP) is generally determined by the maximum depth of the structures to be imaged and must be chosen so that the next pulse is not sent before the echo from the

deepest structure is received from the previous pulse. For example, to receive echoes from a maximum depth of 15 cm, the minimum permissible PRP is about 200 µs. In systems designed for maximum imaging depths of only 5 cm, about 75 µs is the minimum permissible PRP. Typically the PRP is somewhat longer than this minimum to permit additional electronic signals to be generated in preparation for the next pulse.

The pulse repetition frequency (PRF) is often used to describe the rate of transmission of pulses from the pulser to the transducer. The PRF is simply the reciprocal of the PRP (PRF = 1/PRP) and typically varies from 1 to 10 kHz, with the lower PRF required in systems designed to image very deep structures.

THE BEAM FORMER

When multiple-element transducers are used to permit electronic control of beam scanning, beam steering, transmit focusing, and other dynamic functions, the electric voltage pulse from the pulser is actually sent to the beam former rather than the transducer. The beam former then generates multiple pulses (one for each transducer element) at appropriate times and of appropriate amplitudes to accomplish the necessary functions. An example of a beam former is shown in Figure 3-3; it takes a single input pulse, creates nine

Major Components

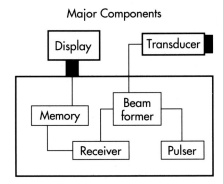

Fig. 3-1. The major components of ultrasonic B-mode imaging systems.

Timing Sequence

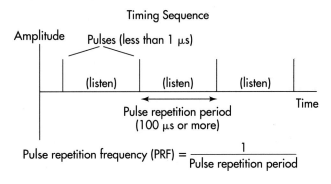

Normal range of PRF is from 1 kHz to 10 kHz

Fig. 3-2. The typical pulser timing sequence used in ultrasonic B-mode imaging systems.

separate pulses, and appropriately delays and changes the relative amplitudes of these pulses so that, when sent to the transducer, they produce a well-focused beam at a given distance from the transducer. As one would expect, the amplitude and intensity of the ultrasound pulses sent into tissue increase as the electric voltage amplitude of the transducer pulses is increased.

In a similar manner, when multiple-element transducers are used to permit electronic control of receive focusing and other dynamic functions, the echoes are also sent to the beam former. The beam former then combines the multiple signals (one from each transducer element) at appropriate times and amplitudes to generate a single pulse, which is then sent to the receiver for further processing.

THE RECEIVER

The receiver performs five important functions that modify the amplitudes and contours of the returning echoes in several ways. These functions are often referred to as amplification, compensation, compression, demodulation, and rejection.

Amplification

The amplifier increases the small voltage levels produced by the transducers in response to the ultrasonic echoes so that larger electrical signals can be obtained for further processing, image display, and storage. This process is illustrated in Figure 3-4. The increase in electrical power achieved by the amplifier (power ratio) is often expressed in decibels (dB). Table 3-1 gives the power ratio in decibels for several commonly discussed power ratios. The power ratio can normally be adjusted by the operator.

Compensation

Ultrasonic attenuation causes echoes arising from deeper structures to have smaller amplitudes at the transducer because of the greater distance they must travel through tissue. It is useful to amplify late-arriving

Transmit Focusing and Apodization

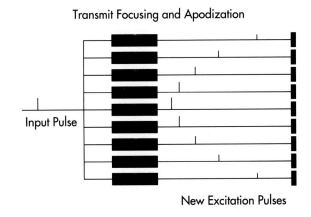

New Excitation Pulses

Fig. 3-3. An example of a simple beam former used to focus the ultrasonic beam from a multielement linear array transducer.

echoes more than early-arriving echoes to make equal-strength echoes appear with equal brightness on the image display. This process is often referred to as time gain compensation (TGC) or depth gain compensation (DGC); it is illustrated in Figure 3-5. In the top row the amplitudes of echoes from identical targets are shown, and they decrease with time due to the attenuation of ultrasonic energy with distance traveled. After passing through the TGC amplifier, which appropriately increases the power ratio with time after the transmit pulse is sent, the amplitudes of the pulses are equalized. This rate of increase can normally be adjusted by the operator.

Compression

The range of echo amplitudes arising from tissue boundaries is very large (approximately 50 dB). Our eyes can "see" brightness levels on an image display over a range of only about 20 dB. The 50 dB dynamic range of the echo amplitudes must be compressed into the 20 dB dynamic range of our vision so we can "see" all of the

Amplification

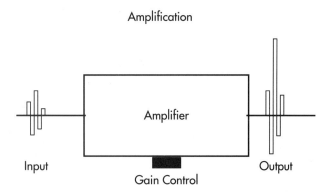

Fig. 3-4. Diagram showing the function of an amplifier in ultrasonic B-mode imaging systems.

Table 3-1. Gain expressed in decibels

Power ratio	Gain (dB)
1 (no gain)	0
2	3
5	7
10	10
1000	30
1,000,000	60

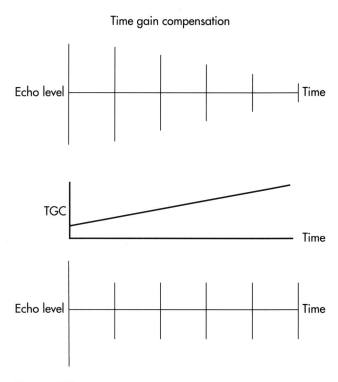

Fig. 3-5. Diagram showing the effect of time gain compensation on echoes arriving at various times from identical targets located at different depths.

echoes on a single display device. The dynamic range of the ultrasonic echoes can be compressed with the use of a nonlinear amplifier, which amplifies the weaker echoes considerably more than the stronger echoes. In Figure 3-6, a graph that illustrates this amplification characteristic is shown. In this example, echoes that are about 10 times stronger than weaker echoes emerge from the compression amplifier only approximately twice as strong as the weaker echoes. Various compression curves can normally be selected by the operator.

Demodulation

We wish to use the electrical signals arising from tissue boundaries to change the brightness of an electron beam in an image display. To change the bidirectional echo signal to a unidirectional signal, the radiofrequency (RF) echo signals are demodulated. This process is illustrated in Figure 3-7. The two-step process involves rectification of the echo signal (during which all the negative going cycles are made positive) and filtering, which smooths the echo contour by removing the high-frequency components of the signal. This unidirectional signal can now be used in forming a B-mode image.

Rejection

Undesired low signal levels from electrical or acoustical noise can be removed from the stream of echo signals by amplifying signals above a certain threshold and rejecting others. This process is illustrated in Figure 3-8. The lowest in amplitude of four signals is considered to be "noise" and a threshold is set by the operator to reject that signal but to allow passage of the other three signals. These three signals will be displayed on the B-mode image, but the rejected signal will not.

THE IMAGE DISPLAY AND MEMORY

To form the B-mode image display, the pulse-echo principle is now used to determine the depths of the targets producing echoes. For each echo pulse, the elapsed time between the sending of the pulse and the receiving of the echo can be accurately measured. If we assume that the average speed of propagation of ultrasound in soft tissues is about 1540 m/s, the depth of the boundary producing each echo can be calculated from the equation.

$$Depth = \frac{(speed \times time)}{2}$$

In Table 3-2 the elapsed times that correspond to various target depths are summarized up to an elapsed time of 200 μs.

A high-quality, real-time, two-dimensional image display must provide about 30 image frames per second or one frame every 33,000 μs. A display highlighting the

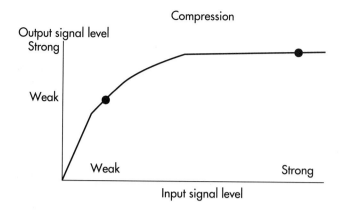

Fig. 3-6. Diagram showing the effect of a compression amplifier on weak and strong input signals.

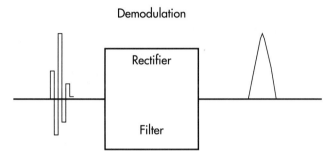

Fig. 3-7. Diagram showing the effect of a rectifier and filter in the demodulation of a radiofrequency echo signal.

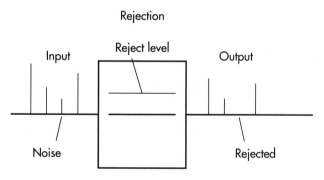

Fig. 3-8. Diagram showing how low-level "noise" signals can be rejected and removed from echo signals used to form B-mode images.

location of one image line is shown in Figure 3-9. Echoes from a 15 cm depth of tissue can be observed in about 200 μs. Thus it is possible to collect information from more than 160 adjacent image lines to make one image frame when imaging is done to a depth of 15 cm. The required frame rate and maximum imaging depth combine to determine the maximum number of lines in an image frame. If the maximum imaging depth is only 5 cm, nearly 500 image lines can be displayed per frame.

The final steps in the formation of a B-mode image are illustrated in the idealized diagrams shown in

Table 3-2. Depth of boundary

Elapsed time (μs)	Depth (cm)
0	0
10	0.77
20	1.54
50	3.85
100	7.70
200	15.4

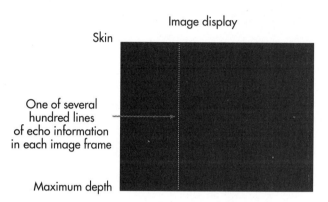

Fig. 3-9. Diagram showing one line of a conventional ultrasonic B-mode image display with the skin surface located at the top and the maximum imaging depth at the bottom.

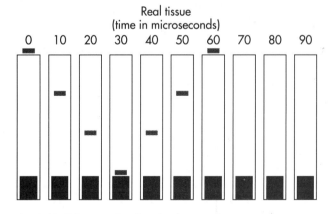

Fig. 3-10. Diagram showing the propagation and reflection of an ultrasonic pulse at successive 10-μs intervals, which should be compared with the corresponding panels in Figure 3-11.

Figures 3-10 and 3-11. The 10 panels in Figure 3-10 show the propagation of a short pulse of ultrasonic energy through tissue at successive 10-μs time intervals. The pulse arrives at a boundary and is reflected at 30 μs. The echo arrives back at the skin surface at 60 μs. This will occur if the reflector is located approximately 5 cm from the skin surface.

Figure 3-11 contains 10 panels, each showing one line of the B-mode image display, corresponding to each of

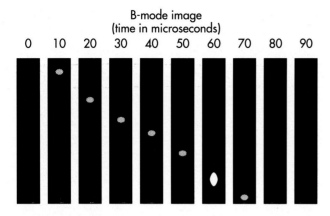

Fig. 3-11. Diagram showing one line of an ultrasonic B-mode image at successive 10-µs intervals, which should be compared with the corresponding panels in Figure 3-10.

the 10 panels in Figure 3-10. At time 0 µs, an electron beam begins to move from the top of the display so that it will move a distance on the display that corresponds to 0.77 cm in each 10 µs. The electron beam is kept very dim (normally not visible, light gray in Fig. 3-11), however, until an echo is received at the skin surface (at 60 µs). At this time, the electrical signal produced by the echo is used to increase the brightness of the electron beam at its current location. The beam remains bright during the pulse duration, after which time the electron beam is once again no longer visible. The "invisible" electron beam continues to move as before until once again turned on by echoes arising from deeper structures, if present.

The amplitudes (often called *gray levels*) of the echoes arising in each image line within very short time intervals

Table 3-3. Gray levels

Bits per pixel	Gray levels
1	2
2	4
3	8
4	16
5	32
6	64
7	128
8	256

(normally corresponding to distance increments between 0.05 and 0.1 mm) can be electronically sampled and stored in digital memory to permit "frozen" images to be replayed at a later time. A typical digital memory divides the image into approximately 250,000 individual pixels (picture elements) and stores, in binary format, the average amplitude of the echoes contained within that pixel. Table 3-3 gives the number of binary digits (bits) that are required to express different numbers of gray (brightness) levels for each pixel. A larger number of gray levels permits a finer gradation of intensity levels to be displayed on the image. Typically, memories are designed to display 256 gray levels, using 8 binary digits, to create the gray-scale B-mode image.

A variety of postprocessing schemes can be used to adjust or filter the relative gray levels in the image to emphasize various image features. Such digital images can also be stored over time to study longitudinal changes in morphology and pathology in studies of disease progression.

4

Color Flow Imaging

Volker A. Knappertz
Charles H. Tegeler

Recently physicians, physicists, and engineers became interested in displaying the vascular physiology of blood flow and blood flow velocities with color-coded images. For many years the Doppler principle has been used to assess flow velocity and to display flow velocities as waveforms. Christian Andreas Doppler originally addressed the color shifts associated with moving targets, relative to an observer (Chapter 2). He described the effect of the frequency shift of a source of waves relative to an observer if either the source, the observer, or the reflector (scatterer) is in motion. Doppler's original observations were derived from the optical spectral changes of fixed stars shifting their emitted light toward the red portion of the visual spectrum, thus increasing the wavelength, signifying movement away from the observer (Doppler effect).[13] Today, this principle is inseparably linked to his name, even as applied to sound waves.

Until recently there has been some confusion regarding the terminology and the usage of the terms *color Doppler* or *color duplex* sonography. Some refer to the color-coded intensity (or decibel) changes in the spectral waveform display, from continuous wave or transcranial Doppler instruments, as color Doppler or color flow imaging (Fig. 4-1; see also Plate 1). Even the color coding of gray scale B-mode images with color (e.g., magenta or rainbow [Fig. 4-2; see also Plate 2]) has been referred to as color duplex imaging. The term *B-mode* may be applied to those images, but when color scale maps are used, the terminology should be modified by a suffix such as B-mode *magenta color scale* images.

The term *color flow imaging* should be reserved for the description of color-coded blood flow velocity information usually superimposed on a B-mode gray-scale ultrasound image of the vessel and the surrounding tissue.

A more recent and alternative approach to depict similar information without use of the Doppler effect and frequency shift is called *time domain processing*. It is based upon pattern recognition of distinct intraluminal targets and the temporal analysis of these clusters of echoes to derive velocity information, which is color coded. The term *color Doppler* therefore is supplemented by *color flow imaging*, which describes the real-time superposition of motion information usually in blood vessels simulating two-dimensional spatial blood flow velocity information.

For clinical purposes color flow imaging was first used in 1983 to analyze blood flow velocities in echocardiography.[36] In 1986 it was introduced to peripheral vascular imaging and in 1987 to general radiology settings. Imaging of the extracranial carotid arteries was

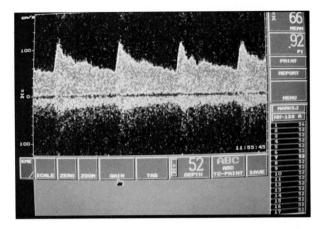

Fig. 4-1. Color spectral display of a fast Fourier transform of the Doppler signal from the middle cerebral artery. Different colors depict differences in power (dB) of the signal. This type of display is especially useful in the detection of high-intensity transient signals (HITS).

first implemented in 1987, and more recently it was applied to vertebral artery scanning.[4,11] Newer applications include transcranial color flow imaging, producing a color flow map of the circle of Willis and the vertebrobasilar circulation.[5]

B-MODE IMAGING WITH ADDED COLOR FLOW IMAGING

Color flow imaging displays Doppler frequency shift or blood flow velocity information, superimposed on a B-mode gray scale image.* Clinicians use color information intuitively. Sonographers trained in B-mode evaluation and Doppler techniques may feel less comfortable with this added information. Most prior training and experience have focused on the B-mode characteristics to steer for angle correction and on high-resolution gray scale B-mode images to evaluate plaque composition and surface features, rather than using color to do so.

Although there might be an intuitive acceptance of the appearance of some of the color flow images because of the resemblance to a mental image of blood flow, an understanding of the physical principles and instrumentation, as well as its strengths and limitations, is mandatory to interpret these images.[28]

PRINCIPLES OF COLOR FLOW IMAGING

B-mode ultrasound imaging takes a three-dimensional ultrasonic data set of a portion of the human body and compresses this information into a two-dimensional display. By adding real-time imaging to that display, the skilled investigator and interpreter then can reconstruct a mental three-dimensional anatomic image and use dynamic information in the analytic process. The addi-

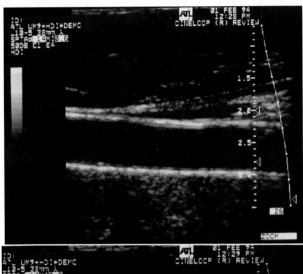

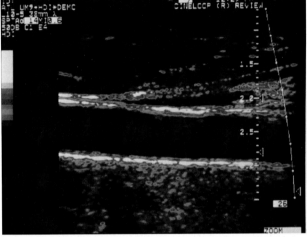

Fig. 4-2. Brightness mode images in magenta (**A**) and rainbow (**B**) maps. These color maps are used to substitute the gray scale map. There is no measurement information added to the image by using color maps.

tion of physiologic information regarding blood flow velocity to the anatomic display introduces another further dimension of simultaneous real-time analysis. Other imaging modalities cannot easily supply a similar amount of information.[31] Dynamic color flow imaging displays blood flow velocities. Therefore, the content of physiologic information is dependent upon the instrument's ability to depict discrete velocity changes in small areas.*

CREATION OF THE COLOR FLOW IMAGE

To create a color flow image involves several steps. The goal is the almost simultaneous real-time acquisition of motion information and anatomic information in a large area of a blood vessel. This involves sampling at multiple sites as well as simultaneous acquisition and

*References 1, 2, 8, 10, 12, 15, 16, 29, 32-34, 40, 46-48.

*References 1, 2, 16, 29, 32-35, 38, 40, 48.

processing of phase shift and B-mode information. The ability to obtain Doppler information at various sites and depths within milliseconds is dependent upon the multigated approach of sampling.[38] A multigated system uses several pulse-listen cycles for each sampling site. It thus obtains Doppler shift information from many adjacent locations, both in width by firing adjacent elements sequentially and in depth. To avoid ambiguity, each site has to be interrogated several times to recreate the phase shift appropriately. This also has to be done serially for each site to avoid range ambiguity. Time is the major limitation and drawback of this method. Time is required for the travel of the ultrasonic beam to the sampling site and for the following listening cycle. As in single-gated pulsed Doppler, information on motion must be detected through changes in phase shift of an echo. This time delay or phase delay reveals motion and direction of motion of a target, with the transducer being the fixed reference point. In color flow imaging, each scan line, or sometimes several scan lines, functions as a pulsed Doppler beam. With the multigated method of firing the beams, various depths can be assessed, although this has to be done serially for each sampling site.[21] Then, each site has to be interrogated several times to reconstruct securely the phase of the Doppler shift.[35] Theoretically, this technique could also produce a spectral display at each sampling site if analyzed with a fast Fourier transform, but there is currently no mode to display that spectral information. The mean of the flow velocity and possibly the variance are therefore encoded in color at each sampling site. After the data have been acquired, they have to be analyzed, processed, and overlaid onto the B-mode image in the instrument. The signal-processing procedure can be twofold: The B-mode and Doppler information can be obtained from the same signal; this is so-called synchronous signal processing. If separate beams are used for the Doppler and gray scale portion of the image, this is termed *asynchronous signal processing*.[38] Most color flow instruments use an asynchronous approach. One of the advantages of this type of data collection is that for most vascular imaging purposes, an angle of insonation has to be established for the flow component, but the B-mode anatomic information is best obtained by perpendicular insonation. This angle of insonation for the color flow (Doppler) portion of the image is created by steering the beams. The center carrier frequencies of the Doppler and B-mode dedicated beams can be different because they are analyzed independently (e.g., a B-mode frequency of 7.5 MHz and a Doppler frequency of 5 MHz). The two entirely different data sets are processed in different memories and are finally overlaid digitally in the scan converter. Because both parts of the image are essentially independently obtained, the overlay process might not completely reach a match. Part of the color flow information might appear outside the B-mode-depicted vessel walls. Computation in most current instruments largely overcomes this matching problem.

INFORMATIONAL CONTENT OF COLOR FLOW IMAGING

The composition of a color map, its vibrancy, its filling of the vessel, and persistence, as well as the shades of color, are all postprocessing features that "smooth" the image and comfort the eye rather than displaying actual measured information from an area of interrogation.

The actual data in a color flow image must be balanced against its aesthetic qualities, the temporal and spatial resolution of flow velocity information superimposed upon anatomic information, and preferably the real-time display of both. This ability determines the quality of an instrument.[28]

Due to physical principles, the penetration of ultrasound into tissue is limited and subject to attenuation and scatter. These principles are partially the basis for how the ultrasonic image is created. Color flow imaging using the Doppler principle is even more limited by attenuation than is B-mode imaging.[28] This is due to the lower reflectivity properties of the blood compared to other tissue, the motion of the reflector, and the high number (7 to 32) of samples to obtain the Doppler frequency shift information. Acoustic penetration may vary greatly with differences in tissue composition, transducer geometry, and instrumentation properties (Fig. 4-3).

A number of factors determine the validity and accuracy of the on-screen representation of a real-time color flow imaging ultrasound display. The interpretation of this on-screen representation, if displayed appropriately, is intuitively easier compared to spectral Doppler information in that it directly resembles the mental concept of vascular physiology. The most important factors affecting the accuracy of the on-screen display are the abilities to distinguish blood flow from wall motion, to distinguish differences of velocities, and to define the temporal relationships of the flow information. These factors depend on the ability of the instrument to discriminate motion, based on the Doppler principle. Spatial resolution is also an important factor. Besides the physical limitations in data acquisition, the processing and handling of this amount of information becomes crucial. A high calculation capacity is required to achieve maximum data display. In a standard color flow imager, each displayed frame contains approximately 250 kilobytes of information. Using a standard frame rate (30 per second), data acquisition results in 7 megabytes per second of information that must be processed and stored temporarily.

In addition, any operator-initiated adjustment, such as setting a focal zone or a color gain adjustment, must

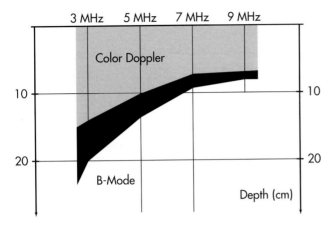

Fig. 4-3. Relative penetration (depth in cm) of color Doppler echoes and B-mode echoes at various center frequencies of the transducer (MHz). The principally lower penetration of color Doppler detection versus B-mode at any given frequency is displayed. This difference is due to the lower reflectivity of blood compared to other tissue, the motion of the reflector, and the required number of samples (7-32) to obtain the frequency shift information. Individual values of penetration may vary greatly with differences in tissue composition, transducer geometry, and instruments.

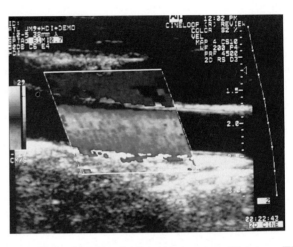

Fig. 4-4. Color bleeding in the common carotid artery. The color assignments signifying blood flow "bleed" over the far wall of the vessel and erroneously suggest flow in this area. Note the clear depiction of the intimal lining and the color flow assignment at the near wall. Bleeding occurs due to low wall filter settings, high color gain settings, long color dwelling time, and high color priority settings.

be translated to multiple parameters, changing B-mode and color flow imaging settings at various stages of the image creation process. The user interfaces in color flow imaging instruments change various settings at multiple levels. For example, if the user wishes to increase the flow velocity information content at a small area within the vessel, numerous changes must be made. Frame rate is increased to improve temporal resolution, which usually decreases the size of the area of interrogation. Then multiple color settings can be adjusted: trade-off between frame rate and color resolution, color gain settings, color velocity scales, persistence time, wall filter settings, and zone focusing, to name a few of the most important. Some systems require all of these adjustments for optimal color imaging, whereas more sophisticated software in other instrumentations allows for reduction of controls and adjusts some of the settings in the background, with the user giving intuitive commands. Expertise in each given instrument and its approaches to image optimization must be attained before color interpretation is feasible.

DISCRIMINATION OF MOTION

Discrimination of motion is twofold: First, it describes the capability of a system to *distinguish moving blood from tissue* (stationary or in motion) within a certain area of the image. It is desirable to depict the blood flow velocities around an atherosclerotic target in a vessel without "bleeding" over the plaque or, by contrast, color coding its comotion with the vessel wall (Fig. 4-4; see also

Plate 3). Second, it denotes the discriminative ability to *differentiate between two distinct but similar flow patterns and velocities* within a vessel or vascularized tissue (compare different velocity scale settings in Fig. 4-5, *A* and *B* of the same vessel; see also Plates 4 and 5). Using a low color velocity scale setting, differences in the central and peripheral segments of the artery are seen. The lower velocities close to the vessel walls are encoded in color. With a high-velocity color scale, there is a uniform color assignment only in the central portions of the vessel. The discriminative power is lost.

An ultrasonic Doppler shift is detected whenever a target in the body scatters an emitted acoustic wave, moving relative to the acoustic source in the transducer. Therefore, a Doppler shift by tissue motion within a certain range of velocities and time might be indistinguishable from a Doppler shift caused by moving blood cells in its vicinity. Such tissue motion occurs constantly within the body, especially close to the heart and to arterial vessels, but also due to respiration, bowel motion, and other muscular contraction. This phenomenon is commonly referred to as a *flash* or *motion* artifact. Color flash artifact has various clinical implications. For example, a lower echogenic signal, as in a cyst or other hypoechoic soft tissue, might not effectively activate the motion-discriminating software, thus resulting in the false impression of flow or vascularization. Color assignment in nonvascular tissue is considered an artifact in the setting of vascular imaging but has actually been proposed to open a new sonographic field, sono-elasticity of tissue. This method uses the low-frequency tissue motion displayed by color imaging to differenti-

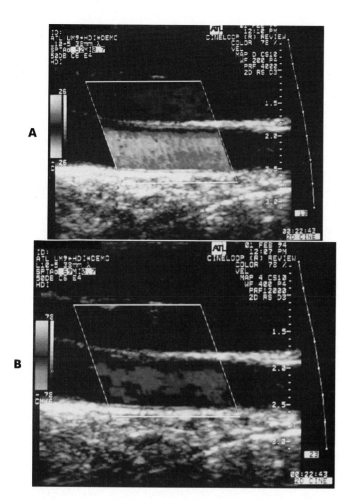

Fig. 4-5. Color velocity scales are + 26 cm/s (**A**) and + 78 cm/s (**B**). **A,** The flow velocities are displayed over the entire vessel lumen. Higher central velocities are seen compared to lower velocities close to the vessel walls. **B,** There is a lack of slow flow detection in the common carotid artery.

ate tissue characteristics, such as tumor from surrounding tissue.[27,37] A small degree of vascular motion over the cardiac cycle, as frequently seen in the carotid systems of younger subjects, leads to displacement of the central high-flow areas over time. Depending on the temporal resolution settings and the enhancement time of the color signal, a displacement or broadening of distinct areas of flow may occur, attributing flow characteristics falsely to certain areas of the vessel.

Most color flow imaging instruments use motion discrimination to distinguish true flow from tissue motion. In the setting of small relative motion of a hypoechoic target, with high color sensitivity settings, as in the attempt to detect residual flow in presumed carotid occlusion, the result is often an artifactual depiction of speckles of color not signifying blood flow and possibly leading to the erroneous conclusion of patency.

An angle of insonation approaching 90° results in directional ambiguity of the flow assignment. Bidirectional color display frequently occurs, and determination of flow direction in this particular segment of the vessel must be attained by shifting the transducer relative to the vessel to create an angle of insonation further away from 90°. Whereas in clinical settings a perpendicular angle is usually undesirable, cross-sectional information including color flow information can yield a better understanding of luminal narrowing. Disregarding velocity estimates and direction, color residual flow can display the functional residual lumen area of a vessel quite accurately.[9,43,44] Additionally, the high sensitivity of current color flow imagers allows for interrogation of minute angle changes around 90°. This may actually assist in the understanding of physiologic flow patterns, such as plug flow, parabolic flow, helical flow, and flow reversal.[18]

TEMPORAL RESOLUTION

The goal of color flow imaging is to attain what is called real-time information. This is largely dependent on the ability to generate multiple images per second. Due to the length and distribution of the cardiac cycle, 20 to 50 frames per second are desirable. Such high frame rates are harder to attain in color imaging than in B-mode imaging; unlike in B-mode imaging, where one pulse echo cycle is sufficient for creating one scan line, a color scan line is created by interrogating motion of blood in the interval between pulses. The number of lines per frame, number of focus areas, and the frame rate all multiplicatively constitute the pulse repetition frequency (PRF). Because time is required for the travel of an ultrasonic beam in tissue (i.e., 13 μs/cm on average), PRF cannot exceed certain values and also trades off depth of penetration if avoiding temporal spatial ambiguity of the echoes. To calculate frequency shifts over a scan line, the instrument must store each scan line and compare it to typically 7 to 32 repeated measurements along that scan line to obtain the desired frequency shift information. The paradigm of the fast Fourier transform (FFT) inherits the uncertainty between accuracy and frequency of multiple sampling, thus resulting in a more exact estimate of velocity with higher frequency of interrogation of a particular scan line.[6,20,28] The spectral display obtained by the FFT is not suitable for implementation with color flow imaging because there is no way to depict the two-dimensional display of this spectral analysis in color-coded flow information. Therefore, an analysis technique called *autocorrelation* is utilized in most color flow imaging instruments. By this method each echo is compared to the corresponding echo of the previous pulse, thus yielding frequency shift information transformable in motion.[20] Each pixel on the color display is encoded with information on direction, mean frequency shift, and possibly variance of frequency shift (see Fig. 4-6 for a color map encoding for

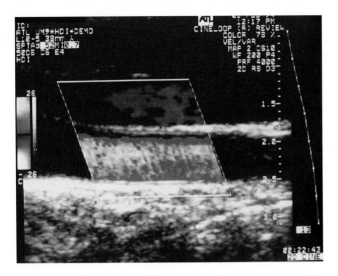

Fig. 4-6. Color velocity scale map encoding for variance. This color map displays velocity information from dark red to light yellow. Increases in the variance of the displayed mean velocities is accomplished by adding green to the color display. In comparison to Fig. 4-4, a slight overall increase in the green content of the colors can be appreciated.

variance; see also Plate 6). Unlike the FFT of one fixed sample volume, the color-coded information does not contain detail on the spectral characteristics but instead provides information about multiple locations within one scan line, although they are only direction, mean velocity, and its variance.[22] Due to these physical and display limitations, potential additional information on flow in the color-coded image, such as width of field and color display lines per second, must be sacrificed to achieve a higher frame rate in color Doppler instruments. Temporal resolution and flow information are juxtaposed, and often one must be sacrificed to optimize the other. They have to be traded off for each other. Frequently, high frame rates of up to 30 Hz are needed to interrogate physiologic flow changes over the cardiac cycle because brief events, such as triphasic flow with a negative flow component at the dicrotic notch, may otherwise be missed in situations of pulsatile flow. The "color box," a region of interest in color interrogation, has therefore been implemented by virtually all color imaging instruments. The smaller the defined area of interest, the higher the temporal resolution and the more acceptable the spatial resolution. Depending on which side of the transducer footprint the elements fire their signals first, a significant time lag between the right and left portions of a color image can occur. A color still frame at a rather slow frame rate setting of, for example, 8 Hz can therefore have a temporal difference of 125 ms between the two sides of the color box, possibly resulting in samples from different parts or different cardiac cycles.[24] Professional interpretation of color imaging can be sufficiently performed only by viewing the area of interest during several cardiac cycles, with knowledge of

the described physical variables. Some systems trade B-mode resolution for temporal color frame rate by doubling color frame rate versus gray scale B-mode frame rate. These complex adjustments have to be software controlled and result in different menus for different clinical settings and organ systems. A "small part" menu or a "carotid" menu is most favorable for interrogation of the extracranial carotid and vertebral arteries and is available with most instruments. For transcranial color imaging, a 2- to 3-MHz probe is frequently used. Sufficient imaging is feasible only with a specialized software adjustment.

SPATIAL RESOLUTION

Color spatial resolution is highly dependent upon the B-mode resolution capacity of a given instrument. The transducer characteristics play the key role in determining this quality. The number of independently operating electronic channels (i.e. independent electronic circuits receiving and transmitting echoes and pulses) determines the lateral resolution of targets by a given system. The transducer has to match these channels to maintain high resolution. Various transducer types are available. The main differences lie in the size of the footprint, surface area, and the geometry of the transducer. Linear array, convex array, annular array, and sector transducers are the most common. For the purpose of color flow imaging, some limitations of nonlinear array transducers are pertinent. Curved-array transducer geometry trades off the favorable increased field of vision with accuracy in flow velocity estimation due to increase of element-to-element scan line angle. Such transducers also have less lateral resolution in the far field.

A theoretical limitation of color spatial resolution is the inverse relationship between the optimal B-mode imaging beam width and the corresponding color imaging beam width. As apparent from spectral Doppler, the size of the sample volume (also sample gate) is directly related to the signal-to-noise ratio in moving targets.[35] The echo of a moving target through a certain beam width produces various amplitudes as it enters and exits the beam. The thinner the beam width, however, the faster this amplitude change is going to occur and the greater the ambiguity of the calculation. This ambiguity between B-mode and color flow imaging resolution might account for the overestimation in measurement of the area of cardiac jets compared to cineangiographic estimates.[17] Some of these trade-offs might be overcome by using the time-domain method of color velocity imaging, which uses the same scan lines for both flow velocity and B-mode imaging information.

COLOR ASSIGNMENT AND GREEN TAGGING

Contemporary color-imaging instruments present a wide variety of color maps, although each of them is limited to display of direction, mean, and possibly variance of relative flow velocity. Frequently, color maps employ two different assignment approaches, first, color changes from one color (e.g. blue), often used by convention for flow toward the probe (positive Doppler shift), to another color (e.g. red) used to depict flow away from the probe (negative Doppler shift). By progressively mixing another color (e.g., green) to the basic color, an impression of a spectral color change (e.g., from blue to lighter blue to green, yellow, and over orange to red) can be created (Fig. 4-5). The second color map approach changes the saturation or the brightness of color to signify different relative frequency or velocity changes. This creates the visual image of more intense flow where there is a higher relative velocity. A third, less frequently used method is to add a color (e.g., green) to the lateral aspect of the color continuous brightness and saturation color bar to signify increase in variance of mean flow velocities in a certain area within the vessel (Fig. 4-6).

An additional method called *velocity tagging,* or, due to the preferred color, green tagging, is available in some instruments.[20] Any chosen range of velocities can be selected and displayed in this color. To demonstrate areas above a critical velocity, for example, all these desired velocities can be green tagged (Fig. 4-7; see also Plates 7 and 8). To depict areas of low flow or zones of flow reversal, velocities close to the baseline can be chosen. This method has some potential to enhance visually and highlight specific features, especially on a still image.

It must be understood that color assignment is a subjective, user-dependent variable, which by itself does not enhance the underlying physical measurement information. For each physiologic and pathologic application, the user has to choose from the abundance of possibilities to try to read the information contained in the color image.

ENHANCING THE COLOR IMAGE

To smooth the appearance of a real-time color flow image, many systems allow the operator to use various time intervals in which the system totally renews the color information. Typically, a dwelling time of 100 to 400 μs is chosen to create the impression of a continuous color filling, or an averaging of multiple frames is implemented. Most instruments allow the accumulation of color information over time. By doing so, the temporal information of color imaging is compromised and substituted for a better color filling of the vessel. At each given time of the cardiac cycle, velocities vary greatly in the vessel. Summation has some potential to create an impression of all velocities over this period of time, although high-flow velocities tend to override low-velocity areas (Fig. 4-8; see also Plates 9 to 13). For many clinical purposes, this seems justified and may facilitate the understanding of the underlying pathophysiology. If

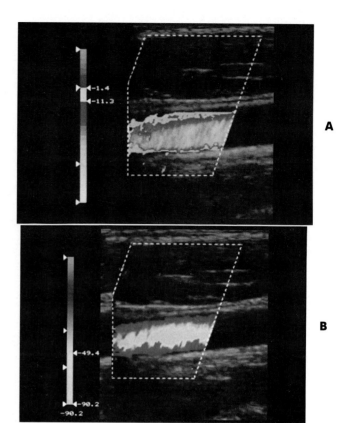

Fig. 4-7. Velocity tagging or green tagging is used in these color flow images. **A,** Low flow velocities ranging from −1.4 to −11.3 cm/s (if angle of insonation and angle of flow are 60° at that area in the vessel). **B,** Areas of higher flow velocities between 49.4 and 90.2 cm/s in the center of the vessel.

quantified analysis of color information is desired, enhancement modes cannot be used.

COLOR ARTIFACTS
Inadequate instrument settings; gain settings

Excessive gain settings mimic, in analogy to spectral Doppler waveforms, the spectral broadening seen in disturbed flow beyond a stenotic segment of the vessel. The color display then contains a variety of frequency shifts within one segment, creating the impression of disturbed, nonlaminar flow. This can also overload the directional circuitry, as observed in spectral Doppler displays, creating a so-called mirror image of the depicted color flow.[19]

Visual control of color gain settings is fairly easy to achieve. Despite this, caution has to be taken not to "undergain" the image. A minimal amount of background noise should be present to ensure adequate color sensitivity. (Not all so-called noise actually resembles noise. Tissue perfusion and tissue motion may well be detected. Focusing only on the preconceived vessel of interrogation might leave out important information.)

When Doppler settings are too low, Doppler shifts may be incompletely displayed or not displayed at all.

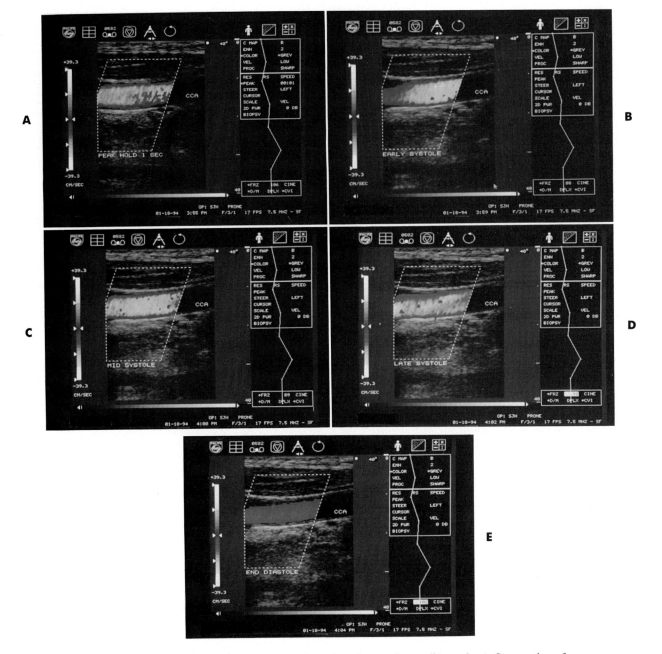

Fig. 4-8. Color velocity summation and single frames over the cardiac cycle. **A,** Summation of color flow velocities over 1 second. **B,** A still frame at early systole; **C,** mid-systole; **D,** late systole; **E,** end diastole. Note how in the early still frame there is still the diastolic component of the previous cardiac cycle visible to the left of the color box. The summation image does not quite reach the peak velocity display as seen in the mid-systole image.

Areas of slow-flow velocities might thus be missed entirely. Gain and velocity scale settings (pulse repetition frequency) must be adjusted to suit the clinical situation being studied (see Fig. 4-5 for various PRF settings in the same vessel). In a suspected pseudo-occlusion or subtotal occlusion of the internal carotid artery, for example, a high color gain, low velocity (pulse repetition frequency) setting might be able to detect minimal residual flow. Similar settings are undesirable in a normal or high flow velocity situation.

Aliasing and color aliasing; angle dependency

Aliasing can occur in pulsed ultrasound studies, mainly in Doppler-based systems (see Chapter 5). Aliasing resembles an artifactual display of frequency shifts, resulting in false velocity readings (Figs. 4-9 and 4-10; see also Plates 14 and 15). If the detected frequency shift exceeds half of the pulse repetition frequency (PRF), which is called the *Nyquist frequency* or *limit,* the reconstruction and display of the frequency or time shift become ambiguous, resulting in false low readings of the

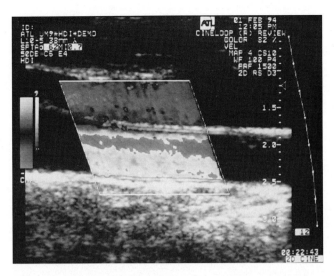

Fig. 4-9. Aliasing in a normal common carotid artery. Jugular vein above; common carotid artery below. Relative flow velocities exceeding 9 cm/s are displayed in cyan. Note how the lower-flow velocities in the jugular vein do not alias.

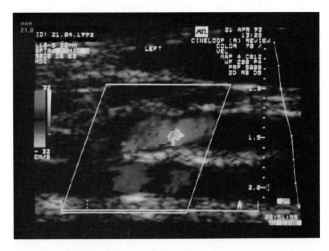

Fig. 4-10. Retrograde flow in the external carotid artery in a common carotid artery occlusion. The upper signal in the color image aliases from cyan to yellow and up to red color codes. It then unaliases "going backward" through the colors red, yellow, cyan, and back to blue.

actual frequency shift.[3] Frequently the spectral display of an aliased signal cluster appears to be cut off at the level of the Nyquist limit and is inserted below the baseline as an inverted Doppler shift.[39]

This phenomenon of aliasing is inherent in the single-gated pulsed-signal echo approach. It therefore equally applies to color-imaging systems that use this method. Color Doppler instruments usually display the frequency shift readings in velocities (i.e., cm/s) to the left of the screen in form of a color bar. The mean velocities displayed here are calculated by using the Doppler equation and assuming an angle of 0°.

Without adequate angle correction, the color velocity reading on the bar does not reflect the real mean velocity. Color aliasing occurs in the form of a wrap-around on the color bar. The color bar can be understood as a linear representation of a three-dimensional circular band. If the upper limit (Nyquist velocity) of the color band is reached and the velocities exceed this limit, the display will switch from the top color of the bar to the bottom color of the bar and display the area in which these velocities occur as high inverted Doppler shifts (Fig. 4-9). If the reverse occurs with normalization of blood flow velocities (e.g., distal to a stenotic segment), this is called *unaliasing* (Fig. 4-10). As opposed to aliasing, color assignments in true flow reversal or change in angle progress through medium-fast velocity colors to slow velocity colors and eventually cross through zero velocity colors (often encoded in black) to inverted low velocity colors, and so forth (Fig. 4-11; see also Plates 16 and 17). These changes in color assignment are not velocity changes but actual directional changes in blood flow. The color assignment signifying true flow reversal—changes in the angle of a vessel or of the

direction of flow in a vessel—is best visually conceived as a stepwise change of color from, for example, the middle of the upper portion of a color bar through the middle of the lower portion of a color bar (Fig. 4-12, aliasing and true flow reversal in the same segment of one vessel; see also Plates 18 and 19). By color interpretation alone, aliasing and true flow reversal can be distinguished on the basis of the different direction of color change over the color bar display. In contrast, true flow reversal and angle-dependent pseudoreversal of flow may be hard to distinguish. This may be especially troubling in the area of the carotid bifurcation, where analysis of flow patterns may be jeopardized by this ambiguity.[45]

In order to obtain accurate information from current high-resolution color flow imaging instruments, precise correction for the angle of insonation is crucial, particularly in areas of change in the direction of flow or anatomic dilatation. Because it is a cosine function, small errors of angle correction such as 3° only marginally influence velocity readings, as long as the angle of insonation is below 65°. With increasing angles, the effect of such an inaccuracy becomes more pronounced so that at 80° the error of the velocity estimate is 30% (Fig. 4-13). Minute changes in the angle of a vessel can result in color assignment reversal (from blue to red) with relative Doppler shifts toward and away from the probe, visually simulating flow reversal.[24] Interpretation of color changes is also complicated by nonlinear array transducer geometry, for which the angulation of the pulse line can lead to erroneous color assignments (Fig. 4-14; see also Plate 20).

Color aliasing can be used to highlight areas of increased velocity or disturbed flow and may help to identify better the functional flow velocity dynamics in

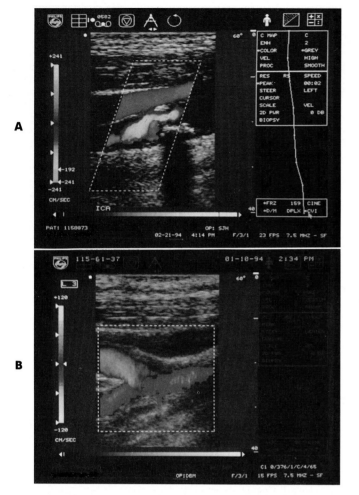

A

B

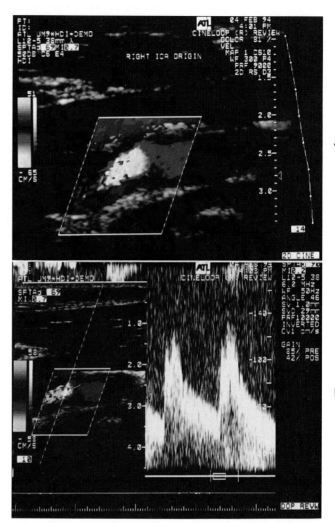

A

B

Fig. 4-11. A, True flow reversal distal to a stenotic segment in the internal carotid artery. Note the change in color assignment from yellow to darker red to black to dark blue to midblue. **B,** Pseudoflow reversal due to change in angle. The color assignment changes follow the same pattern as above. In small areas angle-dependent color changes and true flow reversal might be indistinguishable.

the vicinity of a stenotic plaque. Such information may identify the optimal region for pulsed Doppler measurements (as in Fig. 4-12). Lower pulse repetition frequency settings may improve the filling in of the color assignment over adjacent areas with lower flow velocities, thus increasing color sensitivity in these regions (compare Fig. 4-5 and Fig. 4-9).

Mirror image artifact

Mirror image artifact is often seen in gray scale B-mode imaging. It occurs due to the temporal ambiguity—and the temporal delay—that occurs in specular reflection. If a true target is encountered by a pulsed beam directly, the echo arrival time yields the correct depth. If this same target is encountered by a reflected beam off a strong specular reflector, the later echo arrival time causes the instrument to construct a

Fig. 4-12. Aliasing and true flow reversal in the same segment of a carotid artery. **A,** In the center of the mildly stenotic stenotic jet, areas of cyan indicate aliasing to higher relative flow velocities. Distal to the plaque and inferior to the jet, an area of true flow reversal is noted (color assignment from dark red through black to dark blue). **B,** Color aliasing in the color box with changes from red over yellow and wrap around to cyan. Note that the Doppler spectral waveform display (to the right of the image) does not alias with its baseline at the bottom of the scale.

mirror image with a proportionally deeper location in the image. This image suggests a mirrored image with a proportionally deeper location in the image. This image suggests a mirrored image over the reflector. Mirror images can also occur in color flow imaging of vasculature adjacent to strong reflectors.[23] The subclavian artery mirror image artifact occurs because of its proximity to the pleura-lung interface, which is a strong reflector. The false image then appears to be located intrathoracically (Fig. 4-15). Similar mirror images occur in carotid imaging. The far wall of the common carotid artery may serve as a specular reflector with a mirror

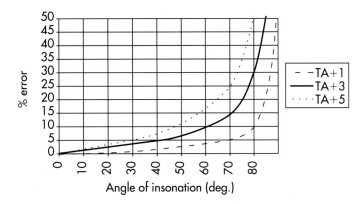

Fig. 4-13. Graph illustrates error in velocity readings in percent at all angles of insonation for deviation from the true angle (TA) of insonation at 1°, 3°, and 5° overestimation. These values are derived from the cosine function and Doppler formula and are therefore theoretical.

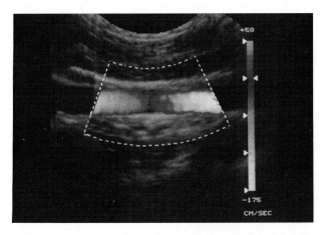

Fig. 4-14. Color assignment changes in a straight vessel due to changes in angle of insonation with different angles of interception in a nonlinear array transducer.

image displayed deep to the vessel. Mirror images might be eliminated by changing the angle of insonation or by different power and gain settings. Under unfavorable conditions, the mirror image might be more prominent than the true image and can be distinguished only by detailed knowledge of regional anatomy, common variations, and the expected ultrasound appearances.[19,26,30,41]

Grating and side lobe artifact

In electronically focused phased-array transducers, additional beams out of the field of the main beam may occur. Each element in such a transducer resembles an aperture through which a source beam is fired. Besides the central beam, diffraction causes side beams or side lobes to occur. They broaden the central beam. They result in echoes out of the intended field of interrogation, which are usually weak. In linear or curved-array transducers a summation of side lobes occurs. They are called *grating lobes*. If those grating lobe beams hit a strong reflector, they may cause the appearance of an object with resultant mislocation of a target. In regular settings with a perpendicular angle of insonation (color box straight), grating lobes can be suppressed to −60 dB below the center lobe power.[38] However, the size of grating lobes increases with steering or angulation of the color box. Lateral resolution is then diminished in these settings. Convexly curved array transducers are especially susceptible to this type of artifact, as are high-frequency linear transducers. Grating lobe artifact has also been recognized as a problem in ultrasound-guided needle biopsy.[25] Although not recognized in the recent literature, side lobe artifacts might also occur in color flow imaging, if a highly vascularized tissue is interrogated.

POWER DOPPLER IMAGING

Color Doppler imaging identifies the mean frequency shift and encodes it into color to display relative motion. Many other parameters can also be displayed and superimposed on the B-mode image. A cornerstone of using mean frequency shifts is the analogy to spectral Doppler information and the straightforward derivation from autocorrelation. Aliasing is an unavoidable limitation of color Doppler imaging, due to the ambiguity of frequency shift analysis. In low-flow situations, which require low PRF settings, discrimination of noise, wall motion, and true flow signals can become increasingly difficult. Angle dependency of the color mean flow Doppler signal introduces additional ambiguity in certain clinical situations. Perpendicular angulations create a signal void, suggesting the absence of flow.

A fundamentally different approach to processing Doppler signals is the derivation of power (intensity) rather than frequency shift information from the autocorrelation function. Power as data, compared to the mean frequency shift, has a far more favorable signal-to-noise ratio. Noise is generally of uniformly low power. By analyzing the power rather than the mean frequency shift and setting the sensitivity of the instrumentation accordingly, a uniform background of noise will be encoded for low intensity, and true blood flow will display significantly more power in the Doppler signal analysis.[42] The power spectrum of a Doppler signal is the integral of the Doppler power curve.[6] Thus, while the frequency shift aliases when half of PRF is exceeded by the mean frequency, the power (intensity) signal does not alias because the integral of the power spectrum will remain virtually unchanged. Then again, Doppler power imaging cannot display velocity or directional changes.

Its future role in clinical settings in neurosonology remains to be determined. This approach may provide more accurate and quicker discrimination of occlusions versus pseudo-occlusion, power analysis of formed-element or gaseous high-intensity transient signals (see Chapters 21 and 22), and possibly perfusion studies in low-flow areas of the brain (Fig. 4-16, transcranial color-coded power Doppler display; see also Plate 21).

COLOR VELOCITY IMAGING

Color velocity imaging (CVI) is a method used to display flow information with a color-encoded duplex mode instrument. At first glance it appears similar to color flow Doppler instruments. The difference lies in the use of time domain processing to evaluate the time shift of backscattered signals to assess motion, rather than the Doppler shift, and thereby velocity. A geometric approach to display flow velocity is utilized rather than the frequency shift approach used by Doppler instruments. An array transducer emits a pulsed beam and identifies a characteristic shape and amplitude of the backscattered signal resembling the texture and position of, for example, an erythrocyte cluster within a

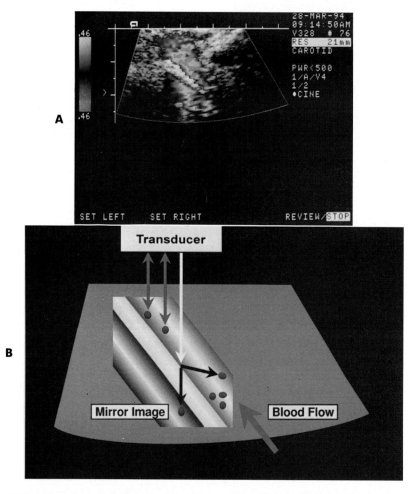

Fig. 4-15. Mirror image artifact **A,** Subclavian artery above the pleural lung interface and mirror image below. **B,** A pulsed echo is reflected at the strong reflecting pleural-lung interface and hits a target on its way back. The instrument assumes this scanline to travel straight and allocates the information deeper in the image, thus creating a mirror image below the reflective structure.

vessel (Fig. 4-17).[49] By repeating this analysis every few microseconds, the stored signature of the preceding backscattered signal is compared to the recent signal signature (cross-correlation). These echo signatures are superimposed by shifting the time intervals until matching is obtained. Small movements of this cluster of red blood cells can be recognized, and differences in signal arrival time can be measured. Thus, the time domain shift can be derived directly from the signal signatures.

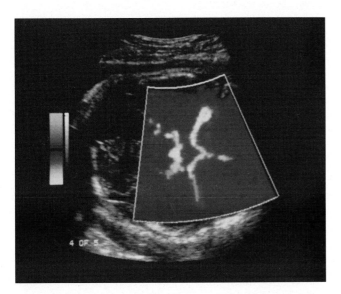

Fig. 4-16. Power image of the circle of Willis. This imaging technique uses the intensity of the signal to display flow. It does not use Doppler shift information and therefore yields neither direction nor velocity information.

Using the known average velocity of ultrasound in soft tissues, the flow velocity is derived:

$$\text{Blood cell velocity} = \frac{\text{distance}}{\text{time}}$$

Because the cosine of the angle of insonation influences the true time shift, much as it influences Doppler shift, it has to be accounted for in the equation, resulting in:

$$V = \frac{D}{T \times \cos}$$

Although this technique does not eliminate the need for angle correction or completely remove the problem of aliasing, it has considerable advantages. Color Doppler instruments must often compromise B-mode scan lines and frame rate in order to increase color Doppler information, reducing the velocity estimate error by averaging a larger number of phases. To maintain temporal resolution and keep an acceptable frame rate, some spatial resolution is sacrificed. This results in the reduction of active color scan lines. The CVI derives both anatomic and motion information from the same echoes, allowing use of all 128 scan lines used for B-mode imaging to create the color velocity image. The gain and threshold settings affect color and B-mode information concurrently rather than trading one for the other. The accuracy of the color-encoded velocities has been confirmed, and an M-mode color display can also be derived to estimate the functional flow lumen and the velocities over the cardiac cycle, yielding a volume flow estimate (see Chapter 11).[14]

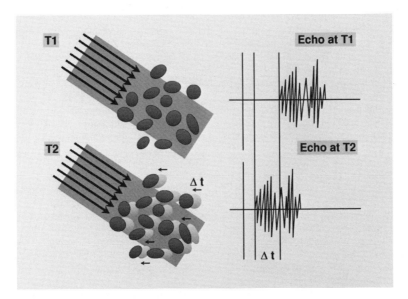

Fig. 4-17. Schematic sketch of the principle of time domain processing. Echo signatures are obtained and matched. If time interval (Δt) and angle of insonation are known, velocity can be calculated.

SUMMARY AND CONCLUSION

Color flow imaging is now available on most vascular and cardiac ultrasound instruments. The color flow display approximates the mental concept of blood flow in a vessel but is only a different way of displaying the physical interrogation. Fast Fourier transform of Doppler data into spectral waveforms yields more functional information in a given sample volume of scrutiny but is a lengthier process because all relevant areas need to be visualized, one after the other. For interrogation of the arteries supplying the brain, color flow imaging is an additional, complementary mode of assessment, which may become a routine method for assessing plaque morphology, identification of areas of high-flow velocities, transcranial real-time imaging with enhanced anatomic information, estimation of volume flow, and detection of low-flow areas by power imaging. The physical derivation of each color flow image must be analyzed and understood before diagnostic decisions are based on it.

ACKNOWLEDGMENTS

We are indebted to Kirsten Spankus, MA, for preparing computer graphic illustrations and to Larry Myers, MBA, BS, RVT, and Dana Meads, RVT, for assisting with color flow image acquisition.

REFERENCES

1. Anonymous: Doppler sonographic imaging of the vascular system. Report of the Ultrasonography Task Force, Council on Scientific Affairs, American Medical Association, *JAMA* 265:2382-2387, 1991.
2. Anonymous: The future of ultrasonography. Report of the Ultrasonography Task Force, Council on Scientific Affairs, American Medical Association, *JAMA* 266:406-409, 1991.
3. Atkinson P, Woodcock JP: *Doppler ultrasound and its use in clinical measurement,* London, 1982, Academic Press.
4. Bartels E, Fuchs H-H, Flugel KA: Duplex ultrasonography of vertebral arteries: examination, technique, normal values, and clinical applications, *Angiology* 43:169-80, 1992.
5. Boghdan U, Becker G, Winckler J, et al: Transcranial color-coded real-time sonography in adults, *Stroke* 21:1680-1688, 1990.
6. Bracewell RE: *The Fourier transform and its application,* ed 2, New York, 1978, McGraw-Hill.
7. Burns PN: The physical principles of Doppler and spectral analysis, *J Clin Ultrasound* 15:567-590, 1987.
8. Cape EG, Jaarsma W, Yoganathan AP: Echo Doppler principles, techniques and applications for the cardiac surgeon (review), *Eur J Cardiothorac Surg* 6 (suppl 1):2-12, 1992.
9. De Bray JM, Lhoste P, Nicoleau S, Saumet JL: Color Doppler imaging (CDI): standard duplex sonography and arteriography of carotid bifurcations, *Stroke* 24:498, 1993 (abstract).
10. De Gaetano AM, Speca S, Summaria V: Combined Doppler US-color-Doppler: physical principles, techniques and hemodynamic considerations (review), *Rays* 16:153-172, 1991.
11. Delcker A, Diener HC: Color-coded duplex sonography in the evaluation of vertebral arteries, *Bildgebung* 59:16-21, 1992.
12. Derchi LE, Rizzatto G, Solbiati L: Color-Doppler instruments: their design principles and modes of use, *Radiol Med (Torino)* 84:523-531, 1992.
13. Doppler CH: Über das farbige Licht der Doppelsterne und einiger anderer Gestirne des Himmels. Versuch einer das Bradley'sche Aberrations-Theorem als integrierenden Theil in sich schließenden allgemeinen Theorie [On the colored light of double stars and some other heavenly bodies. Trial to establish a general theory including Bradley's aberration theorem as an integrated part], *Abh kgl böhm Ges Wiss Prag* 465-482, 1842.
14. Eicke BM, Tegeler CH, Howard G, et al: In-vitro validation of color flow imaging and spectral Doppler for velocity determination, *J Neuroimaging* 3:89-92, 1993.
15. Evans DH: Techniques for color-flow imaging (review), *Clin Diagn Ultrasound* 28:87-107, 1993.
16. Foley WD, Erickson SJ: Color Doppler flow imaging, *AJR Am J Roentgenol* 156:3-13, 1991.
17. Klewer SE, Lloyd TR, Goldberg SJ: In vivo relation between cineangiographic jet width and jet width imaged by color coded Doppler, *Am J Cardiol* 64:1399-1401, 1989.
18. Knappertz VA, Tegeler CH, Kremkau FW, et al: Evidence of helical flow in the human common carotid artery, *Cerebrovasc Disease* 3:11, 1994 (abstract).
19. Kremkau FW, Taylor KJW: Artifacts in ultrasound imaging, *J Ultrasound Med* 5:227, 1986.
20. Kremkau FW: *Diagnostic ultrasound: principles and instruments,* ed 4, Philadelphia, 1993, WB Saunders.
21. Kremkau FW: Modern transducer terminology, *J Diagn Med Sonogr* 6:293, 1990.
22. Kremkau FW: *Principles and instrumentation.* In Merrit CRB, editor: *Doppler color imaging,* New York, 1992, Churchill Livingstone.
23. Kremkau FW: *Principles and pitfalls of real-time color-flow imaging.* In Bernstein EF, editor: *Vascular diagnosis,* St Louis, 1993, Mosby–Year Book.
24. Kremkau FW: Principles of color flow imaging, *J Vasc Technol* 15:104, 265, 325, 1991.
25. Laing FC, Kurtz AB: The importance of ultrasonic side-lobe artifacts, *Radiology* 145:763-768, 1982.
26. Lewandowski BJ, Winsberg F: Echographic appearance of the right hemi diaphragm, *J Ultrasound Med* 2:243-349, 1983.
27. Maresca G, Danza FM, Vecchioli A: Tissue characterization by color-Doppler, *Rays* 16:346-360, 1991.
28. Maslak SH, Freund JG: *Color Doppler instrumentation.* In Lanzer P, editor: *Vascular imaging by color Doppler and magnetic resonance,* Heidelberg, 1991, Springer Verlag.
29. Middleton WD, Middleton MA: Color Doppler ultrasonography, *Curr Opin Radiol* 2:229-236, 1990.
30. Middleton WD, Melson GL: The carotid ghost: a color Doppler ultrasound duplication artifact, *J Ultrasound Med* 9:487-493, 1990.
31. Mistretta CA: Relative characteristics of MR angiography and competing vascular imaging modalities. [Review], *J Magn Reson Imaging* 3:685-698, 1993.
32. Mitchell DG: Color Doppler imaging: principles, limitations, and artifacts, *Radiology* 177:1-10, 1990.
33. Morz R: Color Doppler angiography-technical principles from the clinical viewpoint, limits and possibilities (review, German), *Vasa* 30 (suppl):37-40, 1990.
34. Nolsoe CP, Lorentzen T: Color Doppler ultrasound: principles, technique and clinical use possibilities (review, Danish), *Ugeskr Laeger* 153:3549-3553, 1991.
35. Ommata R, Kasai C: Basic principles of color flow imaging, *Echocardiography* 3:463-477, 1986.
36. Omoto R, editor: *Color atlas of real-time two-dimensional Doppler echocardiography,* Tokyo, 1984, Shindan-To-Chiryo.
37. Parker KJ, Lerner RM: Sonoelasticity of organs: shear waves ring a bell, *J Ultrasound Med* 11:387-392, 1992.
38. Powis RL: Color flow imaging: understanding its science and technology, *J Diagnostic Med Sonography* 4:236-245, 1988.
39. Pozniak MA, Zagzebski JA, Scanlan KA: Spectral and color Doppler artifacts, *Radiographics* 12:35-44, 1992.

40. Ralls PW, Mack LA: Spectral and color Doppler sonography, *Semin Ultrasound CT MR* 13(5):355-366, 1992.

41. Reading CC, Charboneau JW, Allison JW, Cooperberg PL: Color and spectral Doppler mirror-image artifact of the subclavian artery, *Radiology* 174:41-42, 1990.

42. Rubin JM, Adler RS: Power Doppler expands standard color capability, *Diagn Imaging* 66-69, 1993.

43. Sievers C, Knappertz V, Rothacher G, et al: Correlation of color duplex cross section of carotid artery stenosis with pw-Doppler and angiography, *Stroke* 25:749, 1994 (abstract).

44. Sitzer M, Furst G, Fischer H, et al: Between-method correlation in quantifying internal carotid stenosis, *Stroke* 24:1513-1518, 1993.

45. Steinke W, Hennerici M, Rautenberg W, Mohr JP: Symptomatic and asymptomatic high-grade carotid stenoses in Doppler color-flow imaging, *Neurology* 42:131-138, 1992.

46. Sumner DS: Use of color-flow imaging techniques in carotid artery disease, *Surg Clin North Am* 70:201-211, 1990.

47. Taylor KJ, Merritt CR, Hammers L, et al: Doppler color imaging: obstetric and gynecologic applications, *Clin Diagn Ultrasound* 27:195-223, 1992.

48. Taylor KJ, Holland S: Doppler US, part I: basic principles, instrumentation, and pitfalls, *Radiology* 174:297-307, 1990.

49. Tegeler CH, Kremkau FW, Hitchings LP: Color velocity imaging: introduction to a new ultrasound technology, *J Neuroimaging* 1:85-90, 1991.

5

Artifacts

Ward A. Riley

The B-mode image and Doppler information displays provided by diagnostic ultrasound systems are constructed by using a number of basic assumptions about how ultrasonic beams and pulses behave when they travel through and interact with tissue. Often these assumptions are not, in practice, even approximately satisfied. As a consequence, the resulting image or display does not accurately represent the true state of the tissue being examined. These inaccuracies are often referred to as *artifacts,* and they can lead to important errors in the interpretation of the image or display.

There are two general classes of artifacts. In one type, an impression is obtained from the image that a structure is present within the tissue that would be found to be absent at that location in the real tissue. In the other type, an impression is obtained from the image that a structure is absent that would be found to be present in the real tissue. Considerable practical experience and an understanding of the physical principles of ultrasonic imaging are normally required to identify correctly and interpret both classes of artifacts.

This chapter provides a brief introduction to ultrasound artifacts and discusses eight simple but important artifacts that arise in B-mode images. These and additional artifacts are discussed in various chapters of this book as they arise in the discussion of various applications. A more detailed discussion of ultrasound artifacts in medical diagnosis has been provided by Kremkau.[1,2]

BASIC ASSUMPTIONS

A number of important assumptions are made in the design and construction of diagnostic ultrasound system images and displays. Several of the most important are discussed here. Some of them will help us to understand how the simple artifacts discussed in this chapter arise and how they can be easily identified and correctly interpreted.

1. It is normally assumed that ultrasound beams and pulses travel in a straight line once they leave the transducer. In fact, this assumption is only approximately true. The fundamental physical processes of diffraction and refraction can result in focusing, divergence, and bending of the ultrasound beam or pulse from a straight-line path as it travels through tissue. The effects are normally small, but in some circumstances they can manifest themselves in important ways as artifacts.

2. It is normally assumed that ultrasound travels with the same constant propagation speed of 1540 m/s in all soft tissues. This is the average value, but propagation speeds in soft tissue can vary by as

much as ± 10% from this value. Because the pulse-echo principle requires a knowledge of the propagation speed to accurately determine the location of a tissue boundary relative to the transducer, this uncertainty in propagation speed can, on occasion, result in important artifacts.

3. The ultrasound beam is normally assumed to have an infinitesimal lateral dimension and, in the case of ultrasound pulses, an ignorably small spatial extent in the propagation direction. The concept of image resolution is directly related to these assumptions, which are manifestly incorrect in circumstances where considerable image detail is required for correct interpretation of an image. Artifacts related to these incorrect assumptions are frequently present in diagnostic images and information displays.

4. When an echo is received by a transducer, it is assumed to have originated from a tissue boundary located along a line centered and perpendicular to the transducer face. In addition, it is assumed that the transmitted ultrasound pulse traveled along this line on its way to and from the reflecting boundary. Echoes can be received from other locations because of refraction and reflection from multiple boundaries. Thus, this assumption can be incorrect and result in important artifacts.

5. For ultrasound to travel into deeper tissues, reflections from shallower boundaries must remove only a small fraction of the energy from the beam so it can continue to propagate more deeply into the tissues. The ultrasound system normally assumes that reflections are weak and, if this assumption is incorrect, artifacts can result.

EXAMPLES OF ARTIFACTS

Several of the simplest types of B-mode image artifacts are illustrated in Figures 5-1 through 5-8. Each of these simplified diagrams is divided into two halves. The left half shows an ultrasound transducer being scanned across one or more simple real objects, and the right half shows the B-mode image that would result from this scan.

The real objects are assumed to be immersed in a material having the average propagation speed and acoustic impedance of soft tissue through which ultrasonic pulses travel on their way to the object. Echoes may arise only from the boundaries between the object(s) and the surrounding material. The B-mode image is composed of the many vertical lines of echo data received as the transducer is scanned from left to right, with the ultrasound pulses propagating in a vertical direction on each diagram. Reflections from the side and bottom surfaces of the container are assumed to be negligible in these examples.

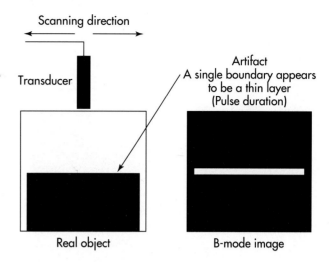

Fig. 5-1. Simplified diagram illustrating the pulse duration artifact. A single boundary appears as a thin white layer on the B-mode image.

Pulse duration artifact

In Figure 5-1, a rectangular object with smooth surfaces and an acoustic impedance different from that of the surrounding material (of a magnitude typical of soft tissues) is imaged. Only the top boundary of the object, radiated by ultrasound propagating in a direction perpendicular to the surface, produces echoes that are received by the transducer.

The received echoes result in bright vertical line segments on the B-mode image beginning at a depth calculated from the pulse-echo principle (Fig. 1-3), using the assumed propagation speed of 1540 m/s and the elapsed time between the transmission and reception of the echoes. The line segments end when the finite duration pulse has been completely received by the transducer.

When interpreted like an ordinary black-and-white optical image, the B-mode image shows what appears to be a thin white layer surrounded by darkness. This is clearly not what the top portion of the real object looks like. The correct location of the top surface of the real object corresponds to the top surface of the "thin white layer" on the B-mode image. The thickness of this layer is an artifact due to the finite duration of the ultrasound pulse.

This thickness artifact would increase if the pulse duration was increased; conversely, it would decrease if the pulse duration was decreased. Normally, a higher-frequency transducer would result in a "thinner" white layer. Axial resolution is directly related to this thickness artifact.

The correct location of the top surface would remain essentially unchanged, however, because it corresponds to the time of arrival of the initial portion of the echo by the transducer. The only real information in the B-mode

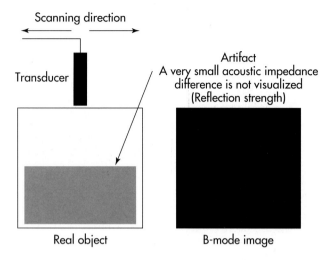

Fig. 5-2. Simplified diagram illustrating the reflection strength artifact. A boundary associated with a very small acoustic impedance difference may not be visualized on the B-mode image.

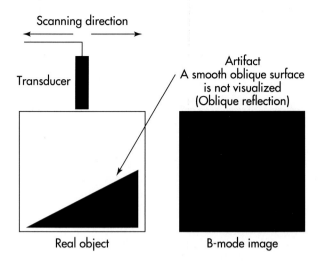

Fig. 5-3. Simplified diagram illustrating the oblique reflection artifact. A smooth surface that is not perpendicular to the ultrasound beam propagation direction may not be visualized on the B-mode image.

image is this location. The location of the lower side of the "thin white layer" is an artifact primarily determined by the transducer characteristics, the ultrasound system, and the instrument control settings.

In high-resolution B-mode imaging of the normal common carotid artery wall, it is not uncommon for the "thin white layer" appearing on a B-mode image — which arises from the echoes originating from the relatively smooth boundary between the blood and the intima — to be interpreted as a representation of the "intimal layer," whose thickness is represented by the thickness of this layer on the B-mode image. This is incorrect, and only the location of the boundary itself can be located from the position of the shallower side of the "thin white layer" on the image.

Reflection strength artifact

The real object shown in Figure 5-2 is identical to that shown in Figure 5-1 with one exception. The acoustic impedance difference between the object and the surrounding material is considerably less in Figure 5-2, closely approaching zero. Consequently, the relative echo strength and brightness of the horizontal lines on the B-mode image in Figure 5-2 are much less than those in Figure 5-1. In fact, to emphasize the effect, the B-mode image "thin white layer" is not even discernible in Figure 5-2. Even though a boundary is truly present, one is unable to visualize it on the B-mode image.

In general, weakly reflecting tissue boundaries may be difficult to "see" on a B-mode image (Fig. 1-2). With experience, one can learn to look more carefully for such boundaries; based upon a knowledge of the anatomy, one would expect such boundaries to be present.

In the common carotid artery, the blood-intima

boundary is often a weakly reflecting surface compared to the adjacent and relatively strongly reflecting media-adventitia boundary. Because of this, it is not uncommon, when the weaker boundary is not well visualized, to identify the arterial lumen as extending as far as the media-adventitia boundary. This is an incorrect identification that is of great importance when one is attempting to measure arterial wall thickness and lumen dimensions accurately.

Oblique reflection artifact

The real object illustrated in Figure 5-3 is a triangle with the top surface making a large angle relative to the horizontal. The acoustic impedance difference is comparable to the object in Figure 5-1.

The echoes from this object are similar in strength to those arising in Figure 5-1. However, because of the oblique (rather than perpendicular) incidence of the ultrasound on this surface and the basic law of reflection from a smooth surface, the reflected pulses travel to the left and are not detected by the transducer. Consequently, because no echoes are received by the transducer, the boundary is not visualized on the B-mode image, even though it is a strongly reflecting boundary similar to that in Figure 5-1. It is not uncommon for smooth boundaries that are weakly reflecting to be absent in an image because precise perpendicular interrogation of the boundary is required for visualization, in addition to the fact that it is difficult to detect the weak echoes.

Ultrasonic beamwidth artifact

The real objects pictured in Figure 5-4 are three objects that are very small compared to the width of the

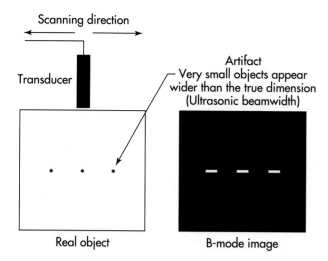

Fig. 5-4. Simplified diagram illustrating the ultrasonic beam-width artifact. The width of very small objects appears larger than their true dimensions on the B-mode image.

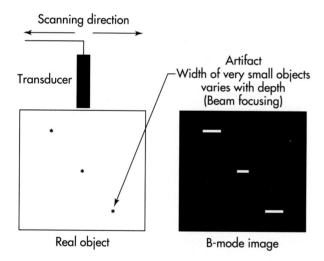

Fig. 5-5. Simplified diagram illustrating the beam focusing artifact. The width of identical very small objects varies with depth on a B-mode image when a focused transducer is used.

transducer face and the wavelength of the ultrasound. The ultrasound is scattered from these objects, and thus receipt of echoes from the objects does not critically depend on the ultrasound interrogation angle.

As the objects are scanned, many positions of the transducer will insonate the objects, and the echoes will be received by the transducer because of the scattered pulses. Consequently, many lines of the B-mode image will contain a white line segment for each object as the entire width of the transducer beam passes by each object. Due to the effect, each object appears to be about as wide as the ultrasonic beam. This is clearly an artifact, and scans of small test objects in imaging phantoms can be used to determine the approximate width and thus the effective lateral resolution associated with the

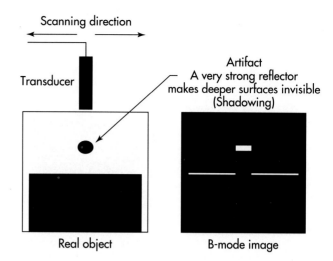

Fig. 5-6. Simplified diagram illustrating the shadowing artifact. A very strong reflector causes deeper surfaces to be invisible on the B-mode image.

ultrasonic beam for the target strength and instrument settings.

This effect also implies that whenever echoes are received from a given depth, all boundaries located at that depth that are also within the beamwidth will contribute to the echo received by the transducer at each moment in time. Consequently, the echo information received from a given depth is a spatial average of those portions of the boundaries insonated by the beam.

Beam focusing artifact

In Figure 5-5, the same objects from Figure 5-4 are moved to three different depths. The imaging of these objects now shows the shallower and deeper objects to appear wider than the one between. This occurs when the transducer beam is focused to have a minimum beamwidth between the top and bottom objects.

Once again the scanning of small test objects in imaging phantoms demonstrates this effect and can be used to study and verify the degree of focusing of the ultrasonic beam. This effect emphasizes the fact that a truer representation of the boundaries at a given depth are obtained when focusing produces the narrowest beam and a smaller region of tissue contributes to the returning echoes.

Shadowing artifact

In Figure 5-6, two objects are examined: the large rectangle discussed in Figure 5-1 and a much smaller object placed between the rectangle and the transducer. The smaller object is assumed to have an impedance considerably different from that of the surrounding material, to scatter ultrasound as do the objects in Figures 5-4 and 5-5, and to attenuate rapidly the ultrasound that passes through it.

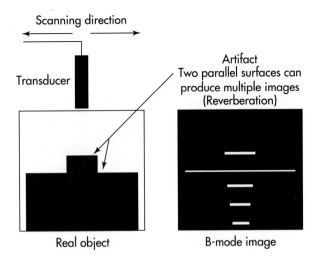

Fig. 5-7. Simplified diagram illustrating the reverberation artifact. Two parallel surfaces with the correct acoustic impedance difference can produce multiple images of the boundaries on the B-mode image.

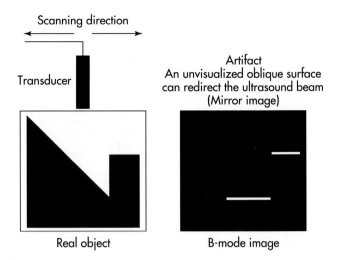

Fig. 5-8. Simplified diagram illustrating the mirror image artifact. A nonvisualized oblique surface can redirect the ultrasound beam to other boundaries and cause them to be visualized in an incorrect location on the B-mode image.

When the transducer scans on the left and on the right of the shallower object, the upper surface of the rectangle is seen on the B-mode image as described in Figure 5-1. When the transducer scans above the shallower object, only the echoes from the shallower object appear on the B-mode images because the ultrasound does not pass through this object. As a consequence, it appears from the B-mode image that two disconnected surfaces at the depth of the rectangle are separated by a "gap" corresponding to the approximate lateral dimension of the shallower object. A way of describing this artifact is to say that the shallower object is casting a shadow on the deeper one. Calcification in an artery wall is the most common source of a shadowing artifact in vascular imaging.

Reverberation artifact

In Figure 5-7, a small rectangle is placed above and in contact with the larger rectangle. The impedances of the two objects are different, as is each impedance from the surrounding material. When the transducer scans on the left or right of the small rectangle, the normal image of the top surface of the rectangle is shown on the B-mode image. If the impedance differences are of the proper magnitude when the transducer is above the small rectangle, the ultrasound pulse can reflect back and forth several times between the top and bottom surfaces and give rise to a series of echoes, equally spaced in time, being received by the transducer. This appears on the B-mode image as a series of equally spaced lines at increasingly greater depths. Equally spaced lines of decreasing intensity are

the characteristics to look for in identifying this common artifact.

Mirror image artifact

The final artifact here involves a more complex object, as shown in Figure 5-8. It consists of an oblique surface that intersects a rectangle whose top surface is perpendicular to the direction of propagation of the ultrasonic beam. As the transducer is scanned from the left, the echoes from the oblique surface do not return to the transducer and thus are not seen on the B-mode image, as discussed in Figure 5-3.

As the transducer approaches the rectangular object, the reflections from the oblique surface strike the left surface of the rectangle and are reflected back to the oblique surface and the transducer so that an echo is received. The elapsed time for this echo is longer than that corresponding to an echo from the oblique surface. The net effect is that the B-mode image displays a horizontal line that is deeper than the oblique surface. This line is effectively a mirror image of the left side of the rectangle as it would appear when viewed from its current position through an optical mirror coincident with the oblique surface. This deeper surface is a mirror image artifact and is clearly not present in the object where it appears in the B-mode image. Similar artifactual displays may be seen with color flow imaging when color is displayed in an inappropriate location outside the vessel.

SUMMARY

Examples of eight common artifacts are described in this chapter. Many others arise in clinical practice in subtle ways and are recognized from an understanding of the physical principles of ultrasound and by practical experience. It is important to understand that they are primarily a result of assumptions used in the design and performance of ultrasound systems that are not satisfied in practice.

REFERENCES

1. Kremkau FW: *Imaging artifacts.* In *Diagnostic ultrasound: Principles, instruments and exercises,* ed 4, Philadelphia, 1993, WB Saunders.
2. Kremkau FW, Taylor KW: Artifacts in ultrasound imaging, *J Ultrasound Med* 5:227, 1986.

6

A Clinical Approach to Hemodynamics

Anne M. Jones

Noninvasive assessment of blood flow provides a method to identify, localize, and quantify stenosis. Accurate completion and interpretation of extracranial physiologic studies require an understanding of fundamental hemodynamic principles. This chapter reviews the relationships that affect flow and the characteristics of normal and abnormal flow states.

BACKGROUND

The definitions used to describe hemodynamic principles, flow characteristics, and noninvasive parameters are often interchanged, creating confusion about terminology. The term *flow* refers to flow rate, or the volume of blood that moves through a vessel per unit time. Flow volume is measured in liters or milliliters. Flow velocity refers to the speed of the flow and is measured in m/s or cm/s. To calculate flow rate or flow velocity, several factors must be known, including arterial pressure, resistance, and vessel radius. These factors are discussed here individually and then collectively.

Pressure is a fundamental component of flow. For flow to occur, there must be a difference in pressure from one end of the artery to the other. Blood flows from the area of higher pressure to the area of lower pressure. The difference in pressure between the two points in the vessel, known as the *pressure gradient,* is the actual force that propels blood through the artery. The pressure gradient (ΔP) can be calculated by subtracting the lower pressure (P2) from the higher pressure (P1).

$$\Delta P = P1 - P2$$

It is the *pressure difference* between the two points in the vessel, rather than the absolute arterial pressure, that determines flow. Another critical component of flow is resistance. Resistance factors are the conditions that impede flow; they include viscosity, vessel length, and vessel radius. Although specific clinical conditions can affect blood viscosity, vessel length and blood viscosity are normally constant and predictable. The vessel diameter can vary significantly, however. In the patient with cerebrovascular disease, a high-grade stenosis can occur before blood volume or velocity are significantly affected and clinical symptoms occur. When the diameter of the carotid artery is reduced by 75%, a "critical stenosis" occurs, causing a profound effect on both flow volume and flow velocity. The effect of a reduction in lumen diameter is demonstrated in Figure 6-1; the graph summarizes the theoretical relationship between flow rate and flow velocity in the presence of arterial stenosis. The reader is encouraged to compare carefully the effect of diameter and cross-sectional area reductions, as the two are not identical.

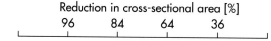

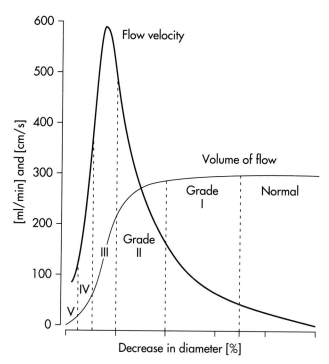

Fig. 6-1. Theoretical relationship between flow velocity and flow rate with varying degrees of stenosis. (From Spencer MP: *Blood flow in arteries.* In Spencer MP, Reid JM: *Cerebrovascular evaluation with Doppler ultrasound,* The Hague, 1981, Martinus Nijhoff; with permission.)

These relationships, described by Spencer,[2] significantly impact hemodynamics and the noninvasive assessment of arterial stenosis. When a stenosis of less than 50% reduction in diameter occurs, it is classified as "nonhemodynamically significant." However, when the diameter is reduced by 75% or more, a "critical stenosis" occurs, and very minor changes in the caliber of the vessel produce significant changes in velocity and flow. Of the three resistance factors—viscosity, vessel length, and vessel radius—vessel radius has the most profound effect on flow. When lumen size increases, flow resistance and flow velocity decrease. Conversely, as lumen size decreases, resistance increases, resulting in increased flow velocity. If the diameter of a vessel is significantly reduced, as in the "critical" stenosis, very minor changes in diameter can create significant changes in flow ve locity as well as flow volume.

The impact of changes in viscosity, vessel length, and vessel radius is described by Poiseuille's law:

$$R = \frac{8l\eta}{\pi r^4}$$

Resistance to flow (R) is directly proportional to viscosity (η) and vessel length (l) and inversely proportional to the fourth power of the vessel radius (r^4).

In order to apply the work of Poiseuille to the arterial circulation, three assumptions are made: laminar flow is present, cardiac output is stable, and arterial pressure is constant. Because these "ideal" conditions are rarely present in the arterial circulation, Poiseuille's law cannot be strictly applied to arterial flow. However, the hemodynamic relationships defined by Poiseuille can be applied to clinical noninvasive testing.

A second example of the relationship between vessel diameter and flow is found in the continuity principle. If the flow rate is constant and the diameter of the vessel increases, the velocity of flow will decrease without affecting the flow volume. In the presence of an arterial stenosis, however, the velocity increases at the site of the stenosis to maintain flow volume. The relationship between velocity and area, described in the continuity principle, is:

$$Q = V_1 \cdot A_1 = V_2 \cdot A_2$$

Flow volume is Q, velocity is V, and area is A. The continuity principle is one of the components that must be considered when assessing flow characteristics in normal and diseased vessels. It helps to explain why the velocities noted in normal segments vary so significantly from velocities at the site of stenosis. The velocity will increase or decrease, according to the dimensions of the vessel in an effort to maintain a constant flow rate.

Pressure, energy, and flow

In a "normal" patient with a stable cardiac output, arterial flow conditions are predictable. The total fluid energy, a combination of kinetic (work) and pressure energy, remains constant. In the presence of a stenosis, the steady flow pattern is disrupted, and flow accelerates at the site of the stenosis; a "pressure drop" occurs because pressure energy must be converted to kinetic energy to maintain flow volume. During this conversion of pressure (potential) energy to kinetic energy, a portion of the potential energy is dissipated as heat, resulting in a pressure drop at the stenosis. Distal to the stenosis, where the lumen diameter normalizes, most of the kinetic energy is converted back to pressure energy, although some energy was lost as heat, as described. This phenomenon of flow acceleration and pressure reduction at the point of stenosis was described by Bernoulli and is often referred to as Bernoulli's principle.

Arterial flow patterns

Fluid is arranged in concentric layers, or laminae, in most major arterial segments. The slowest flow is adjacent to the vessel wall, where flow particles experience resistance, due to the vessel wall. The flow velocity

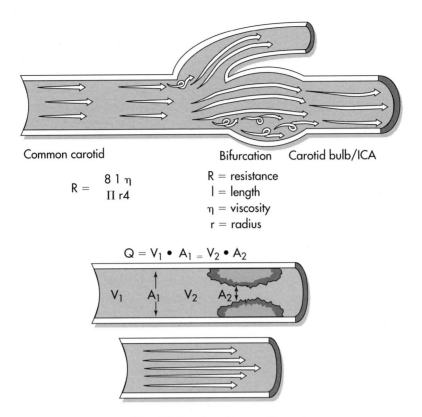

Common carotid   Bifurcation   Carotid bulb/ICA

$$R = \frac{8\,l\,\eta}{\Pi\,r4}$$

R = resistance
l = length
η = viscosity
r = radius

$$Q = V_1 \bullet A_1 = V_2 \bullet A_2$$

Fig. 6-2. Laminar flow profile.

of each layer increases, with the fastest flow center stream. This streamline flow pattern is known as *laminar flow* (Fig. 6-2). Because the layers of flow move at increasing speed, in parallel to one another, a parabolic flow profile occurs. However, the flow profile can be affected by other factors, including flow state and vessel size. Large vessels such as the aorta often have blunt flow profiles because the parallel layers of flow are moving at nearly the same speed. Similar blunted or "plug" flow patterns are noted at vessel origins, where laminar flow has not yet developed. Both plug flow and parabolic flow patterns (Fig. 6-3) are found in normal arteries. An additional finding often noted in normal vessels is the presence of a "helical" flow profile, in which flow layers remain laminar but traverse in a corkscrew fashion through the vessel. This phenomenon, initially documented in flow studies, is frequently noted in the internal carotid artery and may be visible if color flow imaging systems are utilized.

Arterial flow characteristics

Laminar flow occurs most frequently in arterial segments of a constant diameter, with "normal" velocities. The spectral waveform displays a narrow range of velocities, with most of the energy concentrated along the outer envelope of the waveform (Fig. 6-4). The "open" appearance in the lower portion of the spectral

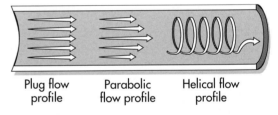

Plug flow   Parabolic   Helical flow
profile   flow profile   profile

Fig. 6-3. Plug, parabolic, and helical flow profiles in normal arteries.

waveform is often referred to as the *window sign.* This descriptive term implies the absence of disturbed or turbulent flow.

Changes in vessel diameter or geometry may create areas of disturbed flow in normal arteries. The disturbed flow pattern is recognized by a widening of the spectral envelope during diastole. Because the flow disturbance is focal and not associated with a stenosis, there is only a minor energy loss, and the laminar flow pattern is quickly resumed. The most common sites of arterial flow disturbances are bifurcations, branches, and curves in arteries. The geometry of branch points and bifurcations creates interesting "entry" and "exit" flow patterns due to changes in vessel diameter and vessel course. Abrupt changes in diameter, often found at the origin of the internal carotid artery, create sites of flow disturbance, often misinterpreted as disease

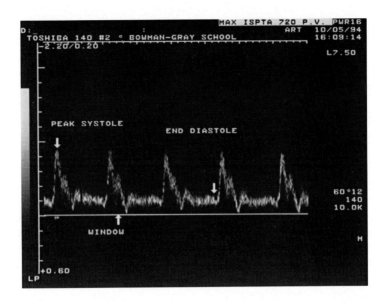

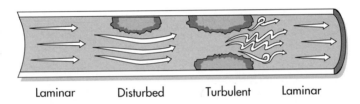

Fig. 6-5. Laminar, disturbed, and turbulent flow patterns in normal and diseased arteries.

rather than as a natural phenomenon due to vessel angle or geometry.

Turbulence verifies a loss of order in the flow profile and most frequently occurs distal to a stenosis, at the point where the high-velocity jet of flow exits the stenosis and suddenly encounters a dilated arterial segment (Fig. 6-5). At the site of turbulence, flow particles move in a random, chaotic fashion, resulting in flow reversals, decreased flow velocity, and reduced pressure.

Turbulence can be predicted by the Reynolds number (Fig. 6-6), a measure that compares vessel diameter, flow velocity, blood density, and viscosity. The tendency for turbulence increases in direct proportion to increasing vessel diameter and flow velocity; it is inversely proportional to viscosity. Turbulence increases in the presence of stenosis because high-velocity flow exits the stenosis and encounters a dilated vessel segment immediately distal to the stenosis. Although turbulence is most frequently associated with significant stenosis, it also occurs at very abrupt changes in vessel diameter or geometry. Tortuous segments or aneurysmal dilatations often exhibit turbulence in the absence of an associated stenosis. Spectral waveform characteristics of turbulent flow usually include an uneven envelope contour, loss of the uniform distribution of velocities ("spectral broadening"), forward and reversed flow components, and a shift in the amplitude toward the lower velocities, creating a concentration of energy along the baseline, often called a *bruit*.

Flow studies by Phillips and colleagues,[1] Giddens and Ku,[9] and others have described complex flow patterns within the carotid artery, particularly at the bifurcation and internal carotid artery origin. As the common carotid artery divides into the internal and external carotids, the vessel dilates. The dilatation usually extends to the origin of the internal carotid artery (carotid bulb). The combination of changing flow rate and vessel geometry results in a unique regional flow pattern producing a boundary layer separation (Fig. 6-7). The flow pattern contains two distinct regions of flow, the faster flow along the vessel axis and the slower flow along the outer wall of the carotid bulb. The distinct changes in the flow pattern are appreciated by stepping a pulsed Doppler across the origin of the internal carotid artery or by using color flow Doppler imaging. The complex flow pattern at the carotid bulb has been implicated in the development of atherosclerotic plaque at the carotid bifurcation. Similarly, Strandness[3] reports that the lack of a boundary layer separation corresponds to the earliest stages of disease at the carotid bulb.

SPECTRAL WAVEFORM CHARACTERISTICS

It is impossible to discuss cerebrovascular hemodynamics without referring in some detail to spectral waveform characteristics of normal and diseased vessels. Interpretation of spectral waveforms is discussed in a later chapter, and only the fundamental elements of waveform recognition are included here.

Under normal conditions, flow to the brain is continuous, or unobstructed, because of the low-resistance distal vascular bed. Unobstructed carotid or vertebral flow is easily recognized by the continuous flow throughout diastole. Systolic acceleration is smooth, with a distinct systolic peak and steady diastolic deceleration. Arterial stenosis in the carotid system will produce changes in waveform characteristics not only at the site of maximum stenosis but also proximal and distal to the lesion. Peak systolic velocity is the primary parameter used to categorize the severity of disease; secondary parameters, such as end-diastolic velocity, diminished diastolic flow, and "spectral broadening" are also useful.

Waveform characteristics change as the status of the distal bed changes. For instance, in the presence of severe internal carotid stenosis, the diastolic component of the common carotid artery is significantly reduced because of the distal obstruction. The external carotid artery, serving as a collateral pathway to the brain, may exhibit an increased diastolic component due to the additional flow volume and the change in its distal perfusion bed from high resistance to low resistance. Flow velocities in the vertebral or contralateral carotid

system may also increase because of the changing hemodynamics associated with occlusion and collateral flow. Changing collateral pathways and resistance patterns can be easily documented and recognized if the hemodynamic principles are applied. At the point of maximum stenosis, flow patterns, although accelerated, are usually laminar. Distal to a significant stenosis, gross turbulence is present and can be recognized by the broad range of velocities contained in the spectral display. Although spectral broadening is often difficult to quantify, it is easily recognized as an abnormal finding by the wide range of velocities and the flow-reversal patterns contained in the waveform. When a stenosis reaches the "critical" level, indicating greater than a 75% reduction in diameter, peak systolic velocities may exceed the display capabilities of the Doppler system, resulting in aliasing or wraparound of the spectral display. In these cases, measurement of the end-diastolic velocity can be helpful for proper categorization of disease severity.

VERTEBRAL ARTERY ASSESSMENT

Because the vertebral arteries supply the posterior circulation, the recognition of abnormal hemodynamics is helpful to the evaluation of the patient with symptoms of posterior ischemia. Assessment of the vertebral arteries should begin with measurement of bilateral brachial blood pressures and auscultation of the supraclavicular vessels. Subclavian stenosis can result in decreased brachial blood pressure and may compromise flow to the vertebral artery. In addition, if the subclavian stenosis is significant, flow direction in the vertebral artery may change direction in a constant or alternating pattern to perfuse the arm. The resulting flow reversal in the affected vertebral artery, referred to as *subclavian steal syndrome,* may cause symptoms of posterior ischemia if the basilar artery is affected.

CONCLUSION

Assessment of extracranial carotid and vertebral artery disease requires an understanding of anatomy, physiology, and the pathophysiology of the disease process. Although duplex instrumentation is used to

$$R_e = \frac{vq^2r}{\eta}$$

V = velocity
q = density of fluid
r = radius of tube
η = viscosity
Reynolds number R_e = Reynolds number

Fig. 6-6. Reynolds number.

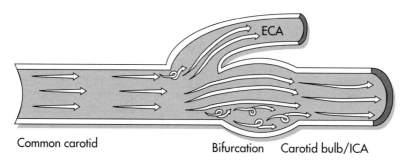

Common carotid   Bifurcation   Carotid bulb/ICA

Fig. 6-7. Boundary layer separation at carotid bulb.

identify, localize, and quantify disease, accurate assessment is impossible without an understanding of the hemodynamic principles. An appreciation of these fundamental physiologic concepts will assist with the recognition of normal and abnormal flow characteristics; because quantification of disease relies on spectral waveform analysis, hemodynamic principles must routinely be applied to the noninvasive and clinical assessment of patients with cerebrovascular disease.

REFERENCES

1. Beach KW: *Evaluating a pulsed Doppler duplex scanner.* In Bernstein EF, editor: *Vascular diagnosis,* ed 4, St Louis, 1993, Mosby–Year Book.
2. Bernstein EF: *Current noninvasive evaluation of extracranial arterial disease.* In Bernstein EF, Callow AD, Nicolaides AN, Shifrin EG, editors: *Cerebral revascularization,* London, 1993, Med-Orion.
3. Bharadvaj BK, Mahon RF, Giddens DP: Steady flow in a model of the human carotid bifurcation; part I: laser-Doppler anemometer measurements, *J Biomech* 15:349-362, 1982.
4. Bharadvaj BK, Mahon RF, Giddens DP: Steady flow in a model of the human carotid bifurcation; part II: laser-Doppler anemometer measurements, *J Biomech* 15:363-378, 1982.
5. Fish PJ: *Doppler methods.* In Hill CR, editor: *Physical principles of medical ultrasonics,* Chichester, 1986, Horwood.
6. Ganog WF: *Review of medical physiology,* Norwalk, Conn, 1991, Appleton & Lange.
7. Guyton AC: *Textbook of medical physiology,* Philadelphia, 1986, WB Saunders.
8. Kremkau FW: *Doppler ultrasound: principles and instruments,* Philadelphia, 1990, WB Saunders.
9. Ku DN, Giddens DP: Pulsatile flow in a model carotid bifurcation, *Arteriosclerosis* 3:31-39, 1983.
10. Phillips DJ, Greene FM, Langlois GO, et al: Flow velocity patterns in the carotid bifurcations of young, presumed normal subjects, *Ultrasound Med Biol* 9:39-49, 1983.
11. Spencer MP: *Blood flow in arteries.* In Spencer PP, Reid JM, editors: *Cerebrovascular evaluation with Doppler ultrasound,* The Hague, 1981, Martinus Nijhoff.
12. Spencer MP: *Hemodynamics of carotid stenosis.* In Spencer MP, Reid JM, editors: *Cerebrovascular evaluation with Doppler ultrasound,* The Hague, 1981, Martinus Nijhoff.
13. Strandness DE: *Doppler ultrasonic techniques in vascular disease.* In Bernstein EF, editor: *Vascular diagnosis,* ed 4, St Louis, 1993, Mosby–Year Book.
14. Strandness DE: *Peripheral arterial disease, a physiologic approach,* Boston, 1967, Little, Brown.
15. Strandness DE, Sumner DS: *Hemodynamics for surgeons,* New York, 1975, Grune & Stratton.
16. Toole JF: *Cerebrovascular disorders,* 4, New York, 1990, Raven.
17. Von Reutern GM, Budigen HJ: *Ultrasound diagnosis of cerebrovascular disease,* New York, 1993, Thieme.arteries.

SECTION TWO

Adult Extracranial Sonography

Doppler Ultrasonography of the Carotid Bifurcation

Jesse Weinberger

Doppler ultrasonography can be used alone[14,17,18] or in combination with B-mode ultrasonography in duplex systems[3,4,7,11] to analyze patterns of blood flow at the carotid bifurcation. Stand-alone Doppler instruments usually use continuous-wave Doppler sonography, whereas duplex systems use pulsed-wave Doppler sonography. These methods allow noninvasive identification and quantification of the severity of carotid stenosis. This chapter emphasizes the clinical use of Doppler methods to study the extracranial carotid artery.

CONTINUOUS-WAVE DOPPLER

A freestanding, portable, continuous-wave Doppler instrument can be used at bedside as part of the clinical examination for cerebrovascular disease.[14-17,19] The transducer frequencies of these instruments are often higher than those used for the Doppler function in duplex systems, in the range of 4 to 10 MHz.[19] Auscultation of the carotid artery bifurcation with these instruments can identify and differentiate the common, internal, and external carotid arteries and the cervical vertebral artery (Fig. 7-1).[14-17] The flow pattern in a normal internal carotid artery has a smooth, gradual runoff in diastole.[15] The flow pattern in the external

carotid artery has a shorter systolic phase and an abrupt drop of frequencies in diastole, whereas the common carotid artery has a flow pattern that is intermediate between the patterns in the internal and external carotid arteries.[15]

Flow direction in the periorbital arteries can also be assessed.[6,15] The supratrochlear artery provides a potential collateral channel between the ophthalmic branch of the internal carotid artery and the external carotid artery. Flow in the periorbital vessels is normally from the internal to the external carotid. In cases of hemodynamically significant obstruction to flow in the internal carotid artery at the bifurcation, flow in the periorbital arteries can become retrograde from the external to the internal carotid artery.[6,15] Flow direction can be assessed along the supraorbital ridge (Fig. 7-1), and the direction of flow can be plotted by a linear recorder (Fig. 7-2). When flow is retrograde from the external to the internal carotid, compression of the superficial temporal or facial arteries can suppress the flow from the external artery.[6] Although not a highly sensitive or specific test for carotid artery disease, the periorbital Doppler examination can assist in the diagnosis of complete occlusions or high-grade stenosis of

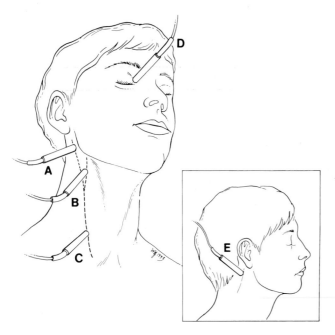

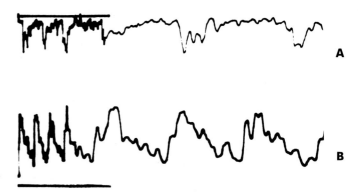

Fig. 7-2. Flow in the supratrochlear artery is antegrade away from the probe (**A**) when flow in the internal carotid artery is not hemodynamically compromised and retrograde toward the probe (**B**) when flow in the internal carotid is hemodynamically obstructed. (From Ringelstein EB: Continuous-wave Doppler sonography of the extracranial brain-supplying arteries. In Weinberger J, editor: *Noninvasive imaging of the cerebral circulation*, New York, 1989, Alan R Liss.)

Fig. 7-1. Flow in the common carotid (*C*), internal carotid (*A*), external carotid (*B*), vertebral (*E*), and supratrochlear (*D*) arteries can be insonated with a freestanding Doppler probe. The external carotid usually lies directly above the common carotid; the internal carotid swings posteriorly and laterally. However, on the right, the internal sometimes lies medial to the external, particularly in women. The vertebral artery can be insonated at the level of the second cervical vertebra, where it leaves the foramen transversarium prior to entering the skull. The supratrochlear artery can be insonated at the medial supraorbital ridge for supraorbital directional Doppler analysis. (Adapted from Ringelstein EB: Continuous-wave Doppler sonography of the extracranial brain-supplying arteries. In Weinberger J, editor: *Noninvasive imaging of the cerebral circulation*, New York, 1989, Alan R Liss.)

the internal carotid artery when duplex diagnosis is equivocal.

When used by an experienced examiner, auscultation of Doppler frequency shifts from the extracranial carotid arterial system with continuous-wave Doppler can identify clinically significant stenosis of greater than 70% with a high degree of accuracy.[2] High frequencies are readily auscultated in the internal carotid artery, and lower-frequency sounds similar to the crashing of plates can be heard in the bifurcation from eddy currents or scattering of soundwaves off calcified plaque.[2,19]

The spectral frequencies recorded with a portable continuous-wave Doppler instrument can be plotted linearly (Fig. 7-3)[16,19] or by spectral frequency analysis.[1,17,18] Peak systolic frequencies recorded in systole correlate accurately with the degree of lumen narrowing in carotid stenosis.[22]

In association with periorbital Doppler examination, most hemodynamically significant lesions in the region of the extracranial carotid bifurcation can be identified by these simple techniques.[19] The information can be employed to decide whether it is necessary to proceed to angiography in patients for whom endarterectomy would be considered.[19]

In our laboratory, auscultation with continuous-wave Doppler is performed on all patients prior to duplex scanning. Flow in the entire region of the bifurcation can be screened to ensure that the appropriate areas of stenosis are identified on B-mode imaging and that spectral analysis measurements are performed at the sites of the most critical stenosis. Color flow duplex sonography now allows screening of the entire artery during the B-mode examination.[11] However, when the bifurcation is tortuous, it is sometimes difficult to follow, even with color flow imaging, and auscultation of the bifurcation with continuous-wave Doppler can still be a useful adjunct.

Some investigators find frequency analysis of continuous-wave Doppler data to be more accurate, compared to angiography, than pulsed Doppler techniques.[6] When the pulse-repetition frequency of the pulsed Doppler instrument is less than twice the frequency shift of the scattered sound waves, aliasing can occur.[3,4,11] The highest-frequency shifts may be recorded in a retrograde direction or lost altogether.[3,4,11] As technology has improved, this has usually not been a significant clinical consideration because the pulse repetition rates can be set high enough to account for all degrees of stenosis. However, sensitivity is sacrificed to some extent, and the highest frequency shifts from a critical stenosis may not be identified. Turbulent flow patterns arising from cardiac valve dysfunction can also more easily be differentiated from carotid stenosis with continuous-wave Doppler so that these findings are not interpreted as an indication of carotid artery stenosis.[20,21]

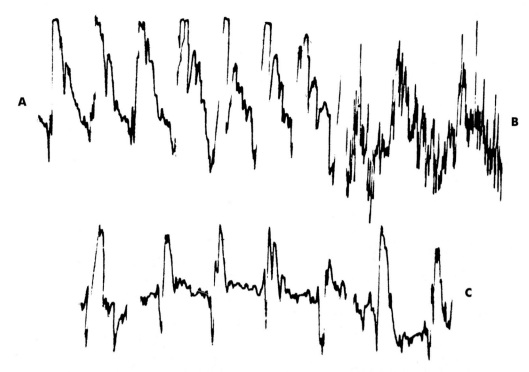

Fig. 7-3. Doppler waveforms can be plotted linearly with a strip chart recorder. The normal flow pattern in the internal carotid (**A**), high-frequency turbulence from a stenotic internal carotid (**B**), and compromised flow in the common carotid artery proximal to a complete occlusion of the internal carotid artery with loss of flow in diastole (**C**), are shown. (From Weinberger J, Biscarra V, Weitzner I, Sacher M: Noninvasive carotid artery testing: role in the management of patients with transient ischemic attacks, *N Y State J Med* 81:1463-1468, 1981.)

SPECTRAL FREQUENCY ANALYSIS OF DOPPLER ULTRASOUND

Spectral analysis of Doppler frequency shifts by fast Fourier transform provides a visual display of the sound auscultated by duplex Doppler.[1,3,4] This method can display either frequency shifts or, if the angle of insonation is known, the flow velocities. Although all frequency shifts (or flow velocities) are displayed on the spectrum, the human ear can differentiate sound qualities that cannot be interpreted by merely reading the spectral display.[2] Therefore, the auditory interpretation of Doppler signals remains a valuable adjunct to quantification by spectral analysis.

The normal internal carotid Doppler signal has a smooth inclination in systole and gradual declination in diastole. The internal carotid is a capacitance vessel, and the signal obtained indicates low-resistance flow to the brain. Spectra of the normal internal carotid measured with continuous-wave and pulsed duplex Doppler methods are shown in Figure 7-4.

The normal external carotid artery Doppler signal has a shorter systolic wave and an abrupt drop-off in diastole because it is a resistance vessel. Peak frequency shifts (flow velocities) are usually higher than in the normal internal carotid artery because the lumen diameter is smaller. Spectra of the normal external carotid measured with continuous-wave and pulsed duplex Doppler methods are shown in Figure 7-5.

The normal common carotid Doppler signal is intermediate between the internal and external carotid signals. There is a less rapid drop-off in diastole than in the external but not as gradual as in the internal (Fig. 7-6). When there is atherosclerotic plaque in the bifurcation without involvement of the internal carotid, peak flow velocities can be normal, but there may be increased intensity and spread of frequencies in the spectra that can be auscultated as a crunching, low-pitched turbulence (Fig. 7-7). When there is plaque at the origin of the internal carotid artery without involvement of the carotid sinus, there may be elevation of the initial systolic peak without spectral broadening (Fig. 7-8 on p. 54). A large proliferative plaque confined to the common carotid may cause no flow disturbance, but a smaller, simple plaque at the origin of the internal carotid artery may cause a severe flow disturbance. Thus, plaque morphology studies with B-mode ultrasonography are important, in addition to the degree of flow disturbance determined by Doppler examination (see Chapter 8).

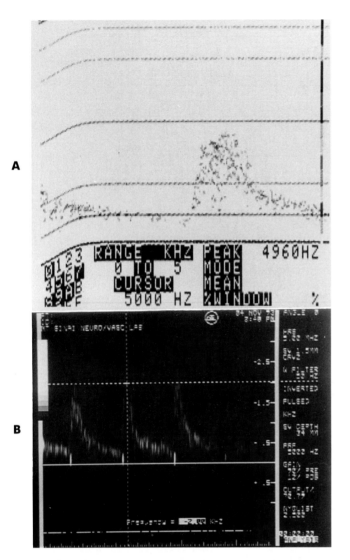

Fig. 7-4. The normal internal carotid artery flow pattern shows a smooth upsweep in systole with a gradual downsweep in diastole. Spectral analyses from a continuous-wave (**A**) and pulsed (**B**) Doppler system are shown. In continuous-wave Doppler, all frequencies encountered by the ultrasound beam are displayed, whereas in pulsed Doppler, the sample is limited by the placement of the Doppler gate to include only flow from the center of the lumen.

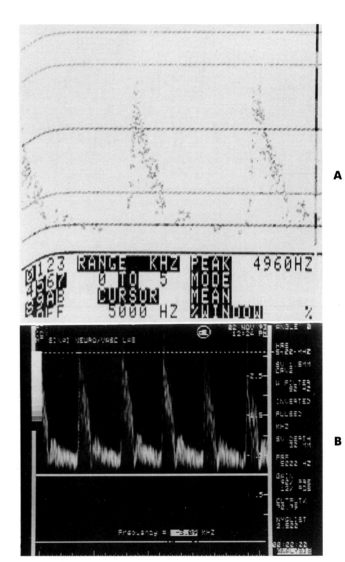

Fig. 7-5. Flow in the normal external carotid artery with continuous-wave (**A**) and pulsed (**B**) Doppler systems. There is a sharp upsweep in systole with a precipitous downsweep into diastole and lower diastolic flow velocity than in the internal carotid artery.

The degree of stenosis at the origin of the internal carotid artery can be categorized into classes. The most commonly used classification for a pulsed Doppler duplex system is A, normal; B, 1% to 15% stenosis; C, 16% to 49% stenosis; D, 50% to 79% stenosis; and D+, 80% to 99% stenosis and complete occlusion (Fig. 7-9 on p. 55).[11] With class B lesions, there is no elevation of the systolic peak, but lower-frequency shifts fill in the window between the maximum systolic waveform and the baseline. With class C lesions, there is moderate elevation of the systolic peak to about 4 KHz, with lower-frequency shifts seen broadening the spectrum. With class D lesions, there is elevation of the systolic peak above 5000 Hz, with spectral broadening of lower-frequency shifts beneath the peak. With class D+ lesions, there is usually such a high elevation of the systolic peak that aliasing occurs, with higher-frequency shifts displayed as retrograde flow below the baseline. With these lesions, there is usually elevation of the end-diastolic frequency shift over 2500 Hz; with a "string" type of lesion, there is total breakup of the waveform, with frequency shifts in diastole approaching frequency shifts in systole.

It has become important to differentiate between a lesion closer to the 50% range and a lesion closer to the 79% range because of the recent findings of the North American Symptomatic Carotid Endarterectomy Trial

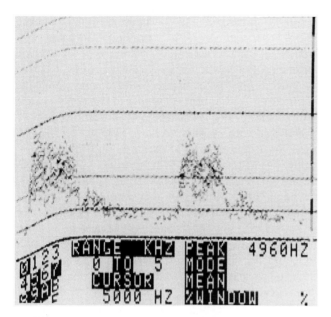

Fig. 7-6. Flow patterns in the common carotid artery are intermediate between the internal and the external, both in the inclination of the slope into systole and the declination into diastole, with intermediate diastolic velocity as well. It is not unusual to encounter a biphasic systole in the normal common carotid artery, but this should not be mistaken for the flow patterns associated with mitral valve dysfunction (see Fig. 7-17).

Collaborators (NASCET) trial of carotid endarterectomy, which demonstrated a beneficial effect of carotid endarterectomy in symptomatic patients with greater than 70% stenosis on arterial angiography.[13] Elevation of end-diastolic frequency shift (velocity) usually suggests a "significant" lesion closer to the 70% range than to the 50% range, when the peak frequency shifts indicate a stenosis of 50% to 79%.[1,11]

Continuous-wave Doppler with spectral analysis can usually be valuable in this assessment.[17,18] The gradations of the degree of stenosis with continuous-wave Doppler spectral analysis are shown in Figure 7-10. Spectral analysis of pulsed Doppler from a color flow duplex system showing high-grade (80% to 99%) stenosis using an "expert" system that broadens the sample volume to approach continuous-wave spectra is shown in Figure 7-11 on p. 57.

The peak frequency shift (velocity) in the normal internal carotid artery distal to the bifurcation is higher than at the origin of the internal carotid artery because the vessel both is narrower and curves away from the probe, changing the angle of insonation. The degree of stenosis as measured by changes in spectral frequency shifts in the distal internal carotid can be exaggerated, compared to the actual degree of stenosis on angiography (Fig. 7-12 on p. 57). Occasionally, severe stenotic lesions in the distal internal carotid can cause elevation of the systolic peak without elevating diastolic frequency

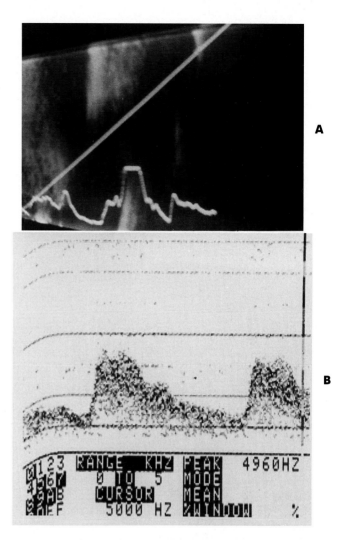

Fig. 7-7. A large plaque is seen in the curvature of the carotid bifurcation on B-mode ultrasound (**A**), but peak velocities in the common and internal carotid arteries are normal (**B**). There is a harsh sound auscultated with continuous-wave Doppler signals in the spectral analysis, even though no changes in velocity are seen.

shifts and causing the waveform to resemble the flow pattern in the external carotid artery (Fig. 7-13 on p. 57). This can lead to a false-negative diagnosis of external carotid artery stenosis. Color flow duplex imaging can often be helpful in differentiating the internal from the external carotid artery by identification of branches from the external. However, it is sometimes necessary to perform arterial or magnetic resonance angiography to be certain whether a stenotic flow pattern is arising from the internal carotid or the external carotid artery when the diastolic flow wave is reduced. It is important to study the distal internal carotid artery even when a plaque with stenosis has been identified at the carotid artery bifurcation because additional plaque with stenosis can arise at the curvature of the distal internal carotid (Fig. 7-14 on p. 58).

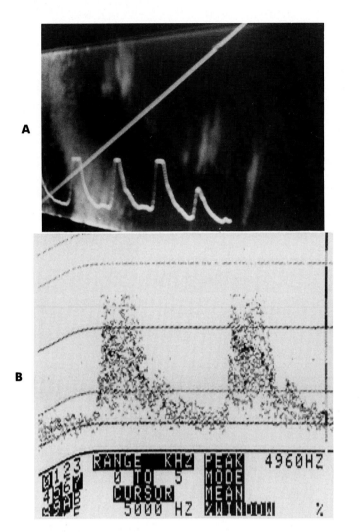

Fig. 7-8. A small, simple plaque at the origin of the internal carotid artery on B-mode ultrasonography **(A)** is causing an elevation of the systolic peak on continuous-wave duplex Doppler in the internal carotid artery, without spread of frequencies **(B).**

The Doppler diagnosis of complete occlusion of the internal carotid artery may be difficult. The characteristic finding is documentation of flow in the external carotid artery and a signal of reflux from the stump of the internal carotid artery with characteristic thumping sound (Fig. 7-15 on p. 58). Sometimes the internal carotid artery is present and cannot be identified because of tortuosity of the vessel, leading to a false-positive diagnosis of complete occlusion. A "normal" internal carotid signal can be obtained in the external carotid artery if the external is providing substantial collateral flow. The ancillary tests of periorbital Doppler, pneumooculoplethysmography,[8] and transcranial Doppler (see Chapter 12) are helpful in establishing the diagnosis of a complete occlusion of the internal carotid artery.

Artifacts from cardiac valve dysfunction, cardiac disease, or cardiac medications can alter the Doppler frequency shift signal and may cause errors in diagnosis. Mitral valve regurgitation, often seen with mitral valve prolapse, produces an initial systolic flow jet that can cause elevation of the initial systolic peak of the carotid waveform. This is associated with a midsystolic dip followed by resumption of systole at a normal velocity (Fig. 7-16 on p. 59). A characteristic flutter turbulence is auscultated with continuous-wave Doppler.[21] The finding of a normal carotid bifurcation on B-mode sonography helps to establish the cardiac origin of the turbulence. Aortic insufficiency can cause an artifact elevating the beginning of the systolic waveform and should be excluded when measuring the peak frequencies or velocities by spectral analysis (Fig. 7-17 on p. 59). This aortic valve artifact is particularly pronounced in dissecting aneurysms of the aorta (Fig. 7-18 on p. 59).[20] Reduced cardiac output can delay the upsweep of systole (flow acceleration) in the common and internal carotid arteries (Fig. 7-19 on p. 59). Cardiac arrhythmias, such as atrial fibrillation, can cause variability in the velocity of blood flow and alter the Doppler waveform (Fig. 7-20 on p. 60). Vasodilator medications such as propranolol can attenuate flow velocities and widen the Doppler waveform (Fig. 7-21 on p. 60). This can lead to underestimation of a stenotic lesion.

CLINICAL APPLICATIONS OF DOPPLER TECHNIQUES

Doppler frequency shift analysis of flow at the carotid artery bifurcation can reliably diagnose lesions causing greater than 50% stenosis of the internal carotid artery with better than 90% accuracy.[1,3,5,18,19,22] The techniques of duplex Doppler with B-mode ultrasonography[7,9,11] and color flow duplex Doppler[11] enhance the accuracy of the technique by demonstrating the location of the turbulence measured with the Doppler spectrum analysis. The degree of frequency shift is proportional to the lumen diameter or residual lumen area. Therefore, Doppler frequency shifts give a more accurate representation of the degree of stenosis and hemodynamic compromise of the artery than visualization of the B-mode image. It also must be remembered that spectral frequency shift analysis gives a more accurate representation of the degree of stenosis than visualization of the lumen diameter with color flow Doppler. The addition of color flow duplex Doppler increases the accuracy of the Doppler study because it shows the regions of turbulence from which the measurements of spectral frequency analysis should be made (see Chapter 9). For all of these Doppler methods, use of standardized protocols and criteria, validation of the same, and ongoing quality improvement are crucial to ensure accurate results.[10]

Patients with symptoms of transient cerebral ischemic attack or amaurosis fugax can be screened by carotid Doppler techniques to identify patients with greater than 50% stenosis. In some laboratories, correlation

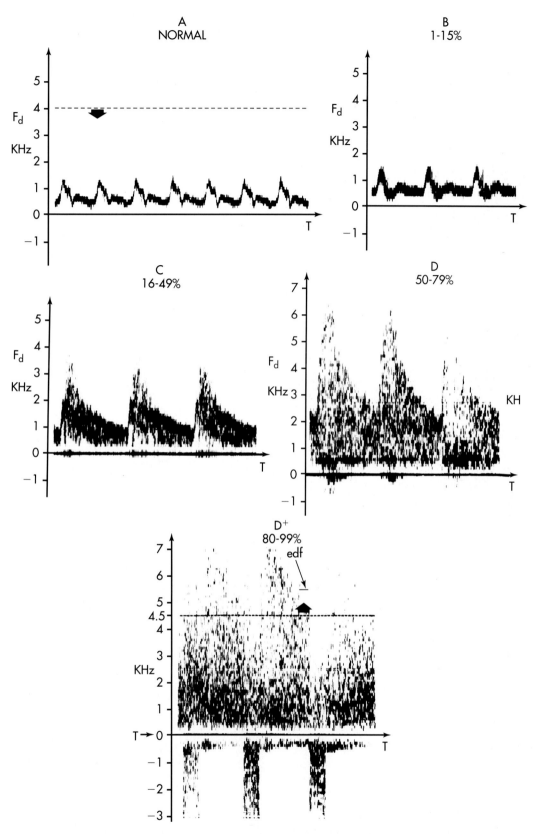

Fig. 7-9. The pulsed Doppler classification of degree of stenosis: **A,** Normal flow; **B,** 1% to 15% diameter reduction with slight spread of frequencies; **C,** 16% to 49% stenosis, with moderate elevation of the systolic peak and more spread of frequencies; **D,** 50% to 79% stenosis; **D+,** Critical stenosis of more than 80% with aliasing of the highest peak velocities showing as a negative deflection. (From Nicholls SC, Zierler RE, Strandness DE Jr: Duplex scanning of the carotid arteries. In Weinberger J, editor: *Noninvasive imaging of cerebrovascular disease,* New York, 1989, Alan R Liss.)

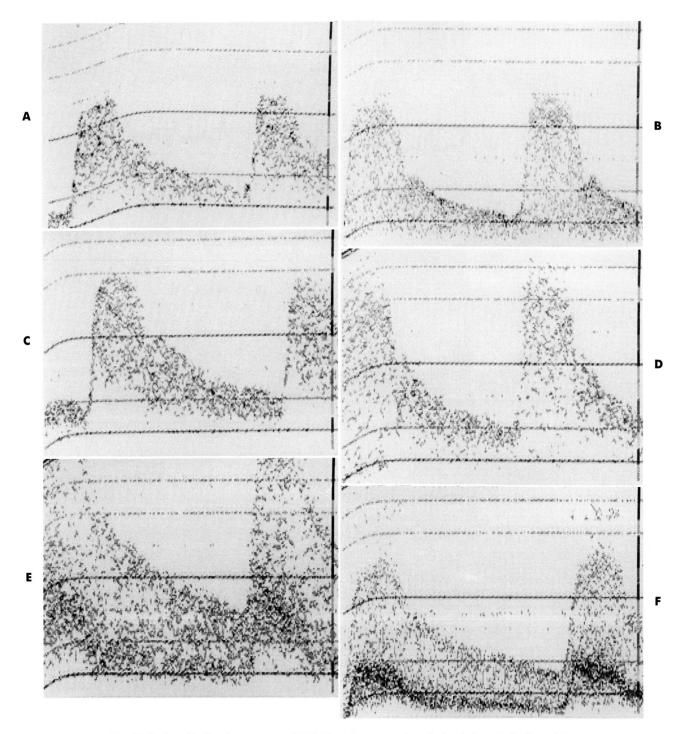

Fig. 7-10. A to **D,** Continuous-wave (CW) Doppler spectral analysis of class A, B, C, and D, D+, lesions. **E,** The systolic peak is elevated to 8000 Hz with no aliasing, and end-diastolic velocities are elevated to 3000 Hz. CW Doppler shows all frequencies encountered. **F,** The velocities just proximal to the severe stenosis appear in the spectrum. The advantage of CW Doppler is that it is more sensitive in detecting the highest-frequency shifts but is less specific than a pulsed duplex system. F is the same spectrum as E, with top of the scale 5000 in E and 10,000 in F.

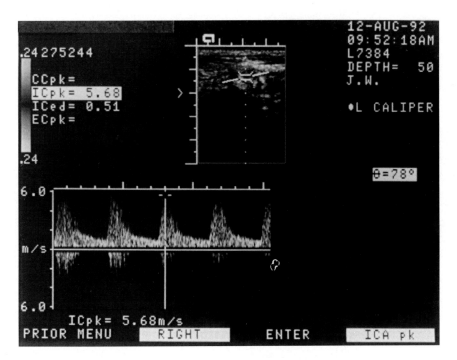

Fig. 7-11. A critical stenosis with a broad, pulsed spectral window showing elevated calculated velocities to 5.6 m/s. The normal range is less than 1 m/s.

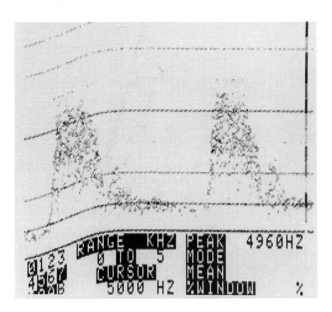

Fig. 7-12. Systolic flow velocities are normally slightly elevated in the distal internal carotid compared to the proximal internal at the origin from the bifurcation.

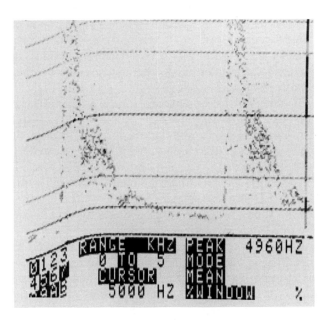

Fig. 7-13. The systolic peak can be elevated without spread of frequencies in diastole in a stenosis of the distal internal carotid.

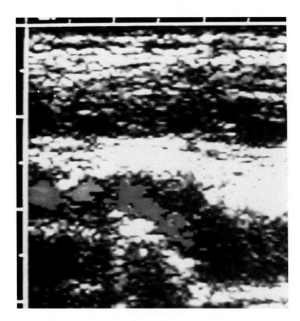

Fig. 7-14. It is important to identify and measure flow in the distal internal carotid even if a lesion is identified proximally, because plaques can form in both locations.

between Doppler findings and angiography can differentiate patients with greater than 70% stenosis from those with 50% to 69% stenosis. When a potentially significant lesion is found, further documentation of the degree of stenosis can be obtained by intraarterial angiography to determine if endarterectomy is indicated. In some instances, magnetic resonance angiography of the carotid bifurcation in combination with duplex Doppler techniques can reliably identify lesions of greater than 70% stenosis in order to determine whether endarterectomy is indicated.

Patients with asymptomatic carotid arterial bruits can also be screened with duplex Doppler flow studies. Doppler can distinguish whether the bruit is caused by atherostenosis of the carotid artery or by a transmitted cardiac murmur. In the past, endarterectomy was not indicated in patients with asymptomatic bruit unless the degree of stenosis was greater than 80%.[12] The Doppler classification shown in Figure 7-9 was designed to identify these patients. A recent clinical advisory from the National Institutes of Health confirmed the need to identify patients with tight asymptomatic carotid stenosis. Results from the Asymptomatic Carotid Artery Study (ACAS) study show that in patients with at least 60% stenosis (measured on cerebral arteriography by the same method used in NASCET), there was a significantly reduced risk of stroke in those having carotid endarterectomy, as compared to medical therapy alone. Due to the method of measurement on the arteriogram, such stenosis likely corresponds to at least a D to D+ lesion, as described earlier. Doppler sonography can also be performed sequentially at 6-month to yearly intervals

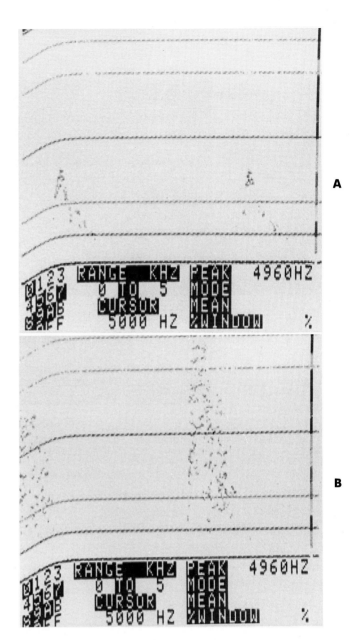

Fig. 7-15. Attenuation of flow in a complete occlusion of the **(A)** internal carotid artery with elevation of flow velocities in **(B)** in the external carotid artery.

in patients with asymptomatic bruit to determine if there is progression of stenosis, which is also associated with a higher incidence of ipsilateral stroke and is considered an indication for carotid endarterectomy.[12]

Doppler sonography is an integral part of the noninvasive carotid artery evaluation for determining the degree of stenosis of the internal carotid artery. However, other factors are important in the pathophysiology of carotid stroke. Real-time B-mode ultrasonography can image the size, morphologic configuration, and constitution of atherosclerotic plaque at the carotid bifurcation, which are also significant factors in the etiology of athe-

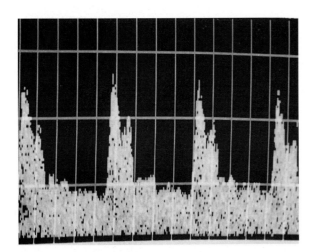

Fig. 7-16. Early systolic flutter turbulence occurs with mitral valve prolapse or regurgitation. There is elevation of the initial systolic peak and a biphasic systole. The auditory findings with CW Doppler are not reflected by spectral analysis and are essential for the diagnosis. The peak elevations from mitral valve dysfunction can lead to a false-positive Doppler diagnosis of carotid stenosis. (From Weinberger J, Goldman M: Detection of mitral valve abnormalities by Carotid Doppler flow study: implications for the management of patients with cerebrovascular disease, *Stroke* 16:977-980, 1985.)

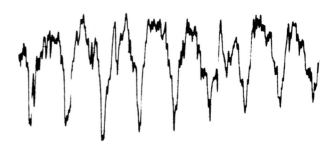

Fig. 7-18. Dissection of the aorta with extension into the internal carotid artery causes a marked artifact in systole, with flow in the true and false lumen. (From Weinberger J: Doppler pulse waveform analysis of carotid artery flow in dissecting aortic aneurysm, *Arch Neurol* 38:256-257, 1981.)

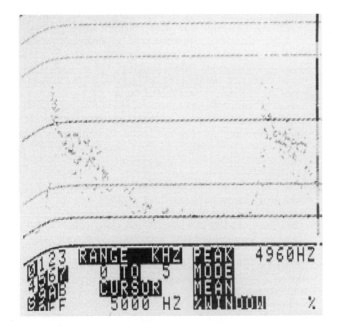

Fig. 7-17. Aortic valve dysfunction can also elevate the initial systolic peak, causing a false positive reading.

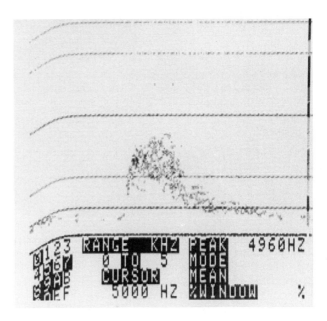

Fig. 7-19. Cardiac failure causes a slow upsweep in systole and can reduce the systolic peak even though there is stenosis. Highest velocity is at the end of systole.

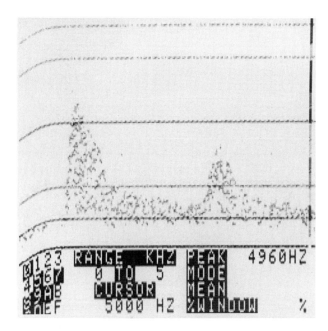

Fig. 7-20. The systolic peak can be variable with cardiac arrhythmias such as atrial fibrillation. With escape beats, there are false-positive peak elevations; with low output beats, there are false-negative peak attenuations.

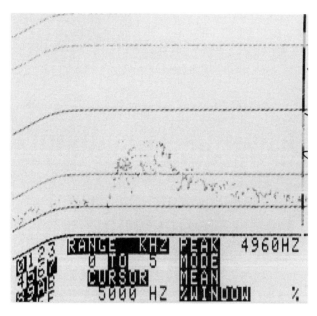

Fig. 7-21. Vasodilator medications such as beta-blockers and calcium channel blockers can prolong the velocity waveform and reduce the peak elevations seen with a stenosis, giving false-negative results.

roembolic stroke (see Chapter 8). The effect of stenosis at the carotid artery bifurcation on the distal cerebral circulation can also be measured by pneumooculoplethysmography, periorbital Doppler, and transcranial Doppler. These studies can yield information in the assessment of patients with atherosclerotic disease at the carotid bifurcation that may be equally as relevant as the determination of the degree of stenosis by Doppler analysis.

ACKNOWLEDGMENTS

Thanks to Lee Mylin and Sam D. Chin for help in preparation of the manuscript.

REFERENCES

1. Bandyk DF, Levine AW, Pohl L, Towne JB: Classification of carotid bifurcation disease using quantitative Doppler spectrum analysis, *Arch Surg* 120:306-314, 1985.
2. Barnes RW, Nixl L, Rittgers SE: Audible interpretation of carotid Doppler signals: an improved technique to define carotid artery disease, *Arch Surg* 116:1185-1189, 1981.
3. Blackshear WM, Lamb S, Murtagh R, et al: Pulsed Doppler ultrasound arteriography and spectrum analysis for quantitating carotid occlusive disease, *J Cardiovasc Ultrasonography* 4:105-112, 1985.
4. Blackshear WM, Thiele BL, Chikos PM, et al: Detection of carotid occlusive disease by ultrasonic imaging and pulsed Doppler spectrum analysis, *Surgery* 86:698-706, 1979.
5. Bloch S, Baltaxe HA, Shoumaker RD: Reliability of Doppler scanning of the carotid bifurcation: angiographic correlation, *Radiology* 132:687-691, 1979.
6. Bone GE, Barnes RW: Clinical implications of the Doppler cerebrovascular examination: a correlation with angiography, *Stroke* 7:271-274, 1976.
7. Fell G, Phillips DJ, Chikos MD, et al: Ultrasonic duplex scanning for disease of the carotid artery, *Circulation* 64:1191-1195, 1981.
8. Gee W, Oller DW, Amundsen DG: The asymptomatic carotid bruit and the ocular pneumoplethysmography, *Arch Surg* 112:1381-1388, 1977.
9. Hennerici M, Freund HJ: Efficacy of CW-Doppler and duplex system examinations for the evaluation of extracranial carotid disease, *J Clin Ultrasound* 12:155-161, 1984.
10. Howard G, Chambless LE, Baker WH, et al: A multicenter validation study of Doppler ultrasound versus angiography, *J Stroke Cerebrovasc Dis* 1:166-173, 1991.
11. Nicholls SC, Zierler RE, Strandness DE Jr.: *Duplex scanning of the carotid arteries.* In Weinberger J, editors: *Noninvasive imaging of cerebrovascular disease.* New York, 1989, Alan R Liss.
12. Norris JW, Zhu CZ, Bornstein NM, Chambers BR: Vascular risks of asymptomatic carotid stenosis, *Stroke* 22:1485-1490, 1991.
13. North American Symptomatic Carotid Endarterectomy Trial Collaborators: Beneficial effect of carotid endarterectomy in symptomatic patients with high-grade carotid stenosis, *N Engl J Med* 325:445-453, 1991.
14. Reid J, Spencer M: Ultrasonic Doppler technique for imaging blood vessels, *Science* 176:1235-1236, 1972.
15. Ringelstein EB: *Continuous-wave Doppler sonography of the extracranial brain-supplying arteries.* In Weinberger J, editor: *Noninvasive imaging of cerebrovascular disease,* New York, 1989, Alan R Liss.
16. Rutherford RB, Hiatt WR, Kreutzer EW: The use of velocity wave form analysis in the diagnosis of carotid artery occlusive disease, *Surgery* 82:695-702, 1977.
17. Spencer M, Reid J, David D, Paulson P: Cervical carotid imaging with a continuous wave Doppler flowmeter, *Stroke* 5:145-54, 1974.
18. Spencer MP, Reid JM: Quantitation of carotid stenosis with continuous-wave (C-W) Doppler ultrasound, *Stroke* 10:326-330, 1979.
19. Weinberger J, Biscarra V, Weitzner I, Sacher M: Noninvasive carotid artery testing: role in the management of patients

with transient ischemic attacks, *N Y State J Med* 81:1463-1468, 1981.

20. Weinberger J: Doppler pulse waveform analysis of carotid artery flow in dissecting aortic aneurysm, *Arch Neurol* 38:256-257, 1981.

21. Weinberger J, Goldman M: Detection of mitral valve abnormalities by carotid Doppler flow study: implications for the management of patients with cerebrovascular disease, *Stroke* 16:977-980, 1985.

22. Zweibel WJ, Zagaebski JA, Crummy AB, Hirscher M: Correlation of peak Doppler frequency with lumen narrowing in carotid stenosis, *Stroke* 13:386-391, 1982.

B-mode Evaluation and Characterization of Carotid Plaque

Edward I. Bluth

Developing a safe and noninvasive, low-cost screening test for the etiologies of stroke is of great importance because stroke continues to be a significant public health problem. Stroke is presently the third leading cause of death (about 150,000 yearly) in the United States. In addition, with modern medical therapies, three times as many stroke victims survive with some residual impairment. As a result, the identification of patients with increased risk to develop stroke is a significant public health concern.

Duplex sonography combining high-resolution imaging and Doppler spectrum analysis has proven to be the best choice for a screening test at the present time. Numerous studies have evaluated and reported that duplex sonography is an effective and accurate means of assessing and detecting arteriosclerotic disease at the carotid bifurcation.[6,16,19] Most recently, reports have shown that the carotid and vertebral arteries can also be accurately assessed with color flow Doppler imaging (CFDI).[5,8,13,27,31]

In the past evaluation for the risk of stroke centered on identifying flow-limited stenosis with oculoplethysmography, periorbital bidirectional Doppler, conven-tional arteriography, or digital vascular imaging.* Identifying flow-limiting stenosis is important because many strokes result from arteriosclerotic stenosis, particularly in the region of the carotid bifurcation. With high-grade stenosis or occlusion, hemodynamic factors and low profusion pressure likely contribute to symptoms. In addition, the presence of high-grade internal carotid stenosis, even in the absence of symptoms, is considered by many to be associated with increased risk for transient ischemic attack (TIA), stroke, and carotid occlusion.

Cerebral embolism is significant cause of stroke and can be due to arteriosclerotic disease of the carotid bifurcation. In fact, it is estimated that 50% to 60% of patients with TIAs have less than 50% stenosis on arteriography. It is known that certain carotid plaques develop hemorrhage, ultimately ulcerate, and, as a result, allow segments to fragment off and travel distally, leading to embolic stroke. With high-resolution imaging, plaque can be characterized into relative risk groups, for containing intraplaque hemorrhage, which is thought by

---

*References 1, 7, 9, 10, 11, 12, 15, 17, 18, 21, 24, 25, 30, 33, 34, 35, 36.

many to be the precursor for plaque ulceration.* In the past, emphasis has been placed on the radiographic diagnosis of flow-limiting stenosis. With the advent of duplex sonography, examiners have been able to investigate both hemodynamic and anatomic features to try to understand the risk of embolic stroke as well.†

TECHNIQUE

The examination is begun with the patient lying supine. The examiner can evaluate the patient either by sitting at the level of the patient's shoulders and approaching the patient directly, in the manner of traditional ultrasound examinations, or by sitting above the patient and reaching over the patient's head to the neck. In any case, it is very important that both examiner and patient are comfortable because the examination usually takes 20 to 40 minutes.

For best visualization, the patient's neck must be hyperextended. Depending on the patient, the carotid vessels can be found by directly scanning the neck with the patient's chin straight or turned in the contralateral direction away from the examiner. On occasion, the vessels can be best approached by scanning from posterior rather than anterior to the sternocleidomastoid muscles. At times both approaches are necessary to evaluate the vessels completely.

It is easiest to scan the patient first in the transverse projection. A rapid transverse scan initially allows the examiner to plan the best approach for obtaining proper sagittal scan planes. It allows one to follow more easily the direction and course of the tortuous vessels. The carotid vessels can be followed from their origin at the innominate or subclavian artery cephalad to its bifurcation. Then, depending on the level of the bifurcation relative to the mandible, 3 to 4 cm of the proximal internal and external carotid arteries can be studied.

Because the carotid vessels are relatively superficial a high-frequency imaging transducer (7.5 to 10 MHz) can be used to visualize the vascular structures. It is important to scan in both transverse and sagittal planes in order to assess properly the relationship of the plaque to the wall and not to identify falsely a sonolucent space between the plaque and the wall caused by a position artifact (Fig. 8-1). Careful attention must also be paid to the sonographic pattern of the tissues and muscles surrounding the vessels. The comparison is very helpful when characterizing plaque and useful in avoiding the false-positive identification of heterogeneous plaque. It is especially important to use optimal gain and flow sensitivity settings. An adequate amount of time must be devoted to characterizing the plaque to do it adequately. Although CFDI aids in the rapid identification of vessels,

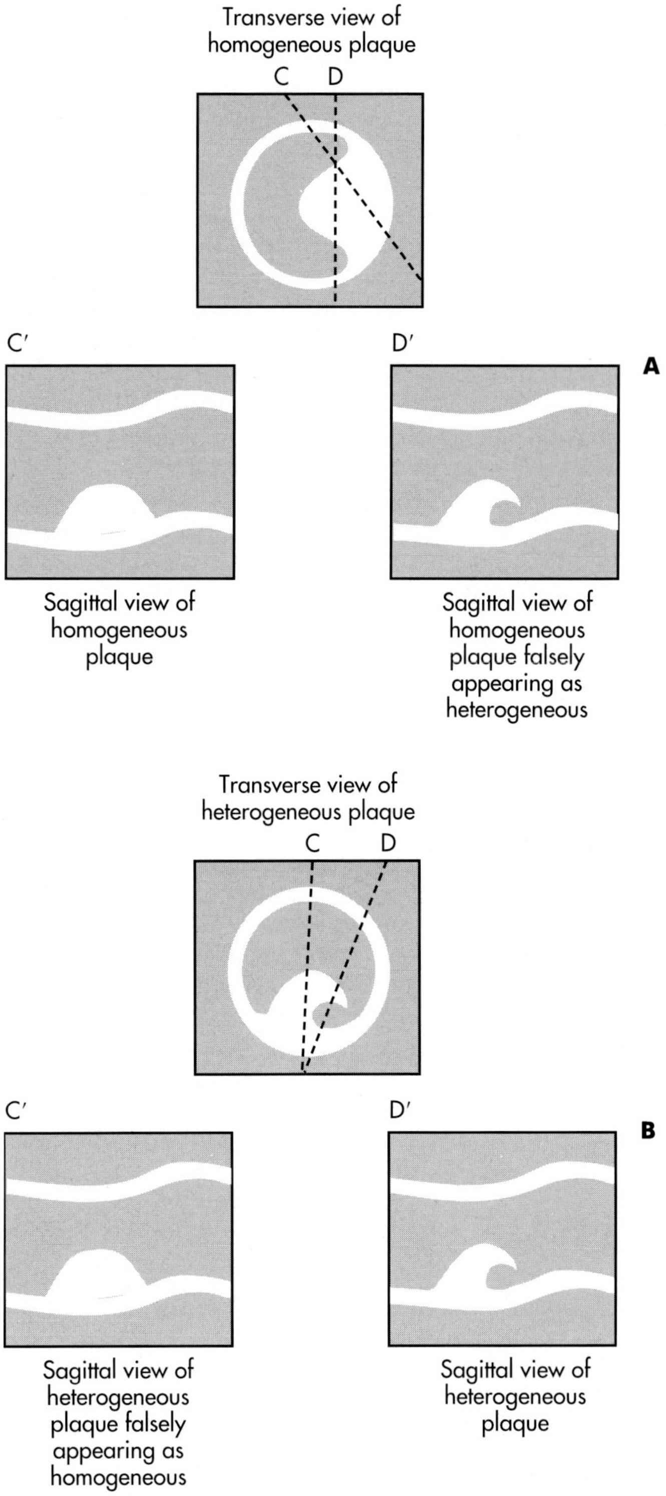

*References 2, 3, 6, 14, 20, 22, 26, 29, 32.
†References 12, 21, 24, 25, 36.

Fig. 8-1. Line diagrams demonstrating the value of obtaining both transverse and sagittal images when characterizing plaque. In the sagittal plane, images can be obtained that would falsely simulate **A,** homogeneous plaque (1B-Scan C′) or **B,** heterogeneous plaque (1A-Scan D′). Correlation in both planes is necessary to be certain that the surface accurately refects a smooth or irregular character.

it frequently makes it more difficult to characterize plaque because the wall margins can become less distinct. As a result, I characterize plaque with gray scale B-mode imaging only and use CFDI to help localize vessels rapidly and determine the optimal location to perform Doppler spectral analysis.

When evaluating plaque, it is important to ascertain which vessel is being studied. Usually the low-resistance pattern of the Doppler spectrum of the internal carotid artery (ICA) is sufficient to enable the examiner to distinguish it from the high-resistance external carotid artery (ECA). The ECA can be further identified by visualizing its branches, a process made much easier with CFDI. It can also be identified, if necessary, by tapping on the temporal artery and noting transmission of sound while viewing the Doppler spectrum. With CFDI, throughout the cardiac cycle, there is usually a continuous color in the ICA, in contrast to intermittent color in the ECA. The ICA usually is larger and located posterolateral to the ECA (Table 8-1). Usually several centimeters of the proximal ICA can be studied. In this manner, the examiner can be certain of the identity of the vessel being studied and direct attention to evaluating the plaque carefully along the vessel's walls.

Table 8-1. Differences between the internal carotid artery and the external carotid artery

	Internal carotid artery	External carotid artery
Size	Larger	Smaller
Location	Posterolateral	Anteromedial
Branches	None	Yes
Waveform	Low resistance	High resistance
Temporal top	Negative	Positive

PLAQUE CHARACTERIZATION

Several vascular surgeons, including Imparato and colleagues[14] and Lusby and associates,[22] have reported finding a significantly increased incidence of intraplaque hemorrhage in the surgical specimens of carotid artery plaque in their symptomatic patients as compared to those who were asymptomatic. As a result, other researchers, using improvements in high-resolution ultrasound, have tried to evaluate carotid plaque in vivo to see if they could identify differences in plaque appearance. This effort has proven to be successful. Bluth and colleagues have shown conclusively that intraplaque hemorrhage can be identified within the vessel wall with an accuracy of 90%, sensitivity of 96%, and specificity of 88%.[2] Others, including Reilly and co-workers[29] and O'Donnell and associates,[26] have shown similar findings.

The ability to identify ulcerations with ultrasound still remains controversial to some. The literature shows that the sensitivity of ultrasound in predicting ulceration ranges from less than 30% to greater than 90% (Table 8-2).[4] In my experience, intraplaque hemorrhage and ulceration are found in those forms of plaque that present a heterogeneous pattern, and the examiner cannot distinguish which patients with heterogeneous plaque have pathologically proven ulcerations.[3] Plaques that are homogeneous in their sonographic appearance contain no pathologic evidence of intraplaque hemorrhage or ulceration. Our studies have shown poor success in identifying ulcerations but excellent results in correctly identifying patients who have intraplaque hemorrhage. If, in fact, it is true that all patients with intraplaque hemorrhage are at greater risk for developing ulcerations, than perhaps it may be of only academic interest to distinguish which patients with intraplaque hemorrhage already have ulcerations.

Table 8-2. Detectability of ulceration with ultrasound

Study (first author)	Number of lesions	Sensitivity	Specificity	Accuracy
Widder, 1990	165	29%	50%	43%
Fischer, 1985	28	30%	58%	42%
O'Leary, 1987	47	39%	72%	60%
Reilly, 1983	50	42%	100%	58%
Comerota, 1990	126	47%*	86%	—
Farber, 1984	29	72%	75%	72%
Ricotta, 1990	1099	72%	32%	—
Widder, 1984	48	75%	83%	79%
O'Donnell, 1985	79	89%	87%	87%
Goodson, 1987	79	90%	89%	91%
Rubin, 1987	32	93%	100%	97%

From Merritt C, Bluth E: *Ultrasound identification of plaque composition.* In Labs K, Jager K, Fitzgerald D, et al, editors: *Vascular ultrasound,* London, 1992, Edward Arnold.
*With stenosis <50%, 77%; 41% with stenosis >50%.

PLAQUE TYPING

Two different forms of plaque can be identified, homogeneous and heterogeneous. Homogeneous plaque (Fig. 8-2) consists of plaque that is relatively uniform in texture, compared to the soft tissues surrounding the vessel wall. It usually contains uniformly low-level echoes. On occasion, uniformly increased echogenicity is seen. The surface of this plaque type is always smooth. Calcification can be present in either form of plaque and does not enter into the scheme of classification. Pathologically, homogeneous plaque corresponds usually to dense, laminated, fibrous connective tissue.

Heterogeneous plaque (Figs. 8-3 and 8-4) has a complex echo pattern that contains at least one well-defined focal sonolucent area. The well-defined sonolucent area should be larger and more distinct than those sonolucent areas that are seen in the surrounding soft tissues and that represent only the limitations of axial resolution. This form of plaque contains areas of intraplaque hemorrhage. The intimal surface of this plaque can be smooth or irregular. When the surface is smooth, it can be either homogeneous or heterogeneous, depending on the presence or absence of a focal sonolucent area within the plaque. Although all ulcerative plaques appear to be heterogeneous, all heterogeneous plaques do not contain ulcerations. There are not sonographic criteria that can separate out those plaques that are heterogeneous and contain ulcerations from those plaques that are heterogeneous and do not pathologically contain ulcerations.[22] Perhaps with the advent of CFDI, some additional criteria may be developed.

SIGNIFICANCE

Although it has been conclusively shown that intraplaque hemorrhage can be sonographically identified, the significance of this finding is still somewhat controversial. It is believed by some that embolization may result when intraplaque hemorrhage of some unknown cause develops within the vessel wall (possibly rupture of the vasa vasorum). The intraplaque hemorrhage is thought to extend to the intimal surface, leading to intimal tears in the vessel lining, initiation of the clotting cascade, and thrombus formation over the tear. The resulting thrombus can then either be incorporated into the vessel wall, resulting in increased stenosis, or break off and embolize into distal vessels of the carotid circulation, leading to stroke.

Others postulate that abnormal blood flow patterns in association with other external factors, such as elevated cholesterol levels or smoking, cause damage to the endothelial surface of the carotid vessels. This leads to unsuccessful attempts to repair the vessel wall and the development of plaque. Ultimately in some patients, because these abnormal flow patterns persist, the surface of the plaque breaks, intraplaque hemorrhage develops, and thrombus forms along the plaque surface as a further attempt at repair. This thrombus can be incorporated into the plaque, causing further flow-limiting stenosis, or it can embolize distally. Perhaps in time, with the more widespread use of CFDI, we will learn more about the mechanism causing the development of intraplaque hemorrhage.

Sterpetti and co-workers have shown in a prospective study that heterogeneous plaque is a significant risk factor for developing subsequent neurologic defects.[32] They analyzed numerous risk factors and found that degree of stenosis and type of plaque were the only statistically significant risk factors for the development of future neurologic events in a group of patients who were followed prospectively for a year. In another study,

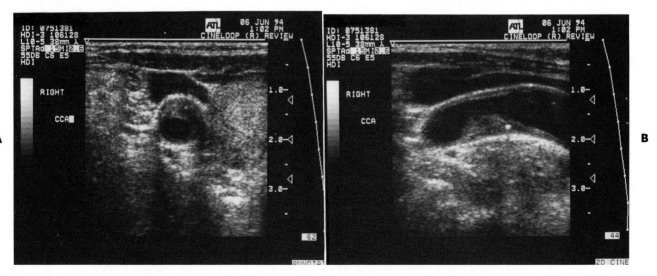

Fig. 8-2. Homogeneous plaque on transverse (**A**) and sagittal (**B**) images. Note the smooth surface and uniform echo pattern. A calcification within the plaque wall is seen.

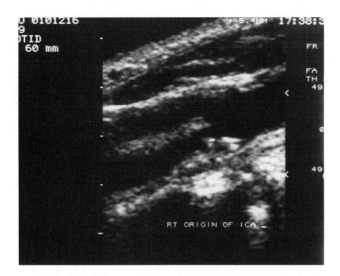

Fig. 8-3. Heterogeneous plaque. Note the irregular surface and large sonolucent area just beneath the plaque's surface.

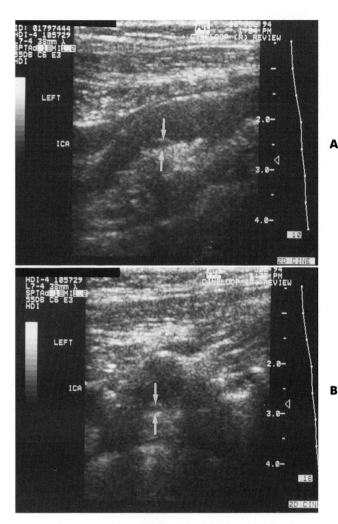

Fig. 8-4. Heterogeneous plaque. Note the sonolucent area beneath the plaque surface on both sagittal (**A**) and transverse (**B**) planes.

Leahy and associates showed that there was a significant increase in ipsilateral cerebral hemispheric symptoms in patients with heterogeneous plaque (50%) compared to patients with homogeneous plaque (22%).[20]

In a more recently published report, Polak, O'Leary, and colleagues characterized the plaque of more than 5200 subjects and made determinations of wall thickness.[28] On initial evaluation, they found that a history of TIAs and stroke was more likely among those patients who, on careful study, had heterogeneous plaque. However, they also noted that the degree of ICA stenosis correlated better with prevalent stroke and TIA than plaque characterization. These patients will be followed by this group for 3 years, at which point it is hoped that additional information regarding the role of plaque characterization in determining the relative risk of stroke will result.

At the present time, however, additional long-term studies are needed to show conclusively that the presence of different forms of plaque leads to a different incidence of neurologic symptoms and stroke before treating patients differently based on plaque characterization will be uniformly accepted. Nevertheless, it is important at the present time to appreciate the differences in plaque features and to categorize plaque whenever possible into these two groupings so that they can be followed for change. At the present time, it would seem logical to follow patients with potentially unstable heterogeneous plaque more closely than patients with homogeneous plaque.

SUMMARY

Duplex sonography, having been shown to be equivalent to arteriography in the evaluation of flow-limiting stenosis, is now a standard part of imaging of the extracranial carotid vessels. Unique to sonography among imaging studies, however, is the ability to evaluate the plaque wall and accurately characterize plaque. Two different patterns for plaque are identified, one homogeneous and the other heterogeneous. Heterogeneous plaque contains areas of intraplaque hemorrhage. Those patients with this form of plaque may be at greater risk for developing embolic stroke. If, indeed, the presence of heterogeneous plaque proves to be, in additional prospective studies, associated with an increased risk of stroke, high-resolution ultrasound will have a uniquely important role in determining which patients fall into this category. As the only noninvasive way to determine this information, it will be important for all performing carotid ultrasound to be knowledgeable in how to accurately characterize plaque. At the present time, in the expectation that this may occur, all interested in carotid ultrasound should learn this methodology.

REFERENCES

1. Blackshear WM, Phillips DJ, Chikos PM, et al: Carotid artery velocity patterns in normal and stenotic vessels, 11:67-71, *Stroke* 1980.
2. Bluth E, Kay D, Merritt C, et al: Sonographic characterization of carotid plaque: detection of hemorrhage, *AJR Am J Roentgenol* 146:1061-1065, 1986.
3. Bluth E, McVay L, Merritt C, Sullivan M: The identification of ulcerative plaque with high resolutions duplex carotid scanning, *J Ultrasound Med* 1:73-76, 1988.
4. Bluth E, Merritt C: Carotid and vertebral arteries. In *Color Doppler Imaging,* New York, 1992, Churchill Livingstone.
5. Bluth E, Merritt C, Sullivan M, et al: The usefulness of duplex ultrasound in evaluating vertebral arteries, *J Ultrasound Med* 8:229-235, 1989.
6. Bluth E, Stavros A, Marich K, et al: Carotid duplex sonography: a multi-center recommendation for standardized imaging and Doppler criteria, *Radiographics* 8:487-506, 1988.
7. Dreisbach JN, Seibert CE, Smazal SF, et al: Duplex sonography in the evaluation of carotid artery disease, *AJNR Am J Neuroradiol* 4:678-680, 1983.
8. Erickson SJ, Mewissen M, Foley W, et al: Stenosis of the internal carotid artery: assessment using color Doppler imaging compared with angiography, *AJR Am J Roentgenol* 152:1299-1305, 1989.
9. Fell G, Phillips DJ, Chikos PM, et al: Ultrasonic duplex scanning for disease of the carotid artery, *Circulation* 64:1191-1195, 1981.
10. Friedman SG, Hainine B, Feinberg AW, et al: Use of diastolic velocity ratios to predict significant carotid artery stenosis, *Stroke* 19:910-912, 1988.
11. Garth KE, Carroll BA, Sommer FG, Oppenheimer DA: Duplex ultrasound scanning of the carotid arteries with velocity spectrum analysis, *Radiology* 147:823-827, 1983.
12. Grant E, Wong W, Tessler F, et al: Cerebrovascular ultrasound imaging, *Radiol Clin North Am* 26:1111-1130, 1988.
13. Hallam M, Reid J, Cooperberg P: Color-flow Doppler and conventional duplex scanning of the carotid bifurcation prospective, double-blind, correlative study, *AJR Am J Roentgenol* 152:1101-1105, 1989.
14. Imparato AM, Riles TS, Mintzer R, et al: The importance of hemorrhage in the relationship between gross morphologic characteristics and cerebral symptoms in 376 carotid artery plaques, *Ann Surg* 197:195, 1983.
15. Jackson VP, Kuehn DS, Bendick PH, et al: Duplex carotid sonography: correlation with digital subtraction angiography and conventional angiography, *J Ultrasound Med* 4:239-249, 1985.
16. Jacobs N, Grant E, Schellinger D, et al: Duplex carotid sonography: criteria for stenosis, accurately, and pitfalls, *Radiology* 154:385-391, 1985.
17. Keagy BA, Pharr WF, Thomas D, Bowles DE: Evaluation of the peak frequency ratio (PFR) measurement in the detection of internal carotid artery stenosis, *J Clin Ultrasound* 10:109-112, 1982.
18. Kotval PS: Doppler waveform parvus and tardus: a sign of proximal flow obstruction, *J Ultrasound Med* 8:435-440, 1989.
19. Langlois Y, Roedever G, Chan A, et al: Evaluating carotid artery disease; the concordance between pulsed Doppler spectrum analysis and angiography, *Ultrasound Med Biol* 9:51-63, 1983.
20. Leahy A, McCollum P, Feeley T, et al: Duplex of ultrasonography and selection of patients for carotid endarterectomy, *J Vasc Surg* 8:558-562, 1988.
21. Loberto F, Nowak M, Quist W: Structural details of boundary layer separation in a model human carotid bifurcation under steady and pulsatile flow conditions, *J Vasc Surg* 2:263-269, 1985.
22. Lusby RJ, Ferrell LD, Ehrenfeld WK, et al: Carotid plaque hemorrhage: its role in production of cerebral ischemia, *Arch Surg* 117:1479, 1982.
23. Merritt C, Bluth E: *Ultrasound identification of plaque composition.* In Labs K, Jager K, Fitzgerald D, et al, editors: *Diagnostic vascular ultrasound,* London, 1992, Edward Arnold.
24. Middleton WD, Foley WD, Lawson TL: Color-flow Doppler imaging of carotid artery abnormalities, *AJR Am J Roentgenol* 150:410-425, 1988.
25. Middleton W, Foley W, Lawson T: Flow reversal in the normal carotid bifurcation: color Doppler flow imaging analysis, *Radiology* 167:207-210, 1988.
26. O'Donnell T, Erodes L, Mackey W, et al: Correlation of B-mode ultrasound imaging and arteriography with pathologic findings at carotid endarterectomy, *Radiology* 157:861, 1985.
27. Polak J, Dobkin G, O'Leary D, et al: Internal carotid artery stenosis: accuracy and reproducibility of color-Doppler-assisted duplex imaging, *Radiology* 173:793-798, 1989.
28. Polak J, O'Leary D, Kronmal R, et al: Sonographic evaluation of carotid artery atherosclerosis in the elderly: relationship of disease severity to stroke and transient ischemic attack, *Radiology* 188:363-370, 1993.
29. Reilly L, Lusby R, Hughes L, et al: Carotid plaque histology using real-time ultrasonography: clinical and therapeutic implications, *Am J Surg* 146:188-193, 1983.
30. Robinson ML, Sack D, Perlmutter GS, Marinelli D: Diagnostic criteria for carotid duplex sonography, *AJR Am J Roentgenol* 15:1045-1049, 1988.
31. Steinke W, Kloetzech C, Hennerici M: Carotid artery disease assessed by color Doppler flow imaging, *AJNR Am J Neuroradiol* 11:259-266, 1990.
32. Sterpetti A, Schultz R, Feldhaus, et al: Ultrasonographic features of carotid plaque and the risk of subsequent neurologic defects, *Surgery* 104:652-660, 1988.
33. Taylor DC, Strandness DE: Carotid artery duplex scanning, *J Clin Ultrasound* 15:635-644, 1987.
34. Vaisman U, Wojciechowski M: Carotid artery disease: new criteria for evaluation of sonographic duplex scanning, *Radiology* 158:253-255, 1986.
35. Withers CE, Gosink BB, Keightley AM, et al: Duplex carotid sonography: peak systolic velocity in quantifying internal carotid artery stenosis, *J Ultrasound Med* 9:345-349, 1990.
36. Zavins C, Giddens D, Bharadvaj B, et al: Carotid bifurcation atherosclerosis: quantitative correlation of plaque localization with flow velocity profiles and wall shear stress, *Circ Res* 53:502-514, 1983.

Color Flow Imaging of the Carotid Arteries

Joseph F. Polak

The first attempts to apply color flow imaging to the carotid arteries were made in the late 1980s. Investigators focused on using the color image of flowing blood to measure directly the residual lumen diameter of stenosis.[8,25,42]

Such an approach has one advantage. The image display resembles the information obtained on a contrast arteriogram. The residual lumen is measured rather than estimated from an increase in blood flow velocity at the stenosis. The process used to create the Doppler color flow image is, however, subject to artifacts. The estimated residual lumen can vary, simply by changing the angle between transducer and stenosis or by changing settings such as the pulse repetition frequency (PRF), various filters, and the overall gain. An alternate approach is to measure the velocity directly from the color flow image. This approach is validated by phantom studies.[21] The irony of the clinical[12] and in vitro studies[21] that use this approach is that they correlate their findings to those of traditional Doppler waveform analysis.

At the time that color flow imaging was introduced, established laboratories were already performing accurate evaluations of carotid artery lesions with the aid of Doppler waveform analysis. Continuous-wave Doppler devices and duplex sonographic devices generate Doppler waveforms that are interpreted with proven and validated diagnostic criteria.[4,40] The early reports that looked at direct sizing of lesion size[8] on the color flow image and stenosis velocity estimates from the color flow map[12] used duplex velocity criteria as a standard. These studies did not reveal any significant differences in the accuracy of these techniques. What was quickly appreciated, however, is the fact that the real-time display of the flow dynamics over distances of 2 to 4 cm permitted a rapid survey of the carotid system. Zones of altered flow dynamics were quickly located, and it therefore seemed feasible to use the color flow map as a means of identifying sites that warranted more careful evaluation with Doppler waveform analysis.[32]

This approach has, over time, become the preferred one. Although it is possible to perform a noninvasive evaluation of the carotid branches by using only color flow maps and appropriate diagnostic criteria — either direct measurement of lumen size or color frequency shifts — the majority of laboratories and practitioners of noninvasive carotid studies still rely on Doppler waveform analysis. These Doppler waveforms are being acquired with the aid of the color flow map. The color

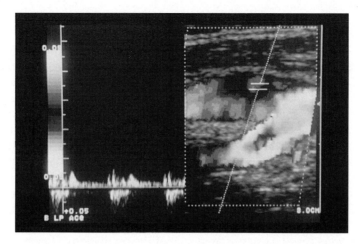

Fig. 9-1. This carotid bifurcation depicts the zone of flow reversal in the proximal internal carotid. The finding on the color flow image is confirmed by the Doppler waveform.

flow image is used to position the Doppler gate and to perform angle correction. This approach may make the velocity measurements as reproducible as those made by arteriography.[32]

There are, however, specific situations in which the color flow map has the potential for improving the accuracy of noninvasive evaluations of the carotids. These are for cases of completely hypoechoic plaques, especially those causing less than 50% diameter narrowing, cases of suspected subtotal occlusion, and, finally, cases in which the velocities are artificially elevated in the carotid contralateral to a high-grade stenosis.

FLOW DYNAMICS: NORMAL CAROTID BIFURCATION

In normal subjects without any atherosclerotic change in the carotid arteries, the color flow image typically shows a zone of flow reversal in the proximal internal carotid artery.[26] This zone of flow reversal and altered flow dynamics is typically located in the distal common carotid opposite to the flow divider between internal and external carotid arteries. It is inherent to the nature of the carotid bifurcation.[20] The color flow image can be used to measure the size of this zone. More importantly, color flow imaging can be used in vivo[26] as well as in vitro[34] to study the factors responsible for this phenomenon. For example, flow separation arises in the absence of pulsatile flow in phantoms with nondistensible walls. It is mostly a reflection of geometry[15] and the proportion of blood flow that is shared between the external and internal carotid branches, as well as their relative sizes.[34]

This flow reversal (Fig. 9-1; see also Plate 22) occurs at the site where the early atherosclerotic plaques are observed. This capability of visualizing a zone of flow reversal in the corresponding portion of the carotid has aided in the understanding of the pathologic mechanism

responsible for early plaque formation. Contrary to hypotheses that suggest that plaque formation is due to increased shearing forces on the endothelium, it appears that areas of decreased shear rates and slow flow encourage the formation of the lesions.[10] This phenomenon can be documented in a consistent fashion in most patients devoid of significant atherosclerotic plaque.[26] The absence of a zone of flow reversal (Fig. 9-2; see also Plate 23) does not, however, appear to have any significant implications on the likelihood that subjects will develop atherosclerotic lesions.

This simple contribution of color flow imaging is probably not relevant to the daily use of this technology in the evaluation of carotid artery disease. It is, however, a reminder that this new technology offers basic physiologic information on the flow dynamics of normal and diseased carotid vessels.

CLINICALLY RELEVANT DIFFERENCES BETWEEN COLOR FLOW AND DUPLEX IMAGING
Distinguishing internal from external carotid arteries

Color flow imaging can distinguish the internal from the external carotid artery by the simple fact that branches arise only from the external carotid. Successful visualization of the external carotid branches can be achieved for patients with, at most, mild carotid disease. The superior thyroidal artery is the first branch that arises at the very origin of the external carotid artery from the common carotid. What follows are a multitude of smaller branches responsible for feeding the face and scalp.

The internal carotid artery tends to have a larger diameter than the external carotid and is also located more laterally. These facts would suggest that there should not be any difficulties in identifying and distinguishing these two carotid branches with color flow imaging alone. This does not appear to be the case in patients with more extensive carotid lesions, in whom such a simple task may become quite difficult.

For example, the color flow signals generated by high-grade lesions of the external carotid artery can mimic those of the internal carotid artery. Quite often, the external carotid side branches may be difficult to identify. The continuity of these branches may be difficult to verify when the arteries lie deep in the soft tissues of the neck. Flow in these small branches may also be due to collaterals when high-grade lesions are present in the external and internal carotid arteries. In these instances, rather than relying on traditional longitudinal plane imaging of the carotid, color flow imaging is done in the transverse plane in an effort to identify the origin of the side branches as they arise from the vessel being studied.

The internal carotid can be consistently distinguished from the external carotid with the aid of duplex

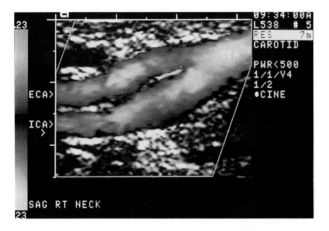

Fig. 9-2. This carotid bifurcation of a young normal volunteer is devoid of a zone of flow reversal.

sonography. Specifically, the external carotid artery Doppler waveform, even when it resembles the internal carotid artery waveform, responds differently to a simple physiologic maneuver. This is achieved with the temporal tap maneuver, which consists of the generation of short impulses or pressure waves by pressing on the preauricular branch of the temporal artery. This creates oscillations on the Doppler waveform sampled within the proximal external carotid artery (Fig. 9-3; see also Plate 24). This oscillatory change in velocity is difficult to perceive on the color flow map but can be readily documented on the Doppler waveform. The reliability of this maneuver increases when a high-grade external carotid artery stenosis is present because the amplitude of the oscillations are magnified. Therefore, even when a high-grade stenosis of the external carotid artery mimics the internal carotid artery, they can still be distinguished from each other with the aid of a temporal tap maneuver.

In summary, the typical location of the internal carotid artery with respect to the external carotid artery and the presence of small branches that arise from the external carotid artery are not consistent enough findings to protect from errors of diagnosis between internal and external carotid arteries. The combination of color flow imaging and the response of the external carotid Doppler waveform to the temporal tap protects against such errors.

Localizing stenotic lesions

Hemodynamically significant stenoses are defined as causing a pressure gradient. This occurs for stenoses that cause at least a 50% narrowing of the lumen diameter. The color flow map can be used to detect the effect of such stenoses on flow dynamics. The velocity of blood

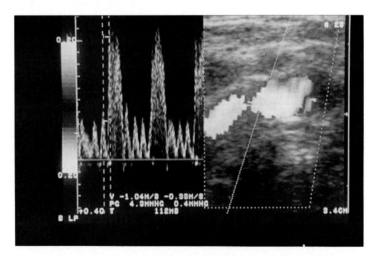

Fig. 9-3. In this patient, the two carotid branches with very similar waveforms. Here, the temporal tap maneuver was administered. It caused prominent oscillations in the Doppler waveform, confirming that this branch was the external carotid artery.

increases as the lumen narrows and is typically the greatest at the point of maximal stenotic narrowing. This is where the color flow map shows the point of maximal velocity.[43] The zone of increased velocity that is established at the point of maximal stenosis can continue as a stenotic jet, typically extending 1 to 2 cm distal to the stenosis (Fig. 9-4; see also Plate 25).[2] The motion of blood, as it decelerates quickly at the boundary of the jet, will become turbulent and cause heterogeneity on the color flow image.[49] There will also be a tendency for blood to reverse direction as the lumen expands distal to the stenotic narrowing and returns to normal. This zone of flow reversal will be seen to the sides of the stenotic jet (Fig. 9-5; see also Plate 26).

Nonlaminar flow is also seen for lesions that do not yet cause a hemodynamically significant narrowing. This causes a spread in the measured velocities of moving blood and is manifest as a broadening of the Doppler spectrum. These may cause zones of altered flow signals on the color flow map, increasing the "variance" of the color flow signal.[43]

After properly adjusting the color flow map for both sensitivity and peak repetition frequency, the sites of stenotic narrowing can therefore be identified by virtue of the increased frequency shifts generated by the rapidly moving red blood cells. If the PRF is set to depict frequency shifts over the normal range of blood flow in the carotid artery, sites of stenotic narrowing show up as points where the color flow signals show aliasing. In addition, as the lesion increases in severity, the stenotic jet that extends downstream from the stenosis will be more easily perceived. The zone of flow reversal that develops to the sides of the stenotic jet is more difficult to show on the color flow map.

These zones—increased frequency shifts at the stenosis and altered flow signals distal to the stenosis—make the color flow map a useful aid for rapidly locating the site of maximal stenotic narrowing. The standard duplex sonographic approach requires the displacement of the Doppler gate, with its sample volume of 1 to 2 mm, along the full length of the artery being studied. This is a time-consuming task made harder when vessels are tortuous, located deep in the soft tissues of the neck, and involved with echogenic atherosclerotic deposits. Because the color flow map depicts long segments of the arteries on one image (Fig. 9-6; see also Plate 27), it makes it possible to rapidly survey large lengths of carotid branches and to detect sites of altered flow dynamics. These sites can subsequently be interrogated with Doppler velocity waveform analysis.

The two alternate ways of using color flow mapping to grade stenosis severity rely on a direct measurement

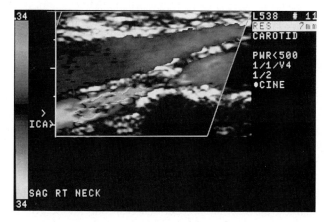

Fig. 9-4. This stenosis in the proximal internal carotid artery causes a zone of flow disturbance that extends at least 1 cm downstream to the stenosis (zone of aliasing is in turquoise).

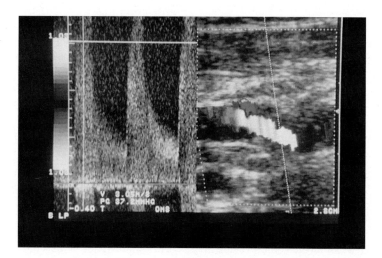

Fig. 9-5. This stenosis is oriented toward the skin. A small zone of flow reversal (blue) is seen distal to the stenotic jet. Proper angle correction was facilitated by the color map.

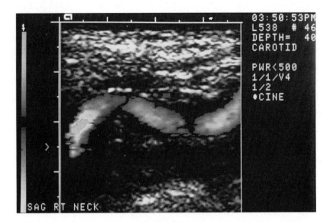

Fig. 9-6. Changes in the direction of the proximal internal carotid artery causes the color map to change colors as the direction of the artery changes. In addition, the sharp angle of the internal carotid artery segment to the left of the image causes a zone of apparent increase in velocity.

made on the color flow image. The first is a direct measurement of the size of the color channel corresponding to the residual lumen of the artery.[8,43] This assumes that the PRF is set high enough and that the specialized filters that are used to process the color flow information are set appropriately. If not, the size of the residual lumen seen on the color flow image will likely be larger than the true lumen because of "bleeding" of the color flow information outside the artery. Under ideal conditions, however, the measured residual "flow lumen" still tends to underestimate the severity of the stenosis with respect to arteriography.[42] The second approach is a direct measurement of the velocity from the frequency shift information on the color flow image. This can be done by determining the point where the color signals alias,[12] or with the aid of a velocity "tag."[21,43] This measurement should ideally be angle-corrected, a condition that is often not met.[12] The velocity estimate obtained in this fashion remains a measurement of the "mean" frequency shift and, after angle correction, of the "mean" velocity. The values will be 30% to 50% lower than the peak velocities measured from the Doppler spectral display. These direct measurements are also hampered by the fact that stenotic lesions may be partly obscured by calcified plaque. They may be missed on the color flow map proper and cannot therefore be graded.[8] However, because the flow disturbance associated with a stenosis extends at least 1 to 2 cm downstream to the lesion,[2,49] the stenotic jet can still be sampled and graded with Doppler waveform analysis. Alternatively, it may be possible to detect a zone of flow reversal downstream to the arterial segment obscured by the calcification. This will at least suggest the presence of a hemodynamically significant lesion whose severity cannot be estimated.

Velocity measurements

Mean versus spectral frequency shift (velocity) measurements. The creation of the color flow map requires enormous mathematical processing of the frequency shift information in the returning echoes.[18] The additional requirements in computer hardware that would be needed to create point-to-point Doppler spectral color maps, although feasible, are well beyond the range of being cost-effective. Instead, the color flow map depicts velocity estimates as a mean value. Velocities measured on the color flow maps are therefore not equivalent to the measurements of peak systolic and peak end-diastolic velocities made on the Doppler waveform display. Instead, a mean or average velocity is obtained. The velocity measurements derived directly from the color flow map will therefore not correlate with the published Doppler velocity criteria used for grading the severity of stenotic lesions.[4]

Aliasing and pulse repetition frequency. Because the color flow image is created over a large field of view, the effective pulse repetition frequency is much lower than that attained with duplex imaging. This has important implications when attempts are made to measure the velocity changes that occur at stenotic lesions.

Because the effective PRF of color flow mapping is lower, aliasing will occur on the color flow map at lower velocities—and therefore lower grades of stenotic narrowing—than what is seen on the Doppler spectrum. This restricts the use of the color flow map to measuring mean velocity at lesions that do not cause an aliased signal. Measurement of the residual lumen diameter of the artery from the color flow map is also complicated by bleeding of the color signals into the surrounding soft tissues. This may be caused by poor gain settings but is also caused by the coarser sampling size of the color Doppler gates as compared to those used to create the gray scale image. For these reasons, the actual size of residual lumen as measured on the color flow image may be overestimated, and the severity of the lesion may be underestimated.[42]

As a general rule, in the presence of aliasing, attempts to estimate directly the stenotic lumen from the color flow map should be done at the highest PRF possible. The selected PRF should be set just short of causing an aliased signal on the color flow image. Aliasing is common when high Doppler frequencies—5 to 7 MHz—are used to create the color flow image. It may be necessary to reduce the color Doppler imaging frequency in order to eliminate aliasing at lower grades of stenotic narrowing.

In general, the PRFs attained with duplex sonography are much higher than what can be achieved with color Doppler imaging. This makes Doppler waveform analysis a more reliable approach for grading stenotic lesion severity based on the frequency shifts detected at the stenotic lesion.

Angle correction. The color flow map cannot reliably be angle corrected. In most instruments, there is an option for interrogating color flow Doppler signals in a vertical direction or angled by 20° to 30° left and right to the vertical. Angling of the color box is useful in those situations where a color Doppler signal cannot be obtained because the artery is perfectly parallel to the transducer surface. If, however, mean velocity measurements are to be made directly from the color flow image, it is necessary to use some form of angle correction. This is normally achieved by using a cursor that can be aligned parallel either to the lumen of the vessel or to the direction of the velocity jet created by a stenotic lesion. This velocity jet need not be parallel to the wall of the artery (Figs. 9-4 and 9-5).

The errors that are made when the angle between ultrasound beam and the direction of flowing blood are above 60° are the same whether color flow mapping or Doppler waveform analysis is used. The angle-corrected velocity measurements become progressively less reliable as the angle increases.

IMAGING PROTOCOL: COLOR FLOW GUIDED DUPLEX SONOGRAPHY
Principle

The clinical use of color flow imaging has evolved so that it serves as a guide for detecting zones of flow abnormality. These are then subjected to further and more careful evaluation of the altered flow dynamics with the aid of Doppler waveform analysis. The evaluation of the carotid system can therefore be referred to as *color flow assisted* or *color flow guided* duplex sonography. Imaging is normally performed in the transverse as well as in the longitudinal plane. Most imaging is, however, conducted in the longitudinal plane, parallel to the artery. This is favored in the vast majority of situations because (1) it depicts flow dynamics over a long segments of the carotid, (2) the transducer must not be displaced needlessly until the flow has been carefully interrogated over the arterial segment in question, and (3) Doppler waveform analysis with appropriate Doppler angle correction can be rapidly done from the same transducer position. Artifacts engendered by the motion of the transducer against the skin are more likely to occur when the transducer is placed in the transverse plane (Fig. 9-7; see also Plate 28) and must then be moved along the course of the artery. Flow signals may be transiently lost and cause some confusion when the transducer is displaced to survey the artery. This may be due to sampling during diastole when the flow velocity is decreased or because of changes in the direction of the vessel.

Color flow imaging can be used efficiently once time

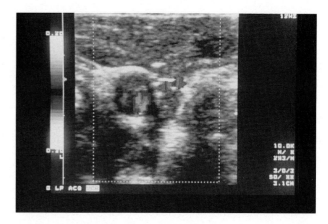

Fig. 9-7. This transverse image of the common carotid artery clearly depicts an eccentric plaque. The color flow lumen contrasts sharply against the plaque (*left*) and the uninvolved wall (*right*).

is taken to select an appropriate baseline velocity range or PRF. This is normally done in the common carotid artery by angling the color flow box 20° to the vertical and angling the transducer in the direction of the artery. The PRF is then adjusted so that the maximal systolic frequency shifts do not alias. The transducer is then displaced in the longitudinal direction along the course of the common carotid artery. The color box is positioned and inverted as needed to depict flow signals within the full lumen of the vessel. Any sites of aliasing are further interrogated with the use of Doppler waveform analysis. Hemodynamically significant focal lesions in the common artery are, however, much less likely than an internal carotid stenosis. The imaging protocol normally requires documenting blood flow velocities with the aid of Doppler waveform analysis at two or three sites in the common carotid.

At the level of the carotid bifurcation, the color flow box is normally angulated in whichever direction that best depicts flow in the selected carotid branch, internal or external. Again, sites of aliasing are searched for and the basic velocity scale or PRF of the color box adjusted with respect to the normal appearing portions of the internal carotid and external carotid lumen. Sampling of the Doppler waveform at sites of aliasing is normally done by positioning the Doppler gate at the site and angle correcting parallel to the velocity jet that is present. If this jet is poorly distinguished, the angle correction is normally made to be parallel with the direction of the vessel at this level.

The altered flow dynamics beyond the stenotic jet are normally documented by sampling the Doppler waveform within the boundary layer of the jet or in the zone of vortical flow outside of the jet. Turbulent flow is normally present at the zone between the reversed and forward flows, as well as at the site of maximal dissipation of the jet energy further downstream from

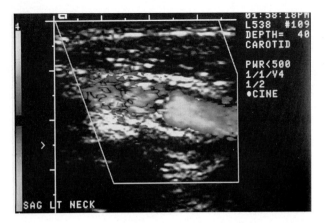

Fig. 9-8. A zone of heterogeneous signals is created to the left of the image by a high-grade lesion in the distal common carotid artery. This correlates with a marked carotid bruit heard on auscultation. It is caused by the vibrations generated in the soft tissues as the jet of blood impacts the wall of the artery.

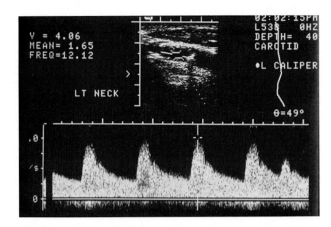

Fig. 9-9. The corresponding Doppler waveform confirms the presence of a high-grade stenosis.

the lesion. The latter may cause a typical vibration in the surrounding soft tissues when the jet impacts on the artery wall (Fig. 9-8; see also Plate 29). A Doppler waveform should also be sampled where the color flow signals become normal more distally (Fig. 9-9; see also Plate 30).

Efficacy

A simple protocol that uses longitudinal color flow imaging to identify possible sites of aliasing, with subsequent Doppler waveform analysis to confirm the severity of the lesion, has been shown to take less time than standard duplex sonography alone.[32] The time taken to obtain the appropriate Doppler spectrum with the aid of the color flow map can be, on average, 40% of what is required when duplex sonography is used alone. Similar time savings are seen if color Doppler is used alone to grade stenosis severity.

Using the color flow map as a means for selecting the site for subsequent Doppler waveform analysis also seems to normalize or standardize the time taken for an examination. For example, with duplex sonography alone, high-grade lesions or complex lesions with calcification, tortuous vessels, and deeper-lying vessels may require a significantly greater amount of time to evaluate than stenotic lesions located in a straight and superficially located carotid artery. Color flow imaging tends to reduce the time taken to evaluate the more difficult cases (Fig. 9-10; see also Plate 31). There does not appear to be any significant advantage in using color flow mapping when an artery is completely normal. An evaluation of a normal carotid bifurcation with color flow mapping requires additional time to determine the proper color flow box position and settings for velocity scales and filters, as well as the color sensitivity.

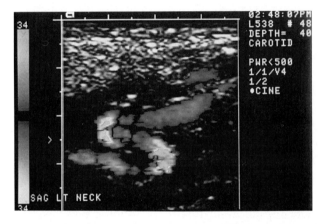

Fig. 9-10. This color flow image depicts a very tortuous internal carotid artery. Without the color map, the artery would be difficult to trace. Sampling with the Doppler gate would be time-consuming. The zones of increased velocity at the outside aspect of the two acute curves in the artery are due to the geometry of the artery and not to the presence of a stenosis.

Another facet of color-guided flow imaging efficacy is the number of patients who ultimately are referred for contrast arteriography. Without appropriate sonographic screening, approximately 50% of patients who undergo arteriography are subsequently shown to have a significant stenosis of more than 50%.[29] With the use of color flow guided duplex sonography, this increases to 90% of the population going to arteriographic evaluation.[32]

Diagnostic criteria

The diagnostic criteria adopted for color flow guided duplex sonography are the same as for the standard duplex sonography. In general, a standard value of 125 cm/s for the peak systolic velocity in the internal carotid artery is believed to correspond to a 50% diameter stenosis. This velocity criterion is adopted with the

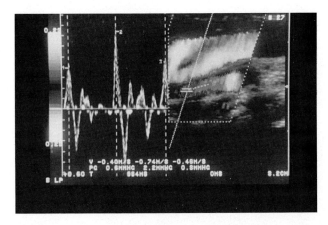

Fig. 9-11. This internal carotid Doppler waveform clearly shows evidence of an arrhythmia. This finding is difficult to appreciate on the color flow image alone. In addition, the waveform shows changes consistent with aortic valve regurgitation.

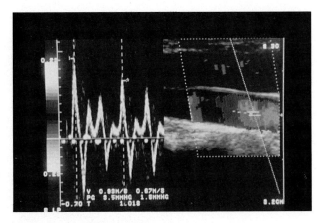

Fig. 9-12. The corresponding common carotid waveform is shown. It depicts a similar increase in velocity for certain cardiac beats. The peak systolic velocity ratio normalizes for these changes in cardiac output. The velocity ratio can also be used to correct for cardiac output changes that might occur over the months or years.

understanding that velocities in the common artery are within normal limits and are not decreased because of (1) a low cardiac output, (2) a high-grade inflow lesion at the origin of the common carotid or innominate artery, or (3) simultaneous high-grade lesions in the external and internal carotid arteries. In these situations, some form of velocity ratio, preferably the peak systolic velocity ratio is preferred. The velocity ratio is also used to compensate for changes in cardiac output, either to arrhythmia or to myocardial or valvular disease (Figs. 9-11 and 9-12; see also Plates 32 and 33). There is still some controversy as to which velocity parameter performs best for evaluating the severity of internal carotid artery stenosis. Although many have adopted the simple peak systolic velocity as a reliable means of quantifying stenotic lesions, others favor the use of peak end-diastolic velocity. The end-diastolic velocity measurements have been shown to have possibly better discriminating power for high-grade stenosis of at least 80% diameter narrowing.[4] The more recent adoption of 70% diameter narrowing as a threshold value for clinically significant carotid stenotic lesions has led to careful analyses of the diagnostic performance of the different criteria and the determination of appropriate threshold values. In one paper, peak systolic velocity appeared to have overall better accuracy than other velocity parameters.[16] In another, the peak systolic velocity ratio of 4 or above seems to discriminate between patients with and without 70% diameter narrowing.[27]

Limitations

The application of color flow mapping assumes that an appropriate imaging window is available and that the segment of the artery being studied is clearly visualized on the color flow map. Calcification that extends over distances of more than 1 cm is an inherent limitation of color flow mapping.[8,32,43] Such calcifications can occur in 9% to 12% of symptomatic patients presenting for noninvasive carotid evaluation.

Velocity patterns in tortuous vessels are very complex and difficult to evaluate, even with color flow maps. The advantage of color flow imaging is, however, the ability to follow the course of these very tortuous vessels. Color flow imaging at sites where the lumen expands—for example, the carotid bulb—typically shows complex flow patterns that may appear difficult to evaluate. The flow separation often intermixes with complex flow patterns that appear confusing when seen in only the one imaging dimension defined by the transducer. In general, however, such situations can be resolved by increasing the PRF and focusing the operator's attention on identifying a distinct velocity jet that would indicate the presence of a high-grade lesion. Confirmation of the altered flow patterns is, however, readily done by simply placing the Doppler gate within the region of complex flow and performing Doppler waveform analysis.

Variance mapping

Variance mapping is a simple method of depicting rapid changes in the direction and pattern of flow as red cells emerge from a stenotic narrowing. Although some laboratories have reported the ability to use variance mapping as a means of better localizing stenotic lesions,[47] others have basically equated the variance map to the site of aliasing.[2]

The reason for this difference is not clear. It may be caused by the algorithms that calculate the variance values within the different sonographic devices. Sites of increased variance can be created at the same location

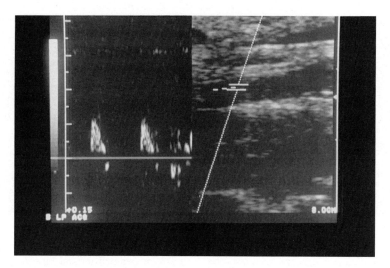

Fig. 9-13. This Doppler waveform is sampled in the internal carotid artery at a point proximal to a high-grade stenosis. There is still mostly antegrade flow despite the loss of diastolic flow.

where aliasing develops by setting the PRF to low values.[2] There does not appear to be any distinct advantage to using this specialized function when performing color flow mapping of the carotid system.

SPECIAL CONTRIBUTIONS OF COLOR FLOW IMAGING

Color flow mapping has made specific contributions to the diagnostic use of Doppler sonography. The technology can help in distinguishing total from subtotal internal carotid artery occlusions and in delineating the presence of hypoechoic plaque. A potential contribution of color flow imaging may be in helping to characterize altered flow dynamics in the carotid bifurcation contralateral to the site of a high-grade stenosis.

Total versus subtotal occlusions

As first described with continuous-wave Doppler, high-grade internal carotid artery lesions, as they become more severe, may cause a decrease in peak systolic velocity rather than an increase.[40] The stenosis reaches such a level of severity that volume flow decreases below a critical value, thereby causing the velocities measured at the stenosis to decrease. This is also likely to occur when complex lesions obstruct the carotid lumen and make it difficult to perform duplex sonography. In essence, the Doppler gate must be positioned over a very small residual lumen in the internal carotid artery and used to sample the length of what is generally a very small residual lumen. This has to be done very meticulously at low PRF and high sensitivity settings.

The Doppler waveform proximal to a subtotal occlusion may indicate a patent artery (Fig. 9-13; see also Plate 34). With color flow imaging, it is possible to use the longitudinal and the transverse planes alternatively

to search for the presence of a very narrowed flow lumen. As is the case with the duplex approach, the PRF should be set at low values and the sensitivities at high levels. In addition, specialized motion discrimination filters should be disabled so that the flow signals are more readily detected. Once a patent lumen is identified, it can be further interrogated with Doppler waveform analysis. In addition, the color flow map can be used to follow the course of the internal carotid to the point just beyond the stenosis, where the flow signals are often distorted and of low amplitude. Doppler waveform analysis can then be used, this time to confirm patency of the internal carotid distal to the subtotal occlusion.

Total occlusions (Fig. 9-14; see also Plate 35), especially if they have occurred recently, cause flow reversal during diastole on the color flow map as well as on the Doppler spectrum sampled just proximal to the occlusion (Fig. 9-15; see also Plate 36). The blood that enters the short segment of the proximal internal carotid artery that is still patent causes to the artery to distend and store some of the blood volume. This is then pushed out of the blind carotid stump when systemic pressures drop during diastole.

The accuracy of duplex sonography in detecting and distinguishing total from subtotal occlusions has been described as being approximately 50% in the early days of carotid Doppler sonography.[55] At first, the introduction of color flow imaging did not appear to have improved the ability to distinguish total from subtotal occlusions.[43] Recent data suggest, however, that color-flow imaging may improve diagnostic accuracy quite significantly.[14] The total number of cases studied in the literature has not made it possible to reach a firm conclusion on the accuracy of the technique.

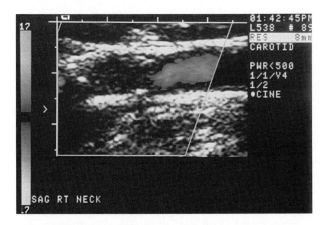

Fig. 9-14. This color flow map shows loss of color flow signals at the site of a total occlusion.

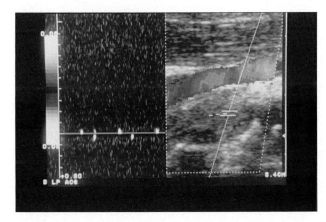

Fig. 9-15. The Doppler waveform sampled in the internal carotid artery at a site proximal to a total occlusion shows a back-and-forth pattern suggesting that blood is entering and leaving this closed system from the proximal internal carotid.

Hypoechoic plaque

Color flow imaging is also very useful in situations where lesions do not cause more than a 50% diameter narrowing. Hypoechoic plaque that is not easily perceived on gray scale image and is difficult to document by Doppler waveform analysis can be quite readily depicted with color flow mapping. The outline of the hypoechoic plaque is clearly shown with color flow mapping, whereas it would not be perceived on the standard gray scale image (Figs. 9-4 and 9-16; see also Plate 37). This is a specific advantage of color flow mapping when compared to traditional duplex sonography.[42,43] This may ultimately be of benefit if, beyond plaque characterization, actual measurements of plaque size become part of the standard clinical examination.

Ulcerated plaque

Gray scale imaging performs poorly in detecting ulcerated carotid plaque.[30] At first impression, color flow

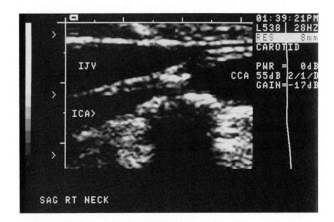

Fig. 9-16. This gray scale image corresponds to the color flow image of Fig. 9-4. Hypoechoic material is not appreciated on this color flow image but is clearly outlined on the color map. The severity of the stenosis would have been underestimated if only the gray scale image would have been used to estimate the severity of the stenosis.

imaging seems unlikely to help with this problem. A localized zone of flow reversal or stagnation of blood flow can be seen in the ulcer crater.[42] This has been reported in the case of very high grade stenoses.[9] Although this sign may be specific, it may not be very sensitive for detecting the presence of ulcerations in lesions that cause a stenosis of less than 50% of the normal lumen diameter.[43] However, the presence of smaller irregularities in the contour of the plaque surface on color flow images appear to correlate with the presence of symptoms.[42]

Contralateral stenosis

The presence of a critical stenosis on one side of the neck appears to have a variable effect on the contralateral carotid system. There is often an increase in the measured velocity on the side contralateral to a high-grade stenosis or total occlusion.[13] This may lead to overestimation of the severity of stenosis on the side contralateral to a high-grade stenosis,[39] an effect that is somewhat inconsistent and difficult to correct for. A measurement of the residual lumen made on the color flow map might help in identifying an inconsistency between the measured Doppler peak systolic velocity and the size of the residual lumen. Again, there are no large studies evaluating how color flow mapping may help in dealing with this problem.

Evaluation of other pathologies

Vasculitis. Takayasu's arteritis causes a diffuse inflammatory process in the media and the adventitia. The subclavian artery and axillary arteries are often involved when the carotid arteries are affected. The pattern seen with vasculitis is quite different from that of atherosclerosis. Atherosclerosis preferentially affects the region of the carotid bifurcation with focal lesions. A diffuse thickening of the arterial wall, often in the common carotid, is more typical of a vasculitis.[6,43]

Radiation. A form of accelerated atherosclerosis can follow neck irradiation. This can also cause a diffuse thickening of the common carotid artery wall with relative sparing of the internal carotid artery bifurcation. Pathologically, this process resembles atherosclerosis and manifests itself within 10 years following irradiation treatment.[7]

Dissection. An aortic dissection can extend into the common carotid artery and end at variable levels in the carotid system. The dissection is best visualized on a longitudinal image.[3,19] A large series that has looked at the outcome of this entity suggests that conservative management is warranted.[54]

Localized internal carotid artery dissection is associated with trauma or is idiopathic and affects young patients. Permanent stroke is the exception rather than the rule. The lesion typically starts in the high portion of the internal carotid artery at the entry into the bony canal. Because of its location, the lesion is often not visualized directly. Flow profiles measured in the more proximal internal carotid artery can show the effect of the more distal outflow obstruction. The waveform tends to be blunted—with signals above and below baseline[45]—or is almost absent. Treatment includes heparinization and observation in that recanalization is quite common.[44]

Pseudoaneurysms and aneurysms. Aneurysms or pseudoaneurysms of the vertebral and extracranial carotid arteries are rare. Their formation may follow trauma due to penetrating injuries. Aneurysms can arise spontaneously within the bifurcation. Carotid sonography can identify the presence of this pathology and determine the level of involvement. Patients typically present with a pulsatile mass.[53]

Most pulsatile masses in patients referred for sonographic studies are shown to be ectatic carotid arteries or slightly enlarged segments of the carotid arteries. True aneurysms of the carotid artery are quite rare.[50]

Neoplasms. Neoplastic lesions involving the carotid bifurcation are rare. Carotid body tumors are extremely hypervascular masses growing in the carotid bifurcation.[41] Other neoplastic masses such as enlarged lymph nodes may involve the contiguous region or may extend into the region of the carotid artery. Neoplastic involvement of the wall of the carotid causes the loss of the interface normally seen between the adventitia and periadventitia of the artery wall.[10]

NEW IMAGING TRENDS

Technologic innovations promise to make color flow imaging less operator-dependent. They include three-dimensional renditions of the color flow information, the use of contrast material to improve lesion perspicuity, and modifications of the color flow map algorithms.

Three-dimensional imaging is achieved by acquiring a series of cross-sectional images. These are reconstructed with the help of a computer. The resulting three-dimensional renditions can then display flow dynamics in the carotid branches.[15,35] This strategy removes some of the sonographer variability and may improve the diagnostic accuracy of color flow imaging.

Modification of the Doppler flow information can also be used to create a "power" display. This is a display of the lumen of flowing blood. The images are less sensitive to angular relationships than the traditional color Doppler images.[37] This technology has yet to be evaluated in any large series.

Color flow mapping can also be achieved without relying on the Doppler effect. Time-domain measurements that correlate with the displacement of small packets of red cells can also be used to create a color flow image.[5] The advantage of this technique is the improved resolution of the color display. The pixel of color information is matched to the gray scale pixel. This may help to decrease the effect of color overflow into the soft tissues surrounding the artery wall. It should minimize underestimation of lesion severity.

The use of contrast agents may also improve the diagnostic accuracy of Doppler sonography or, at the very least, improve precision. It has recently been shown that the margins of the stenotic lumen are much better delineated when a transpulmonary agent is administered.[38]

COLOR FLOW MAPPING FOR IDENTIFYING CANDIDATES FOR CAROTID ENDARTERECTOMY
Screening for "significant" carotid lesions

Carotid sonography is a robust technique capable of screening patients for the presence of significant carotid lesions. Once patients with "significant" stenoses are identified, further evaluation with arteriography will likely lead to an operative intervention, that is, carotid endarterectomy.

The major driving force for the widespread use of carotid sonography has been the need to identify potential candidates for operative intervention. Although carotid endarterectomy has been performed since the mid-1950s, it is only recently that large randomized trials have confirmed the definite benefits derived from the intervention. A large randomized trial has shown a definite benefit for the performance of carotid endarterectomy in patients who have a symptomatic 70% or greater lumen diameter narrowing of the internal carotid artery.[28] The role played by sonography is therefore likely to increase as such symptomatic individuals are screened more aggressively.

The cost-effectiveness of duplex sonography is well recognized when symptomatic individuals are screened. The number of unnecessary angiograms then decreases significantly. For example, the rate of positive angiograms (more than 50% stenosis) increases from 30% to more than 70%.[29] Detection of a 70% or greater stenosis also requires new cutoff values for velocity measurements. In our laboratory, this translates to the adoption of a peak systolic velocity of 2.3 m/s (greater than 70%) instead of 1.25 m/s (greater than 50%).[16] Another possibility is to use a value of 4 or above for the ratio of the peak systolic velocity from the internal carotid to that of the common carotid artery.[27]

This impacts the field of sonography in two ways: (1) the need to distinguish between "hemodynamic significance" and "clinical significance" of stenoses and (2) the pressures from referring physicians who argue that sonography might be used as the sole preoperative examination.

Replacing angiography?

The idea of completely replacing angiography is not new. Such a strategy might be considered in individuals who are studied in vascular laboratories having an excellent track record for consistency and accuracy.[46] It can be estimated that 70% to 80% of carotid artery endarterectomy candidates need not undergo angiography.[36] This approach might be cost-effective[24] but is still subject to sonographer variability. There is, however, another alternative: combining color flow imaging with magnetic resonance angiography.

Magnetic resonance angiography (MRA) appears to threaten the role played by duplex sonography in the evaluation of the carotid arteries. Well recognized as a screening test for the presence of significant stenoses of the carotid arteries, color flow imaging and duplex sonography are not likely to be replaced by MRA. In fact, MRA and duplex sonography, in combination, are replacing arteriography in an increasing fraction of patients undergoing carotid endarterectomy.[33,48]

The more frequently used imaging sequences isolate signals from moving blood while suppressing signals from stationary tissues ("white blood"). The more traditional magnetic resonance imaging techniques visualize the arterial lumen and sites of narrowing by processing more traditional spin echo images ("black blood"). Although the injection of a paramagnetic contrast agent is not needed, its addition can be used to improve visualization of the vessel lumen. Most of the MRA imaging protocols currently rely on the two "white blood" techniques. With the first, the shapes of the applied gradients are preselected so that signal strength is dependent on velocity. This is often referred to as *phase-contrast* MRA. This approach is sensitive to patient motion. It also presupposes that the velocity range is known, a situation difficult to predict when a stenosis is, in fact, present. Because of these two limitations, phase-contrast MRA is not the preferred technique for evaluating the carotid arteries. The alternate type of MRA imaging approach is the time-of-flight MRA. The same type of imaging sequence—gradient refocused sequence—is applied to selected slice locations. However, a series of slice-selective gradients is applied, defining the equivalent of a stack of images oriented perpendicular to the direction of blood flow. The sequence is sensitive to blood entering the imaging plane and, therefore, emphasizes flow that is perpendicular to the imaging plane. A series of images is then acquired as the slice is moved in increments of 1 to 3 mm in the direction perpendicular to the defined imaging plane. This creates the equivalent of a stack of images that can then be processed to create a final image. This display requires the application of a mathematical processing algorithm called the *maximal intensity projection* algorithm. This approach is the one more likely to be used in most applications for the carotid and lower extremity arteries. In general, a series of two-dimensional images is acquired, therefore, the expression 2D time-of-flight angiography. If, however, imaging is conducted over a defined volume, then a data set of three-dimensional time-of-flight images is created. The major limitation of the latter approach is a loss of sensitivity to slowly moving blood as the thickness of the imaging volume increases. An interesting advantage is that flow in curving vessels can be more accurately depicted.

Moving blood causes an increase in signal strength up to a certain maximal velocity. Beyond this, signal is lost due to the effects of turbulence and because of the reconstruction algorithm. This zone of signal loss typically appears when a high-grade stenosis is present and is affected by the sequence used, the length of the refocusing gradient for acquisition of the echo, the pulse repetition rate, and the slice thickness selected. This signal loss is likely to be seen with stenoses of 50% or greater lumen diameter narrowing and is almost always present for stenoses above 70% narrowing.[17]

The sensitivity of 2D time-of-flight sequences approaches 100% in three reported series. The specificity is, however, close to 67% (Table 9-1). If greater care is taken to acquire more complete image sets that include 3D time-of-flight sequences and careful readings performed on the source images before they are processed to form the projection angiograms, then the accuracy increases significantly.[51,52] The penalty is, however, an increase in the imaging time and an increased sensitivity to motion.[22] This problem adds to the current limitations of magnetic resonance imaging, which include patient tolerance to being placed in a small space and subjected

Table 9-1. Accuracy of 2D TOF MRA versus carotid arteriography

Author	Sensitivity	Specificity
Polak et al.	22/23	9/14
Riles et al.	45/45	26/35
Huston et al.	27/27	34/52
Total	94/95 (99%)	69/101 (68%)

to the strong sounds generated by the rapid switching on and off of the gradients used to create the images. In addition, not all patients can be placed in a high-intensity magnetic field. Individuals with pacemakers and other types of indwelling medical devices cannot be safely imaged.

Proposed strategy for evaluating carotid endarterectomy candidates

Doppler sonography and MRA are viewed by many physicians as competitive screening examinations for noninvasively evaluating the carotid arteries. Their traditional role is the screening of the patient with signs or symptoms of TIA or stroke. Contrast arteriography is then normally performed once a patient with a significant carotid lesion is identified. They have also each been proposed as the sole diagnostic test needed for the preoperative selection of endarterectomy candidates. In essence, each has been perceived as a possible replacement for the invasive evaluation with contrast arteriography.

The complementary natures of Doppler sonography and MRA make possible yet another diagnostic strategy. The findings from both techniques, when they concur, are highly accurate in determining the presence or absence of significant lesions. They may be divergent in up to 20% of patients being evaluated. Combining both Doppler sonography and MRA can therefore eliminate the need for contrast arteriography in a significant proportion of patients likely to undergo carotid endarterectomy. An example of the use of this strategy follows: Color flow imaging and Doppler sonography are used to screen the carotid arteries for significant lesions. If there is a need for a further workup, an MRA is obtained to confirm the presence of any significant lesion. If the two techniques give discordant results that cannot be resolved by a combined review of both sets of findings, then an arteriogram can be obtained. The Doppler velocity estimates can be used to grade stenosis severity, and the MRA can be used to assess intracerebral vessels, subtotal versus total occlusions, and the vertebral system. Grading of stenosis severity may be more variable with MRA.[31]

A limitation of this strategy is for the evaluation of the carotid and innominate artery origins. This would require additional MRA imaging sequences, thereby increasing imaging time and cost. The frequency of unrecognized origin stenoses is estimated at 0.6%, and the more significant ones likely cause perturbations in the downstream Doppler waveform in the carotid branches.[1] The intracerebral vessels can also be evaluated with MRA if needed. The presence of tandem lesions that could possibly be missed with this diagnostic strategy likely does not affect outcome following carotid endarterectomy.[23] Significant savings occur because approximately 50% to 70% of angiograms may be replaced by MRA.[33]

CONCLUSION

Color flow imaging is an inherent part of the sonographic evaluation of the extracranial carotid arteries. It helps establish a standardized approach to the evaluation of the carotids and, in doing so, may decrease the amount of operator variability. Future innovations may include the adoption of non-Doppler approaches to measuring flow lumen size or reliance on contrast material to improve the estimates of arterial narrowing.

Today, color flow imaging of the carotid arteries is a powerful noninvasive screening test for detecting the presence of pathology in the carotid arteries. One of its principal tasks is the detection of symptomatic patients who may need carotid endarterectomy. Although it traditionally precedes arteriography, it is increasingly used in combination with MRA or by itself. Which imaging strategy is the best has yet to be determined.

REFERENCES

1. Akers DL, Markowitz IA, Kerstein MD: The value of aortic arch study in the evaluation of cerebrovascular insufficiency, *Am J Surg* 154:230-232, 1987.
2. Baxter GM, Polak JF: Variance mapping in colour flow imaging: what does it measure? *Clin Radiol* 49:262-265, 1994.
3. Bluth EI, Shyn PB, Sullivan MA, et al: Doppler color flow imaging of carotid artery dissection, *J Ultrasound Med* 8:149-153, 1989.
4. Bluth EI, Stavros AT, Marich KW, et al: Carotid duplex sonography: a multicenter recommendation for standardized imaging and Doppler criteria, *Radiographics* 8:487-506, 1988.
5. Bonnefous O, Pesque P: Time domain formulation of pulse-Doppler ultrasound and blood velocity estimation by cross-correlation, *Ultrason Imaging* 8:73-85, 1986.
6. Buckley A, Southwood T, Culham G, et al: The role of ultrasound in evaluation of Takayasu's arteritis, *J Rheumatol* 18:1073-1080, 1991.
7. Chuang VP: Radiation-induced arteritis, *Semin Roentgenol* 29:64-69, 1994.
8. Erickson SJ, Newissen MW, Foley WD, et al: Stenosis of the internal carotid artery: assessment using color Doppler imaging compared with angiography, *AJR Am J Roentgenol* 152:1299-1305, 1989.
9. Furst H, Hartl WH, Jansen I, et al: Color-flow Doppler sonography in the identification of ulcerative plaques in patients with high-grade carotid artery stenosis, *AJNR Am J Neuroradiol* 13:1581-1587, 1992.
10. Glagov S, Zarins C, Giddens DP, et al: Hemodynamics and

atherosclerosis: insights and perspectives gained from studies of human arteries, *Arch Pathol Lab Med* 112:1018-1031, 1988.

11. Gooding GAW, Langman AW, Dillon WP, et al: Malignant carotid artery invasion: sonographic detection, *Radiology* 171:435-438, 1989.

12. Hallam MJ, Reid JM, Cooperberg PL: Color-flow Doppler and conventional duplex scanning of the carotid bifurcation: prospective, double-blind, correlative study, *AJR Am J Roentgenol* 152:1101-1105, 1989.

13. Hayes AC, Johnston W, Baker WH, et al: The effect of contralateral disease on carotid Doppler frequency, *Surgery* 103:19-23, 1988.

14. Hetzel A, Eckenweber B, Trummer B, et al: Color-coded duplex ultrasound in pre-occlusive stenoses of the internal carotid artery, *Ultraschall Med* 14:240-246, 1993.

15. Houi K, Mochio S, Isogai Y, et al: Comparison of color flow and 3D image by computer graphics for the evaluation of carotid disease, *Angiology* 41:305-312, 1990.

16. Hunink MGM, Polak JF, Barlan MM, et al: Detection and quantification of carotid artery stenosis: efficacy of various Doppler velocity parameters, *AJR Am J Roentgenol* 160:619-625, 1993.

17. Huston J, Lewis BD, Wiebers DO, et al: Carotid artery: prospective blinded comparison of two-dimensional time-of-flight MR angiography with conventional angiography and duplex US, *Radiology* 186:339-344, 1993.

18. Kasai C, Namekawa K, Koyano A, et al: Real-time two-dimensional blood flow imaging using an autocorrelation technique, *IEEE Trans Sonics Ultrasound* 32:458-463, 1985.

19. Kotval PS, Babu SC, Fakhry J, et al: Role of the intimal flap in arterial dissection: sonographic demonstration, *AJR Am J Roentgenol* 150:1181-1182, 1988.

20. Ku DN, Giddens DP, Zarins CK, et al: Pulsatile flow and atherosclerosis in the human carotid bifurcation: positive correlation between plaque location and low oscillating shear stress, *Arteriosclerosis* 5:293-302, 1985.

21. Landwehr P, Schindler R, Heinrich U, et al: Quantification of vascular stenosis with color Doppler flow imaging: in vitro investigations, *Radiology* 178:701-704, 1991.

22. Masaryk AM, Ross JS, DiCello MC, et al: 3DFT MR angiography of the carotid bifurcation: potential and limitations as a screening examination, *Radiology* 179:797-804, 1991.

23. Mattos MA, van Bemmelen PS, Barkmeier LD, et al: Routine surveillance after carotid endarterectomy: does it affect clinical management? *J Vasc Surg* 17:819-831, 1993.

24. McKittrick JE, Cisek PL, Pojunas KW, et al: Are both color-flow duplex scanning and cerebral arteriography required prior to carotid endarterectomy? *Ann Vasc Surg* 7:311-316, 1993.

25. Middleton WD, Foley WD, Lawson TL: Color-flow Doppler imaging of carotid artery abnormalities, *AJR Am J Roentgenol* 150:419-425, 1988.

26. Middleton WD, Foley WD, Lawson TL: Flow reversal in the normal carotid bifurcation: color Doppler flow imaging analysis, *Radiology* 167:207-210, 1988.

27. Moneta GL, Edwards JM, Chitwood RW, et al: Correlation with North American Symptomatic Carotid Endarterectomy Trial (NASCET) angiographic definition of 70% to 99% internal carotid artery stenosis with duplex scanning, *J Vasc Surg* 17:152-157, 1993.

28. North American Symptomatic Carotid Endarterectomy Trial Collaborators: Beneficial effect of carotid endarterectomy in symptomatic patients with high-grade stenosis, *N Engl J Med* 325:445-453, 1991.

29. O'Leary DH, Clouse ME, Potter JE, et al: The influence of non-invasive tests on the selection of patients for carotid angiography, *Stroke* 16:264-267, 1985.

30. O'Leary DH, Holen J, Ricotta JJ, et al: Carotid bifurcation disease:

31. Polak JF, Bajakian RL, O'Leary DH, et al: Detection of internal carotid artery stenosis: comparison of MR angiography, color Doppler sonography, and arteriography, *Radiology* 182:35-40, 1992.

32. Polak JF, Dobkin GR, O'Leary DH, et al: Internal carotid artery stenosis: accuracy and reproducibility of color-Doppler-assisted duplex imaging, *Radiology* 173:793-798, 1989.

33. Polak JF, Kalina P, Donaldson MC, et al: Carotid endarterectomy: preoperative evaluation of candidates with combined Doppler sonography and MR angiography, *Radiology* 186:333-338, 1993.

34. Polak JF, O'Leary DH, Quist WC, et al: Pulsed and color Doppler analysis of normal carotid bifurcation flow dynamics using an in-vitro model, *Angiology* 41:241-247, 1990.

35. Pretorius DH, Nelson TR, Jaffe JS: 3-dimensional sonographic analysis based on color flow Doppler and gray scale image data: a preliminary report, *J Ultrasound Med* 11:225-232, 1992.

36. Ricotta JJ, Holen J, Schenk E, et al: Is routine angiography necessary prior to carotid endarterectomy? *J Vasc Surg* 1:96-102, 1984.

37. Rubin JM, Bude RO, Carson PL, et al: Power Doppler US: a potentially useful alternative to mean frequency-based color Doppler US, *Radiology* 190:853-856, 1994.

38. Sitzer M, Furst G, Siebler M, et al: Usefulness of an intravenous contrast medium in the characterization of high-grade internal carotid stenosis with color Doppler-assisted duplex imaging, *Stroke* 25:385-389, 1994.

39. Spadone DP, Barkmeier LD, Hodgson KJ, et al: Contralateral internal carotid artery stenosis or occlusion: pitfall of correct ipsilateral classification—a study performed with color flow imaging, *J Vasc Surg* 11:642-649, 1990.

40. Spencer MP, Reid JM: Quantitation of carotid stenosis with continuous-wave (C-W) Doppler ultrasound, *Stroke* 10:326-330, 1979.

41. Steinke W, Hennerici M, Anlick A: Doppler color flow imaging of carotid body tumors, *Stroke* 20:1574-1577, 1989.

42. Steinke W, Hennerici M, Rautenberg W, et al: Symptomatic and asymptomatic high-grade carotid stenoses in Doppler color-flow imaging, *Neurology* 42:131-138, 1992.

43. Steinke W, Kloetzsch C, Hennerici M: Carotid artery disease assessed by color Doppler flow imaging: correlation with standard Doppler sonography and angiography, *AJR Am J Roentgenol* 154:1061-1068, 1990.

44. Steinke W, Rautenberg W, Schwartz A, et al: Noninvasive monitoring of internal carotid artery dissection, *Stroke* 25:998-1005, 1994.

45. Steinke W, Schwartz A, Hennerici M: Doppler color flow imaging of common carotid artery dissection, *Neuroradiology* 32:502-505, 1990.

46. Thiele BL, Jones AM, Hobson RW, et al: Standards in noninvasive cerebrovascular testing. Report from the Committee on Standards for Noninvasive Vascular Testing of the Joint Council of the Society for Vascular Surgery and the North American Chapter of the International Society for Cardiovascular Surgery, *J Vasc Surg* 15:495-503, 1992.

47. Trattnig S, Schwaighofer B, Hubsch P, et al: Velocity variance function: additional information in color-coded Doppler sonography of the carotids, *Rofo Fortschr Geb Ronaenstr Neuen Bildgeb Verfahr* 153:663-668, 1990.

48. Turnipseed WD, Kennell TW, Turski PA, et al: Magnetic resonance angiography and duplex imaging: noninvasive tests for selecting symptomatic carotid endarterectomy candidates, *Surgery* 114:643-648, 1993.

49. Vattyam HM, Shu MC, Rittgers SE: Quantification of Doppler color flow images from a stenosed carotid artery model, *Ultrasound Med Biol* 18:195-203, 1992.

50. Wang A-M, O'Leary DH: Common carotid aneurysm: ultrasonic diagnosis, *J Clin Ultrasound* 16:262-264, 1988.
51. Wesby GE, Bergan JJ, Moreland SI, et al: Cerebrovascular magnetic resonance angiography: a critical verification, *J Vasc Surg* 16:619-632, 1992.
52. Wilkerson DK, Keller I, Mezrich R, et al: The comparative evaluation of three-dimensional magnetic resonance for carotid artery disease, *J Vasc Surg* 14:803-811, 1991.
53. Wilkinson DL, Polak JF, Grassi CJ, et al: Pseudoaneurysm of the vertebral artery: appearance on color-flow Doppler sonography, *AJR Am J Roentgenol* 151:1051-1052, 1988.
54. Zurbrugg HR, Leupi F, Schupbach P, et al: Duplex scanner study of carotid artery dissection following surgical treatment of aortic dissection type A, *Stroke* 19:970-976, 1988.
55. Zwiebel W, Austin CW, Sackett JF, et al: Correlation of high-resolution B-mode and continuous-wave Doppler sonography with arteriography in the diagnosis of carotid stenosis, *Radiology* 149:523-532, 1983.

Vertebral Sonography

Eva Bartels

The evaluation of the carotid arteries with duplex sonography is widely regarded as a useful procedure.[70] During the last decade, large numbers of publications have dealt with the ultrasonic imaging of common carotid artery bifurcation pathology, whereas duplex sonography of the vertebral arteries has received less attention.[24,32,59] The reasons for this disparity are the anatomic localization of the vertebral arteries, leading to technical problems in their imaging, as well as the fact that surgical intervention has not been as popular a procedure as carotid endarterectomy.

Ischemic events in the vertebrobasilar system, nevertheless, are not rare: In the Duke University study, over a period of 5 years, 22% of cerebral infarctions occurred in the vertebrobasilar territory.[36] In addition, in patients with carotid occlusive processes, the vertebrobasilar circulation plays an essential role in providing collateral flow.[54] It is therefore necessary that, instead of the routine "carotid study," the evaluation of patients with cerebrovascular disorders includes an examination of all extracranial arteries, including the vertebrals.

The first attempts to study the vertebral arteries noninvasively were made using spatial imaging combined with Doppler systems (either continuous or pulsed wave).[67] In 1977, Spencer and colleagues made the first spatial images of the most proximal portion of the vertebral artery, using a continuous-wave imaging system ("Dopscan").[55] In 1978, White and associates modified the commercially available Echoflow equipment by using a pulsed mode with an adjustable time gate, so that they were able to detect the vertebral arteries in the midcervical course.[66] Later, in 1980, Wood and Meire described a technique for imaging the vertebral arteries with pulsed Doppler systems.[29] Using more complex multichannel Doppler instrumentation became possible not only to image the blood vessels in three orthogonal planes but also to display the velocity profiles and to calculate volumetric flow.[68] However, all these systems had various methodologic limitations in regard to the identification of the vessels. Furthermore, they were not capable of imaging the arterial walls as do pulsed-echo techniques.[65]

The introduction of duplex systems, with simultaneous B-mode and flow velocity measurements, considerably reduced some of the technical problems of vertebral sonography. More recently, color Doppler imaging systems have improved even further the accuracy of ultrasonic examinations.[44,45,48,60] They have facilitated the examination of difficult anatomic structures, such as the origin of the vertebral artery from the subclavian artery. Additionally, using color Doppler imaging, the intracranial section of the vertebral artery can also be visualized.

The purposes of this chapter are to describe the

examination technique for the vertebral arteries using duplex sonography and color Doppler imaging, to present the typical pathologic findings in atherosclerotic disease, and to describe the finding in dissection.

ANATOMIC ASPECTS

Basic knowledge of the vertebral anatomy is mandatory in order to effectively study the use of ultrasound. Usually, the vertebral arteries originate from the corresponding subclavian arteries. In about 4% to 6% of patients, the left vertebral artery arises from the aortic arch. In such cases, it is impossible to visualize the origin of the left vertebral artery. Compared with the right, the left vertebral artery origin is situated in a relatively low position, making the visualization rather difficult. Laterally, in close proximity to the vertebral artery, the thyrocervical trunk arises from the subclavian artery. Confusion between the two vessels can easily lead to diagnostic errors. Also, more distally, the branches of the thyrocervical trunk can resemble the vertebral artery. Other branches of the subclavian artery (the costocervical trunk and the internal thoracic artery) do not influence the visualization of the vertebral artery at the origin.

The course of the vertebral artery can be divided into four sections:

1. V1 (pretransverse) segment—between the origin (VO) and entry into the foramen costotransversarium of the C6 vertebra. This part is usually straight but may be tortuous in patients with arteriosclerosis.
2. V2 (transverse) segment—midcervical course in the canalis costotransversarius between the C6 and C2 vertebrae. In both V1 and V2 segments, the vertebral artery is accompanied by the vertebral vein, which courses ventrolaterally parallel to the artery. The examiner must be aware of these anatomic conditions so as not to mistake the artery and the vein, especially during a brief examination.
3. V3 segment—the tortuous course between the C2 vertebra and atlas.
4. V4 segment—the intracranial course of the vertebral artery up to the beginning of the basilar artery.

The vertebral arteries are often unequal in size. As early as 1873, Duret emphasized that the left vertebral artery is, on average, larger than the right vertebral artery.[27] In 400 cases, Krayenbühl and Yasargil found equal width in 26%, a wider left in 42%, and wider right in 32%.[41] According to our results, the average diameter is 3.81 ± 0.46 mm on the left side and 3.88 ± 0.47 mm on the right side.[12]

EXAMINATION TECHNIQUE

Prior to the sonographic examination, the patient's vascular history and the blood pressure on both arms should be noted. In our laboratory, we first perform continuous-wave (CW) Doppler examination of the supratrochlear and carotid arteries as well as of the vertebral arteries at the atlas loop to see if all vessels are present with normal acoustic signal. In general, the results of the CW Doppler study may indicate what to expect from the duplex examination. Particularly, a weaker signal from the vertebral artery, registered at the atlas loop, can indicate that the vessel is either hypoplastic or occluded. In case of occlusion, cervical collaterals can mimic the Doppler signal of the vertebral artery.[50,52] Furthermore, decreased flow secondary to stenosis at the origin can cause a reduced pulsatility of the vertebral signal. All these conditions can then be assessed in more depth by visualization of the vertebral artery using imaging techniques.*

The patient is usually examined in the supine position, with the head in the midline. This contrasts with examination of the carotid artery, during which the head is rotated slightly to the contralateral side. The examiner sits behind the patient's head (Figs. 10-1 and 10-2). Both the examiner and the patient must be comfortable because, particularly in pathologic conditions, the evaluation may take a long time.

Some examiners visualize the vertebral arteries after imaging the carotid artery by angling the transducer laterally. Based on our experience, it is more effective to image the vertebral artery in the midcervical portion initially by placing the transducer paramedian between the trachea and the sternocleidomastoid muscle in the anteroposterior plane. In this transducer position, the transverse processes of the spine, which cause an acoustic shadowing, can be clearly recognized, so that orientation is easier using the B-mode image.[5,6,12] The artery passes straight between the transverse foramina (Fig. 10-3). Then the transducer is moved caudally down to the clavicle for visualization of the origin of the vertebral artery from the subclavian artery. The V1 and V2 segments can be imaged by moving the transducer cephalad in the same anteroposterior plane. An examination in the transverse section can provide further information, although it is necessary only in special conditions, as described later. In contrast, the pretransverse and the intertransverse segments of the vertebral artery should always be imaged in the lateral plane as well. The imaging of the origin in the lateral plane is seldom possible because of anatomic problems.

The V3 segment can be imaged by means of the color Doppler imaging alone. The transducer is placed inferior to the mastoid process, pointing between the patient's contralateral eye and ear. Color Doppler imaging also enables satisfactory visualization of the intracranial V4 segment using the suboccipital ap-

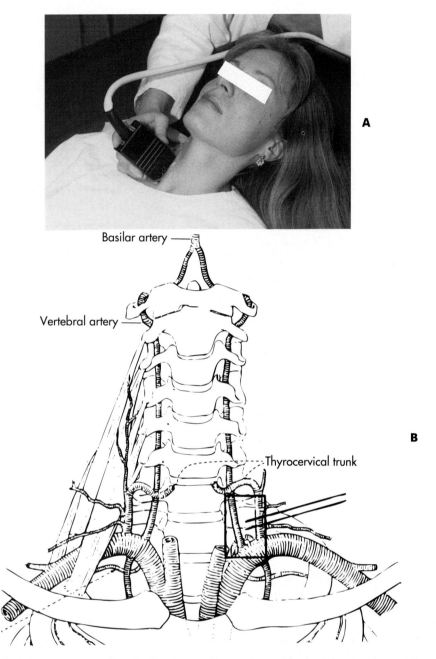

Basilar artery

Vertebral artery

Thyrocervical trunk

A

B

Fig. 10-1. A, Transducer position for the visualization of the vertebral origin; **B,** corresponding anatomic view. Thyrocervical trunk is located laterally from the origin of the vertebral artery.

proach.[17,38,53] The transducer position is similar to that described for transcranial Doppler. Transcranial color Doppler imaging simplifies vessel identification, particularly in patients with tortuous vessels or anatomic variations. In addition, the compression tests at the mastoid (which are nevertheless rarely effective due to the deep location of the vertebral artery) can be eliminated.[11]

After imaging vertebral arteries in the different segments, spectral analysis of the blood flow and velocity

measurements at specific locations must be performed. A correction for the insonation angle must be made to determine the precise velocity.[8] The velocity spectral waveform of the vertebral flow, as illustrated in Figure 10-4, shows a typical low-resistance pattern, with a sharp systolic peak and sustained flow throughout diastole (see also Plate 38). The acoustic signal is similar to that of the internal carotid artery, but with lower intensity.

Both vertebral and transcranial color Doppler sonography require an experienced examiner and good

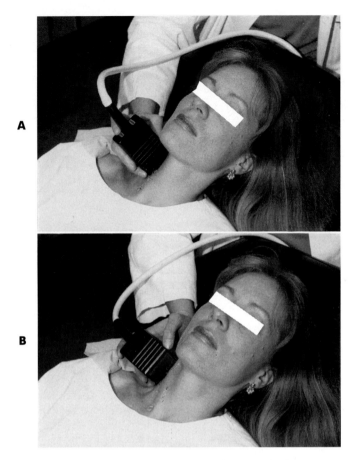

A

B

Fig. 10-2. Transducer position for the visualization of the midcervical portion (segments V1 and V2). **A,** Anteroposterior plane; **B,** lateral plane.

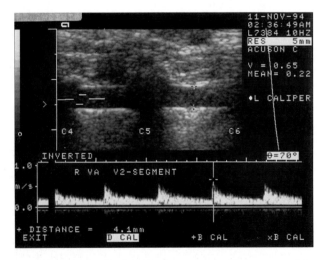

Fig. 10-3. Longitudinal duplex image of the V2 segment of the right vertebral artery *(R VA)* in the anteroposterior plane. The course of the vertebral artery is interrupted by processus transversi of the C4, C5, and C6 vertebrae, causing acoustic shadowing. The diameter of the vessel is 4.1 mm.

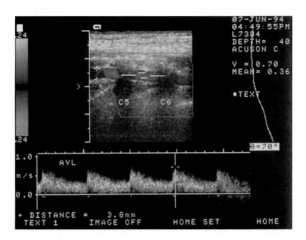

Fig. 10-4. Longitudinal color-coded image of the midcervical course of the left vertebral artery *(AVL).* The sample volume is placed in the section between C5 and C6 vertebrae. The correction for the insonation angle (70°) was done manually. The spectral analysis shows a typical low resistance pattern with high diastolic velocity.

diagnostic equipment. A linear array transducer with 7 MHz imaging frequency and 5 MHz pulsed-wave Doppler frequency is appropriate for vertebral sonography. The transcranial color Doppler imaging can be performed with a color-coded imaging system using a 2 to 2.25 MHz sector transducer.

NORMAL SONOGRAPHIC FINDINGS
Duplex sonography

The combination of two modalities—pulsed-wave Doppler and B-mode imaging—assists in the identification of the artery. The midcervical section of the vertebral artery is easy to image (Figs. 10-3 and 10-4). The identification of the artery is based upon its typical low-resistance Doppler frequency spectrum. The vertebral vein also passes through the transverse foramina of the vertebrae; therefore, spectral analysis is important in order not to confuse one with the other.[6,12] Touboul and colleagues were able to visualize the pretransverse and intertransverse segments in all of 50 examined patients, and we obtained the same results in studying 54 patients.[12,61] The V2 segment is not frequently the site of occurrence of hemodynamically significant arteriosclerotic lesions. Due to its relatively constant lumen, the section is also convenient for the undertaking of diameter measurements and for the evaluation of hemodynamic characteristics.[10] In a study of 42 persons without history of vertebrobasilar symptomatology, peak systolic blood velocity ranged from 19 to 98 (mean 56) cm/s, and peak diastolic blood velocity ranged from 6 to 30 (mean 17) cm/s. Resistive indices ranged from 0.62 to 0.75 (mean 0.69).[63]

An optimal evaluation of the origin is important because it is the most common site of atherosclerotic lesions in the vertebral artery.[47] The transducer position for the insonation of the ostium is shown in Figure 10-1. In this location, an oblique image of the subclavian artery and the vertebral artery origin with the longitudinal image of the proximal V1 segment can be reproducibly obtained. It has already been pointed out that the thyrocervical trunk, which arises from the subclavian artery laterally, can be mistaken for the vertebral artery. To verify the anatomic identification, the transducer is angled slightly to the lateral side, showing the thyrocervical origin. The differentiation between both the vertebral and thyrocervical trunk origin can easily be assessed by spectral analysis. The spectrum of the latter has a higher resistant pattern due to the fact that it provides blood supply to the musculature of the neck.

Conventional duplex sonography is of limited value for the imaging of the vertebral artery in patients with anatomic variations or tortuosity of the VO and V1 segments. Furthermore, visualization in the transverse plane, as well as in the atlas loop region, is not possible with gray scanning alone.[10] Examination in more complicated conditions can be better performed with color Doppler imaging, as described in the following section of this chapter.

Color Doppler imaging

Color Doppler imaging is an ultrasonographic technique that provides real-time information about flowing blood by means of color coding of Doppler frequencies. Its advantages over duplex ultrasonography in the investigation of carotid arteries have been described.[28,34,57] This method is more effective than conventional duplex sonography also in the evaluation of the vertebral arteries, particularly in the imaging of the vertebral origin in difficult anatomic conditions (Fig. 10-5; see also Plate 39).

Compared with the right side, the origin of the left vertebral artery is more difficult to visualize, owing to its rather proximal position. Accordingly, using conventional duplex ultrasonography Touboul and associates were able to identify the vertebral artery ostium in 94% of the cases on the right and in only 60% on the left side.[61] In our study of 60 patients, we were able to image the right vertebral artery origin in 80% and the left in 65% of the cases.[10] In the same patient population, color Doppler imaging improved the detection of the origin: on the right side to 88.3% and on the left side to 73.3%. This method is especially useful in the visualization of tortuous vessels common in elderly patients (Fig. 10-6; see also Plate 40). It has been already pointed out that imaging kinks and coils by using conventional duplex methods can be difficult or even impossible. Nevertheless, in the eventuality of the left vertebral artery arising from the aortic arch or in dorsal or caudal localization of

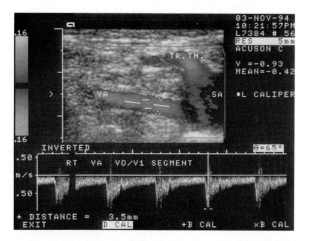

Fig. 10-5. View of the vertebral origin on the right side. The subclavian artery *(SA)* is shown in diagonal plane, and the right vertebral artery *(RT VA)* and the thyrocervical trunk *(TR TH)* in longitudinal plane. The diameter of the vertebral artery is 3.5 mm.

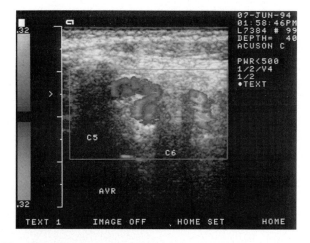

Fig. 10-6. Tortuosity in the V2 segment between C5 and C6 vertebrae, easily recognized by change of the red and blue color coding, indicating different blood flow directions within the kinks.

the ostium, even color Doppler imaging may not be successful.

The examination can be of limited value also in obese patients, with short necks and deeply situated vertebral arteries. In such cases, at least a detection of vertebral flow at the mastoid process using the continuous-wave Doppler examination should be attempted.[50]

Even if the imaging of the midcervical course of the vertebral artery with conventional duplex sonography is easy to perform, the examination is quicker and more effective with color Doppler imaging.[10,63] The differentiation between artery and vein is easier by different color coding of the arterial and venous signal (Fig. 10-7; see also Plate 41).

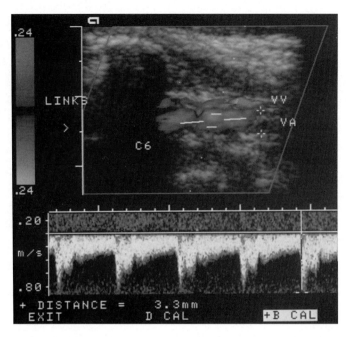

Fig. 10-7. Rostral V1 segment before entry of the vertebral artery *(VA)* into the foramen costotransversarium of C6 vertebra. The vertebral vein *(VV)* situated parallel to the vertebral artery is coded with blue.

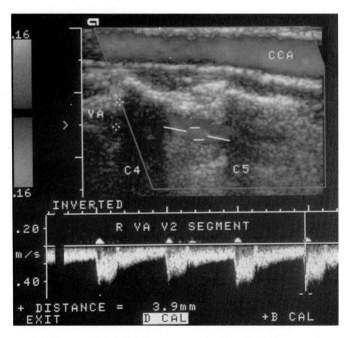

Fig. 10-8. Longitudinal view of the V2 segment of the vertebral artery *(VA)* coded with the same color as the common carotid artery *(CCA)*, demonstrating the orthograde flow in the vertebral artery. (C4 and C5 = cervical vertebrae.)

By comparison with the color coding of the carotid artery, the direction of the blood flow in the vertebral artery can be recognized (Fig. 10-8; see also Plate 42). The flow direction can also be defined in the transverse plane (Fig. 10-9; see also Plate 43). As discussed later,

the assessment of the flow direction in the vertebral artery is essential in diagnosis of steal phenomena.[21,40,49]

Imaging of the vertebral artery at the atlas loop (V3 segment) is rarely successful with duplex scanning because of overlapping of bony structures. Visualization

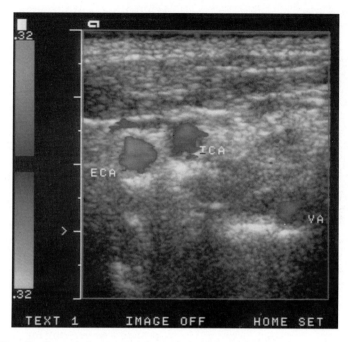

Fig. 10-9. Visualization of the vertebral artery in the transverse plane. The external and internal carotid arteries *(ECA, ICA)* are located medial to the vertebral artery *(VA)*. The same red color coding indicates an orthograde flow direction within the vertebral artery.

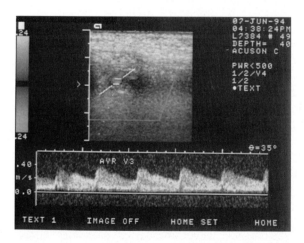

Fig. 10-10. View of the V3 segment (atlas loop) of the right vertebral artery *(AVR)*. The change of the flow direction within the loop is represented by blue and red color coding. The typical low-resistance spectrum with high diastolic velocity avoids a confusion with the occipital artery.

Table 10-1. Visualization of the vertebral artery (60 patients, aged 29 to 77 years; mean age, 51 years)

	Duplex ultrasonography		Color Doppler imaging	
	n	%	n	%
In the pretransverse and in the intertransverse segments C4-5, C5-6				
On the right side	60	100	60	100
On the left side	60	100	60	100
At the atlas loop				
On the right side	11	18.3	52	86.7
On the left side	7	11.7	51	85.0
At the origin				
On the right side	48	80	53	88.3
On the left side	39	65	44	73.3

with color Doppler imaging is significantly better: Trattnig and colleagues were able to display the atlas loop in 76.2% of cases on the right side and in 85.7% on the left (Fig. 10-10; see also Plate 44).[63] In our study, we did not observe any side-to-side differences in detecting the V3 segment of the vertebral artery: Visualization was possible in 86.7% of the cases on the right side and in 85% on the left side (Table 10-1).[10] For an effective examination, however, spectral analysis should be done in order to avoid confusion with the occipital artery.

Using transcranial color Doppler imaging, the intracranial section of the vertebral artery (V4 segment) is accessible by insonation through the foramen magnum.[11,17,38,53] As mentioned earlier, 2 to 2.5 MHz sector transducers are usually optimal for transcranial examination. Using the suboccipital approach, the foramen magnum is first seen on the B-mode image as a hypoechoic circle, surrounded by the hyperechoic line of the occipital bone.[8,38] Subsequently, both vertebral arteries and the basilar artery can be imaged (Fig. 10-11; see also Plate 45). In the case of tortuosity, angling of the transducer position helps to visualize the artery at least in

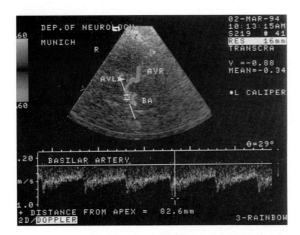

Fig. 10-11. Demonstration of the intracranial V4 segment of the right *(AVR)* and left vertebral artery *(AVL)*, as well as of the basilar artery *(BA)*, using the suboccipital approach. The arteries are coded with blue, according to the flow directed away from the transducer.

several oblique sections. Sometimes a typical **Y** figure at the site of the vertebral junction to the basilar artery can be displayed.[11,53] The depth at which the basilar artery actually begins has long been discussed.[20,51] With the help of color Doppler imaging, the junction site can be clearly recognized in most cases. Schöning and Walter did not find the vertebral junction beyond a depth of 80 mm.[53] In our study, in two patients the basilar artery began at a depth of less than 70 mm.[11]

Transcranial color Doppler imaging simplifies the differentiation between the posterior inferior cerebellar artery (PICA) and the intracranial vertebral artery. Nevertheless, cerebellar arteries can be imaged only under favorable conditions: Kaps and colleagues were able to image the PICA in 50% of 24 healthy individuals, whereas the intracranial vertebral artery could be displayed in 96%.[38]

In comparison with the conventional transcranial method, color Doppler imaging also allows determination of the Doppler angle of insonation, the one resulting in more precise blood flow velocity measurements. However, it is necessary to keep in mind that we do not measure the true angle between the ultrasound beam and the direction of blood flow.[31] The angle, as estimated on color Doppler images, represents a two-dimensional projection of a three-dimensional vector.[45] Therefore, the angle-corrected velocities are proportional — but not equal — to the true velocity. Nevertheless, using conventional transcranial color Doppler imaging, the angle of insonation is not taken into consideration at all, so that the potential measurement error may be greater. Then again, the clinical impact of the angle-corrected blood flow velocities has not yet been investigated.[11]

CLINICAL APPLICATIONS
Vertebral artery stenosis

Severe stenosis in the transverse V2 segment of the vertebral artery seldom occurs. In contrast, the origin of vertebral artery is the second most common stenosis site of the cerebral vessels.[47] The difficulties associated with the imaging of the ostium have already been pointed out. Due to technical problems, it can be difficult to place the sample volume in the narrowest part of the stenosis. Additionally, caliber variations also make the quantification difficult. For this reason, there are no data in the literature concerning the relationship between the actual flow velocity and the grade of the stenosis at the origin of the vertebral artery. In clinical practice, we estimate the grade of stenosis by using a qualitative parameter: We differentiate between nonstenotic plaques and moderate or severe stenosis by the amount of plaque, the presence of aliasing on the color-coded image, increased flow velocity in the site of stenosis, and presence of indirect signs in the poststenotic region (Fig. 10-12; see also Plate 46). The indirect signs are important, especially in cases in which the origin of the vertebral artery cannot be visualized directly: In such conditions, a proximally located severe stenosis can be presumed, based on decreases in both systolic and diastolic velocities, decreased pulsatility (sometimes associated with turbulent flow) revealed in V1 segment, and the presence of cervical collaterals.

In a study of routine duplex investigation of the prevertebral segment of the vertebral artery, Ackerstaff and colleagues showed that duplex scanning of the ostium of the vertebral artery is a reliable test. For the detection of an obstructive lesion with a diameter reduction of 50% or more, they found a sensitivity of 0.8 and a specificity of 0.92.[3]

Vertebral artery occlusion

Contrast angiography is considered the gold standard for the diagnosis of vertebral artery pathology. However, in cases of proximal vertebral artery occlusion, no vessel outline appears on the angiogram. In aplasia of the vertebral artery, the vessel contour is also absent. It is not possible to differentiate between these two conditions with angiography. Nevertheless, duplex ultrasonography can help to clarify this problem.

In a recent occlusion of the vertebral artery at the origin, it is often possible to visualize the echogenic vessel walls with hypoechoic lumen in the V1 and V2 segments, whereas no Doppler signal or color coding of the flow can be detected. Nevertheless, a careful evaluation of the ostium region is important to avoid mistaking the thyrocervical trunk or the vertebral vein for the vertebral artery (Fig. 10-13; see also Plates 47 and 48). A hypoechoic vessel lumen without evidence of blood flow can be sometimes detected

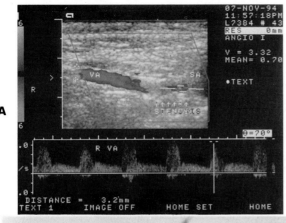

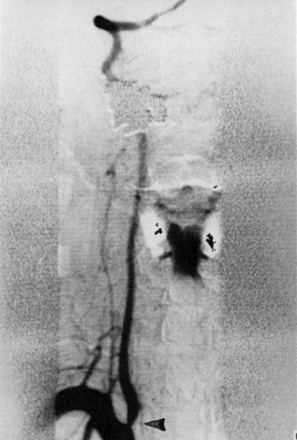

Fig. 10-12. Stenosis of the right vertebral artery *(R VA)* at the origin. **A,** In the stenotic region, a weak color-coded signal with aliasing phenomenon, indicating increased blood flow velocity, can be recognized. Spectral analysis in this area revealed increased systolic velocity (3.32 m/s) with turbulent flow. Subclavian artery *(SA)* is imaged in the diagonal plane. **B,** Arteriographic finding demonstrating the stenosis of the right vertebral artery at the origin.

even several months after the occlusion of the vertebral artery.[5] In contrast, in aplasia of the vertebral artery, no vessel can be visualized.

If an artery has been occluded for a long time, the lumen is filled with echogenic thrombus that cannot be satisfactorily differentiated from the surrounding tissue. Usually, a good formation of cervical collaterals presumes the diagnosis of occlusion in such conditions. By contrast, a good collateralization can sometimes mimic a normal vertebral signal at the atlas loop. To avoid diagnostic errors, it is important to examine the vertebral artery in all segments.

During extracranial evaluation, occlusion of the intracranial vertebral artery or the basilar artery can also be diagnosed based upon indirect signs: A high resistive flow pattern without a diastolic flow component, detected in the midcervical course of a vertebral artery with a normal caliber, is significantly associated with a flow obstruction more distally.[39,50]

Vertebral artery hypoplasia

It has already been pointed out that variations of the vertebral artery caliber are relatively frequent. There is no agreement concerning the definition of vertebral hypoplasia. Delcke and Diener defined hypoplasia by diameters smaller than 2 mm based on a hypoplasia ratio of 1.9%.[26] In postmortem evaluation of 400 cases, Krayenbühl and Yasargil found an extremely thin vertebral artery in 6.2% on the right side and in 4.5% on the left.[41] Accordingly, a similar hypoplasia ratio of 6% was described also by Touboul and associates, based on a diameter criterion for the vertebral artery smaller than 3 mm and measured by the duplex method in 50 patients.[61] In clinical practice, we consider the vertebral artery as hypoplastic if the diameter is smaller than 3 mm and the following criteria are fulfilled: Both the systolic and especially the diastolic velocities are decreased, as well as the presence of a high resistive pattern in the spectral analysis. Additionally, in the majority of cases, the other vertebral artery is dominant with velocities in the upper norm region.[7]

An extremely hypoplastic vertebral artery can make the differentiation between hypoplasia and occlusion difficult or even impossible. The presence of cervical collaterals may indicate an occlusion, but, then again, the thin cervical branches can be mistaken for a hypoplastic vertebral artery.

Diagnostic errors can arise also in the case of a hypoplastic vertebral artery ending in the posterior inferior cerebellar artery. In this relatively frequent anatomic variation, the spectral analysis shows a high resistive pattern, similar to that of an intracranial obstruction of the vertebral artery. The diagnostic criterion is an evident (even if extremely decreased)

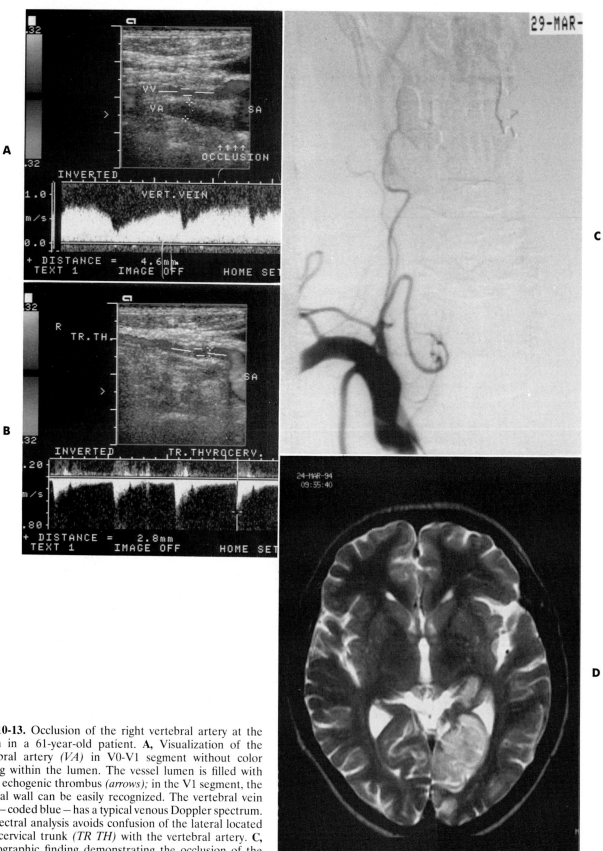

Fig. 10-13. Occlusion of the right vertebral artery at the origin in a 61-year-old patient. **A,** Visualization of the vertebral artery *(VA)* in V0-V1 segment without color coding within the lumen. The vessel lumen is filled with slight echogenic thrombus *(arrows);* in the V1 segment, the arterial wall can be easily recognized. The vertebral vein *(VV)* — coded blue — has a typical venous Doppler spectrum. **B,** Spectral analysis avoids confusion of the lateral located thyrocervical trunk *(TR TH)* with the vertebral artery. **C,** Angiographic finding demonstrating the occlusion of the right vertebral artery. **D,** Magnetic resonance image of the right occipital infarction of this patient.

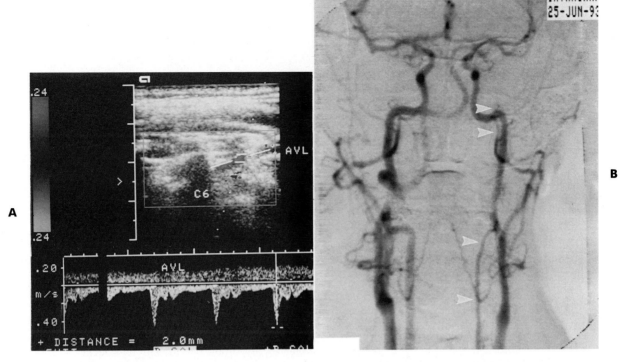

Fig. 10-14. Hypoplastic left vertebral artery *(AVL)* ending in the right posterior inferior cerebellar artery (PICA). **A,** In the rostral V1 segment (before entering in the foramen costotransversarium of the sixth vertebra), a thin artery with a diameter of 2 mm can be imaged. Spectral analysis shows a high resistive pattern with a detectable diastolic flow signal. **B,** Angiographic findings demonstrating a tiny left vertebral artery ending in the PICA (arrows).

diastolic flow in the midcervical course of the vertebral artery, in contrast to the nondetectable diastolic signal in the case of intracranial occlusion (Fig. 10-14; see also Plate 49).

Using the new color-coding modality, based on processing the amplitude signal of the flowing blood (so-called power Doppler, color Doppler energy, or CDE system), seems to improve the detection of extremely hypoplastic arteries with low flow, as demonstrated in Figure 10-15 (see also Plate 50). This color coding is independent of the blood flow velocity and direction, as well as of the angle of insonation. Nevertheless, this is a complementary method, valuable in the assessment of specific questions, that cannot replace the already "traditional" color Doppler imaging.

Subclavian steal syndrome

The subclavian steal syndrome can result from stenosis or occlusion of the subclavian artery or brachiocephalic trunk proximal to the origin of the ipsilateral vertebral artery. In this situation the normal blood supply to the arm is diminished or interrupted, whereby the ipsilateral vertebral artery serves as a collateral pathway around the obstruction. The changes in the blood flow in the vertebral artery depend on the grade of the stenosis of the subclavian artery, resulting in an

incomplete or complete steal effect. In cases of moderate stenosis, only a systolic deceleration of the flow velocity can be observed. In a larger stenosis, the originally orthograde flow becomes alternating (directed toward the arm in systole and toward the brain in diastole) or even retrograde, with flow directed toward the affected arm during the whole cardiac cycle.[21,40,49]

The subclavian steal syndrome can be confirmed using functional tests by means of compression of the upper arm: Decompressing the arm leads to an increased systolic velocity with a reversed flow direction (toward the arm), detected in the vertebral artery, due to the reactive hyperemia after the arm compression.

In a high-grade obstruction, blood can be "stolen" also from the contralateral vertebral artery or from the basilar artery (causing an alternating or reversed flow in the basilar artery or even from the carotid internal artery via the circle of Willis).

Using duplex ultrasonography, the assessment of subclavian steal is easier because the hemodynamic changes mentioned previously can be recorded directly from the lumen of the vertebral artery displayed on the screen. Additionally, using color flow imaging, the reversed flow in the vertebral artery can be detected easily by different color coding of the vertebral artery in

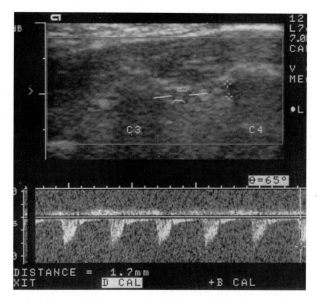

Fig. 10-15. Demonstration of a "color Doppler energy (CDE)" image of a hypoplastic vertebral artery in V2 segment between C3 and C4 vertebrae. CDE is new software in which the color coding is based on processing the amplitude of the Doppler signal, whereby the flow direction cannot be imaged. Using this method, an extremely hypoplastic artery can be visualized. The spectral analysis demonstrates a high resistive flow pattern with an evident diastolic signal. The diameter of the artery is 1.7 mm.

comparison with the ipsilateral carotid artery, so that functional tests are not necessary (Fig. 10-16; see also Plates 51 and 52). Nevertheless, the different color coding of the vertebral artery must be displayed along the whole longitudinal course because, in cases of vertebral tortuosity, kinks and coils can lead to misinterpretations of the flow direction.[10]

Vertebral artery dissection

Extracranial artery dissection has been increasingly reported as a cause of transient ischemic attacks or infarction in young adults.[22,35,43] Arteriography has been long considered as the procedure necessary to establish the diagnosis.[4] Using color Doppler imaging, however, it is possible to recognize dissections noninvasively, not only in the internal carotid artery but also in the extracranial segments of the vertebral artery.[16,56,62] Vertebral artery dissection can occur spontaneously, related to an underlying vascular disorder, or as a result of neck trauma.[23,30,37,42,46,69] During the last 6 years we have followed 18 patients with extracranial vertebral artery dissection, whereby in 72% of the cases the lesion of the vessel was temporally related to trauma.[9]

Ultrasonographic findings in dissection vary from irregular thickening of the vessel wall without hemodynamic alteration, to major structural lesions: intramural hematoma, irregularities of the vessel wall, dissecting membrane, true and false lumen, localized arterial dilation, intravascular echoes, or pseudoaneurysm formation (Figs. 10-17 and 10-18; see also Plates 53 to 56). Tapering stenosis with rostral occlusion is a frequent finding.[18,58] Variable Doppler spectrum waveforms, such as biphasic patterns, resistive patterns, and decreased systolic and diastolic flow velocities, can be observed.

The appearance of the ultrasonographic findings also depends on the site of the dissection. Dissection at the origin or in the V3 or V4 segments can sometimes be assessed by using indirect hemodynamic parameters only, because as mentioned previously, these segments cannot always be visualized.

In our patients, the most common site of a dissection was the distal V1 segment, especially at the point of entry into the foramen costotransversarium of the C6 vertebra (Fig. 10-17).[9] In this region, the artery is possibly exposed to the greatest mechanical injury.[30,37] Particularly this midcervical segment of the vertebral artery is easily accessible for both duplex ultrasonography and color flow imaging, so that the study can be repeated noninvasively as often as necessary. Such follow-up examinations are important for therapeutic decisions, especially in determining the duration of anticoagulant treatment.[9,58]

CONCLUSIONS

Both duplex ultrasonography and color Doppler imaging provide a safe and effective method for the

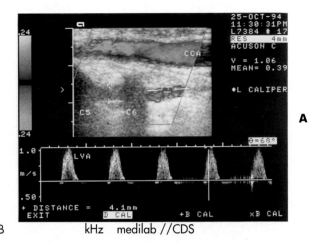

Neurologie KMB   kHz   medilab //CDS

25-Okt-94   11:47

Patient   : medilab //CDS
ARZT   :
GEFÄSS   : VA-L
POWER   : n/a
SONDE   : CW 4 MHz
GAIN   : 20dB
RANGE   : 23dB
WINKEL   : 45 grd
SAMMELV: n/a
FLUSS   : ←□
EMBOLIE   : n/a

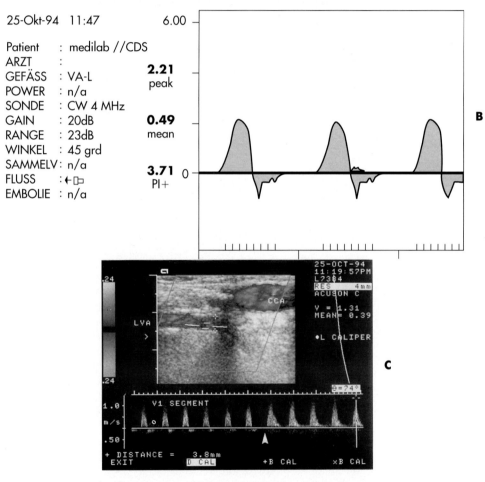

Fig. 10-16. Subclavian steal syndrome. **A,** Longitudinal view of the midcervical course of the left vertebral artery *(LVA)* coded with different color (red) than the common carotid artery (blue, *CCA*), demonstrating the retrograde flow in the vertebral artery. **B,** The spectral analysis indicates a cardiac cycle-dependent alternating blood flow directed toward the arm in systole and toward the brain in diastole. **C,** Functional test: alternating blood flow during the compression of the upper arm. After decompression *(arrow in spectral analysis)*, completely reversed, increased flow (directed toward the arm) can be recorded, due to the reactive hyperemia in the arm.

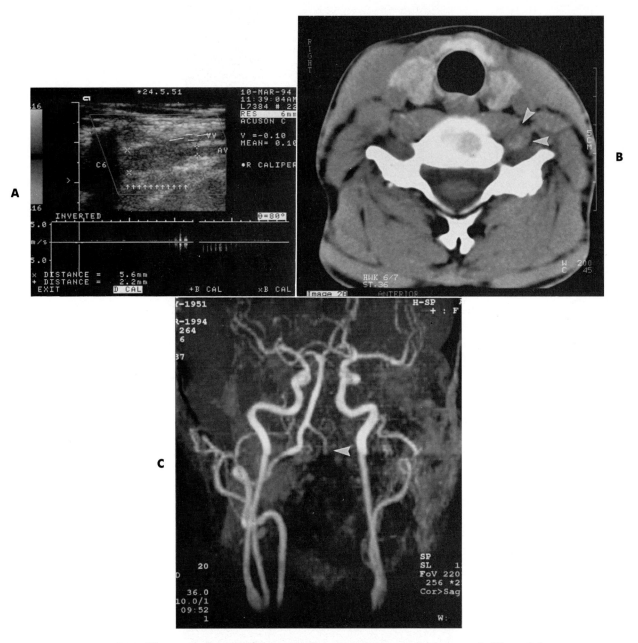

Fig. 10-17. Ultrasonographic finding in the dissection of the vertebral artery. **A,** View of the distal V1 and proximal V2 segment showing a pseudoaneurysm formation *(arrows)* and a dilatation of the vessel at the entrance of the vertebral artery *(AV)* into the foramen costotransversarium of C6 vertebra (diameter proximally 2.2 mm, distally 5.6 mm). In the lumen of the artery no blood flow can be detected. **B,** Admission computed tomography scan at the level of C6-C7 vertebrae, showing the signal-intensive enlarged lumen of the left vertebral artery in the area of the dissection. **C,** Intracranial magnetic resonance angiogram showing an absent left vertebral artery.

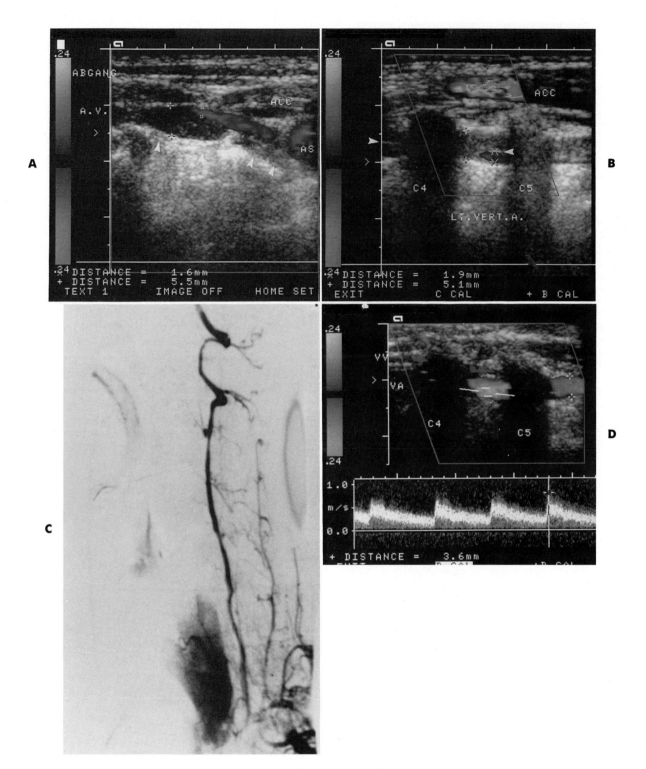

Fig. 10-18. Color flow images of a left vertebral artery dissection in a 33-year-old woman that occurred during a chiropractic manipulation. The dissection is expanding from V0 to the distal V2 segment. **A,** Origin of the left vertebral artery *(A.V.)* from the subclavian artery *(AS)* and the proximal V1 segment. Two intramural hematomas *(arrows)* appear as echolucent longitudinal formations. Reduction of the lumen diameter by 1.6 mm. **B,** More distally in V2 segment (between processus transversi of C4 and C5 vertebrae), two lumina can be seen: the false lumen with blood flow (red coded) is delineated by a dissecting membrane *(arrows)* from the true lumen. The transverse processes C4 and C5 are causing acoustic shadowing. *(ACC = common carotid artery.)* **C,** Admission angiogram of the left vertebral artery dissection showing distinct irregularities of the vessel wall from the origin to the V3 segment. **D,** Follow-up examination 3 years later, showing a good recanalization of the vertebral artery *(VA)* in the V2 segment (between C4 and C5 processus transversi).

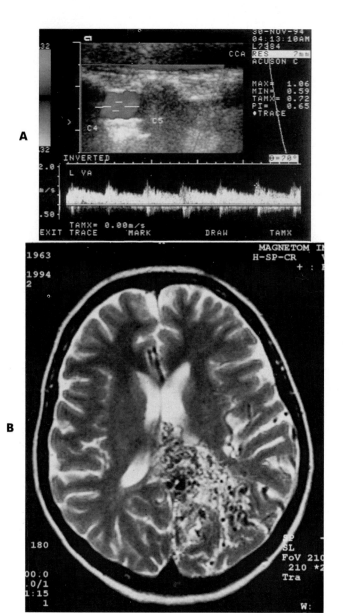

A

B

Fig. 10-19. Arteriovenous angioma (left occipital-parietal) in 31-year-old woman. **A,** View of the midcervical portion of the left vertebral artery *(L VA)* between processus transversi of C4 and C5 vertebrae. The arterial caliber is wide (diameter 5.6 mm); spectral recording shows increased systolic and diastolic velocities with decreased pulsatility index (0.65). All are indirect signs, typical for a feeding artery of an angioma. **B,** Magnetic resonance image of the left occipital-parietal arteriovenous angioma (see box).

noninvasive evaluation of the vertebral arteries (Fig. 10-19; see also Plate 57; box). Conventional duplex ultrasonography is a valuable modality for routine assessment, whereas color Doppler imaging is more suitable for detailed studies in difficult anatomic conditions. During the last decade, the ultrasound technology has improved so much that, in experienced hands, even patients with more complex pathologic findings can be examined satisfactorily. With in-

Vertebral artery hemodynamics

Direct and/or indirect hemodynamic findings in midcervical course of the extracranial vertebral artery:

1. *Normal vertebral artery:* low resistance flow pattern with high diastolic velocity
2. *Occlusion at the origin:* vessel lumen without flow signal (in a recent occlusion); no detection of the vertebral artery in case of an old occlusion, multiple cervical collaterals
3. *Occlusion intracranially:* high-resistance flow pattern with very low diastolic velocity or without diastolic component
4. *Stenosis at the origin*
   Direct signs: visualization of stenotic plaques, aliasing phenomenon, increased flow velocities
   Indirect signs: poststenotic turbulent flow, possible decreased systolic and diastolic velocities in an vertebral artery with normal caliber, cervical collaterals
5. *Stenosis intracranially:* high-resistance flow pattern with low diastolic velocity in an artery with normal caliber.
6. *Hypoplasia:* diameter less than 3 mm, decreased systolic and diastolic velocities, possible higher resistance pattern
7. *Internal carotid artery occlusion or high-grade stenosis:* in case of collateral supply via vertebrobasilar system, hyperperfusion in the vertebral artery (increased systolic and diastolic velocities)
8. *Subclavian steal syndrome:* systolic deceleration, alternating flow or retrograde flow in an artery with a normal caliber
9. *Intracranial angioma:* indirect signs indicating vertebral artery as an angioma-feeder: high systolic and diastolic velocities, decreased pulsatility index (see Fig. 10-19)

creased knowledge and development of new instrumentation, further improvement in the accuracy of performed examinations can be expected. In summary, vertebral sonography is a practical noninvasive method that should become a routine part of each cerebrovascular study.

REFERENCES

1. Ackerstaff RGA, Eikelboom BC, Moll FL: Investigation of the vertebral artery in cerebral atherosclerosis, *Eur J Vasc Surg* 5:229-235, 1991.
2. Ackerstaff RGA, Grosveld WHJM, Eikelboom BC, Ludwig JW: Ultrasonic duplex scanning of the prevertebral segment of the vertebral artery in patients with cerebral atherosclerosis, *Eur J Vasc Surg* 2:387-393, 1988.
3. Ackerstaff RGA, Hoeneveld H, Slowikowski JM, et al: Ultrasonic duplex scanning in atherosclerotic disease of the innominate, subclavian and vertebral arteries: a comparative study with angiography, *Ultrasound Med Biol* 10:409-418, 1984.

4. Anson J, Crowell RM: Cervicocranial arterial dissection, *Neurosurgery* 29:89-96, 1991.
5. Bartels E: Duplexsonographie der Vertebralarterien, 2.Teil: Klinische Anwendungen, *Ultraschall Med* 12:63-69, 1991.
6. Bartels E: Duplexsonographie der Vertebralarterien, 1.Teil: Praktische Durchführung, Möglichkeiten und Grenzen der Methode, *Ultraschall Med* 12:54-62, 1991.
7. Bartels E: Farbkodierte Dopplersonographie der Vertebralarterien. Vergleich mit der konventionellen Duplexsonographie, *Ultraschall Med* 13:59-66, 1992.
8. Bartels E: Transkranielle farbkodierte Duplexsonographie: Möglichkeiten und Grenzen der Methode im Vergleich zu der konventionellen transkraniellen Dopplersonographie, *Ultraschall Med* 14:272-278, 1993.
9. Bartels E, Flügel KA: Ultrasonic findings in traumatic dissection of extracranial carotid and vertebral arteries, (abstract). *J Neuroimaging* 2:218, 1992.
10. Bartels E, Flügel KA: Advantages of color Doppler imaging for the evaluation of vertebral arteries, *J Neuroimaging* 3:229-233, 1993.
11. Bartels E, Flügel KA: Quantitative measurements of blood flow velocity in basal cerebral arteries with transcranial duplex color-flow imaging, *J Neuroimaging* 4:77-81, 1994.
12. Bartels E, Fuchs HH, Flügel KA: Duplex ultrasonography of vertebral arteries: examination technique, normal values and clinical applications, *Angiology* 43:169-180, 1992.
13. Bendick PJ, Glover JJ: Vertebrobasilar insufficiency: evaluation by quantitative duplex flow measurements, *J Vasc Surg* 5:594-600, 1987.
14. Bendick PJ, Jackson VP: Evaluation of the vertebral arteries with duplex sonography, *J Vasc Surg* 3:523-530, 1986.
15. Bluth EI, Merritt CRB, Sullivan MA, et al: Usefulness of duplex ultrasound in evaluating vertebral arteries, *J Ultrasound Med* 8:229-235, 1989.
16. Bluth EI, Shyn PB, Sullivan MA, Merritt CRB: Doppler color flow imaging of carotid artery dissection, *J Ultrasound Med* 8:149-153, 1989.
17. Bogdahn U, Becker G, Winkler J, et al: The transcranial color coded real-time sonography in adults, *Stroke* 21:1680-1688, 1990.
18. deBray JM, Dubas F, Joseph PA, et al: Etude ultrasonique de 22 dissections carotidiennes, *Rev Neurol (Paris)* 45:702-709, 1989.
19. deBray JM, Maugin D, Jeanvoine H, et al: Etude prospective sur la valeur clinique de l'exploration echotomographique des artères vertebrales, *J E M U* 7:80-85, 1986.
20. Büdingen HJ, Staudacher T: Die Identifizierung der Arteria basilaris mit der transkraniellen Doppler-Sonographie, *Ultraschall Med* 8:95-101, 1987.
21. Büdingen HJ, Staudacher T, Stoeter P: Subclavian steal: Transkranielle Doppler-Sonographie der Arteria basilaris, *Ultraschall Med* 8:218-225, 1987.
22. Caplan LR, Amarenco P, Rosengart A, et al: Embolism from vertebral artery origin occlusive disease, *Neurology* 42:1505-1512, 1992.
23. Caplan LR, Baquis GD, Pessin MS, et al: Dissection of the intracranial vertebral artery, *Neurology* 38:868-877, 1988.
24. Carroll BA: Carotid sonography, *Radiology* 178:303-313, 1991.
25. Davis PC, Nilsen R, Braun IF, Hoffman JC: A prospective comparison of duplex sonography vs angiography of the vertebral arteries, *AJNR Am J Neuroradiol* 7:1059-1064, 1986.
26. Delcke A, Diener HC: Die verschiedenen Ultraschallmethoden zur Untersuchung der Arteria vertebralis—eine vergleichende Wertung, *Ultraschall Med* 13:213-220, 1992.
27. Duret H: Sur la distribution des artères nourricières du bulb rachidien, *Arch Physiol* 5:97, 1873.
28. Erickson SJ, Mewissen MW, Foley WD, et al: Stenosis of the internal carotid artery: assessment using color Doppler imaging compared with angiography, *AJNR Am J Neuroradiol* 152:1299-1305, 1989.
29. Fish PJ: *Multichannel, direction resolving Doppler angiography.* In Kazner E, de Vlieger M, Müller HR, McCready VR, editors: *Ultrasonics in medicine,* Amsterdam, 1975, Excerpta Medica.
30. Friedman DP, Flanders AE: Unusual dissection of the proximal vertebral artery: description of three cases, *AJNR Am J Neuroradiol* 13:283-286, 1992.
31. Giller CA: Is angle correction correct? *J Neuroimaging* 4:51-52, 1994.
32. Gomez RC: Carotid plaque morphology and risk for stroke, *Stroke* 24:25-29, 1989.
33. Grant EG, White EM: *Duplex sonography,* New York, 1988, Springer.
34. Hallam MJ, Reid JM, Cooperberg PL: Color-flow Doppler and conventional duplex scanning of the carotid bifurcation: prospective, double-blind, correlative study, *AJR Am J Roentgenol* 152:1101-1105, 1989.
35. Hart RG, Easton JD: Dissections, *Stroke* 16:925-927, 1985.
36. Heyman A, Wilkinson WE, Hurwitz BJ, et al: *Clinical and epidemiologic aspects of vertebrobasilar and nonfocal ischemia.* In Berguer R, Bauer RB, editors: *Vertebrobasilar occlusive disease,* New York, 1984, Raven.
37. Josien E: Extracranial vertebral artery dissection: nine cases, *J Neurol* 239:327-330, 1992.
38. Kaps M, Seidel G, Bauer T, Behrmann: Imaging of the intracranial vertebrobasilar system using color-coded ultrasound, *Stroke* 23:1577-1582, 1992.
39. Kazumi K, Yasaka M, Moriyasu H, et al: Ultrasonographic evaluation of vertebral artery to detect vertebrobasilar axis occlusion, *Stroke* 25:1006-1009, 1994.
40. Klingelhöfer J, Conrad B, Benecke R, Frank B: Transcranial Doppler ultrasonography of carotid-basilar collateral circulation in subclavian steal, *Stroke* 19:1036-1042, 1988.
41. Krayenbühl H, Yasargil MG, editors: *Die vaskulären Erkrankungen im Gebiet der Arteria vertebralis und Arteria basilaris,* Stuttgart, 1957, Thieme.
42. Leys D, Lesoin F, Pruvo JP, et al: Bilateral spontaneous dissection of extracranial vertebral arteries, *J Neurol* 234:237-240, 1987.
43. Mas JL, Bousser MG, Hasboun D, Laplane D: Extracranial vertebral artery dissections: a review of 13 cases, *Stroke* 18:1037-1047, 1987.
44. Merritt CRB: Doppler color flow imaging, *J Clin Ultrasound* 15:591-597, 1987.
45. Mitchell DG: Color Doppler imaging: principles, limitations, and artifacts, *Radiology* 177:1-10, 1990.
46. Mokri B, Houser OW, Sandok BA, Piepgras DG: Spontaneous dissections of the vertebral arteries, *Neurology* 38:880-885, 1988.
47. Moosy J: *Morphology, sites and epidemiology of cerebral atherosclerosis.* In Milliken C, editor: *Cerebrovascular disease,* Baltimore, 1986, Williams & Wilkins.
48. Omoto R, Kaisai C: Basic principles of Doppler color flow imaging, *Echocardiography* 3:463-473, 1986.
49. Von Reutern GM, Büdingen HJ, Freund HJ: Dopplersonographische Diagnostik von Stenosen und Verschlüssen der Vertebralarterien und des Subclavian-Steal-Syndroms, *Arch Psychiat Nervenkr* 222:209-228, 1976.
50. Von Reutern GM, Büdingen HJ: *Ultraschalldiagnostik der hirnversorgenden Arterien,* Stuttgart, 1989, Thieme.
51. Ringelstein EB, Kahlscheuer B, Niggermeyer E, et al: Transcranial Doppler sonography: anatomical landmarks and normal velocity values, *Ultrasound Med Biol* 16:745-761, 1990.
52. Ringelstein EB, Zeumer H, Poeck K: Non-invasive diagnosis of intracranial lesions in the vertebrobasilar system. A comparison of Doppler sonographic and angiographic findings, *Stroke* 16:848-855, 1985.

53. Schöning M, Walter J: Evaluation of the vertebrobasilar-posterior system by transcranial color duplex sonography in adults, *Stroke* 23:1280-1286, 1992.

54. Sindermann F: Krankheitsbild und Kollateralkreislauf bei einseitigem und doppelseitigem Carotisverschluβ, *J Neurol Sci* 5:9-25, 1967.

55. Spencer MP, Reid JM, Brockenbrough EC, Thomas GI: *Noninvasive cerebrovascular evaluation,* Seattle, 1977, Institute of Applied Physiology and Medicine.

56. Steinke W, Schwartz A, Hennerici M: Doppler color flow imaging of common carotid artery dissection, *Neuroradiology* 32:502-505, 1990.

57. Steinke W, Kloetzsch C, Hennerici M: Carotid artery disease assessed by color Doppler flow imaging: correlation with standard Doppler sonography and angiography, *AJNR Am J Neuroradiol* 11:259-266, 1990.

58. Sturzenegger M: Ultrasound findings in spontaneous carotid artery dissection. The value of duplex sonography, *Arch Neurol* 48:1057-1063, 1991.

59. Taylor CD, Strandness DE: Carotid artery duplex scanning, *J Clin Ultrasound* 15:635-644, 1987.

60. Tegeler CH, Kremkau FW, Hitchings LP: Color velocity imaging: introduction to a new ultrasound technology, *J Neuroimaging* 1:85-90, 1991.

61. Touboul PJ, Bousser MG, Laplane D, Castaigne P: Duplex scanning of normal vertebral arteries, *Stroke* 17:921-923, 1986.

62. Touboul PJ, Mas JL, Bousser MG, Laplane D: Duplex scanning in extracranial vertebral artery dissection, *Stroke* 18:116-121, 1987.

63. Trattnig S, Hübsch P, Schuster H, Pölzleitner D: Color-coded Doppler imaging of normal vertebral arteries, *Stroke* 21:1222-1225, 1990.

64. Visonà A, Lusiani L, Castellani V, et al: The echo-Doppler (duplex) system for the detection of vertebral artery occlusive disease: comparison with angiography, *J Ultrasound Med* 5:247-250, 1986.

65. White DN: *Vertebral ultrasonography.* In Zwiebel WJ, editor: *Introduction to vascular ultrasonography,* New York, 1986, Grune & Stratton.

66. White DN, Curry GR, Stevenson RJ: *Recording vertebral artery blood flow.* In White DN, Lyons EA, editors: *Ultrasound in medicine,* New York, 1978, Plenum.

67. White DN, Ketelaars CEJ, Cledgett PR: Noninvasive techniques for the recording of vertebral artery flow and their limitations, *Ultrasound Med Biol* 6:315-327, 1980.

68. Wood CP, Meire HB: A technique for imaging the vertebral artery using pulsed Doppler ultrasound, *Ultrasound Med Biol* 6:329-339, 1980.

69. Youl BD, Coutellier A, Dubois B, et al: Three cases of spontaneous extracranial vertebral artery dissection, *Stroke* 21:618-625, 1990.

70. Zwiebel WJ: *Introduction to vascular ultrasonography,* New York, 1986, Grune & Stratton.

Ultrasonic Quantification of Blood Flow Volume

B. Martin Eicke
Charles H. Tegeler

The detection of extra and intracranial disease of the vascular system is the main focus of neurosonology. The high incidence of vascular disease with all its devastating medical and economical consequences underlines the need for a noninvasive, inexpensive, and reliable diagnostic method. Many of the clinically significant questions can be answered by modern ultrasonic devices. For a sufficient diagnosis of cerebrovascular disease, hemodynamic and morphologic information are required.

Hemodynamic information is obtained by Doppler instruments. This technique measures the blood flow velocity within a vessel. Guidelines have been established to differentiate between normal and abnormal flow velocities.[24,33] Stenotic lesions can be identified by the presence of accelerated flow velocities. The shape of the velocity profile provides information about vascular resistance not only in the area of insonation, but also about further distal and proximal in the vessel system. Turbulent or disturbed flow can be identified, indicating vascular disease in specific areas.

B-mode imaging allows an accurate morphologic evaluation of extracranial vascular disease, identifying atherosclerotic plaques of different composition, and determining the residual lumen in a stenotic vessel.

Duplex instruments combine the potentials of B-mode imaging and Doppler systems. With these instruments it is possible to identify extracranial stenoses more accurately. Using low frequency transducers, reliable localization of the intracranial vessels is possible.

All these diagnostic tools help the physician to identify high risk patients and to interpret the extent of vascular disease. However, the potentially most important factor of cerebral hemodynamics, the estimation of the cerebral flow volume, is often neglected. *How much* blood and oxygen are pumped to the brain? The identification of velocity accelerations or plaque at a stenotic site is helpful, but may not be sufficient. Criteria used today may not adequately address the effect of cerebrovascular lesions on overall cerebral hemodynamics and often deal superficially with morphologic data.

The following two examples illustrate some potential diagnostic problems:

Case 1. In a young adult, high flow velocities are measured at the origin of the internal carotid artery, and some small atherosclerotic plaques are identified in this area. The interpretation of these data may be difficult. They may represent a completely normal hemodynamic finding with some physiologically increased flow velocities for which the small plaques have no hemodynamically important effect. The same findings might also be interpreted as a significant stenosis caused by the atherosclerotic material. Last but not least, these findings may also be seen with a distally located arteriovenous malformation causing increased flow volume and velocity in the more proximal conduit vessel sections. All these interpretations are plausible, and the diagnosis may remain unclear. Specific ratios like the internal carotid artery (ICA)–common carotid artery (CCA) velocity ratio may be helpful but may not be completely satisfactory.

Case 2. On the B-mode image, a large plaque is seen at the origin of the ICA. The flow velocities, however, do not exceed the normal limits. Again, three different diagnostic conclusions are possible. These findings can be interpreted as a hemodynamically nonstenotic lesion with some plaques. A second interpretation might be a very high-grade stenosis with dampened flow velocities. Finally, depending on the analysis of the contralateral side and the vertebral arteries for potential collateral flow, it may be interpreted as a moderate stenosis. Again, the diagnostic meaning may remain unclear.

Quantification of the volume flow rate might allow a more accurate and reliable diagnosis in both cases. Diameter of the residual lumen and flow velocity are valuable but may be insufficient parameters. The key functional question remains: How much blood is supplying the brain?

CLINICAL IMPORTANCE AND POTENTIAL APPLICATIONS

From a neurologic perspective, information on the actual volume flow rate may become important in a variety of different clinical circumstances (Table 11-1) including patients with both symptomatic and asymptomatic atherosclerotic cerebrovascular disease. Vessels of interest are not only on the affected side but also contralateral, so that collateral flow may also be

assessed. Volume flow rate information may help differentiate various subtypes of dementia (e.g., dementia of Alzheimer's type versus multiinfarct). Some arteriovenous malformations are characterized by hyperemia, and evaluation of the effect of therapy should include the estimation of this extra blood flow volume. Monitoring during treatment with drugs that may affect cerebral perfusion may become a major application of cerebral volume flow rate measurements. These include substances having specific interaction with neurotransmitters, antihypertensive drugs, and medications used primarily for cardiac applications.

METHODS

Several methods have been used to measure volume flow rate:

Electromagnetic flow meters
Ultrasonic devices
    Range gated Doppler measurements
    Combination of A-mode scanner with Doppler elements
    Multirange-gated duplex scanning (color flow M-mode)
    Power-based flow estimations
MR Imaging

Electromagnetic flow meters

Electromagnetic flow meters were introduced in the mid-1960s[26] and are still the most accurate and reliable method to measure flow volume. These instruments are clamped around the vessel, and constant flow measurements can be taken. The method is based on the magnetic induction principle: Blood as a conductor of electricity has a voltage generated in it when it moves through a magnetic field, cutting the lines of magnetic force. Flow volume is proportional to this induced voltage. These systems, including transsonic flowmeters,

Table 11-1. Applications of volume flow determination

Clinical problem	Question
Stroke, transient ischemic attacks	Degree of a stenotic lesion
	Extent of collateral flow
	Overall cerebral perfusion
Dementia	Differentiation of vascular dementia and other forms of dementia
	Extent of the perfusion deficit in vascular dementia
Migraine	Differentiation of hypervolemic and hypovolemic forms or stages of migraine
Arteriovenous malformation	Extent of the shunt volume
	Extent of the potential volume deficit in other vessels
Cardiac failure	Extent of a potential cerebral flow volume deficit
Drug monitoring	Effect of:
	Thrombolytic therapy
	Antithrombotic therapy
	Cardiac therapy
	Vasoactive drug therapy
	Antihypertensive drug therapy

require an invasive procedure and are therefore predominantly used in animal models or intraoperatively in vascular surgical procedures like carotid endarterectomy. Their use in daily practice for physicians not performing surgical procedures is limited.

Noninvasive ultrasound devices

Area and velocity based calculations. Ultrasonic devices have been used to determine flow volume in humans since the early 1970s. The physical equations and explanations of flow on which these methods are based are discussed in the following paragraphs.

Flow volume is the product of flow velocity and the area in which this velocity occurs.

$$\text{Flow volume (m}^3\text{/s)} = \text{flow velocity (m/s)} \times \text{area (m}^2)$$

For accurate measurements, both parts of this equation, velocity and area, have to be calculated simultaneously. In clinical practice, several different approaches are used to obtain these two parameters.

Velocity determination. Most instruments utilize the Doppler technique for flow velocity determination. The measured Doppler frequency shifts are used to calculate flow velocities in relation to the transmitting and receiving probe. There is a direct correlation of higher frequency shifts with the relative speed of the moving targets toward or away from the transducer, with higher frequency shifts representing higher flow velocities. Continuous-wave (cw) Doppler instruments provide excellent sensitivity. All flow velocities along the scan line are detected and displayed in a spectrum, with the lower flow velocities representing the blood flow near the vessel wall and the higher flow velocities, blood flow in the center of the vessel (Fig. 11-1). Pulsed-wave (pw) Doppler probes also provide information on the depth of insonation. The sample volume is usually positioned in the center of the vessel to detect the highest flow velocities (Fig. 11-2). In cw and pw Doppler instruments, the envelope of the maximum frequency shift over time is used for further calculations. However, this requires

some important assumptions: To estimate the mean spatial velocity across the entire vessel diameter, symmetric, parabolic, laminar flow has to be present. Only in this case is the following equation valid.

$$\text{Mean spatial velocity (m/s)} = \frac{1}{2}\text{ peak velocity (center)}$$

This assumption, however, does not completely apply to multigated pulsed instruments. These instruments display information not from one specific depth but from multiple depths. The easiest format to handle this extensive information is by color coding the velocity information, as used in color duplex instruments, which are rapidly becoming the gold standard for clinical ultrasound scanning in the neck.[8] In these instruments the color coded flow velocities at specific depths are superimposed on the vessel morphology in the gray scale image. A major pitfall of this technique is the difficulty to insonate structures at deeper depths as the color sensitivity is dropping dramatically with increasing depth of insonation. This is a severe problem with attempted insonation of all intracranial vessels and the vertebral arteries. Velocity assessment in color duplex instruments can also be done using other approaches besides the conventional frequency domain based Doppler technology. A new technology, color velocity imaging (CVI), utilizes a time domain rather than a frequency domain based approach to obtain flow velocity data[4] and has proven to be accurate for in vivo[33] and in vitro evaluations.[7] Potential advantages are an improved spatial color resolution and independence from the effect of the operating frequency, which may cause problems in a conventional Doppler instrument using broad-band frequency transducers.[4,28] Using time domain processing, the mean spatial velocity can be calculated more accurately because the flow velocity profile identifies the highest flow velocities all along a scan line continuously. This peak is not necessarily localized in the center of the vessel. Such an asymmetric parabolic flow pattern can be quantified (Fig. 11-3).

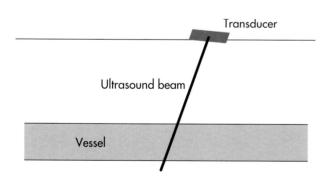

Fig. 11-1. Continuous-wave (cw) Doppler: All flow velocities along the scan line are displayed in the spectrum.

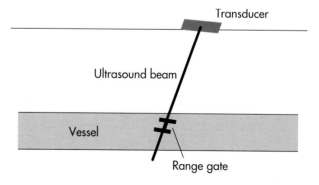

Fig. 11-2. Pulsed wave (pw) Doppler: Only the velocities from a specific sample volume, depending on the preset range gate, are displayed.

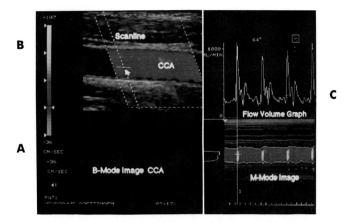

Fig. 11-3. A, Color duplex B-mode image. The velocity information is color coded and superimposed on the gray scale image. **B,** Color duplex image. A specific scan line (for M-mode display) is chosen from the B-mode image and tracked over time. **C,** M-mode display. The velocity profile demonstrates asymmetric parabolic flow. Once the velocity peak within the vessel has been determined, the mean spatial velocity can be calculated, assuming asymmetric parabolic flow (CVI-Q).

$$\text{Mean spatial velocity (m/s)} =$$
$$\frac{\tfrac{1}{2} \text{ peak velocity} \times y_1 + \tfrac{1}{2} \text{ peak velocity} \times y_2}{y_{1+2}}$$

Volume flow rate measurements require, as indicated by the SI unit m^3/s, not only average spatial velocity information but also average data over a period of time. By tracking the mean spatial velocity over a period of time and averaging the data from diastole and systole, the temporal mean velocity can be calculated. This can be achieved by averaging the data from the Doppler display or in color duplex instruments tracking color (velocity) information along one scan line (M-mode).

$$\text{Mean temporal velocity (m/s)} =$$
$$\frac{\Sigma(n) \text{ Velocities (systolic, diastolic)}}{n}$$

A serious problem in all instruments is angle correction. This information is required to convert the relative blood flow velocities toward or away from the transducer to absolute flow velocities of the moving blood in the vessel. To calculate the absolute velocity of flow within a vessel, angle correction is required. The more perpendicular the vessel is located in the neck, the more important this cosine function becomes. Exact knowledge of this angle is required for reliable and accurate calculations.

All duplex instruments allow adjusting for the correct angle, based on the appearance in the B-mode image.

Doppler-only instruments do not obtain any direct information on the position of the vessel in situ. However, the simultaneous use of two or more Doppler transducers can help to minimize this problem. These transducers are fixed to each other in a specific angle.

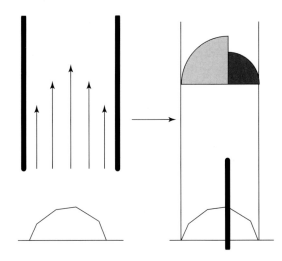

Fig. 11-4. Angle correction in CW Doppler. In this setting, two receiving probes are used simultaneously. Depending on the angle of insonation, there will be a difference in the reflected frequency shifts at the two receiving transducers. Using trigonometric equations, it is possible to correlate this difference in frequency shifts to the actual angle of insonation, with bigger differences occurring at angles closer to 90°.

The volume flow meter (VFM) probe used by Uematsu and colleagues[30] has three elements, one transmitting and two receiving. By the amount of the difference of the frequency shifts detected by the receiving elements, the angle of insonation can be trigonomically calculated (Fig. 11-4), and conversions to absolute velocities can be performed. This kind of instrumentation is used by several other authors.[3,5,17,18,32] Payen and associates use only two probes.[20] With this system it is possible to find the appropriate position of the transducer in relation to the vessel, only in this case the reflected frequency shifts are equal, one with positive and the other with negative frequency shifts (Fig. 11-5).

Area information. In case of a circular vessel, the area can be calculated by measuring the diameter of the vessel.

$$\text{Area (m}^2) = [\text{diameter/2 (m)}]^2 \times \pi$$

For this reason, volume flow rate measurements cannot be performed in many regions of potential interest like the carotid bifurcation or vessels affected by an acircular plaque formation. There are different approaches to estimate the diameter in a specific vessel:

1. Pulsed Doppler (range gate): Pulsed Doppler instruments transmit ultrasonic waves at determined intervals. Knowing the round-trip travel time of the ultrasound beam in soft tissue from the transducer to a reflecting target at a specific depth and back to the receiving element, it is possible to accurately localize and differentiate vessels along the scan line. By minimizing the time gate for processing of the returning ultrasound beam,

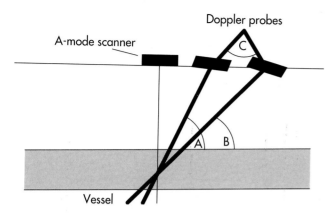

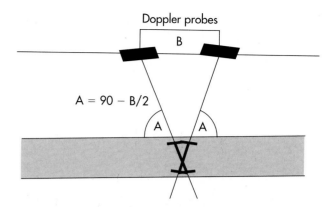

Fig. 11-5. Angle correction in pw Doppler: By using two transmitting and receiving transducers, the actual angle of insonation can be determined, when the occurring frequency shifts at both receiving elements are equal.

Fig. 11-6. Difference of functional and anatomic vessel diameter. This example shows a very pulsatile CCA of a patient with an occluded ICA on the same side. The anatomic vessel diameter does not change very much over the cardiac cycle. Color is indicating flow, which is easy to identify in systole throughout the vessel diameter. In diastole, however, flow is identified only in the center of the vessel. With no flow detected near the vessel walls, the functional vessel lumen is smaller than the anatomic diameter.

information from a very small sample volume can be obtained. By placing this tiny sample volume carefully at different depths along the scan line and searching for flow, the near and far walls of the vessel can be identified. This technique does not provide information concerning diameter changes over the cardiac cycle. Most authors using this technique consider the changes of diameter over the cardiac cycle to be less than 10% and therefore negligible.[22,23] The accuracy of these systems depends on the minimal size of the sample volume.

2. Imaging methods are helpful to track the diameter continuously over time. The use of an amplitude-mode (A-mode) system allows detection of changing vessel diameter over the cardiac cycle.[31] The display of data from an A-mode scan line over time is called M-mode (motion mode sonography). Gray scale only instruments track the anatomic diameter.[18,30-32] The introduction of color duplex instruments allows a differentiation between functional and anatomic diameter. In these instruments with multirange gated pulsed Doppler (or time domain) elements, diameter calculation can be performed by using the outline of the color-coded flow information (color M-mode).[7,15] Especially in vessels with pulsatile flow characteristics, the functional flow diameter may be smaller than the anatomic diameter (Fig. 11-6). The exact importance of this difference as a source of error is unclear.

3. A rather simple approach to determine the vessel diameter is to use the B-mode image. Assuming a stable vessel diameter, these calculations can be performed in virtually all commercially available duplex instruments.[2] Some authors determine the systolic and diastolic vessel diameter and average these two data.[12] These measurements can be performed for the anatomic diameter, using the

gray scale image, or for the functional vessel diameter, using the color flow data.

There are systems commercially available that integrate velocity and diameter information. Some instruments are equipped with a set of double or triple Doppler elements plus an A-mode scanner.[30] In some duplex instruments, the diameter information as measured by the B-mode image is combined with the velocity measurements. In these instruments the volume flow rate is calculated as the product of the present fixed diameter and the actual Doppler information. The most elegant solution is a color M-mode system, which provides simultaneous information about functional diameter and multirange gated velocity information. These systems are available for color Doppler[5] and time domain signal processing (CVI).[7] In some of these instruments, postprocessing on a separate computer is required; in some systems the information can be processed by the system software itself (CVI-Q, color velocity imaging quantify). All systems described were tested in vivo and in vitro. Acceptable accuracy data with errors between 6% and 13% were reported.[7,8,35]

Power (intensity) and velocity based volume calculations. A very different ultrasonic technique to determine the flow volume is based on the assumption of increased Doppler echo reflections with increased flow volume.[16] The product of flow velocity and echo intensity is used to estimate the flow volume without information of the diameter.

Flow volume (m³) ≈ intensity (W) × flow velocity (m/s)

This technique is accurate in vitro and is of specific interest in transcranial Doppler sonography, where diameter information is not available because of insuf-

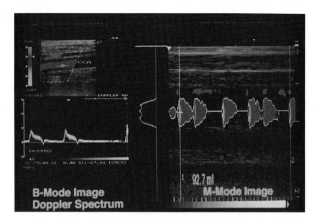

Fig. 11-7. Influence of the angle of insonation on potential angle correction errors. In this example a 2° angle correction error is assumed. At low angles of insonation, the occurring velocity error is negligible; the diameter error, however, is significant, as is the volume flow error. For angles of insonation close to 90°, the occurring diameter error is negligible; flow velocity and volume flow are unacceptable. Thus, the acceptable range for volume flow measurements is an angle between 30° and 70°.

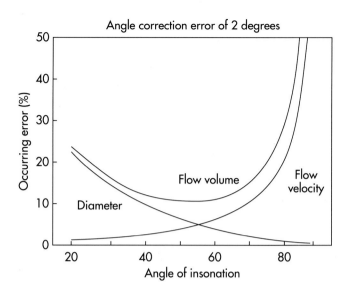

Fig. 11-8. Volume flow rate and off-axis error. An off-axis error produces a velocity and a diameter underestimation. This example is based on an 8-mm vessel and an infinitely thin beamwidth. The actual volume flow errors are smaller, depending on the beamwidth (usually around 1 mm).

ficient resolution of the morphologic structures by color pixels or the B-mode gray scale image. The amount of the reflected power is dependent on the penetration of the ultrasound beam in tissue. As this penetration may be very different in individual patients, absolute numbers of flow cannot be given, and this technique is limited to relative flow volume changes.

Potential errors in ultrasonic flow volume determination. There are more problems to be considered for use of ultrasound technology for flow volume determination.

Angle correction. As explained previously, there are several techniques to assess the actual angle of insonation. Angle correction is essential for flow velocity and diameter calculations: Detected frequency shifts (kHz) can be converted into determinations of the actual blood flow velocity (cm/s) in these instruments. This is a cosine-dependent function. Also, the calculation of the vessel diameter requires the information of the actual angle of insonation; in this case, it is a sine-correlated function. Angle correction is easy to perform under standardized in vitro conditions. For in vivo studies it is more difficult to perform perfect angle correction within a range of ± 2°. A 2° error at an angle of insonation around 60° will cause a volume flow rate error of approximately 10%. The same 2° error at an angle of insonation of 30° or 70° will cause a flow volume error of 18%. Thus, if possible, no measurements should be taken with an angle of insonation of less than 30° or more than 70°, as the risk for unavoidable errors rapidly increases outside this range (Fig. 11-7). This problem applies only to those techniques in which the absolute values are of relevance.

Relative changes (%) are not influenced by inaccurate angle corrections.

Off-axis error. Off-axis error may be a severe problem, especially in patients with respiratory movements of the carotid or vertebral vessel system. An off-axis error simultaneously causes a velocity error by missing the peak flow velocities in the center of the vessel and underestimation of the actual vessel diameter (Fig. 11-8). In this example of an 8-mm vessel, 1 mm of off-axis error produces a 10% error, and a 2-mm off-axis error produces a 30% underestimation of the actual volume flow rate. Relative and absolute values are influenced by an intermittent, unpredictable off-axis error due to respiratory movements. Constant off-axis errors do not influence relative changes of flow volume.

Circular vessel. The assumption of a circular vessel is essential for the calculation of the area from the measured diameter information. It is of clinical importance because the carotid system in the area of the bifurcation is not circular, and measurements should not be taken at this site. In the presence of an acircular atherosclerotic plaque, the same problem occurs. In case of doubt, an initial transverse B-mode study can prove or disprove the circularity of the vessel. With the other techniques, the relative values are not altered as long as the same position of the probe is used and an identical error occurs for all measurements.

Turbulent flow. Turbulent, disturbed flow remains a major problem for ultrasonic flow volume determination. It is virtually impossible to calculate the volume flow rate in the presence of turbulent flow. This excludes the bifurcation and areas of stenotic or immediate

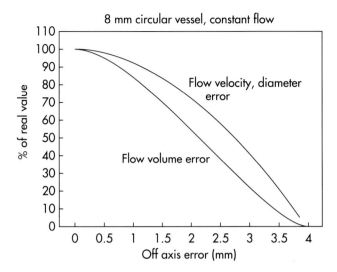

Fig. 11-9. Flow profiles over one cardiac cycle in a normal 30-year-old person. **A,** Parabolic flow profile in late diastole; **B,** Plug flow in early systole; **C,** M-shape flow in mid-systole; **D,** Symmetric parabolic flow in mid-diastole.

poststenotic flow from such calculations. Measurements have to be taken either proximal or far distal to the site of the stenotic lesion. Careful observation of the flow profile is required. Not only absolute but also relative values are influenced by turbulence: With increased volume flow rate, flow velocity may increase, the critical Reynolds number may be exceeded, and turbulence may occur. Because the absolute volume flow rate calculation may be inaccurate for this second measurement, the relative change is also influenced by this error. Volume flow rate calculations in the presence of turbulent flow are virtually impossible and any measurement should be rejected.

Nonparabolic flow. The flow profile in the common carotid artery may not fulfill the criteria for laminar parabolic flow and may change rapidly over the cardiac cycle (Fig. 11-9). The spatial flow velocity profile may appear as a M-shaped function with two symmetrical off-center velocity peaks. Plug flow may also occur. Especially in the presence of helical flow, this kind of flow disturbance will occur with the higher flow velocities closer to the vessel wall.[20] Under these circumstances, the equation for the average spatial flow velocity no longer applies. This is a problem for most scanning techniques and, to a lesser extent, also applies for color M-mode systems.

Tracking the anatomic vessel diameter. Some of the methods listed (especially single range-gated Doppler) do not take into account potential changes of the diameter over the cardiac cycle. Physiologic anatomic diameter in systole or diastole is believed to be less than 10% of the entire vessel diameter. Because the diameter measurement will be converted to an area calculation, this may result in a flow volume error of up to 20% in

diastole. Additional gray scale A-mode scanning for tracking the diameter over time may help to minimize this problem.

Tracking of the functional vessel diameter. Color M-mode displays show a discrepancy of anatomic and functional vessel lumen particularly in vessels with higher pulsatility. This differentiation of anatomic and functional vessel diameter may be an unrecognized problem with gray scale A-mode scanners. This phenomenon occurs predominantly in diastole when the detectable flow velocities are strictly localized in the center of the vessel. In such cases, no flow is detected near the vessel walls. The diastolic volume flow may be overestimated. Lack of color sensitivity in color duplex instruments may cause an underestimation of volume flow. Other potential problems of this assumption have been discussed previously.

A summary of potential advantages of the different ultrasound techniques is given in Table 11-2.

MR imaging

Phase-sensitive MR imaging may help to quantify the flow volume not only in the carotid arteries but also the intracranial vessels.[1] This technique helps to estimate the functional diameter of the vessel and the flow velocity[8] simultaneously. Potential problems with this method are the duration of the acquisition time with potential artifacts due to movements and time intensive off line analysis.

NORMAL VALUES

Normal values of blood flow in the common carotid and vertebral arteries were initially established in the 1960s using xenon radionuclide methods. The blood flow in the common carotid was estimated to be around 350 ml/min[13] and in the vertebrals approximately 100 ml/min.[14]

Values around 380 to 520 ml/min were reported for the individual common carotid artery (Table 11-3) with different ultrasound techniques. These absolute numbers have to be judged carefully. Previous methods have used either a constant vessel diameter over the entire cardiac cycle or have assumed a functional vessel diameter according to the anatomic diameter. This may cause overestimation of volume flow rates, especially the diastolic component. Age appears to be a significant factor. Newborns have an average volume flow of 96 ml/min; at the age of 1 month, it is 234 ml/min. By the age of 3 years the average flow increases to 444 ml/min and reaches a maximum between the ages of 5 and 20 years (486 ml/min).[31] The same author showed decreased flow volume in the age group between 40 and 60 years (402 ml/min). In a different study, slightly lower flow volumes were reported in patients older than 45 years (385 ml/min), as compared to patients younger than 45 years

Table 11-2. Potential problems of ultrasound techniques

Problem	Single range gate (Doppler only)		Doppler plus gray scale A-mode		Gray scale Duplex (B-mode)		Color duplex (M-mode)		Power weighted
	Absolute	Relative	Absolute	Relative	Absolute	Relative	Absolute	Relative	Relative
Angle correction	+/−	−	+/−	−	+/−	−	+/−	−	−
Off-axis error	+	−	+/−	−	+/−	−	+/−	−	−
Circular vessel	+	−	+	−	−	−	−	−	−
Turbulent flow	+	+	+	+	+	+	+	+	+
Laminar parabolic flow	+	+/−	+	+/−	+	+/−	+/−	−	−
Change of anatomic diameter	+	+/−	−	−	+/−	−	−	−	−
Insonation at deeper depths	+/−	+/−	+/−	+/−	+/−	+/−	+	+/−	+/−

−, no problem; +/−, potential problem; +, definite problem.

Table 11-3. Common carotid artery flow volume rate in normal populations

Author	n	Flow (ml/min)
Benetos 1986 (3)	18	429 ± 21
Bouthier 1985 (5)	38	396 ± 19
Eicke 1995 (6)	125	330 ± 60 women 375 ± 70 men
Hamada 1993 (12)	28	564 ± 120
Meyd 1992 (18)	40	513.6 ± 92.4
Payen 1982 (23)	21	387 ± 183
Uematsu 1983 (30)	120	456 ± 66
Uematsu 1985 (31)	27	402 ± 29 women 480 ± 90 men

(410 ml/min).[5] In a recent trial in normal subjects we found age and gender to be the two most decisive factors of the volume flow rate with a 15% higher volume flow in men. Blood pressure, heart rate, smoking, body weight, body surface, and educational degree were not significant factors. In the presence of essential hypertension, flow volume is reported to be decreased by about 10% to 15%, particularly in the elderly.[3,5]

Few ultrasound data are available concerning the vertebral arteries. Bendick and Glover reported a flow volume for most vertebrals in the range of 50 to 150 ml/min based on the range-gated Doppler technique.[2]

Clinical applications

To date, the clinical applications of volume flow rate measurements include stroke and cerebrovascular disease, dementia, and arteriovenous malformations. Such data might also be extremely useful for monitoring drug effects.

Ischemic strokes result from embolic mechanisms, hemodynamic mechanisms, or a combination of both. Although most are believed embolic, it is often difficult to understand or document the ischemic mechanism for an individual patient. Retrospective data such as the infarct pattern on computed tomographic (CT) brain scan may help to distinguish hemodynamic from embolic stroke.[25] However, it remains problematic to predict which patients are at excess risk for a specific type of stroke.

The presence of extracranial carotid stenosis is known to confer an increased risk for stroke, but the mere presence of such a lesion may not be the most important pathophysiologic factor because not all patients with tight stenosis will experience stroke or transient ischemic attack (TIA). There may be more specific markers of increased risk for individual patients.

Neurologically speaking, three key questions must be asked following the identification of cerebrovascular stenosis: (1) Is the stenotic lesion generating emboli? (2) How does the lesion affect volume flow rate? (3) When the lesion reduces volume flow rate distally, are these changes compensated for by collateral flow from extraintracranial anastomoses, the contralateral carotid system, or the vertebrobasilar system? The first question can now be addressed by Doppler sonography. The other questions may be addressed by quantitative flowmetry. The answers to the second and third questions may play a key role in distinguishing between high- and low-risk lesions. However, volume flow rate information has been difficult to acquire noninvasively.

Rather limited data are available regarding volume flow rate in the clinical setting of cerebrovascular disease. Wada and colleagues showed an inverse correlation between severity of atherosclerotic disease identified by autopsy and CCA volume flow rate.[32] This study calculated the severity score from aggregate data regarding 10 different unilateral sites, including the external carotid and the anterior cerebral arteries. Uematsu reported decreased volume flow rate in the ipsilateral CCA of 27 patients with angiographically proven carotid disease.[31] Flow volume rate in the ipsilateral CCA, proximal to greater than 90% stenosis, was about half of normal values (210 ml/min versus 486 ml/min). However, the exact location of the stenosis was not mentioned.

Benetos and associates also reported decreased volume flow rate in the ipsilateral CCA, depending on the degree of ICA stenosis.[3] This study included 24 patients with ICA stenosis between 40% and 100% on angiography, 14 of whom were normotensive and 10 hypertensive, and the correlation was significant in both groups. In addition, for comparable degrees of stenosis, the volume flow rate in the hypertensive group was less than for normotensive patients.

Meyd and colleagues studied the effect of stenosis both ipsilaterally and contralaterally to assess for collateral flow effects.[18] Volume flow rates were compared in patients having greater than or less than 70% stenosis. Ipsilateral volume flow rate was only slightly decreased in those patients with less than 70% stenosis, compared to controls (473 versus 513 ml/min). However, with more than 70% stenosis, volume flow in the ipsilateral CCA was decreased to 360 ml/min. The contralateral CCA showed increased volume flow rate only in the group with more than 70% stenosis (649 ml/min). Patency of the anterior communicating artery was not mentioned, but these results suggested an ability to document and study collateral flow extracranially for individual patients. In fact, the ratio of flow volume in the contralateral-ipsilateral CCA of greater than 1.4 had a positive predictive value of 100% for identifying stenosis greater than 70%.

Tegeler and co-workers used time domain processing to determine volume flow rates in the CCA in patients with cerebrovascular disease; they found significant relationships between the severity of stenosis and both the ipsilateral and contralateral volume flow rates.[29]

Bendick and Glover reported the evaluation of collateral flow via the vertebral arteries in patients with high-grade carotid stenosis.[2] Subjects were normal, had mild atherosclerosis, or had tight carotid stenosis. They reported combined volume flow in the vertebrals of more than 200 ml/min as much more frequent in those with tight carotid stenosis.

The quantitative effect of collateralization via the anterior or posterior communicating arteries or the ophthalmic arteries is uncertain. Likewise, the clinical importance of such measurements has not been prospectively confirmed. An integrated approach using extracranial volume flow rate measurements, transcranial Doppler sonography, and reactivity testing may provide a much clearer assessment of the real hemodynamic impact of cerebrovascular disease and might allow more precise identification of those patients at highest risk for clinical events.

The clinical features of patients with dementing illnesses may offer few clues as to the exact cause of the clinical syndrome. Ultrasound has been used to try to differentiate vascular from nonvascular dementias. Increases in the velocity pulsatility index reportedly correlate with vascular dementias.[21] Volume flow rate measured by color flow imaging also appeared to correlate with vascular causes of dementia.[9] Using the latter approach, up to 90% of demented patients could correctly be classified. An inverse relationship has also been suggested between carotid volume flow rate and the severity of dementia.[17] Finally, age may play a more important role in volume flow rate in demented patients than in normal patients.[31]

Intracranial arteriovenous malformations (AVM) can often be identified by transcranial Doppler (TCD) sonography. Characteristic findings include increased blood flow velocities with decreased pulsatility indices.[10] Conventional angiography, TCD, or MR angiography can help to identify supplying vessels. However, the actual shunt flow volume, which may be quite important in the setting of superselective embolization procedures, can only be estimated by such methods. Using duplex sonography, Lin and colleagues found increased volume flow rate in the ICA (945 to 1680 ml/min) in patients with a direct communication between ICA and a cavernous fistula.[16] In three of four cases of cavernous sinus fistulae, supplied by dural branches of the external carotid artery, the volume flow rate was increased in this extracranial vessel. But when dural ICA branches fed the fistula, no increased volume flow was seen in the ICA. Flow volume measurements may help to document treatment effect noninvasively during therapeutic embolizations or during the follow-up period. Based on limited clinical work, volume flow rates greater than 500 ml/min in the CCAV (CVI-Q technique) are quite unusual in normal subjects and, as an isolated finding, should raise suspicions of an AVM.

An exciting potential use for volume flow rate measurement is monitoring drug effects. Many drugs have the potential to alter the cerebral circulation and perfusion. Such effects may be variable and unpredictable for individual patients. For example, vasoactive drugs such as the calcium channel blockers, alpha- and beta-mimetics or blockers, serotonin active agents, or nitroglycerin, as well as drugs with primarily cardiac clinical uses, may also have profound effects on cerebral hemodynamics. The use of cerebrovascular volume flowmetry may allow objective monitoring of such and also offer an opportunity to confirm the effect of drugs claiming to improve cerebral hemodynamics.

CONCLUSION

Volume flow rate may be the most clinically important parameter for understanding cerebral hemodynamics in specific patients. Volume flow rate is the final product from integration of many other factors, including flow velocity, percent stenosis, vessel morphology, and the potential for collateral function. As such, it may be a more precise or accurate way to gain an overall assessment of function and risk for individual patients.

Clinical applications have been reported in normals, atherosclerotic disease, a.v. malformations, and dementia. However, earlier data were cumbersome to obtain or interpret and required some questionable assumptions. The availability of color duplex M-mode systems and time domain processing has helped to accelerate data acquisition time and increased the accuracy and reliability of these measurements. Depending on the depth of insonation and specific vessel characteristics, either cw Doppler in combination with an M-mode scanner, gray scale duplex, or color M-mode systems are applicable. Not all limitations of this method have been overcome. Insonate of the intracranial vessels, the vertebral, and the internal carotid arteries remain dificult for many clinical applications. Ongoing studies may lead to new understanding, classification, and management especially of cerebrovascular disease, based on volume flow rate changes. Such methods may provide important new insights for the other clinical situations mentioned previously and many more yet to be identified.

REFERENCES

1. Bendel P, Buonocore E, Bockisch A, Besocci MC: Blood flow in carotid arteries: quantification by using phase-sensitive MR imaging, *AJR Am J Roentgenol* 152:1307-1310, 1989.
2. Bendick PJ, Glover JL: Vertebrobasilar insufficiency: evaluation by quantitative duplex flow measurements: a preliminary report, *J Vasc Surg* 5:594-600, 1987.
3. Benetos A, Safar ME, Laurent S, et al: Common carotid blood flow in patients with hypertension and stenosis of the internal carotid artery, *J Clin Hypertens* 1:44-54, 1986.
4. Bonnefous O, Pesque P: Time domain formulation of pulsed-Doppler ultrasound and blood flow velocity estimation by cross correlation, *Ultrasonic Imaging* 8:73-85, 1986.
5. Bouthier J, Benetos A, Simon A, et al: Pulsed Doppler evaluation of diameter, blood velocity and blood flow of common carotid artery in sustained essential hypertonus, *J Cardiovasc Pharmacol* 7:99-104, 1985.
6. Eicke BM, Tegeler CH: Ultrasonic quantitative flow volumetry of the carotid arteries: initial experience with a color flow M-mode system, *Cerebrovasc Dis* 1995.
7. Eicke BM, Tegeler CH, Howard G, et al: In-vitro validation of Color Velocity Imaging and spectral Doppler for velocity determination, *J Neuroimaging* 3:89-92, 1993.
8. Firmin DN, Nayler GL, Klipstein RH, et al: In vivo validation of MR velocity imaging, *J Comput Assist Tomogr* 11:751-756, 1987.
9. Gill RW: Measurement of blood flow by ultrasound: accuracy and sources of error, *Ultrasound Med Biol* 11:625-641, 1985.
10. Giller CA: Arteriovenous malformations. In Babikian VL and Wechsler LR, editors: *Transcranial doppler ultrasonography,* St. Louis, 1993, Mosby.
11. Görtler M, Niethammer R, Widder B: Differentiating subtotal carotid artery stenoses from occlusions by colour-coded duplex sonography, *J Neurol* 241:301-305, 1994.
12. Hamada T, Takita M, Kawano H, et al: Difference in blood flow volume of the common carotid artery between vascular and nonvascular dementia detected by colour duplex sonography, *J Neurol* 240:191-194, 1993.
13. Hardesty WM, Roberts B, Toole JF, Royster HP: Studies of carotid-artery blood flow in man, *N Engl J Med* 263:944-946, 1960.
14. Hardesty WM, Whitacre WB, Toole JF, Royster HP: Studies on vertebral artery blood flow, *Surg Forum* 13:482-483, 1962.
15. Juul R, Slørdahl SA, Torp H, et al: Flow estimation using ultrasound imaging (color M-mode) and computed postprocessing, *J Cereb Flow Metabol* 11:879-882, 1991.
16. Lin HJ, Yip PK, Liu HM, et al: Noninvasive hemodynamic classification of carotid-cavernous sinus fistulas by duplex carotid sonography, *J Ultrasound Med* 13:105-113, 1994.
17. Matsumoto M, Sekimot H, Goriya Y, et al: Relationship between carotid blood flow volume and degree of dementia in the elderly studied with a two-dimensional echographically guided ultrasonic Doppler flow volumeter: a pilot study, *J Cardiovasc Ultrason* 7:315-320, 1988.
18. Meyd CJ, Abu-Shakra S, Bleecker ML: Carotid high-low flow ratio most accurately predicts significant stenosis, *Arch Neurol* 864-869, 1992.
19. Minnich LL, Snider AR, Meliones JN, Yanock C: In vitro evaluation of volumetric flow from Doppler power-weighted and amplitude-weighted mean velocities, *J Am Soc Echocardiogr* 6:227-236, 1993.
20. Nichols WW, O'Rourke ME: *The nature of flow of a fluid.* In *McDonald's blood flow in arteries,* ed 3, London, 1990, Edward Arnold.
21. Norris JW, Zhu CZ, Bornstein NM, Chambers BR: Vascular risks of asymptomatic carotid stenosis, *Stroke* 22:1485-1490, 1991.
22. Olson RM, Cooke JP: Human carotid artery diameter and flow by a noninvasive technique, *Medical Instrumentation* 9:99-102, 1975.
23. Payen DM, Levy BI, Menegalli DJ, et al: Evaluation of human hemispheric blood flow based on noninvasive carotid blood flow measurements using the range-gated Doppler technique, *Stroke* 13:392-398, 1982.
24. Ries F: Differentiation of multiinfarct and Alzheimer dementia by intracranial hemodynamic parameters, *Stroke* 24:228-235, 1993.
25. Ringelstein EB, Koschorke S, Holling A, et al: Computed tomographic patterns of proven embolic brain emboli, *Ann Neurol* 26:759-765, 1989.
26. Spencer MP, Denison AB: The square-wave electromagnetic flowmeter: theory of operation and design of magnetic probes for clinical and experimental applications, *IRE Transactions on Medical Electronics* 220-228, 1959.
27. Strandness DE: Ultrasound in the study of atherosclerosis, *Ultrasound Med Biol* 12:435-464, 1986.
28. Tegeler CH, Kremkau FW, Hitchings LP: Color velocity imaging: introduction to a new ultrasound technology, *J Neuroimaging* 1:85-90, 1991.
29. Tegeler CH, Knappertz VA, Eicke BM, et al: Carotid artery volume flow rate correlates with severity of stenosis, (Abstract) *Radiology* 193:231, 1994.
30. Uematsu S, Yang A, Preziosi TJ, et al: Measurement of carotid blood flow in man and its clinical application, *Stroke* 14:256-266, 1983.
31. Uematsu S, Folstein MS: Carotid blood flow measured by an ultrasonic volume flowmeter in carotid stenosis and patients with dementia, *J Neurol Neurosurg Psychiatry* 48:1230-1233, 1985.
32. Wada T, Kodaira K, Fujishiro K, Okamura T: Correlation of common carotid flow volume measured by ultrasonic quantitative flowmeter with pathological findings, *Stroke* 22:319-322, 1991.
33. Westkott HP, Andreesen H: Frequency domain (pw-Doppler) versus time domain (color velocity imaging) method: velocity measurements in superficial arteries, *J Ultrasound Med* 12:S2, 1993 (abstract).
34. Withers CE, Gosink BB, Keightley AM, et al: Duplex carotid sonography: peak systolic velocity in quantifying internal carotid artery stenosis, *J Ultrasound Med* 9:345-349, 1990.
35. Zierler BK, Kirkman TR, Kraiss LW, et al: Accuracy of duplex scanning for measurement of arterial volume flow, *J Vasc Surg* 16:520-526, 1992.

SECTION THREE

Adult Transcranial Doppler

The Transcranial Doppler Examination: Principles and Applications of Transcranial Doppler Sonography

Shirley M. Otis
E. Bernd Ringelstein

The assessment of the extracranial cerebral vessels by Doppler ultrasonography was first reported by Miyazaki and Kato in 1965.[31] Despite the rapid development of this technique extracranially, it was not applied to the intracranial arteries in that it was generally assumed that the cranium was largely impenetrable to ultrasound. However, in 1982 Aaslid, Markwalder, and Nornes developed a transcranial Doppler device with a pulse sound emission of 2 MHz that could penetrate the skull successfully and accurately measure both blood flow direction and velocities in the basal cerebral vessels and in the circle of Willis.[6] During the last several years, this technique has turned out to be an increasingly useful tool in the whole field of neurosonology. With the introduction of this intracranial ultrasound technique, it became possible to record intracranial blood flow velocity directly. Thus, transcranial Doppler (TCD) became an important noninvasive method for assessing cerebral hemodynamics and for evaluating intracranial cerebral vascular disease.

Although the relationship remains unclear between actual cerebral blood flow and the flow velocities measured by TCD within the basal cerebral arteries, this limitation can be overcome as relative changes in blood flow velocity reflect the relative changes in regional cerebral blood flow.[26,39] In addition to its noninvasive character and low cost, TCD offers the advantages that relative changes in cerebral blood flow can be measured objectively, immediately, as often as desired, and for as long as necessary.[3,11] The abrupt or short- and long-lasting effects of any external mechanical manipulation or functional stimulation of the intracranial circulation can be assessed in real time as can the pathophysiology of cerebral circulation in acute stroke.[10,45] This makes TCD an attractive tool for monitoring, particularly during neurosurgical, cardiac, and cerebrovascularization operations, both for knowledge of the immediate status of cerebral blood flow and for reducing the occurrence of postoperative cerebral complications.[19,29,30,37] The box lists the already established

---

Clinical applications of transcranial Doppler

- Diagnosis of intracranial occlusive disease (individual and epidemiologic aspects)
- Auxiliary test for extracranial occlusive disease in inconclusive extracranial tests
- Evaluation of hemodynamic effects of extracranial occlusive disease on intracranial blood flow (e.g., internal carotid artery occlusion, subclavian steal)
- Detection and identification of feeders of arteriovenous malformations
- Preoperative compression tests for evaluation of collateralizing capacities of circle of Willis
- Detection of right-to-left shunts in the heart (e.g., patent foramen ovale) and paradoxical embolism
- Intermittent monitoring and follow-up of
    - Vasospasm in subarachnoid hemorrhage and migraine
    - Spontaneous or therapeutically induced recanalization of occluded vessels
    - Establishment of collateral pathways after occluding interventions
    - Occlusive disease during anticoagulative or fibrinolytic therapy
- Continuous monitoring during
    - Neuroradiologic interventions (e.g., balloon occlusion, embolization)
    - Short-term pharmacologic trials of vasoactive drugs and anesthetics
    - Carotid endarterectomy (shunt)
    - Cardiac surgery (ischemic encephalopathy? embolism?)
    - Increasing intracranial pressure
    - Evolution of brain death
- Functional tests
    - Stimulation of cerebral vasomotors with CO_2 or other vasoactive drugs (e.g., acetazolamide)
    - External stimulation of visual cortex
- Neuropsychologic tasks for hemispheric dominance (with simultaneous bilateral and TCD recording)

---

applications of TCD sonography in clinical and experimental settings.

EXAMINATION TECHNIQUES
General requirements

Like every other ultrasound technique, TCD ultrasonography is based on the physics and principles that apply to any ultrasound device and can be affected by various conditions. The laboratory room used should be situated in an area that is quiet and comfortable and where extraneous noise will not interfere with the examination. The patient should be comfortable and warm, and the examination table should support the patient's head comfortably. In order to facilitate relax-

ation of the patient, a short explanation of the purpose of the examination and the techniques of the examination to be used should be given.

Absolute prerequisites

Before a TCD examination is performed, two prerequisites should be fulfilled: (1) The status of the extracranial arteries must be completely known, and (2) the patient must be lying supine and comfortably to preserve a stable position of the probe and to avoid major fluctuations in the carbon dioxide pressure. The examiner must also deal with two main anatomic considerations: The number and extent of so-called acoustic windows or foramina within the skull that can be penetrated with the ultrasound beam are sometimes limited and/or not easily identified, and the arteries of the base of the skull are extremely variable in respect to size, development, site, and course.*

Acoustic properties of the skull

The problem of acoustic properties of the skull has been well studied, and transmission of the ultrasound beam through the cranium depends on the structure of the skull itself.[48] The skull consists of three layers of bone, each of which influences the beam in a different manner. The middle layer (diploë) has the most important effect on the attenuation and scattering of the sound, whereas the outer and inner tables, made of so-called ivory bone, are more important for refraction. Because of the essential absence of bony spicules in the temporal region, this is an attractive area for ultrasound evaluation. Grolimund has performed a number of in vitro experiments to determine the effect of the skull bone on Doppler ultrasound.[18] His experiments have shown that a wide range of energy loss occurs in different skull samples and that the power loss depends on the thickness of the skull. In no case was the power measured behind the skull greater than 35% of the transmitted power. He further showed that the skull has the effect of an acoustic lens and that the refraction of the beam depended more on variation of bone thickness than on the angle of insonation. His data suggested that it would be advantageous to use ultrasound lenses with longer focal lengths to improve the sensitivity, particularly at depths of 5 and 10 cm.

Transcranial Doppler devices

Commercial systems that use a 2-MHz Doppler ultrasound device of pulsed, range-gated design and with good directional resolution are available. For transcranial application the primary consideration is a good signal-to-noise resolution. This is one reason the available instruments developed for transcranial application

---

*References 6, 7, 36, 37, 38, 45.

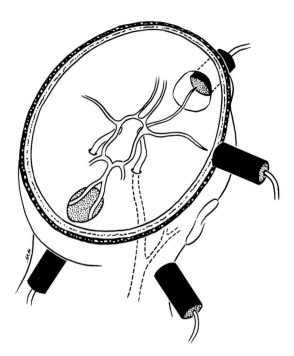

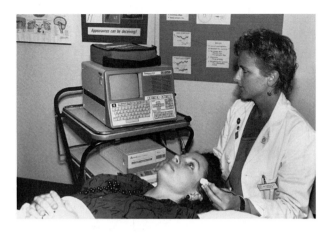

Fig. 12-2. Transtemporal approach for insonation of the middle cerebral artery (M1 and M2 segments), anterior cerebral artery (A1 segment), distal carotid siphon, posterior cerebral artery (P1 and P2 segments), top of the basilar artery, and the posterior communicating artery if it is acting as a collateral channel.

Fig. 12-1. Relationship of the ultrasound probes at the available acoustic windows and their relationship to the basal cerebral arteries.

have larger and less defined sample volume than most other pulsed Doppler instruments. The former have a decreased bandwidth in an attempt to improve the signal-to-noise ratio. Additional requirements are transmitting power between 10 and 100 mW/cm^2/s, adjustable Doppler gate depth, pulse repetition frequency up to 20 kHz, focusing of the ultrasonic beam at distances of 40 and 60 mm, and on-line, time-averaged velocity and peak systolic velocity produced by spectroanalysis of backscattered Doppler signals.[2] Instruments include the first commercially available transcranial Doppler, TCD-64 (Eden Medical Electronics Überlingen, Germany), and the recently developed Transpect Transcranial Doppler (Medasonics, Mountainview, California). Both systems include a special 2-MHz transducer for continuous monitoring that can be attached to the head by a specially developed headband or helmet. Also available is the TransScan (Eden Medical Electronics, Überlingen, Germany), a three-dimensional transcranial imaging system with velocity color-coding and mapping capabilities.[2] Recently, B-mode imaging with duplex systems has become available to visualize both the intracranial arteries and the surrounding brain tissue.[8,9,12,43]

Acoustic windows

A complete TCD examination evaluates the ophthalmic (OA), intracranial internal carotid (ICA), middle cerebral (MCA), anterior cerebral (ACA), posterior cerebral (PCA), basilar (BA), intracranial and extracranial vertebral (VA), and submandibular carotid

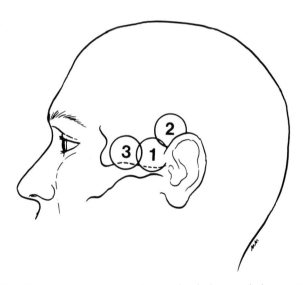

Fig. 12-3. Available temporal acoustic windows and placement of the probe: *1,* preauricular position; *2,* posterior window; and *3,* anterior window. The probe should be placed first in the preaural region to identify the middle cerebral artery. Subtle meandering movements of the probe should be performed in each position. If position 1 is not successful, position 2 should be tried before position 3.

arteries. This is made possible by taking advantage of the anatomic skull foramina. Four different approaches have been described to insonate the intracranial arteries: transtemporal, transorbital, suboccipital, and submandibular (Fig. 12-1).[2,38]

Transtemporal approach. In the transtemporal approach, the probe is placed on the temporal plane, cephalad to the zygomatic arch and immediately anterior and slightly superior to the tragus of the ear conch (Figs. 12-2 and 12-3, *1*). This site is usually the most promising.

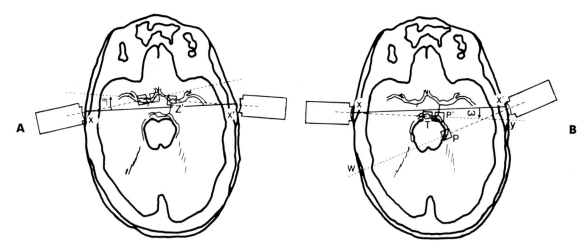

Fig. 12-4. Position of the probe in the temporal region to insonate the anterior and posterior part of the circle of Willis. **A,** Line *XX'* indicates a frontal plane that runs through the regular placement of the probe on either side and, simultaneously, perpendicular to the sagittal midline of the skull. *Z'* indicates the site of the intracranial bifurcation of the internal carotid artery. The *XZ'* distance was 63 ± 5 mm. μ indicates the angle with which the probe is more anteriorly aimed at the middle and anterior cerebral arterial segments. This angle was 6° ± 1.1°. **B,** ω indicates the angle with which the beam is directed more posteriorly to insonate the top of the basilar artery *(T)* and the P1 segments *(P')* on both sides. This angle was 4.6 ± 1.2°. The bifurcation of the basilar artery could be insonated at depths of 78 ± 5 mm, corresponding to the distance *XT* or *X'T,* respectively. *Y* indicates the fictional point where the pathway of the beam then transits the contralateral skull (i.e., approximately 2 to 3 cm behind the external acoustic meatus). The P2 segments *(P)* also can be insonated if the beam is directed even more posteriorly and slightly caudally (line *X,P*). W lies approximately 5 cm behind the contralateral external acoustic meatus.

A more posterior window immediately over and slightly dorsal to the first one may be more appropriate in a minority of cases; this is the optimal site for insonation of the P2 segment of the PCAs (Fig. 12-3, *2*). In some patients, more frontally located temporal windows may be present (Fig. 12-3, *3*). With these preauricular, transtemporal approaches, the beam can be angulated anteriorly or posteriorly relative to a frontal plane running through the corresponding probe positions on either side of the head. The anterior orientation of the beam allows insonation of the M1 and M2 segments of the MCA, the C1 segment of carotid siphon, and the A1 segment of the ACA, including the anterior communicating artery (ACOA) (Fig. 12-4, *A*). The posteriorly angulated beam insonates the P1 and P2 segments of the PCA, the top of the BA, and the posterior communicating arteries (PCOA) (Fig. 12-4, *B*).

Transorbital approach. The ophthalmic artery can be insonated at depths of 45 to 50 mm, whereas the C3 segment (anterior knee of the carotid siphon) is normally met at insonation depths of 60 to 65 mm (Figs. 12-5 and 12-6, *A*). At slightly greater insonation depths of 70 to 75 mm, the C2 segment shows flow away from the probe (downward deflection), and the C4 segment shows flow toward the probe (upward deflection), provided that the angulation of the beam is nearly sagittal via the supraorbital fissure or via the infraorbital fissure, with a

slightly oblique approach (Fig. 12-6, *B*). When the probe is placed at the superior outer quadrant of the eyelids and the beam angulated medially, the ultrasound beam penetrates the optic canal and is aimed at the contralateral arteries (i.e., ACA, supraclinoidal carotid siphon, proximal MCA). Typical insonation depths are listed in Table 12-1.

Suboccipital approach. The suboccipital approach is essential for screening the vertebrobasilar system in its whole length (Fig. 12-7, *A*). The probe is placed exactly between the squama occipitalis and the palpable spinous process of the first cervical vertebra, with the beam aimed at the bridge of the nose and an insonation depth of 65 mm. The patient may be seated with the head flexed or lying with the head turned laterally (Fig. 12-8). The distal VAs are tracked in both directions with small insonation depths (35 to 50 mm); by angulating the beam strongly to one side, the examiner can screen the extradural part of the VAs on the posterior arch of the atlas (flow toward the probe). The top of the BA is normally reached at depths of 95 to 125 mm, with flow directed away from the probe (Fig. 12-7, *B*).

Submandibular approach. The submandibular approach completes the examination in the sense that the retromandibular and more distal, extradural parts of the ICA (C5-C6 segment) can be evaluated (Fig 12-9, *A*). This particular examination is helpful as a complemen-

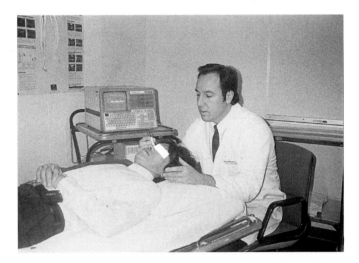

Fig. 12-5. Transorbital approach for insonation of the various segments of the carotid siphon (C1-C4), the ophthalmic artery, and, via the optic canal, the contralateral anterior cerebral artery.

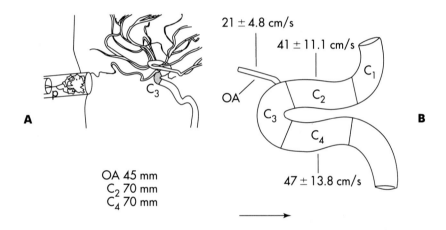

Fig. 12-6. Insonation of the ophthalmic artery *(OA)* and carotid siphon via the transorbital approach. **A,** Probe location and relationship to the ophthalmic artery and carotid siphon. Representative insonation depths are also given. **B,** Normal flow velocity values within the various segments of the carotid siphon and ophthalmic artery.

tary test to extracranial studies and helps avoid overlooking chronic occlusions of the ICA in cases with abundant collateralization via the external carotid artery. The beam is directed slightly medially and posterior to the longitudinal axis of the body, where the ICA regularly can be tracked up to 80 to 85 mm, where it bends medioanteriorly to form the siphon (Fig. 12-9, *B*).

Diagnostic measurements

The primary diagnostic measurements for identifying cerebral arteries are (1) the insonation depth, (2) the direction of blood flow at that depth, (3) the flow velocities (mean time of flow velocity and systolic or diastolic peak flow velocities), (4) site of the probe's position (temporal, orbital, suboccipital, and

submandibular), (5) direction of the ultrasonic beam (posterior, anterior, caudad, or cephalad), (6) the "traceability" of vessels, and (7) response to carotid compression.[2,37]

Initial examination. Generally, it is most convenient to start with the MCA on either side at an insonation depth of 50 to 55 mm and then to track the basal arterial network step by step in various directions. Proof of traceability of the MCA is decisive for its unequivocal identification. This is also true for the other basal arterial vasculature. Traceability refers to the fact that the MCA (and usually other arteries) can be tracked in incremental steps from more shallow depths (e.g., 35 mm) to deeper sites (e.g., 55 mm) without changes in the character of the flow profile and direction. When the

Table 12-1. Normal values of mean blood velocity (cm/s) for cranial arteries

Age (yr)	Middle cerebral artery (M1)	Anterior cerebral artery (A1)	Posterior artery (P1)	Basilar artery	Vertebral artery
10-29	70 ± 16.4	61 ± 14.7	55 ± 9	46 ± 11	45 ± 9.8
30-49	57 ± 11.2	48 ± 7.1	42 ± 8.9	38 ± 8.6	35 ± 8.2
50-59	51 ± 9.7	46 ± 9.4	39 ± 9.9	32 ± 7	37 ± 10
60-70	41 ± 7	38 ± 5.6	36 ± 7.9	32 ± 6.7	35 ± 7
Insonated depth (mm)	50-55	60-65	60-65	90-95	60-65

Velocities are given as means plus or minus the standard deviation.

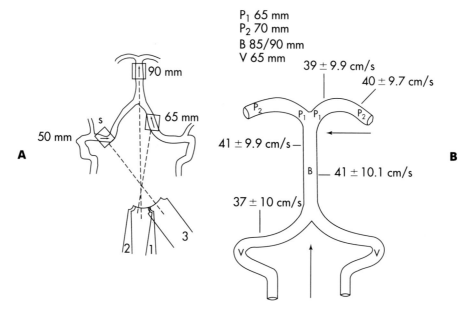

Fig. 12-7. A, Transcranial Doppler sonography of the vertebral system via the suboccipital approach. **B,** Representative insonation depths and normal flow velocity values within the distal vertebral arteries and the basilar trunk. The P1 and P2 velocities are measured transtemporally.

MCA is tracked medially (65 to 70 mm), an abrupt change in the direction of flow indicates insonation of the A1 segment of the ACA. Flow toward the probe at this step is usually registered from the carotid siphon (Fig. 12-10).

When the beam is angulated more posteriorly during a transtemporal approach, the P1 segment of the PCA can be picked up most readily at an insonation depth of 65 to 70 mm and can then be tracked over the top of the BA (75 mm) to the contralateral PCA (P1, 80 to 85 mm). The criteria of traceability include display of a bilateral blood flow at the top of the BA and the change of flow direction within the contralateral PCA. These are important features for identification of the PCA without resorting to the use of compression tests. Generally, depending on the clinical situation being evaluated,

examinations via the orbital, suboccipital, or submandibular pathways follow.

Flow velocity measurements. The mean flow velocities and standard deviations of various vessel segments at representative insonation depths are shown in Table 12-1 for different age groups. Normal flow velocity values in adults show good interobserver correlation (Table 12-2).* In normal subjects the highest velocities are almost always found in the MCA or ACA. The PCAs and the BAs have lower Doppler shifts than the MCA. This variation, however, does not reflect differences in cerebral blood flow but differences in the ratios of territorial blood flow and diameter of the feeding artery.[17]

*References 5, 7, 16, 20, 38, 42.

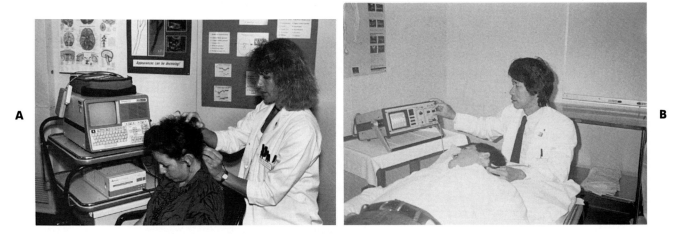

Fig. 12-8. The suboccipital approach for insonation of the distal vertebral arteries and the basilar trunk. **A,** Patient in the sitting position with head forward flexed. **B,** Alternative method of examination with the patient supine and head turned comfortably to one side.

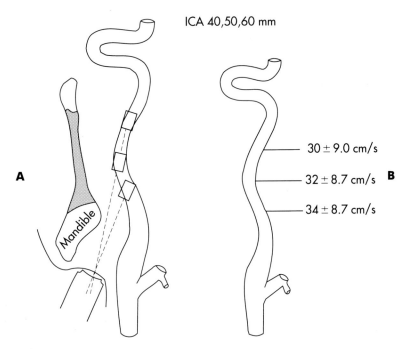

ICA 40,50,60 mm

30 ± 9.0 cm/s

32 ± 8.7 cm/s

34 ± 8.7 cm/s

Mandible

Fig. 12-9. A, Transcranial Doppler sonography of the petrous portion of the internal carotid artery (ICA) via the submandibular approach. The ICA can be tracked from depths of 25 to 80 mm corresponding to the C4 and C5 segments of the ICA. **B,** Representative insonation depths and normal flow values within the distal intracranial ICA.

Flow velocities in the basal cerebral arteries show a consistent decrease with increasing age (Table 12-1).[19,21,40] These findings correlate well with age-related changes seen in studies of cerebral blood flow.[24,25] This underlines the validity and sensitivity of the ultrasound method as an intraindividually close semiquantitative estimate of cerebral blood flow on the basis of velocity data.

Vessel identification. Identification of vessels is primarily based on the window or foramen used, the angulation of the beam, the depth of insonation, the direction of blood flow relative to the probe, and the traceability of the vessel segments. However, in pathologic conditions and in many individuals, particularly the elderly, compression tests may be required for the unequivocal identification of certain arterial segments.[6,28,33,38] Compression tests during TCD examinations can be performed on the common carotid arteries (CCA), low in the neck (with two fingers) (Fig. 12-11, *A*), or on the VAs at the mastoidal slope (Figs. 12-11, *B;* and 12-12). Little risk of creating embolism from plaques in the carotid arteries exists if compression is performed only after knowledge of B-mode imaging of the carotid arteries and by an experienced investigator.[44,46] Generally, compression maneuvers

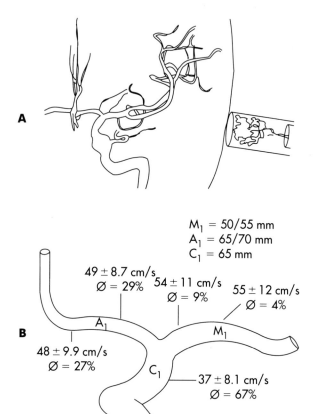

Fig. 12-10. Temporal placement of the probe and its relationship to the middle cerebral artery (MCA). **A,** The beam axis is in line with the M2, M1, and A1 segments of the cerebral vasculature. **B,** Representative insonation depths and normal flow values within the MCA, the anterior cerebral artery, and the distal part of the internal carotid artery.

strictly for arterial identification are not necessary; however, these compression maneuvers are extremely valuable in the assessment of collateral pathways. Figures 12-13 and 12-14 show the ways flow is affected in intracranial arteries during compression maneuvers. Responses include (1) no reaction at all, (2) increase of flow velocity, (3) decrease of flow velocity, (4) reversal of flow, (5) alternating flow direction (to and fro), and (6) cessation of flow (Table 12-3).

Three-dimensional localization

Because of the variability and complexity of the vessels that comprise the circle of Willis, handheld TCD devices are subject to problems of vessel identification and documentation; furthermore, TCD does not provide morphologic information about the basal vessels. These problems significantly limit conventional TCD sonography. Aaslid developed the first mapping device designed to minimize technical difficulties associated with TCD sonography. From an early two-dimensional device, the instrument has evolved to a three-dimensional system (Fig. 12-15).[1,2,4,34,35] This multiprojection sample volume unit produces a composite diagram of patent intracranial vessels (Fig. 12-16). This vascular map is produced by plotting the Doppler sample volume locations. Velocity and direction of flow are color coded for each distinct point of insonation. For each point, velocity is indicated by color, and the strength of the signal is indicated by the size of the dot. The memory in the system can recall the location of the ultrasonic windows and the positions from which the signals were obtained. These capabilities permit easy identification of cranial landmarks and provide the ability to use the stored information for follow-up studies. The three-dimensional (3D) technique provides a visual map that aids the operator in locating the intracranial vessels.

As with the conventional TCD (handheld probe), the patient is supine, but with the 3D device the head is held with a headpiece that feeds the *x, y,* and *z* coordinates of transducer position into a computer. The 3D ultrasonic map of the intracranial vessels is then reconstructed from these coordinates. The locations of the MCA, ACA, terminal ICA, and PCA are

Table 12-2. Normal values of mean blood velocity (cm/s) for the middle, anterior, posterior, and basilar arteries

Author	Middle	Anterior	Posterior	Basilar
Aaslid, Huber, Nornes[5]	62 ± 12	51 ± 12	44 ± 11	48 mean
DeWitt, Wechsler[14]	62 ± 12	52 ± 12	42 ± 10	42 ± 10
Harders[19]	65 ± 17	50 ± 13	40 ± 9	39 ± 9
Hennerici, et al.[21]	58 ± 12	53 ± 10	37 ± 10	36 ± 12
Ringelstein, et al.[38]	55 ± 12	49 ± 9	40 ± 10	41 ± 10
Russo, et al.[42]	65 ± 13	48 ± 20	35 ± 18	45 ± 10

Values are given as means plus or minus the standard deviation.

mapped bilaterally. Identification of the PCA, which is often a difficult vessel to locate, is made easier by using the map as a guide.

One of the important advantages of 3D TCD is its ability to discriminate between the anterior and posterior parts of the circle of Willis (both of which are insonated from the temporal region). A second advantage is the identification of the carotid siphon, with flow both toward and away from the probe. In addition, the vertebrobasilar system may be displayed in both the lateral and horizontal planes, which helps determine the probe-to-vessel angle more accurately. This angle is often difficult to measure because of the small size, tortuosity, and possible congenital abnormalities of the basilar vessels. A comparative study of conventional handheld TCD and 3D TCD monitoring revealed that visual mapping improves the operator's accuracy and shortens examination times.[23]

The three-dimensional transcranial imaging system is subject to certain disadvantages, however. Inadequate positioning of the patient's head may lead to significant error. The posterior vessels are often hidden behind the carotid system, and misinterpretation of insonated vessels because of anatomic variations or collateral flow remains a problem, as it does with conventional, handheld TCD. When the PCOA and ACOAs act as collaterals, they may be misinterpreted as focal areas of stenosis in the carotid siphon or ACA, respectively. These limitations, however, are less apt to happen with the mapping technique than with handheld TCD.

DIAGNOSTIC PARAMETERS
The Doppler spectral waveform

The Doppler shift recorded from the intracranial arteries is not a single pure frequency such as that from a single moving reflector. The signal received is a mixture of different frequency components coming from reflectors moving at different velocities. The spectral broadening effect is therefore even more prominent in the TCD recordings than in the cervical or peripheral sampling due to the large sample volume size compared to the dimensions of the intracranial artery. Frequently, not only is the entire cross-sectional lumen of an artery

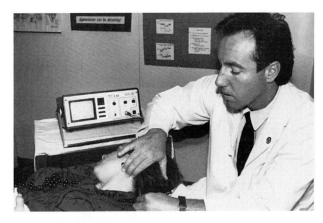

Fig. 12-12. Supine patient with head turned and neck flexed, allowing access to the intracranial vertebral by way of the foramen magnum, and the compression of the vertebral artery at the mastoid.

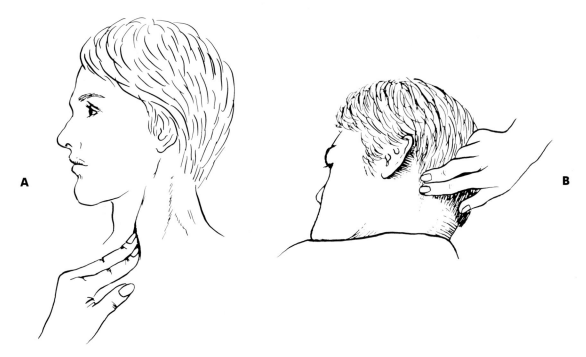

Fig. 12-11. Compression tests. **A,** Compression of the common carotid artery low in the neck. **B,** Compression of the vertebral artery at the mastoid slope.

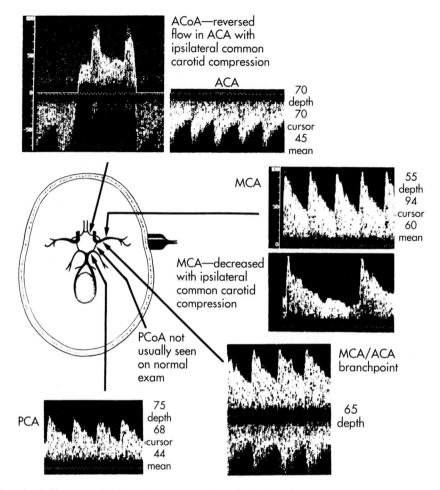

Fig. 12-13. Transcranial Doppler sonography of the basal intracranial arteries from the transtemporal approach, their normal location, and their response to compression of the common carotid artery.

insonated but also other arteries and different segments of nearby vessels may contribute to the Doppler signal. Despite these problems, the intracranial spectral waveform is very similar to that seen in the cervical ICA. Both of these waveforms reveal a high diastolic flow component and a major concentration of flow forward, resulting in a continuous type of Doppler signal. As in extracranial vessel analysis, the intracranial spectral waveform evaluates the peak systolic and diastolic and mean flow velocities. Of particular importance is the evaluation of the systolic upstroke, pulsatility, direction of flow, and spectral distribution. In TCD instruments, the mean flow velocity is calculated and displayed automatically and refers to a time mean of the peak velocity envelope, with the envelope being a trace of the peak flow velocities as a function of time.

The typical features of a circumscribed stenosis of a large basal cerebral artery are similar to those of the extracranial arteries and include acceleration of flow (increased flow velocity), disturbed flow (spectral broad-

ening and enhanced systolic low-frequency echo components), and covibration phenomena (vibration of vessel wall and surrounding soft tissue).[27,41] As in extracranial disease, mild stenosis increases peak velocity with little change in the rest of the Doppler pattern, whereas moderate or severe stenosis leads to greater increase in peak velocity with spectral broadening, increased diastolic velocity, and turbulent flow. A poststenotic drop in peak velocity is usually seen as well.

Functional tests

Because of its excellent time resolution of flow velocity measurements, TCD is ideal for functional tests with rapid changes of cerebral perfusion. Such tests are aimed primarily at the evaluation of the reserve mechanism of the cerebral vasculature by using various stimuli such as hypocapnia or hypercapnia, increased or reduced systemic arterial pressure, and hypoxia.

Intactness of vasomotor reserve implies that a drop in perfusion pressure can be counterbalanced by vasodila-

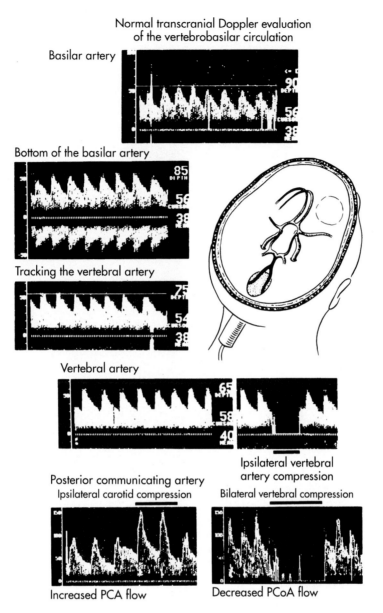

Fig. 12-14. Transcranial Doppler examination of the vertebrobasilar circulation, normal vessel location, and the effects of compressive maneuvers.

tation of cortical arterioles to maintain a sufficient blood supply. Carbon dioxide reactivities permit the study of the reaction of cerebral arteries in different pathologic situations and measurement of cerebral vascular reserve. These tests are useful in evaluating the hemodynamic impact of extracranial occlusive carotid disease and other conditions of reduced cerebral perfusion; they are discussed in detail in Chapter 14.

Effects of extracranial occlusive disease

Because of the ability of TCD to identify collateral flow, the various pathways and number of functional collaterals can be assessed. The patency of the circle of Willis can be tested by recording the changes in blood velocity and flow direction in the basal cerebral arteries in response to compression of the CCA. Significant changes occur in the intracranial circulation because of extracranial flow-limiting disease. Velocity in the MCA decreases ipsilateral to severe carotid stenosis or occlusion, and the pulsatility index* generally decreases because of the vasodilatation in the distal arterial

*The pulsatility index (PI) is a common measure for describing the shape of signal waveforms. PI is derived by the formula $PI = \frac{PSV - EDV}{MV}$ where PSV = peak systolic velocity, EDV = end diastolic velocity, and MV = mean velocity.

Table 12-3. Effects of compression tests of the common carotid arteries on various vessel segments and their diagnostic meanings

Insonated vessel segment	Findings at rest	Effect of ipsilateral CCA compression test	Effect of contralateral CCA compression test	Functional meaning of compression test
MCA (M1/M2)	Normal flow velocity, flow toward probe	↓ or ↓↓ or [ ]	0 or [↓]	Confirmation of vessel identity
ACA (A1)	Normal flow velocity flow away from probe	[↓↓] or [ ] or with D	[0] or ↑ or ↑↑ with or without D	Confirmation of vessel identity, presence or absence of potential anterior collateral pathway
ACoA	No signal available	[↑↑ with D and flow toward probe]	↑↑ with D and flow away from the probe	Confirmation of existence of ACoA
	Indistinguishable from contralateral ACA	0 or ↑ or ↑↑	[↓↓] or [ ] or with D	See ACA
	Indistinguishable from ipsilateral ACA	See ACA	0 or ↑ or ↑↑	See ACA
PCA (P1)	Normal flow signal, flow toward probe	0 or ↑ or ↑↑	0 or ↑	Confirmation of vessel identity, presence or absence of potential posterior collateral pathway
PCA (P2)	Normal flow signal, flow away from probe	0 or ↑, or ↓↓ or [ ] if ICA supplied	0 or [↓]	Confirmation of vessel identity and type of PCA supply, differentiation of basilar and/or ICA blood supply
PCoA (transtemporal or transorbital)	No signal available. Indistinguishable from PCA or MCA branches without compression maneuvers. Alternating flow	In nonembryonal type: with D or ↑↑ with D. With flow toward probe in vicinity of PCA. With flow toward probe during transorbital insonation. In embryonal type: ↓ or ↓↓ or ↓↓ or ↓. 0 or ↑	No reactions thus far	Confirmation of existence of PCoA, differentiation of posterior and anterior collateral pathway, differentiation of basilar or ICA blood supply
DVA	Normal flow signal away from probe	0 or ↑	0 or ↑	Confirmation of existence of vessel
BA conclusive insonation	Normal flow signal away from probe	0 or ↑ or [↑↑]	0 or ↑ or [↑↑]	Confirmation of existence of posterior collateral pathway, differentiation from carotid vascular tree within large depths
ICA, C2-C4 segments of collateral siphon, (transorbital approach)	Normal flow toward probe, away from probe, or bidirectional	[ ] or ↓↓ and/or [↑↑ with D]*	0 or ↑	Exclusion of silent ICA occlusion, analysis of potential pathways
ICA-C1 (transtemporal approach)	Low-frequency flow toward probe. Indistinguishable from MCA (M1)	[ ] or ↓↓	0 or ↑	Analysis of potential collateral pathways, differentiation from MCA often possible

CCA, Common carotid artery; MCA, middle cerebral artery; ↓, slight decrease of flow velocity; ↓↓, strong decrease of flow velocity; [ ], very rare event; 0, no effect; ACA, anterior cerebral artery; ↓, reversal of flow toward or away from transducer; D, local distortion of blood flow due to relative stenosis; ↑, slight increase of flow velocity; ↑↑, strong increase of flow velocity; ACoA, anterior communicating artery; PCA, posterior cerebral artery; P1, precommunicating part of PCA; P2, postcommunicating part of PCA; ICA, internal carotid artery; ↓, alternating flow; DVA, distal vertebral artery; BA, basilar artery. This list reflects our present experience but may not be complete. It refers to findings in normal subjects.

*Due to jet of PCoA collateral channel, overlap of ↓ and ↑↑ signals is possible.

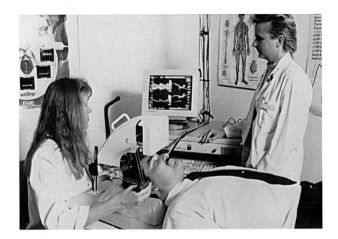

Fig. 12-15. Three-dimensional transcranial Doppler mapping in a normal volunteer using a headpiece with *x, y,* and *z* coordinates, which allow a three-dimensional reconstruction of the intracranial vessels. (Courtesy of Trans-Scan, Eden Medical Electronics, Überlingen, Germany.)

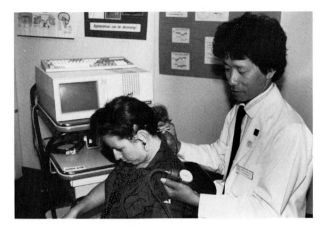

Fig. 12-17. Position of the probe and patient for the suboccipital monitoring of the vertebrobasilar arteries during hyperemic testing for subclavian steal syndrome.

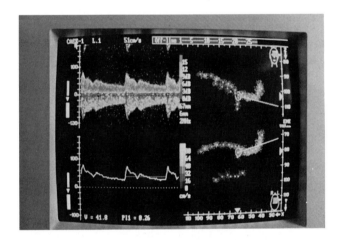

Fig. 12-16. Three-dimensional transcranial Doppler mapping of a normal volunteer, right temporal approach. The upper left quadrant displays the spectral waveform from the juncture of the anterior and middle cerebral arteries. The upper right quadrant shows the coronal image projection, and the bottom right quadrant is the horizontal image display.

circulation ipsilateral to the stenosis.[20,27,47] Increased velocities and turbulence in the collateral arteries are accentuated during compression of the CCA. A functional ACOA can be shown by reversal in flow direction in the proximal ACA ipsilateral to a significant stenosis. Increased velocity in the ACA contralateral to the stenosis in the ICA with reversal of the direction of flow in the ipsilateral ACA suggests collateral circulation from the contralateral ICA via the ACOA. Similar findings are shown in the PCA, revealing functional collateral flow from the posterior circulation via the PCOA. These findings have also been recorded in the BA in patients with severe bilateral carotid disease, with

collateral flow being supplied by both hemispheres from the posterior circulation. Correlation with angiography is basically good; however, angiography may not functionally show reversal of flow, depending on the pressure of injection of contrast material.[27] Many researchers believe that TCD may provide a much more accurate indication of functional collateral flow.

Evaluation of hemodynamic disturbances within the ICA-MCA pathway is of particular interest in patients with subtotal stenosis or occlusions of the ICA, both unilaterally and bilaterally. Although the main mechanism of stroke is thromboembolism rather than low flow, a small subgroup of patients do experience transient ischemic attacks, permanent stroke, or progressive ischemic eye disease because of critically reduced blood flow.[12,13,39,40]

Subclavian steal mechanism is the classic paradigm to study hemodynamic disturbance in the vertebrobasilar system in man. Rapid flow changes due to any kind of restriction of blood flow in the VA can be measured directly within the BA. Under resting conditions, blood flow within the BA is rarely critically impaired, even if the steal is continuous. However, if the contralateral feeding VA is also diseased, blood flow in the BA may become reduced. During hyperemia testing of the stealing arm, velocity and direction of flow within the basilar trunk may become less or more affected (Figs. 12-17 and 12-18). Essentially, subclavian steal is a benign condition; even in patients with symptoms, most vertebrobasilar symptoms are caused by cerebral microangiopathy rather than flow disturbance.[36] Blood flow in the BA is extremely resistant to any critical changes due to subclavian steal mechanism. In rare cases, however, TCD has convincingly identified individuals for beneficial recanalizations.

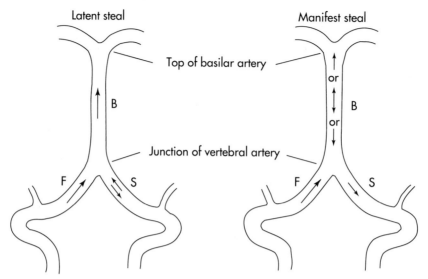

Subclavian steal mechanism

Latent steal

Manifest steal

Top of basilar artery

B

or

or

B

Junction of vertebral artery

F   S

F   S

F = Contralateral feeding VA   S = Homolateral stealing VA   B = Basilar trunk

Fig. 12-18. Schematic drawing of the flow conditions in the various vertebrobasilar vessel segments in patients with subclavian steal mechanism. With latent steal, flow in the feeding vertebral artery *(F)* is increased during brachial hyperemia and is normal in the basilar trunk *(B)*. By contrast, the blood column shows an alternating flow direction in the stealing vertebral artery *(S)*. During manifest steal, blood flow in S is continuously reversed. This leads to unaffected, alternating, or reversed blood flow within the basilar trunk. During transcranial Doppler sonography, each of the three vessel segments can be differentiated clearly by means of the segment's characteristic flow changes during brachial hyperemia. (From Ringelstein EB: *A practical guide to transcranial Doppler sonography.* In Weinberger J, editor: *Noninvasive assessment of the cerebral circulation in cerebrovascular disease,* New York, 1988, Alan R Liss.)

PITFALLS IN TRANSCRANIAL DOPPLER EXAMINATIONS

The principles of Doppler technique are equally applicable to the intracranial and extracranial cerebral arteries; however, because the examiner is not able to image these arteries, specific limitations are inherent. Transcranial Doppler ultrasonography is strongly dependent on the examiner, who must thoroughly understand anatomic landmarks and have the ability to visualize in three dimensions. The examiner must also possess the technical skills to optimize the position and angle of the probe so that the arterial signals from different parts of the circle of Willis can be properly identified. Because this identification is primarily based on anatomic knowledge and sample volume position, variation in the normative data and anatomy must be understood. As a result of these variabilities and the complexity of the vessels that comprise the circle of Willis, TCD ultrasonography is subject to unique problems of vessel indentification and documentation.

Other difficulties exist as well. Without imaging, the probe-to-vessel angle is impossible to determine. Sample volume-to-vessel size is relatively large, and congenital anomalies and tortuosity of the basal cerebral vessels are extensive. These technical problems may lead to misinterpretation and confusion. Collateral flow acceleration in the communicating arteries may be confused with stenosis. The PCA and ACA may be small, congenitally absent, or stenotic. Displacements of the basal arteries caused by mass lesions may easily lead to the misdiagnosis of occlusion. Additional physical limitations of ultrasound absorption and reflection—skull thickness, availability of adequate bony windows—further complicate diagnosis. Methodologic errors may also result with failure to detect low-grade stenosis and lesions in distal vessel branches. Common sources of error and trouble spots are listed in the box.

Many of these problems have been alleviated with newer instrumentation and increasing experience. Yet little information is available on the sensitivity and specificity of TCD ultrasonography. A major problem has involved the marked variation in its sensitivity and specificity from one arterial segment to another. Accuracy parameters have to be calculated separately for the

---

Common sources of error and trouble spots

Anatomic

Variations and incomplete circle of Willis
Missing or hypotrophic anterior cerebral artery
Posterior cerebral artery stemming directly from the internal carotid artery
Atretic vertebral artery

Technical

Absent temporal windows
Not identifying the best temporal window
Small temporal window
Too transparent a temporal window

Instrumentation

Large sample volume
Exceeds Nyquist limits
Improper use and adjustment of gain control
Unknown Doppler angle

Interpretive errors

Misinterpretation of hyperdynamic collateral channels as stenosis
Displacement of arteries caused by space-occupying lesions
Misdiagnosis of vasospasm as stenosis
Poor gold standard of angiography

---

carotid siphon; the various segments in the MCA, ACA, and PCA; and, in particular, the VA and BA. In spite of these problems, TCD ultrasonography has emerged as an important new diagnostic tool.[31] For further, more detailed discussion see Otis, 1993.[31]

CONCLUSION

The tremendous potential of TCD is becoming more apparent as more and more investigators from different backgrounds are reporting on its uses in different clinical settings. Because of its noninvasive characteristics and excellent time resolution, detailed and repeated investigations of intracranial cerebral blood flow can be monitored.

Like other freehand ultrasound examinations, TCD is operator-dependent, and the new examiner is dependent on a learning curve before becoming proficient. Many of the pitfalls of this technique can potentially be overcome with the new advances now enabling clinicians to penetrate the available ultrasound window and skull foramen with B-mode imaging. This represents a major breakthrough in intracranial arterial diagnosis and allows a combination of the anatomic imaging information and Doppler physiologic flow information. This duplex color system promises to have the same dramatic effect on intracranial vessel identification and diagnosis

as it has in the extracranial carotid examination and is discussed in Chapter 19.

REFERENCES

1. Aaslid R: *Transcranial Doppler flow mapping,* Proceedings of Ultrasound Diagnosis of Cerebrovascular Disease Symposium, Seattle, May 1985.
2. Aaslid R: *Transcranial Doppler sonography,* Vienna and New York, 1986, Springer-Verlag.
3. Aaslid R: Visually evoked dynamic blood flow response of the human cerebral circulation, *Stroke* 18:771-775, 1987.
4. Aaslid R: *Five years of TCD: look back. Two years of TCD scanning: Look forward.* Paper presented at International Workshop on 3-D Transcranial Doppler Scanning, Bonn, November 1987.
5. Aaslid R, Huber P, Nornes H: Evaluation of cerebrovascular spasm with transcranial Doppler ultrasound, *J Neurosurg* 60:37-41, 1984.
6. Aaslid R, Markwalder TM, Nornes H: Noninvasive transcranial Doppler ultrasound recording of flow velocity in basal cerebral arteries, *J Neurosurg* 57:769-774, 1982.
7. Arnolds B, von Reutern GM: Transcranial Doppler sonography: examination technique and normal reference values, *Ultrasound Med Biol* 12:115, 1986.
8. Becker G, Greiner K, Kaune B, et al: Diagnosis and monitoring of subarachnoid hemorrhage by transcranial color-coded real-time sonography, *Neurosurgery* 28:814-820, 1991.
9. Becker G, Perez J, Krone A, et al: Transcranial color-coded real-time sonography in the evaluation of intracranial neoplasms and arteriovenous malformations, *Neurosurgery* 31:420-428, 1992.
10. Biniek R, Ringelstein EB, Brückmann H, et al: Recanalization of acute middle cerebral artery occlusion monitored by transcranial Doppler sonography. In Hacke W, et al, editors: *Thrombolytic therapy in acute ischemic stroke,* Berlin, 1991, Springer-Verlag.
11. Bishop CFR, Powell S, Insall M, et al: The effect of internal carotid artery occlusion on middle cerebral artery blood flow at rest and response to hypercapnia, *Lancet* 1:710-712, 1986.
12. Bogdahn U, Becker G, Winkler J, et al: Transcranial color-coded real-time sonography in adults, *Stroke* 21:1680-1688, 1990.
13. Caplan LR, Sergay S: Positional cerebral ischemia, *J Neurol Neurosurg Psychiatry* 39:385-391, 1976.
14. Carter JE: Chronic ocular ischemia and carotid vascular disease, *Stroke* 16:721-728, 1985.
15. DeWitt LD, Wechsler H: Transcranial Doppler, *Stroke* 19:915-921, 1988.
16. Edelmann M, Ringelstein EB, Richert F: Transcranial Doppler sonography for monitoring of the middle cerebral blood flow velocity during carotid endarterectomy, *Rev Bras de Angiol e Clint Vasc* 16:96-100, 1986.
17. Frackowiak RSJ, Lenzi GL, Jones T: Quantitative measurements of cerebral blood flow and oxygen metabolism in man using 15-oxygen and positron emission tomography. Theory, procedure and normal values, *J Comput Assist Tomogr* 4:727-732, 1980.
18. Grolimund P: *Transmission of ultrasound through the temporal bone.* In Aaslid R, editor: *Transcranial Doppler sonography,* Vienna and New York, 1986, Springer-Verlag.
19. Harders A: *Monitoring of hemodynamic changes related to vasospasm in the circle of Willis after aneurysm surgery.* In Aaslid R, editor: *Transcranial Doppler sonography,* Vienna and New York, 1986, Springer-Verlag.
20. Harders A: *Neurosurgical applications of transcranial Doppler sonography,* Vienna and New York, 1986, Springer-Verlag.
21. Hennerici M, Rautenberg W, Schwartz A: Transcranial Doppler ultrasound for the assessment of intracranial arterial flow velocity, part II, *Surg Neurol* 27:523-532, 1987.
22. Hennerici M, Rautenberg W, Sitzer G, et al: Transcranial Doppler ultrasound for the assessment of intracranial arterial flow velocity,

part I: examination technique and normal values, *Surg Neurol* 27:439-448, 1987.

23. Katz ML, Smalley KJ, Comerota AJ: Transcranial Doppler: prospective evaluation of hand-held vs. mapping technique, *J Vasc Surg* 14:69-71, 1990.

24. Kennedy C, Sokoloff L: An adaptation of the nitrous oxide method to the study of the cerebral circulation in children: normal values for cerebral blood flow and cerebral metabolic rate in childhood, *J Clin Invest* 36:1130-1135, 1957.

25. Kety SS: Human cerebral blood flow and oxygen consumption as related to aging, *J Chronic Dis* 3:478-486, 1956.

26. Kety SS, Schmidt CF: The effects of altered tensions of carbon dioxide and oxygen on cerebral blood flow and oxygen consumption of normal young men, *J Clin Invest* 27:484-492, 1948.

27. Ley-Pozo J, Ringelstein EB: Noninvasive detection of occlusive disease of the carotid siphon and middle cerebral artery, *Ann Neurol* 28:758-765, 1990.

28. Lindegaard R, Bakke SJ, Grolimund P: Assessment of intracranial hemodynamics in carotid artery disease by transcranial Doppler ultrasound, *J Neurosurg* 63:890-898, 1985.

29. Lundar T, Lindegaard K, Froysaker T: Cerebral perfusion during nonpulsatile cardiopulmonary bypass, *Ann Thorac Surg* 40:144-150, 1985.

30. Lundar T, Lindegaard K, Froysaker T: Cerebral carbon dioxide reactivity during nonpulsatile cardiopulmonary bypass, *Ann Thorac Surg* 41:525-536, 1986.

31. Miyazaki M, Kato K: Measurement of cerebral blood flow by ultrasonic Doppler technique, *Jpn Circ J* 29:375-379, 1965.

32. Otis SM: *Pitfalls in transcranial Doppler diagnosis.* In Babikian VL, Wechsler LR, editors: *Transcranial Doppler ultrasonography,* St Louis, 1993, Mosby–Year Book.

33. Padayachee TS, Kirkham FJ, Lewis RR, et al: Transcranial measurement of blood velocities in the basal cerebral arteries using pulsed Doppler ultrasound: a method of assessing the circle of Willis, *Ultrasound Med Biol* 12:5-14, 1986.

34. Ries F: *Three-dimensional transcranial Doppler scanning.* In Bernstein EF, editor: *Recent advances in noninvasive diagnostic techniques in vascular disease,* St Louis, 1990, Mosby–Year Book.

35. Ries F, Solymosi L, Horn R, et al: Evaluation of the hemodynamic effect of extra- and intracranial cerebrovascular lesions by 3-D transcranial Doppler scanning, *J Cardiovasc Ultrasonogr* 7:78, 1988.

36. Ringelstein EB: *Transcranial Doppler monitoring.* In Aaslid R, editor: *Transcranial Doppler sonography,* New York, 1986, Springer-Verlag.

37. Ringelstein EB: *A practical guide to transcranial Doppler sonography.* In Weinberger J, editor: *Noninvasive imaging of cerebral vascular disease,* New York, 1989, AR Liss.

38. Ringelstein EB, Kahlscheuer B, Niggemeyer E, et al: Transcranial Doppler sonography: anatomical landmarks and normal velocity values, *Ultrasound Med Biol* 16:745-761, 1990.

39. Ringelstein EB, Sievers C, Ecker S, et al: Noninvasive assessment of CO_2-induced cerebral vasomotor response in normal individuals and patients with internal carotid artery occlusions, *Stroke* 19:963-969, 1988.

40. Ringelstein EB, Zeumer H, Angelou D: The pathogenesis of strokes from internal carotid artery occlusion: diagnostic and therapeutical implications, *Stroke* 14:867-875, 1983.

41. Ringelstein EB, Zeumer H, Korbmacher G, et al: Transkranielle Dopplersonographie der hirnversorgenden Arterien: atraumatische Diagnostik von Stenosen und Verschluessen des Carotissiphons und der A. cerebri media, *Nervenarzt* 56:296-306, 1985.

42. Russo G, Profeta G, Acampora S, et al: Transcranial Doppler ultrasound. Examination technique and normal reference values, *J Neurosurg Sci* 30:97, 1986.

43. Schöning M, Buchholz R, Walter J: Comparative study of transcranial color duplex sonography and transcranial Doppler sonography in adults, *J Neurosurg* 78:776-784, 1993.

44. Silverstein A, Doniger D, Bender MB: Manual compression of the carotid vessels, carotid sinus hypersensitivity, and carotid artery occlusions, *Ann Intern Med* 52:172, 1960.

45. Spencer MP, Whisler D: Transorbital Doppler diagnosis of intracranial arterial stenosis, *Stroke* 17:916-921, 1986.

46. Webster JE, Gurdjian FJ: Observation upon response to digital carotid artery compression, *Neurology* 7:757, 1957.

47. Wechsler LR, Sekhar LN, Luyckx K, et al: The effects of endarterectomy on the intracranial circulation studied by transcranial Doppler, *Neurology* 37 (suppl I3):317, 1987.

48. White DN, Curry GR, Stevenson RJ: The acoustic characteristics of the skull, *Ultrasound Med Biol* 4:225-252, 1978.

13

Transcranial Doppler Indices of Intracranial Hemodynamics

Maura Bragoni
Edward Feldmann

The basic features of intracranial hemodynamics measured by transcranial Doppler ultrasound (TCD) are the velocity and direction of blood flow. The TCD blood flow velocity data can also be employed to calculate unique indices that enhance our understanding of normal and abnormal cerebrovascular physiology. These indices may be measured directly by TCD equipment and its software or calculated by hand from primary data collected by the instrument. The indices discussed in this chapter are listed in Table 13-1.

Ultrasonographers may routinely apply several of these indices to the evaluation of patients with common cerebrovascular disorders. For example, the hemispheric index (VMCA/VICA) is helpful in discriminating vasospasm from hyperemia in patients who have had subarachnoid hemorrhage. Pulsatility index (PI) and flow acceleration (FA) can indirectly assess the severity of extracranial internal carotid artery (ICA) stenosis.

Many more applications of these indices remain under active investigation. For example, the resistance index (RI) provides indirect information about intracranial pressure (ICP). The PI and RI have been applied to cerebral perfusion pressure (CPP) monitoring, hydrocephalus monitoring in children and neonates,[25] and the study of head trauma and brain death. The PI may be

able to distinguish different forms of migraine headache.[60,61]

This chapter defines the indices under study, explores how systemic endogenous and exogenous factors affect their measurement, and illustrates normal and pathologic values of the indices for various neurologic disorders.

DEFINITIONS

Because most TCD indices are based on velocity measurements, the various intracranial blood flow velocities must first be defined. Two basic velocity measurements made by TCD are illustrated in Figure 13-1. The peak systolic flow velocity (PV) is defined as the maximum value of flow velocity in systole, at the apex of the waveform. The end-diastolic flow velocity (EDV) is defined as the velocity measured at end diastole, usually at the lowest point before a new waveform begins.

The mean flow velocity (MV) may be measured either by the TCD equipment software or by hand. The internal software of the TCD device calculates the MV as the average of the edge frequency over a cardiac cycle; the edge frequency is the envelope of instantaneous peak velocities throughout the course of a cardiac cycle. One method of hand measurement (Fig. 13-2) results in an

Table 13-1. Transcranial Doppler indices

Index	Meaning	Source
PI	Pulsatility index	Gosling, King, 1974
PTI	Pulsatility transmission index	Lindegaard et al, 1985
RI	Resistance index	Pourcelot, 1976
FA	Flow acceleration	Kelley et al, 1990
D-MCA	Delta-middle cerebral artery: side-to-side MCA velocity difference	Babikian et al, 1989
VMCA/VICA	MCA/ICA velocity ratio (hemispheric index)	Lindegaard, et al, 1989
VMCA/VACA	MCA/ACA velocity ratio	Adams, et al, 1992
ACAVR	ACA velocity ratio: ACA velocity ipsilateral to MCA stenosis divided by contralateral ACA velocity	Brass et al, 1989

ICA, Internal carotid artery; *MCA*, middle cerebral artery; *ACA*, anterior cerebral artery.

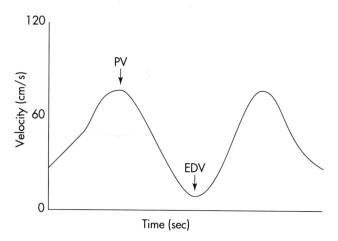

Fig. 13-1. Transcranial Doppler tracing of middle cerebral artery velocity over two cardiac cycles. (*PV*, peak systolic flow velocity; *EDV*, end-diastolic flow velocity.)

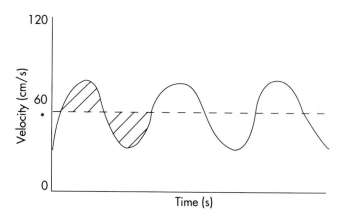

Fig. 13-2. Transcranial Doppler tracing of middle cerebral artery velocity over three cardiac cycles. The mean velocity (MV) may be estimated by drawing an horizontal line that divides the area under the velocity curve of one cardiac cycle above and below the horizontal line into two approximately equal parts. Asterisk represents the intersection of this line on the ordinate, an estimate of mean velocity.

MV approximating that calculated by the internal software.[1,19] It may also be calculated as follows:

$$MV = (PV + 2EDV) / 3$$

Pulsatility index

The pulsatility index (PI) describes the shape of the waveforms as displayed by TCD equipment. Gosling and King first described a formula to calculate PI:[26]

$$PI = PV - EDV / MV$$

A rounded waveform has a lower PI, whereas a more peaked waveform has a higher PI,[22] as shown in Figure 13-3.

The pulsatility index is believed to represent an estimate of downstream vascular resistance. Low-resistance vascular beds have higher diastolic flow velocities than high-resistance vascular beds.[34] Thus, low-resistance vascular beds have low PI, whereas high-resistance beds have high PI.[36]

The low pulsatility of the cerebral vasculature reflects the brain's unique metabolic needs. The brain requires continuous blood flow throughout the cardiac cycle. This is physiologically accomplished by high diastolic flow associated with low downstream resistance and, consequently, low pulsatility. Consider the ophthalmic (OA) and internal carotid artery (ICA) siphon waveforms. The OA waveform is characterized by a low diastolic flow velocity and high downstream resistance, with a high PI (Fig. 13-4, *A*). In contrast, the ICA siphon waveform is characterized by comparatively high diastolic flow velocity with low downstream resistance, resulting in a low PI (Fig. 13-4, *B*).

Pulsatility transmission index

The pulsatility transmission index (PTI) was invented in order to avoid the great individual variations in PI due to systemic cardiovascular factors such as heart rate, blood pressure, aortic abnormalities, vascular compliance and arterial PCO_2 levels. It is calculated with the following formula[37]:

$$PTI = PI \text{ (study vessel)} / PI \text{ (reference vessel)} \times 100\%$$

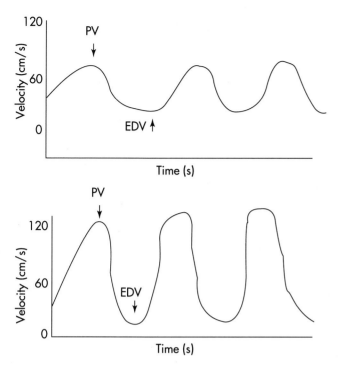

Fig. 13-3. Two different transcranial Doppler tracings of middle cerebral artery velocity. **A,** A more rounded waveform with a relatively low pulsatility index. **B,** A more peaked waveform with a higher pulsatility index. (*PV,* Peak systolic flow velocity; *EDV,* end-diastolic flow velocity.)

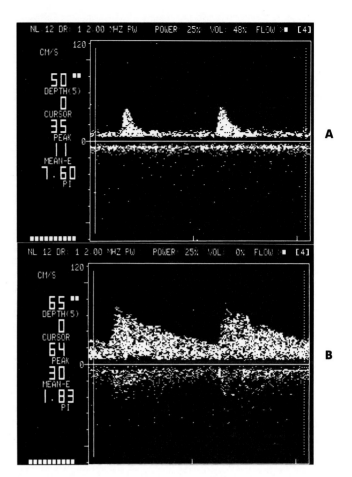

Fig. 13-4. **A,** Transcranial Doppler (TDC) waveform of an ophthalmic artery, characterized by a higher pulsatility index (PI) **B,** TCD waveform of a carotid siphon, characterized by a lower PI.

Thus, the PI of the study vessel is normalized with respect to a presumably unremarkable reference vessel. Unfortunately, this index contains a potential source of error because the assumption that the pulsatility of the reference intracranial artery is normal is not readily demonstrable and may not be correct.[33]

Resistance index

Resistance index (RI), first introduced by Pourcelot,[48] is another presumptive measure of downstream vascular resistance. It is calculated with the following formula:

$$RI = PV - EDV / PV$$

Like PI, increased RI is believed to reflect increased downstream vascular resistance. For example, patients with raised intracranial pressure harbor increased resistance to blood flow.[25] These patients exhibit reduced diastolic flow velocities and increased RI on TCD.

Flow acceleration

Flow acceleration (FA) is the inclination or slope of the systolic upstroke of the waveform (Fig. 13-5). The following formula is used to calculate FA:

$$FA = PV - EDV / \text{time differential}$$

A low middle cerebral artery (MCA) FA is found in conditions associated with increased upstream resistance, such as severe proximal ICA stenosis or aortic stenosis.[33,50]

Delta middle cerebral artery

Side-to-side MCA flow velocity difference, or delta-MCA (D-MCA), is calculated as the difference between the MCA peak systolic flow velocity ipsilateral to an extracranial ICA stenosis and the contralateral MCA peak systolic flow velocity[8]:

$$D - MCA = MCAPV \text{ (ipsilateral to ICA stenosis)} - \\ MCAPV \text{ (contralateral to ICA stenosis)}$$

The absolute value of D-MCA increases when there is a severe proximal stenosis in one internal carotid artery.[8,14] The physiologic explanation is that a lower volume of blood flow reaches the middle cerebral artery ipsilateral to ICA stenosis. Because MCA velocity depends on both MCA diameter and flow volume, a lower flow volume will result in a lower MCA velocity if MCA diameter remains constant.

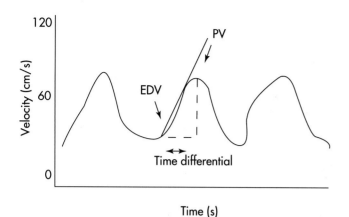

Fig. 13-5. Transcranial Doppler tracing over three cardiac cycles. Flow acceleration is calculated by the following formula: $FA = (PV - EDV) / time\ differential$. (*FA,* Flow acceleration; *PV,* peak systolic flow velocity; *EDV,* end-diastolic flow velocity.)

Hemispheric index

The middle cerebral artery–internal carotid artery flow velocity ratio (VMCA/VICA), the so-called hemispheric index or Lindegaard index,[40] distinguishes vasospasm from states of systemic hyperemia. To calculate this index, the ICA blood flow velocity must be measured from the neck, below the angle of mandible. A 2-MHz pulsed-wave Doppler probe is aimed cranially, insonating at a depth of 40 to 50 mm, in order to achieve a small angle of insonation between the ultrasound beam and the distal extracranial portion of the ICA.

Physicians caring for patients with subarachnoid hemorrhage must commonly distinguish between states of systemic hyperemia and cerebral vasospasm, both of which are associated with elevated MCA velocities. These patients are often treated with hypervolemic therapy and also undergo frequent venipuncture, resulting in increased cerebral blood volume and decreased hematocrit, respectively. These situations represent systemic hyperdynamic states, and both VMCA and VICA will increase, but their ratio remains unchanged. In contrast, patients with vasospasm show an increased MCA velocity out of proportion to any increased ICA velocity, resulting in an increased VMCA/VICA ratio.[5]

Arterial velocities ratio

The MCA/anterior cerebral artery (ACA) velocity ratio (VMCA/VACA) is utilized in the study of MCA territory infarcts.[5] The MCA velocity is physiologically higher than the ACA velocity.[58] Thus the normal MCA/ACA velocity ratio is greater than 1.2. An increased ACA velocity with a lower ratio has been observed in patients with MCA territory infarction due to occlusion of an MCA branch vessel.[42] The relatively high ACA velocity suggests the presence of compensa-tory collateral flow via leptomeningeal channels from the ACA to the MCA territory.[10]

The side-to-side ACA velocity ratio (ACAVR) is calculated as the ACA velocity ipsilateral to MCA stenosis divided by the ACA velocity contralateral to MCA stenosis (ACAVx/ACAVref).[10] This index increases with ipsilateral MCA stenosis or occlusion, presumably because of high ACA velocities associated with collateral flow via leptomeningeal collaterals to the underperfused MCA territory downstream from the MCA stenosis.[10]

PHYSIOLOGIC DETERMINANTS OF BLOOD FLOW VELOCITY AND INDICES

The indices previously defined are calculated by using blood flow velocity measurements. The velocity of cerebral blood flow is influenced by numerous systemic and technical factors that must be assessed for proper interpretation of TCD. The effect of these factors on TCD indices of intracranial hemodynamics is unpredictable, however; the indices are derived from velocity differences and ratios that may not be affected by changes in velocities. There are few published data detailing the effect of systemic factors on TCD indices of intracranial hemodynamics.

Age

Cerebral blood flow velocity decreases with age.[6,27,35] Several explanations have been offered, including reduced cerebral blood flow (CBF),[5,57] increased vascular resistance downstream from insonated vessels, and decreased vascular compliance.[2] The effect of age on PI and RI is controversial. According to some authors, older patients show both increased PI and RI;[2,63] others found no such relationship.[59] For the other indices, no data on age effects are available.

Gender

Cerebral blood flow velocity has been reported to be 3% to 5% higher in females than in males.[5] This difference may be due to the capacity of estrogen to lower vascular resistance, resulting in an increased blood flow velocity.[53] Women and men over age 50 do not show any difference in CBF velocity, PI, or RI,[2] indirectly implicating an effect by estrogen that presumably abates with menopause. Further data related to estrogens is presented in the Medication section later in this chapter.

Vessel diameter

There is an inverse relationship between blood flow velocity and vessel diameter in the presence of constant cerebral blood volume (CBV). Wide interindividual variability in vessel diameter has been described in normal subjects.[17,54] This may explain the wide range of velocity values recorded in the basal cerebral arteries in normal subjects.[39]

Blood pressure

Increases in PV and PI have been described in the carotid arteries of patients with increased blood pressure.[67] Increased blood pressure is associated with a more marked increased in systolic flow velocity than diastolic flow velocity, explaining the increased pulsatility. The mechanism is not clear. Blood pressure increases may cause cerebral artery constriction and an associated increased blood flow velocity, as suggested by Lindegaard and colleagues, who described MCA vasoconstriction with incremental changes in blood pressure in patients undergoing carotid endarterectomy.[39]

Blood pressure variations, as well as ICP B waves,[23,43] are believed to cause variation in TCD velocities in normal subjects and in neurosurgical patients. To detect these velocity variations, which may be as large as 40% in neurosurgical patients and 20% in normal subjects, TCD monitoring of a single location in a single vessel for at least 3 to 5 minutes is necessary.[23]

In our practice, we do not monitor every location in each vessel for this length of time, but we report the highest mean velocity value recorded. We believe this practice is useful in repetitive studies, such as in patients with vasospasm after subarachnoid hemorrhage (SAH), where comparison of serial velocity values is clinically important.

Cardiac physiology

The dependence of cerebral blood flow velocity on cardiac output is not completely understood. Variability in intracranial velocity values has been described in normal subjects in association with different degrees of physical exercise. The MCA velocity increases after mild to moderate physical exercise but decreases after vigorous exercise, even in the presence of increasing blood pressure and heart rate. The MCA velocity increase observed with moderate exercise is believed to be due to an initial blood pressure and heart rate increase; the drop in MCA velocity with vigorous exercise is believed to follow the ensuing vasoconstriction of cerebral resistance vessels secondary to hyperventilation, also resulting in an increase in PI.[29]

The effect of heart rate on PI is unpredictable. Some authors found that a decreased heart rate was associated with an increased PI;[5,37,59] others found that an increased heart rate was associated with an increased PI.[67]

An increased PI has been described in patients with either aortic valve incompetence or diminished cardiac output.[5] Both situations are characterized by an almost absent diastolic flow compared to flow during systolic ejection.[67]

A decreased FA has been described in patients with aortic stenosis and other causes of myocardial dysfunction.[68] In aortic stenosis, FA decreases because of the prolonged time required to complete left ventricular systolic ejection.[50]

Cerebral blood volume

In patients with arteriovenous malformations (AVMs), an increased cerebral blood volume (CBV) in the vascular malformation is associated with increased velocity values recorded in feeding arteries, despite their enlarged diameter.[38] The PI values are decreased in AVM feeding vessels because of their typically low vascular resistance.[38] The literature provides no data describing the effects of CBV on other TCD indices of intracranial hemodynamics.

Hematocrit

Hematocrit (Hct) and cerebral blood flow velocity are inversely proportional[6]; CBF measurements and Hct have a similar relationship.[12] Increased velocities have been recorded in patients with sickle cell anemia, whereas decreased CBF and velocities have been recorded in patients with polycythemia.[5,6,13]

Interpretation of such changes in intracranial velocities may be complicated by the presence of associated disorders. For example, elevated velocities in sickle cell anemia cannot be assumed to be due to anemia, as intracranial occlusive disease occurs in these patients. An MCA velocity greater than 170 cm/s in sickle cell anemia is considered a sign of MCA stenosis and is believed to be a risk factor for stroke.[3,4]

Fibrinogen

Fibrinogen levels and cerebral blood flow velocity are also inversely proportional.[6] Increased fibrinogen levels have been associated with increased plasma viscosity. High viscosities are associated with high resistance and low velocities.[6] One would hypothesize that PI and RI would be affected by the changes in vascular resistance associated with variations in fibrinogen and hematocrit, but little data exist to support this theory.[12]

Carbon dioxide

Transcranial Doppler recordings are made proximal to the brain's resistance vessels. Consequently, when Pco_2 increases, vasodilatation of resistance vessels results in increased CBF and increased velocities recorded in the proximal basal cerebral arteries.[9] When Pco_2 decreases, vasoconstriction of resistance vessels results in decreased CBF and decreased velocities recorded in the proximal basal cerebral arteries.[17,51] The integrity of cerebral autoregulatory vascular capacity may be tested through the CO_2 response. The role of carbon dioxide in TCD evaluation is detailed in Chapter 14 of this book.

As a consequence of these changes in vascular resistance in response to Pco_2 changes, an inverse correlation between Pco_2 and PI is found, both in normal subjects[31] and in patients undergoing anesthesia.[62] Data on other indices are lacking.

Medications

Blood flow velocity may also be influenced by drugs. A decreased MCA velocity and an increased PI have been observed with thiopentone administration.[62] This phenomenon has been referred to as *vasoconstrictor barbiturate capacity,* with resistance vessel constriction resulting in lower upstream velocities and higher PI, much like the response to hypocapnia. Low doses of halothane, isuflurane, and enflurane produce no velocity changes from that in the awake state. By contrast, high doses of each drug produce variable changes. A marked increase in velocity was observed in the normoventilating group given high doses of halothane; in the high-dose isoflurane and enflurane groups, only a slightly increased velocity was recorded.[62]

A decreased blood flow velocity has been associated with calcium antagonists such as nimodipine, used for vasospasm after subarachnoid hemorrhage,[56] or nifedipine, used in systemic hypertension.[18] Presumably, the drugs dilate basal cerebral arteries, lowering blood flow velocity.

Nitroglycerin, a vasodilating agent, has been tested in normal subjects and in patients affected by migraine without aura. The migraine patients showed a greater decrease in mean and peak systolic MCA velocities than the control group. A decreased PI was observed only in the migraine group. No changes in blood pressure or heart rate were seen. According to the authors, these changes were consistent with a more marked MCA vasodilatory effect by the drug in the migraine patients.[66]

A complex relationship exists between estrogen level and PI. During menopause, an increased PI has been observed, presumably due to a low level of estrogen. The PI normalizes after estrogen replacement in these postmenopausal women.[20] These findings are consistent with a direct effect of estrogen on intracranial resistance vessels. An increase in middle cerebral artery peak systolic velocity has been observed during estrogen therapy in catamenial migraine patients.[11] Also, an increased FA has been found in postmenopausal women after estrogen replacement therapy.[47] The authors speculated that the increased FA represented a positive inotropic effect of the estrogen.

Insonation angle and examiner variability

Cerebral blood flow velocity measured by transcranial Doppler depends on insonation angle,[17,41] as demonstrated by the Doppler equation[65]:

$$F_D = 2F_0 V \cos \emptyset / c$$

where F_D is the Doppler shift frequency, F_0 is the emitted Doppler frequency, V is the velocity of the blood in the vessel, c is the sound propagation speed, and $\emptyset$ is the Doppler angle. When the angle between the ultrasound beam and the vessel is 0°, the cosine will be

1 and the recorded velocity will be the actual velocity of the blood. When the angle between the ultrasound beam and the vessel is 90°, the cosine will be 0 and the recorded velocity will be 0. At insonation angles between 0° and 90°, recorded velocities will underestimate true velocities and should be angle corrected, if possible.

The PI is not influenced by insonation angle[26] because PI represents a ratio of three velocities, all measured at the same insonation angle. One would hypothesize that other indices employing multiple velocities in their formulae are similarly independent of insonation angle.

The skill of the examiner and an adequate window of insonation are essential to optimal TCD testing. In the presence of a tiny window, the study may be difficult to perform,[41] and follow-up results will be variable. In the presence of an inadequate window, the intensity of the signal may be so poor that it is impossible to measure PV and EDV reliably. Consequently, it will be difficult to calculate indices. Higher power output capabilities on newer equipment may help to avoid this problem.

NORMAL AND PATHOLOGIC VALUES
Pulsatility index

Normal values for PI and PTI have been reported in several studies[30,38,59] (Table 13-2). A pathologic increase in PI has been found in association with increased ICP[24,28,31] and decreased CPP. In increased ICP, both systolic and diastolic flow velocity are decreased,[15] but the latter more than the former, producing a marked increased in PI.[16,31]

A clinical role for serial PI measurements has been proposed in hydrocephalic children developing increased ICP. Changes in PI may help define the optimal time for shunting. Lower flow velocities and higher PI are found in hydrocephalus with higher ICP.[44] A precise cutoff value of PI determining the need to shunt has not yet been established. However, hydrocephalic children with clinical signs of increased ICP have a mean PI of 1.72, compared to a mean PI of 1.06 in hydrocephalic children without clinical signs of increased ICP. After shunting in the former group, PI decreases to values found in patients without clinical signs of increased ICP.[44]

The use of PI monitoring in patients with hydrocephalus and intracranial hypertension varies across institutions, as does the use of any of the indices discussed in this chapter. A paucity of prospective data, as well as the management philosophy of neurosurgeons, limits the role of PI monitoring in patients with ICP elevation in our institution to isolated cases where a neurosurgeon experienced with TCD seeks to add noninvasive laboratory support to the decision-making armamentarium. The use of PI monitoring in patients with increased ICP is clearly neither routine nor widespread.

In patients with presumptive brain death, an in-

Table 13-2. Normal values of PI and PTI
in intracranial and extracranial arteries

	PI (SD)	PTI (%)
MCA	0.54-0.89 (0.02)	93-107
ACA	0.84-0.88 (0.02)	NA
ICA	0.95-0.96 (0.02)	NA

PI, Pulsatility index; *PTI*, pulsatility transmission index; *MCA*, middle cerebral artery; *ACA*, anterior cerebral artery; *ICA*, extracranial internal carotid artery; *NA*, data not available; *SD*, standard deviation. Data from Hennerici M, Rautenberg W, Sitzer G, et al: Transcranial Doppler ultrasound for the assessment of intracranial arterial flow velocity, part 1: examination technique and normal values, *Surg Neurol* 27:439-448, 1987; Lindegaard KF, Grolimund P, Aaslid R, et al: Evaluation of cerebral AVMs using transcranial Doppler ultrasound, *J Neurosurg* 65:335-344, 1986; and Steinmeier R, Laumer R, Boudár G, et al: Cerebral hemodynamics in subarachnoid hemorrhage evaluated by transcranial Doppler sonography, part 2: pulsatility indices: normal reference values and characteristics in subarachnoid hemorrhage, *Neurosurgery* 33:10-19, 1993.

Table 13-3. Mean flow acceleration and pulsatility index versus angiographic internal carotid artery stenosis

Carotid angiography (% stenosis)	Flow acceleration mean value cm/s² (95% CI)	Pulsatility index mean value (95% CI)
<70%	380 (335, 425)	0.96 (0.91, 1.01)
≥70%	194 (155, 233)*	0.71 (0.63, 0.78)*

*Differs from number above, $p < 0.0001$.

creased PI together with a progressive decrease in diastolic flow velocity, reversal of blood flow in diastole and, ultimately, an almost absent systolic flow velocity have been described.[46] However, TCD patterns recorded during brain death are not 100% specific and must be used in conjunction with clinical and other laboratory markers of brain death. In our institution, the demonstration of absent CBF is not required for the diagnosis of brain death, which is a clinical diagnosis. However, in patients whose families and physicians are inexperienced with the concept of brain death, additional noninvasive data obtained by TCD may bolster confidence in this difficult diagnosis. In hospitals where a demonstration of poor cerebral perfusion is a required adjunct to clinical criteria for diagnosis, TCD may be routinely performed.[46] In no instance should the diagnosis of brain death be made with only TCD data, unsupported by rigorous satisfaction of clinical criteria. Increased PI and PTI, measured in a structurally normal ICA, have been associated with ipsilateral middle cerebral artery occlusion.[42]

Several authors have described a decreased PI in the MCA ipsilateral to a severe extracranial ICA stenosis, presumably because downstream dilatation of resistance vessels to improve CBF lowers vascular resistance.[7,37,55] Others could not confirm this finding.[33] Thus, changes in PI alone are not considered specific or sensitive for diagnosis of extracranial carotid stenosis.

However, PI may serve a useful role as part of a battery of TCD indices used to predict the angiographic severity of extracranial ICA stenosis identified by carotid duplex ultrasound. The TCD battery used in our laboratory consists of the following seven parameters: reversed flow in the ipsilateral ophthalmic artery, re-

versed flow in the ipsilateral anterior cerebral artery, elevated flow velocity (greater than 80 cm/s) in the contralateral anterior cerebral artery, absence of Doppler signal in the ipsilateral ophthalmic artery or carotid siphon, and diminished PI and FA in the ipsilateral middle cerebral artery. The presence of any one of these parameters makes the battery "positive." The TCD battery has a 95% sensitivity for identifying greater than 70% ICA stenosis as measured by the North American Symptomatic Carotid Endarterectomy Trial (NASCET) method on conventional angiography. Table 13-3 shows the correlation of PI and FA with ICA stenosis in 84 vessels studied angiographically. Thus, FA and PI, as part of a larger battery, help gauge the severity of ICA stenosis and predict the need for angiography.

A decreased PI has been described in feeding arteries of AVMs.[27,38,45] Simultaneous PI and mean flow velocity measurements have been employed during and after surgical resection of AVMs in order to detect incomplete obliteration of the feeding arteries. With removal of feeders, PI increases and mean flow velocity decreases in the upstream vessels. When new feeders are recruited, PI decreases and mean flow velocity increases to preoperative values, alerting the physician that further treatment is necessary.[32] Neurosurgeons in our institution do not use TCD to identify AVMs or gauge their response to surgical or radiation therapy.

Arteries exhibiting vasospasm secondary to subarachnoid hemorrhage are found to have a decreased PI. The decrement in PI is proportional to the degree of vasospasm.[22] In our practice, the diagnosis of vasospasm depends exclusively on velocity elevation, and PI changes are not routinely employed in diagnosis.

A decreased PI and an increased MV have been observed in the headache-free period of migraine patients, at rest.[60] Migraine patients and controls have also had posterior cerebral artery (PCA) monitoring performed during exposure to daylight and during eye closure. A marked decrease in MV and an increase in PI were recorded in the PCA during eye closure, compared to that in normal subjects. The authors hypothesized a greater vascular reactivity in migraine patients.[60]

Table 13-4. Normal values of resistance index in intracranial and extracranial arteries

Artery	Mean (SD)
Middle cerebral artery	0.56 (0.07)
Anterior cerebral artery	0.56 (0.07)
Extracranial internal carotid artery	0.58 (0.07)

Data from Steinmeier R, Laumer R, Boudár G, et al: Cerebral hemodynamics in subarachnoid hemorrhage evaluated by transcranial Doppler sonography, part 2: pulsatility indices: normal reference values and characteristics in subarachnoid hemorrhage, *Neurosurgery* 33:10-19, 1993.

Table 13-5. Delta-MCA in normal persons and patients with internal carotid artery stenosis

ICA angiographic residual lumen	Number of patients	D-MCA (SD) (cm/s)
Normal residual lumen	15	8.7 (5.9)
Stenosis; residual lumen >1 mm	16	16.4 (11.7)
Stenosis; residual lumen ≤1 mm	21	26.6 (25.4)
Occlusion; no residual lumen	14	38.7 (19.4)

D-MCA, Delta middle cerebral artery velocity; *ICA*, extracranial internal carotid artery; *SD*, standard deviation.
Data from Cantelmo NL, Babikian VL, Johnson WE, et al: Correlation of transcranial Doppler and noninvasive tests with angiography in the evaluation of extracranial carotid disease, *J Vasc Surg* 11:786-792, 1990.

Distinguishing migraine with aura and migraine without aura cannot be reliably performed by TCD during the headache-free period but may be possible during headache,[61] when migraine with aura is associated with a decreased PI and increased MV, while migraine without aura is associated with increased PI and decreased MV.[61] Distinguishing these two forms of migraine, however, remains a clinical rather than a TCD task. Perhaps TCD research in this field will help physicians predict which drugs are more likely to induce beneficial clinical responses in particular patients.

Resistance index

Normal RI values for cerebral arteries are presented in Table 13-4.[59] Pathologically elevated RI has been observed during increased ICP, suggesting increased resistance to flow.[25] Presumably, ICP has a greater influence on diastolic blood flow velocity, whereas systolic blood flow velocity is influenced more by systemic blood pressure.[31] Thus, increases in ICP would selectively decrease diastolic velocities more than systolic velocities and raise RI.

We and others have used RI to help diagnose vasospasm after subarachnoid hemorrhage. Patients with severe spasm and ischemia commonly develop secondary elevation in ICP. Increased ICP will elevate RI to values above 0.6. Ultimately, velocity values decrease in this situation, as perfusion of the swollen brain becomes progressively difficult. It is important to recognize that this decrement in velocities is not a sign of improved spasm. The ultrasonographer is alerted to this situation by detecting a high RI (greater than 0.6) in association with decreased cerebral artery velocities.[34] We interpret this finding as equivocal, as the increased RI may mask elevated intracranial velocities and make spasm hard to detect. Increased RI may also be a marker of brain death, a condition in which all resistance indices are increased.

Then again, patients with progressive vasospasm but normal ICP may have a diminished RI (less than 0.5). Presumably, as a compensatory response to maintain adequate CPP, arterioles distal to spastic vessels dilate and reduce RI.[34] It is this compensatory response that may prevent increased ICP in these patients.

Flow acceleration

Normal values for flow acceleration have not been published in large series of subjects. Kelley and colleagues found mean values of 592 ($\pm$200) cm/s^2 in 12 normal subjects.[33]

A decreased value of FA has been described in the MCA ipsilateral to a severe flow-limiting extracranial ICA stenosis. Values of 229 ($\pm$115) cm/s^2 have been reported in patients with 75% to 100% extracranial ICA stenosis.[33] The FA can be used as part of a battery of TCD indices to help predict the angiographic severity of an extracranial ICA stenosis, as discussed previously.

Delta middle cerebral artery

Delta-MCA has been employed as a marker of internal carotid artery stenosis, either in the extracranial segment or in the siphon. The D-MCA increases as ICA residual lumen decreases, as illustrated in Table 13-5. An overall accuracy of 65% was found for D-MCA in detecting severe carotid artery disease. However, a linear regression analysis found that such TCD measurements were not considered helpful in adding significant information to duplex scanning in the evaluation of carotid artery stenosis.[14]

Hemispheric index

Normal values of VMCA/VICA are illustrated in Table 13-6.[40] An increased index of at least 3 is consistent with angiographic vasospasm in the MCA in patients with subarachnoid hemorrhage.[40] Severe angiographic spasm has been associated with a ratio of at least 6.[40]

Weber and associates used the hemispheric index as a marker of vasospasm in severe head injury patients.[64] Unfortunately, only a few angiograms were performed in order to confirm the diagnosis of vasospasm. Serial measurement of the index has also been utilized in the follow-up of vasospasm patients treated with angioplasty, in order to distinguish between hyperemia and recurrent vasospasm.[21] The index remains normal in patients with cerebral hyperemia, where elevated velocities in both MCA and ICA occur.

We recommend use of this index in patients with SAH in whom "triple-H" (hypervolemia, hypertension, and hemodilution) therapy has been administered or in whom severe anemia or other potential causes of a systemic hyperdynamic state are present.

Arterial velocities ratio

The normal mean value of VMCA/VACA is 1.27 (0.12). This index may be applied to the study of middle cerebral artery territory infarction due to MCA branch occlusion.[5,27] A decreased MCA velocity together with an increased ipsilateral ACA velocity (so that the inverted ratio is greater than 1.2) have been recorded in these patients.

Normal values of the side-to-side ACA velocity ratio (ACAVR) are 1.04 (range 0.76 to 1.19).[10] An increased ACAVR of 1.34 (range 1.15 to 1.74) has been observed in middle cerebral artery stem occlusion or stenosis in patients whose ICA was normal.[10]

The arterial velocities ratios are markers of leptomeningeal collateral flow from ACA to MCA territory. Until such collateral flow is linked to improvements in outcome or the decision to administer thrombolytic therapy or is used to help evaluate the effect of thrombolysis in patients with MCA occlusive disease, we do not routinely use these ratios.

Table 13-6. Hemispheric index (VMCA/VICA): normal and pathologic values

	Normal mean (standard deviation)	Pathologic values
VMCA/VICA	1.76 (0.10)	>3

VMCA/VICA, Middle cerebral artery mean flow velocity/internal carotid artery mean flow velocity.
Data from Lindegaard KF, Nornes H, Bakke SJ, et al: Cerebral vasospasm diagnosis by means of angiography and blood velocity measurements, *Acta Neurochir* 100:12-24, 1989.

Table 13-7. Abnormalities in transcranial Doppler indices, by neurologic disease

Neurologic disease	Index increased	No change	Index decreased
Brain death	PI PTI RI		
Increased ICP	PI PTI RI		
Decreased CPP	PI PTI RI		
Arteries feeding territory of cerebral infarction			PI PTI
MCA territory infarct			VMCA/VACA
MCA stenosis or occlusion	ACAVR PI PTI (recorded in extracranial ICA)		
Vasospasm	VMCA/VICA	RI	RI PI PTI
Hyperemia		VMCA/VICA	
AVM feeding vessels			PI PTI
Severe extracranial ICA stenosis	D-MCA		FA
Migraine with aura and without aura (headache-free period)			PI PTI
Migraine with aura (during headache)			PI PTI
Migraine without aura (during headache)	PI PTI		

ICP, Intracranial pressure; *CPP,* cerebral perfusion pressure; *SAH,* subarachnoid hemorrhage; *AVM,* arteriovenous malformations; *ICA,* intracranial carotid artery; *MCA,* middle cerebral artery; *ACA,* anterior cerebral artery; *ACAVR,* ACA velocity ratio; *VMCA/VICA,* hemispheric index; *VMCA/VACA,* MCA/ACA velocity ratio; *PI,* pulsatility index; *PTI,* pulsatility transmission index; *RI,* resistance index; *FA,* flow acceleration; *D-MCA,* delta middle cerebral artery.

OVERVIEW

A summary of the alterations in TCD indices in various neurologic disorders is presented in Table 13-7.

The clinical utility of these indices depends on their reliability in detecting a host of varied neurologic disorders. Unfortunately, the indices are not always specific in detecting particular neurologic diseases. For example, PI and RI are increased in brain death but also in other clinical situations as illustrated in Table 13-7.

The identification of a gold standard to assess the accuracy of the indices would help define their clinical role. However, gold standards for these indices are uncommon and impractical. For example, an increased RI presumably secondary to increased ICP may be indirectly confirmed with intracranial pressure monitoring, but no gold standard exists that can easily and directly measure intracranial vascular resistance.

When a gold standard does not exist, changes in these indices must be correlated with clinical events and indirect laboratory markers of the disease in question. For example, TCD indices are correlated with clinical brain death criteria to see how well the indices predict brain death. However, severe increased ICP may give rise to changes in TCD indices similar to those seen in brain death, confounding the accurate diagnosis of brain death based on TCD alone.[49,52]

Further investigations are needed to collect more data on TCD indices of intracranial hemodynamics and their utility in normal and pathologic conditions. Careful studies of clinical outcomes and treatment effects are needed before the indices can enjoy more widespread, routine use.

REFERENCES

1. Aaslid R, Markwalder TM, Nornes H: Noninvasive transcranial Doppler ultrasound recording of flow velocity in basal cerebral arteries, *J Neurosurg* 57:769-774, 1982.
2. Ackerstaff RGA, Keunen RWM, van Pelt W, et al: Influence of biological factors on changes in mean cerebral blood flow velocity in normal aging: a transcranial Doppler study, *Neurol Res* 12:187-191, 1990.
3. Adams RJ, Aaslid R, Gammal TE, et al: Detection of cerebral vasculopathy in sickle cell disease using transcranial Doppler ultrasonography and magnetic resonance imaging, *Stroke* 19:518-520, 1988.
4. Adams RJ, Mekie V, Nichols F, et al: The use of transcranial ultrasonography to predict stroke in sickle cell disease, *N Engl J Med* 326:605-610, 1992.
5. Adams RJ, Nichols FT, Hess DC: *Normal values and physiological variables.* In Newell DW, Aaslid R, editors: *Transcranial Doppler,* New York, 1992, Raven Press.
6. Ameriso SF, Pagauiui-Hill-A, Meiselmau HJ, et al. Correlates of middle cerebral artery blood velocity in the elderly, *Stroke* 21:1579-1583, 1990.
7. Babikian VL: *Transcranial Doppler evaluation of patients with ischemic cerebrovascular disease.* In Babikian VL, Wechsler LR, editors: *Transcranial Doppler ultrasonography,* St Louis, 1993, Mosby–Year Book.
8. Babikian VL, Araki C, Ahern G, et al: The delta middle cerebral artery flow velocity: an index of extracranial carotid artery stenosis severity, *J Cardiovasc Technol* 8:162-163, 1989.
9. Bishop CCR, Powell S, Rutt D, et al: Transcranial Doppler measurement of middle cerebral artery blood flow velocity, *Stroke* 17:913-915, 1986.
10. Brass LM, Duterte DL, Mohr JP: Anterior cerebral artery velocity changes in disease of the middle cerebral artery stem, *Stroke* 20:1737-1740, 1989.
11. Brass LM, Kisiel D, Sarrel PM: A correlation between estrogen and middle cerebral blood velocity at different times in the menstrual cycle in women with catamenial migraine, *J Cardiovasc Technol* 9:68, 1990.
12. Brass LM, Panlakis SG, DeVivs D, et al: Transcranial Doppler measurement of the middle cerebral artery: effect of hematocrit, *Stroke* 19:1466-1469, 1988.
13. Brass LM, Prohovmik I, Panlakis SG, et al: Middle cerebral artery blood velocity and cerebral blood flow in sickle cell disease, *Stroke* 22:27-30, 1991.
14. Cantelmo NL, Babikiau UL, Johnson WC, et al: Correlation of transcranial Doppler and noninvasive tests with angiography in the evaluation of extracranial carotid disease, *J Vasc Surg* 11:786-792, 1990.
15. Cardoso ER, Kupchak JA: Evaluation of intracranial pressure gradients by means of transcranial Doppler sonography, *Acta Neurochir Suppl (Wien)* 55:1-5, 1992.
16. Chan KH, Dearoleu MN, Miller JD, et al: The effect of changes in cerebral perfusion pressure upon middle cerebral artery blood flow velocity and jugular bulb venous oxygen saturation after severe brain injury, *J Neurosurg* 77:55-61, 1992.
17. DeWitt LD, Rosengart A, Teal PA: *Transcranial Doppler ultrasonography: normal values.* In Babikian VL, Wechsler LR, editors: *Transcranial Doppler ultrasonography,* St Louis, 1993, Mosby–Year Book.
18. Fagan SC, Bimdlish V, Rdseu S, et al: Transcranial Doppler to evaluate the effects of antihypertensive medication on cerebral blood flow velocity, *J Clin Pharmacol* 32:66-69, 1992.
19. Fujioka KA, Douville CM: *Anatomy and freehand examination techniques.* In Newell DW, Aaslid R, editors: *Transcranial Doppler,* New York, 1992, Raven Press.
20. Gangar KG, Vyas B, Whitehead M, et al: Pulsatility index in internal carotid artery in relation to transdermal oestradiol and time since menopause, *Lancet* 338:839-842, 1991.
21. Giller CA, Batjir HH, Kopitmi K, et al: Persistent high TCD velocities in arterial segments following angioplasty or dilatation with papaverine: evidence for hyperemia? *Stroke* 25:755, 1994.
22. Giller CA, Hodges K, Batjer HH: Transcranial Doppler pulsatility in vasodilatation and stenosis, *J Neurosurg* 72:901-906, 1990.
23. Giller CA, Lam M, Roseland A: Periodic variations in transcranial Doppler mean velocities, *J Neuroimaging* 3:160-162, 1993.
24. Giulioni M, Urisino M, Alvisi C: Correlations among intracranial pulsatility, intracranial hemodynamics, and transcranial Doppler waveform: literature review and hypothesis for future studies, *Neurosurgery* 22:807-810, 1988.
25. Goh D, Minns RA, Pye SD: Transcranial Doppler (TCD) ultrasound as a noninvasive means of monitoring cerebrohaemodynamic change in hydrocephalus, *Eur J Pediatr Surg* 1(suppl):14-17, 1991.
26. Gosling RG, King DH: Arterial assessment by Doppler-shift ultrasound, *Proc R Soc Med* 67:447-449, 1974.
27. Grolimund P, Seiler RW, Aaslid R, et al: Evaluation of cerebrovascular disease by combined extracranial and transcranial Doppler sonography: experience in 1,039 patients, *Stroke* 18:1018-1024, 1987.
28. Hassler W, Steinmetz H, Gawlowski J: Transcranial Doppler ultrasonography in raised intracranial pressure and in intracranial circulatory arrest, *J Neurosurg* 68:745-751, 1988.

29. Hellstrom G, Wahlgren NG: Physical exercise increases middle cerebral artery blood flow velocity, *Neurosurg Rev* 16:151-156, 1993.

30. Hennerici M, Rautenberg W, Sitzer G, et al: Transcranial Doppler ultrasound for the assessment of intracranial arterial flow velocity, part 1: examination technique and normal values, *Surg Neurol* 27:439-448, 1987.

31. Homburg AM, Jakobsen M, Enevoldsen E: Transcranial Doppler recordings in raised intracranial pressure, *Acta Neurol Scand* 87:488-493, 1993.

32. Kader A, Young WL, Massaro AR, et al: Transcranial Doppler changes during staged surgical resection of cerebral arteriovenous malformations: a report of three cases, *Surg Neurol* 39:392-398, 1993.

33. Kelley RE, Nemon RA, Shing-Her-Juang, et al: Transcranial Doppler ultrasonography of the middle cerebral artery in the hemodynamic assessment of internal carotid artery stenosis, *Arch Neurol* 49:960-964, 1990.

34. Klingelhofer J, Sander D, Holzgraefe M, et al: Cerebral vasospasm evaluated by transcranial Doppler ultrasound at different intracranial pressures, *J Neurosurg* 75:752-758, 1991.

35. Ley-Pozo J, Ringelstein EB: Noninvasive detection of occlusive disease of the carotid siphon and the middle cerebral artery, *Ann Neurol* 28:640-647, 1990.

36. Lindegaard KF: *Indices of pulsatility.* In Newell DW, Aaslid R, editors: *Transcranial Doppler,* New York, 1992, Raven Press.

37. Lindegaard KF, Bakke SJ, Grolimund P, et al: Assessment of intracranial hemodynamics in carotid artery disease by transcranial Doppler ultrasound, *J Neurosurg* 63:890-898, 1985.

38. Lindegaard KF, Grolimund P, Aaslid R, et al: Evaluation of cerebral AVMs using transcranial Doppler ultrasound, *J Neurosurg* 65:335-344, 1986.

39. Lindegaard KF, Lundar T, Wiberg J, et al: Variations in middle cerebral artery blood flow investigated with noninvasive transcranial blood velocity measurements, *Stroke* 18:1025-1030, 1987.

40. Lindegaard KF, Nornes H, Bakke SJ, et al: Cerebral vasospasm diagnosis by means of angiography and blood velocity measurements, *Acta Neurochir (Wien)* 100:12-24, 1989.

41. Maeda H, Etami H, Hauds N, et al: A validation study on the reproducibility of transcranial Doppler velocimetry, *Ultrasound Med Biol* 16:9-14, 1990.

42. Mattle H, Grolimund P, Huber P, et al: Transcranial Doppler sonographic findings in middle cerebral artery disease, *Arch Neurol* 45:289-295, 1988.

43. Newell DW, Aaslid R, Steoss R, et al: The relationship of blood flow velocity fluctuations to intracranial pressure B waves, *J Neurosurg* 76:415-421, 1992.

44. Norelle A, Fischer AQ, Flannery AM: Transcranial Doppler: a noninvasive method to monitor hydrocephalus, *J Child Neurol* 4:S87-S89, 1989.

45. Petty GW, Massaro AR, Tatewichi TK, et al: Transcranial Doppler ultrasonographic changes after treatment for arteriovenous malformations, *Stroke* 21:260-266, 1990.

46. Petty GW, Wiebers DO, Meissner I: Transcranial Doppler ultrasonography: clinical applications in cerebrovascular disease, *Mayo Clin Proc* 65:1350-1364, 1990.

47. Pines A, Fisman EZ, Leno Y, et al: The effects of hormone replacement therapy in normal postmenopausal women: measurements of Doppler-derived parameters of aortic flow, *Am J Obstet Gynecol* 164:806-812, 1991.

48. Pourcelot L: *Diagnostic ultrasound of cerebral vascular diseases.* In Donald I, Levi S, editors: *Present and future of diagnostic ultrasound,* Rotterdam, 1976, Kooyker.

49. Powers AD, Graeber MC, Smith RR: Transcranial Doppler ultrasonography in the determination of brain death, *Neurosurgery* 24:884-889, 1989.

50. Rahimtoola SH: *Valvular heart disease.* In Stein JH, editor: *Internal medicine,* St Louis, 1994, Mosby–Year Book.

51. Ringelstein EB, Otis SM: *Physiological testing of vasomotor reserve.* In Newell DW, Aaslid R, editors: *Transcranial Doppler,* New York, 1992, Raven Press.

52. Ropper AH, Kehene SK, Wechsler L: Transcranial Doppler in brain death, *Stroke* 37:1733-1735, 1987.

53. Sarrel PM: *Blood flow.* In Lobo RA, editor: *Treatment of the postmenopausal woman: basic and clinical aspects,* New York, 1994, Raven Press.

54. Saver JL, Feldmann E: *Basic transcranial Doppler examination: technique and anatomy.* In Babikian VL, Wechsler LR, editors: *Transcranial Doppler ultrasonography,* St Louis, 1993, Mosby.

55. Schneider PA, Rossman ME, Bernstein EF, et al: Effect of internal carotid artery occlusion on intracranial hemodynamics: transcranial Doppler evaluation and clinical correlation, *Stroke* 19:589-593, 1988.

56. Seiler RW, Newell DW: *Subarachnoid hemorrhage and vasospasm.* In Newell DW, Aaslid R, editors: *Transcranial Doppler,* New York, 1992, Raven Press.

57. Shaw TG, Moztel KF, Stirling Meyer J, et al: Cerebral blood flow changes in benign aging and in cerebrovascular disease, *Neurology* 34:855-862, 1984.

58. Sorteberg W, Laugmoeu JA, Linolegaard K-F, et al: Side-to-side differences and day-to-day variations of transcranial Doppler parameters in normal subjects, *J Ultrasound Med* 9:403-409, 1990.

59. Steinmeier R, Laumer R, Boudar J, et al: Cerebral hemodynamics in subarachnoid hemorrhage evaluated by transcranial Doppler sonography, part 2. pulsatility indices: normal reference values and characteristics in subarachnoid hemorrhage, *Neurosurgery* 33:10-19, 1993.

60. Thie A, Fuhlendorf, Spitzer K, et al: Transcranial Doppler evaluation of common and classic migraine, part I: ultrasonic features during the headache-free period, *Headache* 30:201-208, 1990.

61. Thie A, Fuhlendorf, Spitzer K, et al: Transcranial Doppler evaluation of common and classic migraine, part II: ultrasonic features during attacks, *Headache* 30:209-215, 1990.

62. Thiel A, Zickmann B, Hempelmann G: Transcranial Doppler sonography: effects of halothane, enflurane and isoflurane on blood flow velocity in the middle cerebral artery, *Br J Anaesth* 68:388-393, 1992.

63. Titianova EB, Velcheva IV, Mateev PS: Effects of aging and hematocrit on cerebral blood flow velocity in patients with unilateral cerebral infarctions: a Doppler ultrasound evaluation, *Angiology* 44:100-106, 1993.

64. Weber M, Grolimund P, Seiler RW: Evaluation of posttraumatic cerebral blood flow velocity by transcranial Doppler ultrasonography, *Neurosurgery* 27:106-112, 1990.

65. Zagzebski JA: *Physics and instrumentation in Doppler and B-mode ultrasonography,* In Zwiebel WJ, editor: *Introduction to vascular ultrasonography,* Toronto, 1992, WB Saunders.

66. Zanette EM, Aguoli A, Cerbo R, et al: Transcranial Doppler (TCD) after nitroglycerin in migraine without aura, *Headache* 31:596-598, 1991.

67. Zwiebel WJ: *Doppler evaluation of carotid stenosis.* In Zwiebel WJ, editor: *Introduction to vascular ultrasonography,* Toronto, 1992, WB Saunders.

68. Zwiebel WJ: *Spectrum analysis in Doppler vascular diagnosis.* In Zwiebel WJ, editor: *Introduction to vascular ultrasonography,* Toronto, 1992, WB Saunders.

14

Cerebral Blood Flow and Cerebrovascular Physiology

Viken L. Babikian
Jens J. Schwarze

The ability to monitor cerebral blood flow (CBF) is appealing to clinicians because various cerebrovascular and systemic disorders can disrupt CBF and cause cerebral damage. Several technologies, including xenon-133 inhalation or intravenous administration, xenon-computerized tomography (xenon CT), single photon emission computed tomography (SPECT) and positron emission tomography (PET) are available today to measure CBF and assess cerebrovascular physiology.[118] However, each of these methods has various limitations, and all are considered to be invasive because they rely on the administration of radioactive markers.

The introduction of transcranial Doppler ultrasonography (TCD) to clinical use in 1982 provided for the first time the ability to monitor CBF noninvasively and during prolonged periods of time. TCD has been extensively utilized since, both in the laboratory and at the bedside, and it is now clear that in addition to its many advantages, the technique also has significant limitations. In this chapter, TCD studies of CBF and cerebrovascular physiology are critically reviewed.

TRANSCRANIAL DOPPLER ULTRASONOGRAPHY AND CEREBRAL BLOOD FLOW

Transcranial Doppler's ability to monitor arterial flow has led investigators to question whether TCD indices, such as peak systolic or mean flow velocity (FV), can be used to assess CBF. Several studies have compared FVs from cerebral arteries at the level of the circle of Willis to simultaneously measured CBF values from cerebral regions corresponding to the arterial territories. CBF was measured in these investigations by either the xenon-133 inhalation or intravenous administration methods[11,13,22,105] or by single photon emission tomography.[121] In young, healthy subjects, a significant correlation between baseline FV and CBF values is present for the middle (MCA), posterior (PCA), and anterior (ACA) cerebral arteries and the internal carotid artery (ICA); the correlation coefficient is highest for the PCA and lowest for the ICA.[105] Findings have been mixed for individuals with cerebrovascular disease. Although Brass and colleagues[13] reported a linear relationship between peak systolic FV and CBF and Zanette and

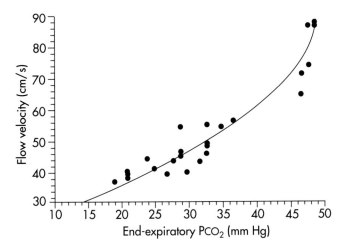

Fig. 14-1. Relationship of the end-expiratory P_{CO_2} and the middle cerebral artery mean flow velocity in a healthy, young subject. Other investigators have described linear and biasymptotic equations.

associates[121] found a significant correlation in acute stroke, most studies suggest that baseline FVs do not correlate[88] or correlate poorly[11,21] with flow values. The cause(s) of this discrepancy in results is not known.

Because CBF changes in response to variations in arterial CO_2 concentration, the relationship between arterial or end-expiratory CO_2 pressure and peak FV has been studied extensively (Fig. 14-1). A linear relationship with a slope of 2.9% per mm Hg change has been reported by Kirkham and associates for the MCA over the end-expiratory CO_2 pressure range of 20 to 60 mm Hg.[49] The value of the slope is similar to results from CBF measurements, suggesting that MCA FV changes parallel changes in CBF.[49] A linear relationship has also been reported by other investigators,[40,82] but Hartmann and associates found only a "fair" correlation for normal patients and a poor one for patients with cerebrovascular disease.[40] The finding of exponential[73] and biasymptotic[94] equations raises a question regarding the exact relationship and illustrates some of the limitations inherent to the methods of measurement. These limitations are reviewed in subsequent sections of this chapter. Interestingly, FV changes obtained after the administration of other vasoactive stimulants, such as acetazolamide, also correlate closely with changes in CBF[11,49,88] and support the notion of a close correlation. It should be noted that the FV-CBF correlation is dependent on the regional CBF level and that it is strong at CBF values less than 20 ml/100 g per minute but weak if the CBF exceeds that level.[39] Flow velocity changes tend to be smaller than CBF changes, and the discrepancy increases at high CBF values.[83]

Based on theoretical considerations, Sorteberg and colleagues have established a formula that describes the relationship between flow velocity in an artery (V in cm/s), the regional CBF (rCBF in cm^3/100 g brain tissue/s), the artery's perfusion territory (T in 100 g brain tissue), and its luminal area (A in cm^2)[105,106]:

$$V = \frac{1}{60} (rCBF) \, T \, (A)^{-1}$$

The formula suggests that for FV to be representative of rCBF, the artery's perfusion territory and its diameter must remain constant during the period of measurement. The following review of the formula highlights some limitations when FVs are used as indices of CBF:

- In healthy subjects and individuals with no known cerebrovascular disease, the main limitation concerns congenital variations of the circle of Willis that determine an artery's perfusion territory. For example, in subjects with hypoplastic ACA A1 segments, a "normal" variant present in 2% to 12% of the general population, the perfusion territory of the contralateral ICA is significantly increased, because the latter supplies both ACAs. [99] As a result, the resting FV in the supraclinoid ICA is slightly elevated, even though rCBF values are unchanged. In addition, small variations in arterial diameter size in normal patients introduce an additional variable in this population. The variations are usually small for the PCA and may be more marked for the ACA.[10] The preceding variables may partially explain the wide range of baseline FV values in normals.[24]

- In individuals with acute cerebrovascular disease, arterial diameter and perfusion territory are in a dynamic condition, and other factors have to be taken into consideration. For example, due to vasospasm, the arterial diameter can change in the days following aneurysmal subarachnoid hemorrhage. Similarly, in patients with embolic MCA trunk occlusions, recanalization frequently occurs along with gradual changes in arterial diameter.[36] Another consideration in this group concerns transient changes in collateral flow because they affect the artery's perfusion territory.

- In patients undergoing surgery, the arterial diameter can change because of the effect of anesthetic agents and the response to changes in blood pressure or arterial CO_2 or O_2 pressure (respectively, $PaCO_2$ and PaO_2). In addition, arterial perfusion territory can change postoperatively as a result of surgical procedures. For example, the perfusion territories of an operated carotid may increase following endarterectomy without a measurable increase in corresponding CBF values;[12] it can also change following clamping or resection of arterial or venous segments during arteriovenous malformation surgery.

- In addition to the preceding considerations, several,

usually unaccounted for, factors may affect the relationship of baseline FVs with CBF. Variables, such as vasoactive medications and small changes in blood pressure or $Paco_2$, can affect FVs without simultaneously having an effect on CBF. These factors can elicit compensatory arterial changes that affect TCD measurements while CBF remains constant.

- Variations in the angle of insonation among individuals constitute a correctable limitation. They introduce an error in the determination of FVs that depends on the cosine of the angle.[24] Fluctuations in heart rate and cardiac output also have an effect on CBF and FV. These are reviewed later in this chapter.

The peak systolic and mean FVs are the two TCD indices most frequently used in the preceding studies, but whether other indices derived from raw TCD data may be more accurate is unknown.[22,121] The respective advantages and disadvantages of mean and peak systolic FVs have not been adequately studied. Although most investigators seem to prefer the mean FV in flow determinations because it may be a better approximation of velocities throughout the cardiac cycle, there are few data to support this contention.[56]

In summary, the use of FV as an index for CBF is based on the assumption that arterial diameter, perfusion territory, and several hemodynamic parameters are stable during the period of measurement.[56] When these premises are verified, FV may be a useful index of CBF. For example, in patients with low-flow cerebral infarction distal to an occluded cervical ICA, the ipsilateral MCA's perfusion territory and M1 segment diameter are likely to be stable during prolonged periods of time. Similarly, when anesthetic agents have reached steady-state concentration during surgery, the variables are expected to be reasonably stable. Under these and similar conditions, changes in FV correlate with changes in CBF, and the correlation is stronger at low CBF values. In most clinical settings, however, variations of factors such as blood pressure and $Paco_2$ occur during the testing period and invalidate the preceding assumptions. As noted in the subsequent sections, when these variations are of limited amplitude, the introduced error may be small enough for TCD measurements to be acceptable for clinical use.

Whether FV is an accurate index of arterial flow volume has also been reviewed. A study by Lindegaard and associates suggests it may be.[66] These investigators measured flow with cuff probes and, during carotid endarterectomy or nonpulsatile cardiopulmonary bypass, found a linear relationship between ICA flow volume and ipsilateral MCA FV. Others have taken a different approach to arterial flow measurements.[100, 122] Flow velocity (in cm/s) in an arterial segment is proportional to flow (Q in cm^3/s) when the artery's luminal area (A in cm^2) does not change. This can be expressed as

$$Q = A \text{ (FV)}$$

and can be used to assess flow noninvasively in selected arterial segments. B-mode instruments permit measurement of the internal diameter of an artery, thus allowing measurement of its area. An average of the mean velocity over an interval of time can be obtained with Doppler instruments.[122] A high correlation between volumes measured by duplex scanning and timed blood collections exists in laboratory animals for the systemic circulation.[122] Measurements of ICA and vertebral artery (VA) diameters can be performed with some duplex instruments. Using a color duplex instrument, Schöning and colleagues also measured angle-corrected and time-averaged velocities and calculated flow volumes in these arteries in healthy adults.[100] The preceding measurements cannot be extended to intracranial arteries at the present time because of the inability to determine their diameters reliably with available TCD duplex instruments. Technical innovations may help overcome these limitations in the future.

Another approach to the same problem relies on the determination of signal power. Measurement of the frequency shift averaged over the power density of a received signal can help estimate the instantaneous average blood velocity over a cross-section of the artery.[7] As a result, changes in an artery's cross-sectional area are expected to cause a proportional increase in signal power.[1] Measurements of signal power and its changes have already been used to assess changes in arterial cross-sectional area in physiologic testing of healthy subjects.[1]

TRANSCRANIAL DOPPLER ASSESSMENT OF CEREBROVASCULAR PHYSIOLOGY

The regulation of CBF is accomplished through several mechanisms that respond to specific stimuli.[77] A detailed review of these mechanisms is out of this chapter's scope but has been presented elsewhere.[26] These processes are of interest in the context of the present chapter for the following two main reasons: First, because changes in blood pressure and in Pao_2 and $Paco_2$, as well as the corresponding responses in arterial diameter, can affect TCD measurements. In addition, disease states can impair these mechanisms. Second, TCD studies have permitted limited assessment of these pathways and have shed some new light on our understanding of the way they function. The following paragraphs summarize autoregulation and vasoreactivity studies pertinent to TCD measurements. The effect of cognitive tasks on CBF and TCD measurements is presented in Chapter 18.

Autoregulation

Introduced by Fog in 1938[29] and further developed by Lassen in 1959,[61] the concept of cerebral autoregulation now refers to the intrinsic ability of the brain to maintain CBF constant during changes of arterial and cerebral perfusion pressure.[18,85] In normotensive individuals, the approximate upper and lower limits of the mean arterial blood pressure (MABP) within which autoregulation is effective are 60 and 150 mm Hg, respectively. The ability to maintain flow constant in a cerebral artery in spite of blood pressure changes depends to a large degree on the modulation of vascular resistance. This is summarized by Ohm's law:

$$Q = \Delta P/R$$

where Q represents blood flow, ΔP is the pressure gradient between the two ends of the vessel, and R is the resistance to flow. Because a vessel's resistance to flow is inversely related to the fourth power of its radius (Poiseuille's law), changes in cerebrovascular resistance are accomplished in most physiologic conditions by constriction and dilation of cerebral arteries. As discussed earlier, any change in arterial diameter is a major concern when prolonged or repeated TCD testing is performed because TCD measurements are based on the assumption that the insonated artery's diameter does not vary significantly during the period of measurement. Whether this assumption can be justified is reviewed in the following paragraphs. In subsequent parts of this section, TCD studies of normal and abnormal autoregulation are presented.

Autoregulation and the different cerebral arterial segments. Most of the peripheral vascular resistance in humans resides in small arteries and arterioles 8 to 50 μm in diameter. A definitive anatomic site for cerebrovascular resistance has not yet been identified, but observations in laboratory animals suggest that arterioles less than 400 μm in diameter are its main contributors. According to Kontos and associates, cerebrovascular resistance is not exclusively limited to one segment of the arterial tree in the cat, and autoregulatory responses are MABP dependent.[58] The aorta and large extracranial vessels leading to the circle of Willis do not change significantly with variations of blood pressure and comprise approximately 17% of the cerebrovascular resistance at a MABP of 120 mm Hg.[58] Vessels of the circle of Willis and large cerebral surface vessels more than 200 μm in diameter undergo autoregulatory adjustments in response to MABP variations ranging between 110 and 160 mm Hg and are the primary segments that accommodate for pressure changes in that range; when the MABP is 120 mm Hg, they contribute 26% of the total cerebrovascular resistance. Small cerebral surface and intracerebral arterioles less than 100 μm in diameter start dilating only when the MABP

is less than 90 mm Hg, and their dilatation becomes more marked at MABP values less than 70 mm Hg; they contribute approximately 32% of the total cerebrovascular resistance. The remaining resistance is provided by capillaries. Other investigators have reported slightly different findings.[68]

The significance of the preceding and other animal studies to cerebral autoregulation in humans is not entirely clear. Diameters of human circle of Willis arteries and the first segments of the MCA, ACA, and PCA, which are insonated with TCD, usually exceed 1 mm.[10,30,99] First branches of these segments, such as the orbitofrontal, central sulcus, and angular arteries, have diameters in the 0.5 to 1.3 mm range.[10] Perforating branches of the MCA have diameters that range between 80 and 840 μm with means of 280 μm and 510 μm for the medial and lateral perforators.[72] Although these arteries and their immediate branches are thought to behave like vessels of a similar size in animals, the human cerebral circulation may not function as predicted from observations of pial vessel in animals,[2] and significant differences in cerebrovascular regulation may exist among species.

Some studies in humans also support the notion of the ICA and basal cerebral arteries being mainly "conductance" arteries. Giller and colleagues measured the diameters of cerebral arteries during craniotomy and monitored the effect of MABP changes of approximately 30 mm Hg from normotensive or slightly hypotensive levels.[33] The mean diameter change from baseline was approximately 4% for the ICA, MCA M1 segment, and VA and in excess of 20% for the ACA and MCA M2 segment; arterial segments with smaller diameters had more vigorous responses.[33] It should be noted that these measurements were obtained while the patients were anesthetized with isoflurane and N_2O, agents that can impair cerebrovascular responsiveness, at least to some degree[54] (Fig. 14-2). Intraarterial pressure measurements during surgery also show that, although the pressure within the supraclinoid ICA and proximal ACA and MCA is similar to that of the cervical ICA, it drops to 83% of the cervical ICA's pressure in small arteries and arterioles with an average diameter of 400 μm.[8]

When taken together, the preceding findings suggest that autoregulatory responses to small alterations in blood pressure seem to involve mainly arterioles equal to or less than 400 μm in diameter and that changes in distal ICA and proximal MCA diameters are relatively small. This implies that FVs constitute an acceptable index for flow in these arterial segments during small blood pressure changes and that they can be used to assess autoregulatory changes in the distal arterial bed as long as the other factors presented in the preceding cerebral blood flow section remain constant during the period of measurement.

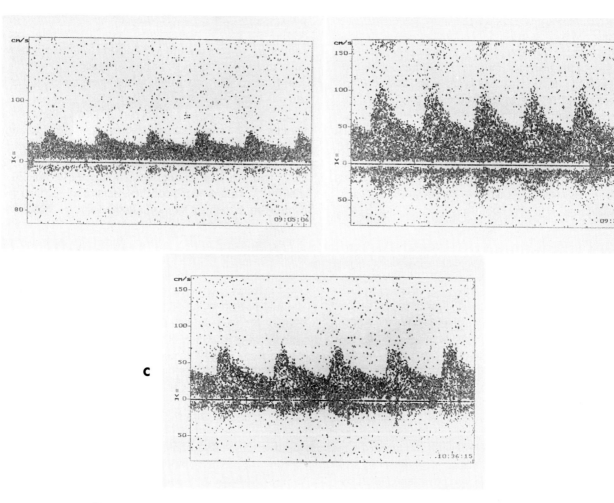

Fig. 14-2. Middle cerebral artery flow velocity changes in a patient with impaired cerebrovascular autoregulation following the administration of anesthetic agents during surgery. **A,** The systemic blood pressure is 87/43 mm Hg, and the mean flow velocity is approximately 36 cm/s. **B** and **C,** The respective blood pressure and flow velocity readings are 206/88 mm Hg and 68 cm/s and 136/63 mm Hg and 45 cm/s.

The preceding conclusion is contradicted by results from mainly animal studies, indicating that the major basal cerebral arteries, vessels with a tunica media composed predominantly of smooth muscle layers,[26] can dilate and constrict in response to various stimuli and contribute significantly to cerebrovascular resistance. In the cat, intravascular measurements show that the pressure in large arteries at the base of the brain, such as the basilar artery, is approximately 80% of aortic pressure.[28] At a systolic pressure of 50 mm Hg, 39% of the loss of pressure head occurs in arteries upstream from 300 μm surface vessels;[108] in addition, resistance shifts with the systolic pressure: At 180 mm Hg the upstream pressure loss decreases to 33%.[108] In the mongrel dog, stepwise changes in the inlet pressure applied at the ICA origin result in corresponding changes in the ICA's resistance but no pressure varia-

tions at the level of the circle of Willis.[78] Underlining the relative importance of the "conductance" vessels in the regulation of CBF, Mchedlishvili and colleagues suggested that similar constriction of smaller brain arteries occurs only when changes in systemic arterial pressure are large and overcome the autoregulatory ability of the ICA.[78] Calf MCAs, "large" vessels when compared to human arteries, dilate and constrict when submitted to different pressures.[114] Note should also be made that pathologic processes such as atherosclerosis and chronic hypertension can increase overall cerebrovascular resistance, including resistance in large arteries.[28]

In summary, our present understanding of human cerebral autoregulation and vascular resistance remains limited. Available data suggest that autoregulatory responses to most blood pressure changes involve all levels of the cerebral arterial tree; the level of involvement and its extent probably vary with the blood pressure and from one circulatory or metabolic disturbance to the other. At MABP values in the 85 to 125 mm Hg range, the major adjustments in cerebrovascular resistance seem to occur in pial arterioles 200 to 400 μm in diameter and in precapillary parenchymal arterioles. Variations in blood pressure within that range are likely to elicit more significant changes in arteriolar than arterial diameter, and changes in the latter are more marked for the ACA than the MCA M1 segment and ICA. As a result, when TCD is used to assess flow or autoregulatory changes, the inability to correct for small variations in the insonated artery's diameter during the study will introduce an error, the extent of which remains undetermined when using instruments available today. The error is likely to be smallest for the MCA and ICA. However, in spite of this error, given the noninvasive nature of ultrasonic testing and the limitations of other technologies available today, TCD measurements may be acceptable to clinicians and investigators when small blood pressure changes are taken into consideration.

Assessment of normal autoregulation. The relationship between autoregulatory responses and the diameter of Willisian arteries in humans has also been studied with TCD. Aaslid and associates studied the effect of rapid, 20 mm Hg step drops in blood pressure within the physiologic range and used signal power analysis to investigate changes in arterial cross-sectional area.[1] An abrupt drop in blood pressure was associated with an almost simultaneous drop in FV; although the pressure remained low for 10 to 15 seconds, FVs returned to control levels within approximately five heartbeats that lasted 8 seconds. This was thought to represent the speed of the autoregulatory response. In addition, because there was no change in signal power during hypocapnia, and because the change in power during normocapnia was lower than changes in blood pressure and FV, Aaslid and colleagues concluded that the arterial diameter does not change significantly during small changes in blood pressure.[1] Giller and associates studied normotensive hypovolemia induced in healthy volunteers during graded lower body negative pressure. They found that the ratio of MCA to systemic arterial pulsatility indices increased by 22% and suggested that sympathetic activation induced by hypovolemia causes vasoconstriction of intracranial small vessels, presumably distal to the MCA M1 segment.[32] A fast autoregulatory response is also present in human venous beds.[2]

Other TCD studies suggest that the arterial diameter responds to pharmacologic agents or to changes of blood pressure. Indirect evidence, based on measurements of TCD signal power obtained from healthy individuals subjected to tilt-table testing, suggests that in this group the M1 segment also dilates.[81] Similarly, in the study by Giller and colleagues quoted in the preceding para-

graph, normotensive hypovolemia in healthy volunteers leads to a drop in the mean FV of approximately 16%, raising the possibility of a small M1 segment change that does not reach the amplitude of the more distal small vessel vasoconstriction in response to sympathetic activation.[32] Combined TCD and SPECT studies indicate that sublingual nitroglycerin reduces MCA FVs without concurrently changing CBF in the region corresponding to the artery, suggesting dilatation of the M1 segment.[20] Although the action of nitroglycerin on the cerebral vasculature does not qualify as an example of autoregulatory response, the results of the study confirm the ability of the basal cerebral arteries to dilate in response to specific stimuli.

Most noradrenergic nerves supplying major vessels at the base of the brain originate at the superior cervical sympathetic ganglia.[26] Fibers in the walls of the MCA, ACA,[116] and pial vessels extend to arterioles in the brain parenchyma.[18] When stimulated, they have a variable vasoconstrictive effect on cerebral arterioles and arteries[117] and do not cause a consistent decrease of regional CBF.[18] The principal function of adrenergic fibers may be to protect the cerebral vasculature from marked increases in blood pressure by causing a constriction of inflow vessels and larger arterioles. Stimulation of the upper thoracic sympathetic chain causes a marked and rapid increase of the MCA mean FV in humans, even when blood pressure changes remain in the autoregulatory range.[116] Changes in heart rate and blood pressure precede the FV response, suggesting that the cerebral hemodynamic changes are primarily "a heart mediated response" rather than a direct effect of the sympathetic stimulation on cerebral arterial diameter.[116]

Assessment of autoregulation: disease states

Ischemic cerebrovascular disease. Cerebral autoregulation is impaired in acute conditions such as hypertensive encephalopathy, cerebral infarction, trauma, and intracranial infection.[85] In these conditions, vasomotor paralysis may be temporary. Hypertension[28] and diabetes mellitus,[9] risk factors associated with arterial disease, can induce chronic changes in vasomotor tone.

In patients with extracranial carotid artery severe stenosis, a sudden drop in systemic pressure of 20 to 40 mm Hg is followed by an abrupt fall in MCA FVs of approximately 25%; unlike normal individuals, in whom these changes are corrected in 5 to 8 seconds, FVs return to pretest values after 20 to 60 seconds, indicating an exhausted vasomotor response.[93] The autoregulatory impairment is not detected in all patients. In approximately 55% of those with cervical ICA severe stenosis or occlusion, MCA FVs on the side of the lesion are not significantly lower than FVs in the contralateral MCA. Compensatory collateral flow and cerebral autoregulation are considered to be adequate in these cases.[84] However, in patients with multiple, flow-limiting le-

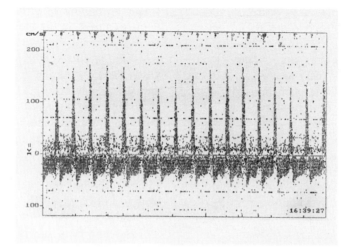

Fig. 14-3. Effect of increased intracranial pressure on flow velocities. When the intracranial pressure reaches the diastolic pressure level, mean and diastolic velocities drop. In this case, blood flow is retrograde during diastole.

sions or incompetent collateral channels, compensatory mechanisms can be overwhelmed and CBF can fall.[3]

Subarachnoid hemorrhage. Autoregulation is often impaired following subarachnoid hemorrhage.[41,46] For obvious reasons, TCD studies of autoregulation during the acute stage following hemorrhage are limited. A more thorough understanding of the cerebrovascular response to cerebral perfusion pressure changes in this context would be clinically useful because therapeutic manipulations of blood pressure during the acute course of the illness may have unexpected effects. For example, cerebral ischemia may be inadvertently accentuated during surgery or when using agents, like nitroglycerin or nimodipine, with a potential for arterial vasodilatation and hypotension. These measures can divert blood from the territories of arteries with vasospasm and impaired autoregulation to territories with intact autoregulatory mechanisms.

Trauma. The neurologic outcome of head-injured patients is determined by the direct effects of trauma on the brain and its secondary complications such as increased intracranial pressure. The latter is caused not only by mass lesions but also by an alteration in the volume-pressure relationships and by changes in cerebrospinal fluid volume and in brain stiffness. As a result of brain injury, two main determinants of CBF—cerebral perfusion pressure and cerebral autoregulation—can be severely altered.

Cerebral autoregulation is impaired in patients with head trauma.[85] The extent and severity of this impairment are not totally clear. Pressure passive FV changes can be found throughout the cerebral perfusion pressure range in less than 25% of patients with increased intracranial pressure, but in the majority of cases these changes do not occur until the perfusion pressure drops

below a threshold of 45[67] or 70 mm Hg,[17] suggesting that autoregulation is active above the threshold. Even in those with relatively preserved autoregulation, however, when the intracranial pressure reaches the level of diastolic pressure, the mean and diastolic FVs drop in spite of maximum distal vasodilatation[103] (Fig. 14-3). Impaired autoregulation is associated with hyperperfusion, vasospasm, and decreased CO_2 reactivity. Not surprisingly, it is also associated with an unfavorable outcome.[107]

Orthostatic hypotension and syncope. In patients with multiple system atrophy or autosomally inherited dopamine-β hydroxylase deficiency—both diseases associated with autonomic nervous system failure—a clinically asymptomatic orthostatic MABP drop of approximately 20% causes a 16% decrease of the MCA mean FV but no CBF changes.[15] This suggests reactive vasodilatation of the M1 segment and reduction of cerebrovascular resistance.[15] Autoregulation is also intact in the Shy-Drager syndrome,[14] a condition associated with orthostatic hypotension and syncope. The TCD findings suggest that in symptomatic patients with these disorders, severe blood pressure drops can overcome cerebral autoregulatory mechanisms. Figures 14-4 and 14-5, respectively, present TCD findings following postural changes in a healthy subject and in a patient with symptomatic orthostatic hypotension.

Combined tilt-table and TCD testing results suggest that patients with syncope of unknown etiology can be divided into at least three subpopulations:[34] (1) patients with drops in MABP and mean FV and an increase (or no change) in the heart rate during testing, presumed to have vasodepressor syncope; (2) subjects with drops of MABP, pulse, and mean FV, categorized of having vasovagal syncope; and (3) patients without a drop in

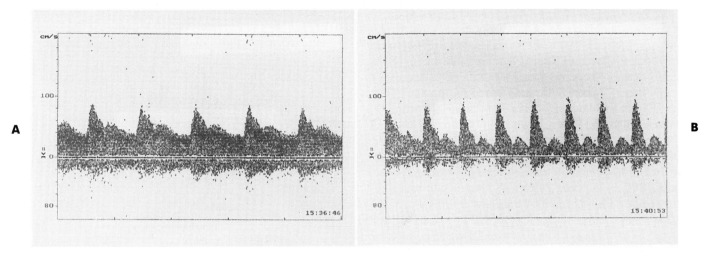

Fig. 14-4. Effect of postural changes on intracranial blood flow in a healthy control. The middle cerebral artery is insonated. **A,** The subject is supine and the blood pressure is 110/70 mm Hg. **B,** Twenty seconds after resumption of the upright position, the blood pressure is 110/90 mm Hg, diastolic flow has decreased and the pulsatility index has increased, indicating an active autoregulatory response.

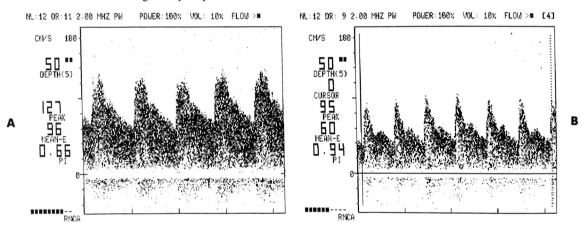

Fig. 14-5. Effect of postural changes on intracranial blood flow in a patient with autoimmune autonomic neuropathy and symptomatic orthostatic hypotension. The middle cerebral artery is insonated. **A,** The patient is supine and the blood pressure is 120/70 mm Hg. **B,** The recording was obtained approximately 60 seconds after the patient stood up from a lying position; the corresponding blood pressure was 85/50 mm Hg. (Courtesy of Dr. F. Romanul.)

MABP but with a significant decrease of mean FV. The mechanism of disease in the third subgroup has been described as "cerebral syncope" by Gomez and colleagues.[34] The last subgroup is of special interest because the laboratory findings are consistent with a primary disorder of cerebral autoregulation.

Sudden increases in intracranial pressure. In normal individuals, a cerebral perfusion pressure of approximately 70 to 85 mm Hg is sufficiently large to permit adequate CBF. However, in some clinical settings, the MABP can drop or the intracranial pressure can increase, causing a reduction of cerebral perfusion pressure. The effects of conditions such as head trauma, leading to prolonged increased intracranial pressure on

CBF and TCD parameters, are reviewed in Chapter 17. Transient, marked increases in intracranial pressure causing loss of consciousness can also be seen in cough syncope and in subarachnoid hemorrhage at the time of aneurysmal rupture.[27,37,76] The circulatory arrest and subsequent intracranial flow changes have been monitored with TCD.[37,76]

Vasoreactivity

Cerebrovascular reactivity refers to the responses of the cerebral arterial tree and the CBF to specific vasoactive substances. In individuals not receiving vasoactive pharmacologic agents, the major physiologic modulators of cerebrovascular resistance are CO_2[62] and

O_2.[69] As discussed earlier in this chapter, hypercapnia is a strong stimulus that can markedly increase CBF: At $Paco_2$ levels in the 38 to 42 mm Hg range, CBF increases by about 4% for each 1 mm Hg increase of $Paco_2$; flow drops of the same range correspond to similar decreases of the $Paco_2$. According to Lassen and Astrup, the effect of CO_2 is mediated by the pH of arteriolar smooth muscle cells. The latter depends on the blood CO_2 and intracellular HCO_3^- contents.[62] Because CO_2 easily diffuses through the endothelial cell membrane and hydrogen and bicarbonate ions cannot do so, intravascular CO_2 is a major determinant of cerebrovascular resistance. Using cerebral angiography, Huber and Handa have shown that, in response to a $Paco_2$ drop from 39 to 25.2 mm Hg, arteries 2.5 mm or more in diameter do not significantly change, whereas arteries with diameters of 0.5 to 2.5 mm have a mean narrowing of 8%.[45] They also reported that basal cerebral arteries with diameters exceeding 2.5 mm do not dilate when the Pao_2 is increased from 39.7 to 57.4 mm Hg. However, arteries with diameters of 2 to 2.5 mm and 1.5 to 2 mm dilate by 3.8% and 5%, respectively, and arterioles 0.5 to 1 mm, the smallest vessels that can be identified by angiography, dilate by 22.5%.[45] Variations in Pao_2 have the opposite effect to those in $Paco_2$. Although moderate changes do not affect cerebrovascular resistance, $Paco_2$ levels below approximately 50 mm Hg cause dilatation of pial arterioles 25 to 300 μm in diameter.[55,57] In summary, CBF responses to changes in $Paco_2$ or Pao_2 are predominantly mediated through dilatation or constriction of pial arteries and arterioles rather than the large arteries at the base of the brain.[18]

The cerebral arterial tree is also sensitive to a variety of chemical agents. They include medications such as nitroglycerin, which can vasodilate the proximal segments of intracranial arteries causing a drop in FVs,[20] and sumatriptan, which can increase FVs[16] but whose exact mechanism of action is not well understood. Acetazolamide, a carbonic anhydrase inhibitor, increases arterial CO_2 content and may also have a direct action on vascular smooth muscle cells,[43,110] thereby vasodilating cerebral vessels.[43] It is frequently used when cerebral arterial tone and vasoreactivity are tested. The precise effect of acetazolamide on the different cerebral vessels remains relatively unknown, but most investigators agree that it causes dilatation of small cerebral resistance arteries and arterioles. However, larger arteries may also respond to acetazolamide. Muller measured the MCA Doppler signal power and suggested that acetazolamide may cause dilatation of the MCA trunk.[80] Sorteberg and associates have compared FV and CBF changes after acetazolamide administration and, finding a larger increase in MCA, ACA and PCA FVs than in CBF in cerebral regions corresponding to these arteries, have

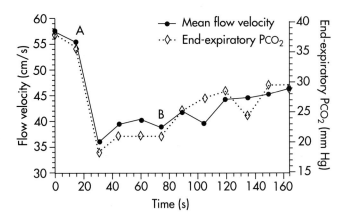

Fig. 14-6. Flow velocity response to Pco_2 changes following hyperventilation in a healthy subject. Note the tight coupling between changes in end-expiratory Pco_2 and middle cerebral artery mean flow velocity. *A* corresponds to the beginning and *B* to the end of hyperventilation.

suggested that the drug has a constricting effect on first segments of these arteries.[106]

As indicated in the preceding paragraphs, cerebrovascular reactivity is frequently tested following CO_2 or acetazolamide administration. Each of these methods has inherent limitations that restrict its applicability. Contradictory findings regarding the caliber of vessels most responsive to acetazolamide raise a question regarding the reliability of vasoreactivity testing with that medication. The relative stability of basal cerebral arteries following moderate changes of $Paco_2$ suggests that FV changes in the studied arterial segments correlate closely with CBF changes in the artery's territory. When the two methods are compared, CO_2 has a more powerful vasoactive effect.[50] For these reasons, CO_2 stimulation is the preferable method for assessment of cerebrovascular reactivity in patients who can cooperate.

In the following paragraphs, investigations of cerebral vasoreactivity based primarily on TCD technology are reviewed. Some feel that the results of cerebrovascular reactivity tests based on acetazolamide or CO_2 administration can be clinically helpful, for example, when selecting candidates for superficial temporal artery to MCA bypass surgery.[48,80] However, conclusive data showing that cerebrovascular reserve, as assessed by TCD, is a useful index of clinical outcome are available in only selected conditions.[51]

Assessment of normal vasoreactivity. In normal subjects, FVs decrease within 15 seconds from the onset of hyperventilation (Fig. 14-6)[71] and can drop by 35.3% from baseline values (Figs. 14-6 and 14-7).[94] They increase by as much as 52.5% during hypercapnia (Fig. 14-7). An exponential function[70,73] or a biasymptotic

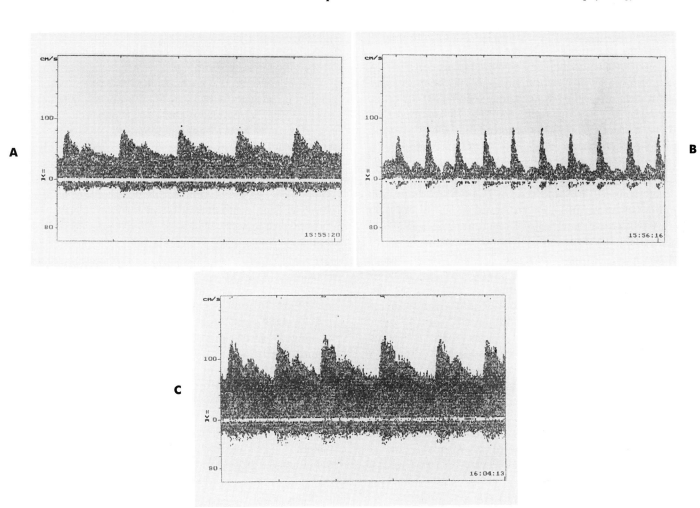

Fig. 14-7. Effect of P_{CO_2} changes on flow velocities in a healthy subject. **A,** The end-expiratory P_{CO_2} is 35 mm Hg, and the mean velocity is approximately 50 cm/s. **B,** The end-expiratory P_{CO_2} is 21 mm Hg after 45 seconds of hyperventilation, and the mean velocity is 33 cm/s. **C,** The recording was obtained after inhalation of 5% CO_2. The end-expiratory P_{CO_2} is 49 mm Hg, and the mean velocity is 88 cm/s.

curve[94] best describe the MCA FV and Pa_{CO_2} relationship (Fig. 14-1). Interestingly, the response to hypocapnia is enhanced after age 60.[6]

When administered intravenously, the effect of a 1000 mg acetazolamide bolus can be observed within less than 3 minutes, with FVs reaching a plateau within 10 minutes;[23] the latter is approximately 35% higher than the baseline MCA FV,[23,88,106] lasts more than 30 minutes,[88] and gradually decreases afterward. Increased FVs persist for 60 to 120 minutes.[23]

Assessment of vasoreactivity: disease states

Ischemic cerebrovascular disease. Cerebrovascular reactivity has been extensively studied with TCD in patients with risk factors for cerebral arterial disease. A significant FV increase from baseline is detected in insulin-dependent diabetics following intravenous acetazolamide administration, and mean FVs in these pa-

tients are lower than those of controls at all times.[23] Chronic hypertensives have baseline FVs similar to those of controls,[71,109] a diminished vasodilatory response to hypercapnia,[6] a greater vascular resistance,[109] and a rapid recovery of FVs from hypocapnia.[71] Interestingly, early-stage hypertensives demonstrate higher FVs than chronic hypertensive or normotensive subjects and have nearly normal arterial resistance.[109] A recent report by Rubba and colleagues also shows that, when compared to age- and sex-matched healthy controls, individuals with familial hypercholesterolemia have low baseline FVs and mildly increased pulsatility indices; FVs increase within 24 hours from low-density lipoprotein apheresis that does not have a significant effect on cardiac output, systemic vascular resistance, and viscosity.[96] When taken together, the preceding studies suggest that vascular risk factors have a chronic effect on the cerebral vasculature that precedes the development of symptoms of cerebral ischemia.

That cerebrovascular reactivity is impaired in patients with symptoms of cerebral ischemia has been demonstrated by extensive studies using xenon-133 and other methods.[84,85] Resting CBF is frequently decreased in these patients[3,84] on the symptomatic side.[84] A good correlation between TCD and SPECT assessment of vasoreactivity in patients with cerebrovascular disease[22] has prompted several TCD studies as well. Hemodynamic changes are detected by TCD in asymptomatic patients with carotid stenosis[19] and are more severe in those who have symptoms of cerebral ischemia.[19,94] In the latter, impairment in vasomotor reactivity is more severe on the symptomatic side.[79] The main finding in these patients consists of a reduction, when compared to normal patients, of FV changes in response to the vasoactive agents (see Plates 58 to 61). Because acetazolamide and hypercapnia are potent arteriolar vasodilators, the reduction implies that these arterioles undergo chronic autoregulatory vasodilatation[11] with a subsequent drop in vascular resistance and reduction of autoregulatory range. Decreased pulsatility and resistivity indices distal to carotid occlusion further confirm the notion of arteriolar vasodilatation and reduced cerebrovascular resistance.[101] Positron emission tomography studies indicate that this state of vasodilatation is consistent with the finding of increased cerebral blood volume distal to occluded arteries[31] and that it is accompanied by an increased oxygen extraction fraction.[47] As a result of vasodilatation, a significant redistribution of blood flow in favor of the nonoccluded side can occur following acetazolamide injections, with a drop in CBF distal to the stenosed ICA.[115] This has also been described as a steal phenomenon.[88]

The finding of severe impairment of vasoreactivity in a higher proportion of patients with borderzone rather than "territorial" cerebral infarcts[91] provides further support to the traditional notion of hemodynamic compromise in these individuals. Vasoreactivity is impaired distal to cervical ICA lesions, causing occlusion or more than 70% stenosis.[19,48,70,91,94] In spite of this, not all cervical ICA stenoses cause distal hemodynamic compromise, and the severity of extracranial occlusive disease does not reliably identify patients with impaired vasoreactivity.[65] It has been suggested that collateral flow through the circle of Willis is a useful predictor of the cerebral perfusion reserve.[19] Interestingly, collateral flow through the ophthalmic artery is identified more frequently ipsilateral to hemispheres with impaired rather than intact vasoreactivity.[53] These TCD findings are confirmed by PET studies and indicate that although ICA stenosis can impair CO_2 reactivity,[64] severity of stenosis and residual carotid artery lumen are not

reliable indices of the cerebral circulation's hemodynamic status.[90] Rather, PET findings suggest that collateral flow is the primary determinant of cerebral perfusion pressure.[90] The presence of reduced vasoreactivity in patients with lacunar infarction[70] indicates, however, that hypertensive changes at the level of small arterioles may be an independent contributor to impaired reactivity unrelated to the presence of carotid stenosis.

The clinical significance of impaired cerebral perfusion reserve has been examined in several recent studies. Using TCD to evaluate perfusion reserve, Kleiser and Widder prospectively followed 85 patients with ICA occlusion for a mean interval of 38 months.[51] A significantly increased incidence of transient ischemic attack and cerebral infarction was present in those patients with an exhausted reserve at the time of enrollment. In another study of patients with more than 70% stenosis or occlusion of an ICA, vascular reserve was assessed by the xenon-CT method, and those with a compromised reserve and relatively low baseline CBF had a higher rate of stroke ipsilateral to the compromised territory.[120] These findings are contradicted by a small PET study not showing a consistent correlation between cerebral hemodynamic impairment and subsequent infarction.[89] In spite of these limitations, decreased CBF and impaired cerebrovascular reserve capacity have been used as clinical indices to select candidates for superficial temporal artery to MCA anastomosis,[48,59,115] and an increase in regional vasodilatory capacity has been shown in the majority of patients following surgery,[48,115] even when CBF is not increased.[119] Vasoreactivity also returns to normal following carotid endarterectomy.[79,97] However, whether these measures are effective in reducing the risk of subsequent ipsilateral infarction remains unknown. It should also be noted that the methodologic limitations presented in the beginning sections of this chapter are seldom taken into account in most of these studies.

Intracerebral hemorrhage. Cerebral vasoreactivity is also reduced in patients with intracerebral hemorrhage.[52] It is slightly decreased when the intracranial pressure increase is only mild or moderate, and it is severely impaired in those with marked pressure elevations. Marked reductions in reactivity are associated with a poor outcome.[52]

Subarachnoid hemorrhage. In addition to a global reduction of CBF that can be seen during the first 10 days after aneurysmal subarachnoid hemorrhage,[75] most patients develop focal areas of low perfusion. The latter has been attributed to vasospasm and is present in 77% of Hunt and Hess grades I and II patients and in 100% of those in grades III, IV, and V.[104] Low perfusion areas become more prominent between days 9 and 14 and gradually resolve afterwards.[104] The extent of flow reduction is less and its duration is shorter in patients with good outcomes.

Clinical[104] and laboratory[83] studies show that cerebrovascular reactivity is impaired following subarachnoid hemorrhage. With increased severity of vasospasm, there is a gradual reduction of the arterial response to $Paco_2$ changes.[42] In most of these patients, although the reaction to hypocapnia is normal, the hypercapneic response is weak because of chronic, maximal vasodilatation of small arteries and arterioles compensating for ischemia. The response to acetazolamide is blunted as well.[44] These findings are confirmed by PET studies showing elevated cerebral blood volume in grade III and IV patients.[38] The course of impaired vasoreactivity usually parallels that of vasospasm: Vasoreactivity declines before ischemic symptoms are clinically evident[44] and returns to normal usually within 4 to 6 weeks from the onset of hemorrhage. Nimodipine, a frequently used calcium channel blocker, has been known to have no effect on CO_2 reactivity.[102]

As noted in the Autoregulation section, there is an increased risk of hypotensive episodes during the weeks following aneurysmal hemorrhage. The decreased vasomotor reserve is of concern in this context because of the risk of ischemic complications with hypotension. In the animal model, a pressure-passive fall in CBF but not FV has been shown at an MABP of 100 mm Hg or less.[83] Whether such a high MABP threshold is also valid at the bedside is not known, but the laboratory findings emphasize the need to maintain the MABP within narrow limits in these patients.

TCD studies of cerebrovascular reactivity in patients with arteriovenous malformations are limited in number.[25,74] Resistance is reduced in feeding arteries.[74] Flow through these vessels is pressure passive because the malformation's nidus lacks resistance arterioles. In spite of these findings, FVs are increased, and vasoreactivity is frequently decreased in these arteries.[25] Vasoreactivity may also be reduced in nonfeeding arteries ipsilateral or contralateral to the malformation.[25]

Trauma. The intracranial hemodynamic sequelae of head injury include vasospasm, luxury perfusion, and impaired autoregulation and vasoreactivity. Not all patients with head trauma have impaired vasoreactivity.[67,103] The latter is frequently decreased in individuals with severe neurologic deficits[67,103] who have a Glasgow Coma Scale score of 5 or less;[103] it returns to nearly normal values with improvement of the scores, usually after the first week following trauma. Whether reduced vasoreactivity is of prognostic value is not clear: Although severe impairment has also been associated with poor outcome,[67] some degree of impairment seems to be present in all outcome groups.[107] Reduced CO_2 reactiv-

ity correlates with hyperperfusion and decreased autoregulation but not vasospasm.[107]

EFFECT OF CARDIAC DISORDERS ON TRANSCRANIAL DOPPLER MEASUREMENTS

Transcranial Doppler studies of CBF are usually performed with the assumption that pulse and cardiac output are stable or vary minimally during the testing period. Although this assumption is justified in the majority of patients, persistent cardiac dysrhythemias can introduce an additional variable in TCD measurements that limits the use of standard TCD indices. The effect of selected cardiac disorders on CBF and TCD measurements are reviewed in the following paragraphs.

Although the majority of cardiac rhythm changes of short duration are not associated with clinically detectable neurologic dysfunction, severe bradycardia and some tachydysrhythmias can induce dizziness or syncope.[113] The impact of cardiac dysrhythmias of short duration on cerebral circulation has been difficult to assess and is not well understood because of technical limitations. However, the impact of chronic dysrhythmias has been assessed previously.[63,87] For example, CBF is decreased in patients with atrial fibrillation who are not in heart failure[63,87] and increases by 3.6% at 24 hours and 10.1% at 30 days from cardioversion to sinus rhythm.[87] TCD studies show that in atrial fibrillation the peak and mean FVs are lower than those of controls.[5] In addition, there is an increased beat-to-beat variation in FVs (Fig. 14-8) and in the pulsatility index.[5] FVs corresponding to premature ventricular contractions are also more than 30% lower than velocities of beats that precede or follow them.[4] During ventricular fibrillation, FVs decay more rapidly than the systemic pressure, falling to zero within 14 seconds.[60] Interestingly, in patients with ventricular tachycardia, FVs can remain unchanged or drop without reaching zero.[60] In addition, TCD has been used to assess the effect of cardiopulmonary resuscitation following cardiac arrest:[35,112] Although antegrade flow is detected with adequate chest compressions, in most patients, either no signal is detected or a to-and-fro pattern is seen between compressions, indicating inadequate cerebral perfusion.[112] Unfortunately, the preceding preliminary observations have not been confirmed by large studies. The effect of cardiac dysrhythmias should be taken into account in interpreting TCD results.

As discussed in the Autoregulation section, according to the traditional notion of cerebral autoregulation, CBF does not significantly change when the MABP fluctuates within certain limits. This concept may not be valid in some disease states. In the animal model, although CBF is not affected by manipulations of the cardiac output in normals, it varies directly with cardiac output in animals with ischemic brains.[111] Baseline CBF can also be

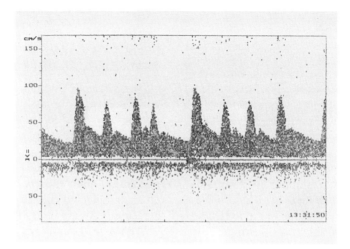

Fig. 14-8. Middle cerebral artery Doppler spectra in a patient with atrial fibrillation. Note the beat-to-beat variation in flow velocities.

decreased in patients with severe congestive heart failure but does not change[86] or improves[92] after the administration of antihypertensive agents, even when the blood pressure drops.[86,92] In addition, PET shows that in congestive heart failure, the local cerebral metabolic rate for glucose is approximately one third of the normal value; it increases significantly in the cortical gray matter after a dobutamine infusion, which causes an increase in cardiac output and oxygen delivery.[95] TCD studies of patients with congestive heart failure show a drop in peak and mean FVs when compared to controls,[5] possibly reflecting the decreased cardiac index[98] and its effect on CBF.[85,92]

CONCLUSION

Transcranial Doppler ultrasonography's ease of use, noninvasiveness, and versatility have permitted its utilization in the monitoring of cerebral hemodynamic changes in a variety of clinical and research settings. The findings of this review indicate that established TCD applications include the assessment of CBF and cerebrovascular physiology. However, significant theoretical considerations and technical limitations restrict these applications. When these limitations are taken into account, TCD can provide useful information.

This review also shows that the number of TCD studies of CBF and cerebrovascular physiology with a potential for an impact on patient care remains limited. It is hoped that the introduction of new technical developments and the completion of well-designed studies will provide new information that can be used to improve patient well-being.

REFERENCES

1. Aaslid R, et al: Cerebral autoregulation dynamics in humans, *Stroke* 20:45-52, 1989.

2. Aaslid R, et al: Assessment of cerebral autoregulation dynamics from simultaneous arterial and venous transcranial Doppler recordings in humans, *Stroke* 22:1148-1154, 1991.
3. Ackerman RH, et al: Extracranial vascular disease and cerebral blood flow in patients with transient ischemic attacks, *Acta Neurol Scand Suppl* 60(suppl 72):442-443, 1979.
4. Ameriso SF, Sager P, Fisher M: Effect of premature ventricular contractions on middle cerebral artery blood flow velocity, *J Neuroimaging* 1:129-133, 1991.
5. Ameriso SF, Sager P, Fisher M: Atrial fibrillation, congestive heart failure, and the middle cerebral artery, *J Neuroimaging* 2:190-194, 1992.
6. Ameriso SF, et al: Age, hypertension, and cerebral vasomotor reactivity, *Ann Neurol* 34:254, 1993, (abstract).
7. Arts MGJ, Roevros JM: On the instantaneous measurement of bloodflow by ultrasonic means, *Med Biol Eng* 10:23-34, 1972.
8. Bakay L, Sweet WH: Cervical and intracranial intra-arterial pressures with and without vascular occlusion, *Surg Gynecol Obstet* 95:67-75, 1972.
9. Bentsen N, Larsen B, Lassen NA: Chronically impaired autoregulation of cerebral blood flow in long term diabetics, *Stroke* 6:497-502, 1975.
10. Bing BA, Waddington MM: Intraluminal diameters of the intracranial arteries, *Vasc Surg* 1:137-151, 1967.
11. Bishop CCR, et al: Transcranial Doppler measurement of middle cerebral artery blood flow velocity: a validation study, *Stroke* 17:913-915, 1986.
12. Boysen G, et al: Cerebral blood flow and internal carotid flow during carotid surgery, *Stroke* 1:253-260, 1970.
13. Brass LM, et al: Middle cerebral artery blood velocity and cerebral blood flow in sickle cell disease, *Stroke* 22:27-30, 1991.
14. Briebach T, Laubenberger J, Fischer PA: Transcranial Doppler sonographic studies of cerebral autoregulation in Shy-Drager syndrome, *J Neurol* 236:349-350, 1989.
15. Brooks DJ, et al: The effect of orthostatic hypotension on cerebral blood flow and middle cerebral artery velocity in autonomic failure, with observations on the action of ephedrine, *J Neurol Neurosurg Psychiatry* 52:962-966, 1989.
16. Caekebeke JF, et al: Antimigraine drug sumatriptan increases blood flow velocity in large cerebral arteries during migraine attacks. *Neurology* 42:1522-1526, 1992.
17. Chan KH, et al: The effect of changes in cerebral perfusion

pressure upon middle cerebral artery blood flow velocity and jugular bulb venous oxygen saturation after severe brain injury, *J Neurosurg* 77:55-61, 1992.

18. Chehrazi BB, Youmans JR: *Cerebral blood flow in neurosurgery.* In Youmans JR, editor: *Neurological surgery,* Philadelphia, 1990, WB Saunders.

19. Chimowitz MI, et al: Transcranial Doppler assessment of cerebral perfusion reserve in patients with carotid occlusive disease and no evidence of cerebral infarction, *Neurology* 43:353-357, 1993.

20. Dahl A, et al: Effect of nitroglycerin on cerebral circulation measured by transcranial Doppler and SPECT, *Stroke* 20:1733-1736, 1989.

21. Dahl A, et al: Vasoreactivity assessed by transcranial Doppler ultrasound and regional cerebral blood flow measurements, *Stroke* 24:498, 1993 (abstract).

22. Dahl A, et al: Cerebral vasoreactivity in unilateral carotid artery disease, *Stroke* 25:621-626, 1994.

23. De Chiara S, et al: Cerebrovascular reactivity by transcranial Doppler ultrasonography in insulin-dependent diabetic patients, *Cerebrovasc Dis* 3:111-115, 1993.

24. DeWitt LD, Rosengart A, Teal PA: *Transcranial Doppler ultrasonography: normal values.* In Babikian VL, Wechsler LR, editors: *Transcranial Doppler ultrasonography,* St Louis, 1993, Mosby–Year Book.

25. Diehl RR, et al: Blood flow velocity and vasomotor reactivity in patients with arteriovenous malformations, *Stroke* 25:1574-1580, 1994.

26. Edvinsson L, MacKenzie ET, McCulloch J: *Cerebral blood flow and metabolism,* New York, 1993, Raven Press.

27. Eng CC, et al: The diagnosis and management of a perianesthetic cerebral aneurysmal rupture aided with transcranial Doppler ultrasonography, *Anesthesiology* 78:191-194, 1993.

28. Faraci FM, Heistad DD: Regulation of large cerebral arteries and cerebral microvascular pressure, *Stroke* 66:8-17, 1990.

29. Fog M: The relationship between the blood pressure and the tonic regulation of the pial arteries, *J Neurol Psychiatry* 1:187-197, 1938.

30. Gabrielsen TO, Greitz T: Normal size of the internal carotid, middle cerebral and anterior cerebral arteries, *Acta Radiol* 10:1-10, 1970.

31. Gibbs JM, et al: Evaluation of cerebral perfusion reserve in patients with carotid artery occlusion, *Lancet* 1:310-314, 1984.

32. Giller CA, et al: The cerebral hemodynamics of normotensive hypovolemia during lower-body negative pressure, *J Neurosurg* 76:961-966, 1992.

33. Giller CA, et al: Cerebral arterial diameters during changes in blood pressure and carbon dioxide during craniotomy, *Neurosurgery* 32:737-742, 1993.

34. Gomez CR, Janosik DL, Lewis LM: *Transcranial Doppler in the evaluation of global cerebral ischemia: syncope and cardiac arrest,* In Babikian VL, Wechsler LR, editors: *Transcranial Doppler ultrasonography,* St Louis, 1993, Mosby–Year Book.

35. Gomez CR, et al: Assessment of the cerebral hemodynamic effect of CPR using transcranial Doppler, *Neurology* 40:145, 1990 (abstract).

36. Gomez CR, et al: Transcranial Doppler findings in acute spontaneous recanalization of middle cerebral artery embolism, *J Neuroimaging* 1:63-67, 1991.

37. Grote E, Hassler W: The critical first minutes after subarachnoid hemorrhage, *Neurosurgery* 22:654-661, 1988.

38. Grubb RL, et al: Effects of subarachnoid hemorrhage on cerebral blood volume, blood flow, and oxygen utilization in humans, *J Neurosurg* 46:446-453, 1977.

39. Halsey JH, et al: Blood velocity in the middle cerebral artery and regional cerebral blood flow during carotid endarterectomy, *Stroke* 20:53-58, 1989.

40. Hartmann A, et al: Correlation of regional cerebral blood flow and blood flow velocity in normal volunteers and patients with cerebro-vascular disease, *Neurochirurgia (Stuttg)* 34:6-13, 1991.

41. Hashi K, et al: Cerebral hemodynamics and metabolic changes after experimental subarachnoid hemorrhage, *J Neurol Sci* 17:1-14, 1972.

42. Hassler W, Chioffi F: CO_2 reactivity of cerebral vasospasm after aneurysmal subarachnoid hemorrhage, *Acta Neurochir (Wien)* 98:167-175, 1989.

43. Hauge A, Nicolaysen G, Thoresen M: Acute effects of acetazolamide on cerebral blood flow in man, *Acta Physiol Scand* 117:233-239, 1983.

44. Hiramatsu K, et al: The evaluation of the cerebrovascular reactivity to acetazolamide by transcranial Doppler ultrasound after subarachnoid hemorrhage, *Stroke* 21:69, 1990. (abstract).

45. Huber P, Handa J: Effect of contrast material, hypercapnia, hyperventilation, hypertonic glucose and papaverine on the diameter of cerebral arteries, *Invest Radiol* 2:17-32, 1967.

46. Ishii R: Regional cerebral blood flow in patients with ruptured intracranial aneurysm, *J Neurosurg* 50:587-594, 1979.

47. Kanno I, et al: Oxygen extraction fraction at maximally vasodilated tissue in the ischemic brain estimated from the regional CO_2 responsiveness measured by positron emission tomography, *J Cereb Blood Flow Metab* 8:227-235, 1988.

48. Karnik R, et al: Evaluation of vasomotor reactivity by transcranial Doppler and acetazolamide test before and after extracranial-intracranial bypass in patients with internal carotid artery occlusion, *Stroke* 23:812-817, 1992.

49. Kirkham FJ, et al: Transcranial measurement of blood velocities in the basal cerebral arteries using pulsed Doppler ultrasound: velocity as an index of flow, *Ultrasound Med Biol* 12:15-21, 1986.

50. Kleiser B, Scholl D, Widder B: Assessment of cerebrovascular reactivity by Doppler CO_2 and diamox testing: which is the appropriate method? *Cerebrovasc Dis* 4:134-138, 1994.

51. Kleiser B, Widder B: Course of carotid artery occlusions with impaired cerebrovascular reactivity, *Stroke* 23:171-174, 1992.

52. Klingelhöfer J, Sander D: Doppler CO_2 test as an indicator of cerebral vasoreactivity and prognosis in severe intracranial hemorrhages, *Stroke* 23:962-966, 1992.

53. Knop J, et al: ^{99m}Tc-HMPAO-SPECT with acetazolamide challenge to detect hemodynamic compromise in occlusive cerebrovascular disease, *Stroke* 23:1733-1742, 1992.

54. Kofke AW: *Transcranial Doppler ultrasonography in anesthesia.* In Babikian VL, Wechsler LR, editors: *Transcranial Doppler ultrasonography,* St Louis, 1993, Mosby–Year Book.

55. Kogure K, et al: Mechanisms of cerebral vasodilatation in hypoxia, *J Appl Physiol* 29:223-229, 1970.

56. Kontos HA: Validity of cerebral arterial blood flow calculations from velocity measurements, *Stroke* 20:1-3, 1989.

57. Kontos HA, et al: Role of tissue hypoxia in local regulation of cerebral microcirculation, *Am J Physiol* 234:H582-H591, 1978.

58. Kontos HA, et al: Responses of cerebral arteries and arterioles to acute hypotension and hypertension, *Am J Physiol* 234:H371-H383, 1978.

59. Kuroda S, et al: Acetazolamide test in detecting reduced cerebral perfusion reserve and predicting long-term prognosis in patients with internal carotid artery occlusion, *Neurosurgery* 32:912-919, 1993.

60. Lash SR, et al: Continuous transcranial Doppler monitoring during ventricular fibrillation and ventricular tachycardia in humans, *Stroke* 23:467, 1992 (abstract).

61. Lassen NA: Cerebral blood flow and oxygen consumption in man, *Physiol Rev* 39:183-238, 1959.

62. Lassen NA, Astrup J: *Cerebral blood flow: normal regulation and*

ischemic thresholds. In Weinstein PR, Faden AI, editors: *Protection of the brain from ischemia,* Baltimore, 1990, Williams & Wilkins.

63. Lavy S, et al: Effect of chronic atrial fibrillation on regional cerebral blood flow, *Stroke* 11:35-38, 1980.

64. Levine RL: Blood flow reactivity to hypercapnia in strictly unilateral carotid disease: preliminary results, *J Neurol Neurosurg Psychiatry* 54:204-209, 1991.

65. Ley-Pozo J, Willmes K, Ringelstein EB: Relationship between pulstatility indices of Doppler flow signals and CO_2 reactivity within the middle cerebral artery in extracranial occlusive disease, *Ultrasound Med Biol* 16:763-772, 1990.

66. Lindegaard KF, et al: Variations in middle cerebral artery blood flow investigated with noninvasive transcranial blood velocity measurements, *Stroke* 18:1025-1030, 1987.

67. Lundar T, Lindegaard KF, Nornes H: Continuous recording of middle cerebral artery blood velocity in clinical neurosurgery, *Acta Neurochir (Wien)* 102:85-90, 1990.

68. MacKenzie ET, et al: Effects of hemorrhagic hypotension on the cerebral circulation, *Stroke* 10:711-718, 1979.

69. Macko RF, et al: Arterial oxygen content and age are determinants of middle cerebral artery blood flow velocity, *Stroke* 24:1025-1028, 1993.

70. Maeda H, et al: Reactivity of cerebral blood flow to carbon dioxide in various types of ischemic cerebrovascular disease: evaluation by the transcranial Doppler method, *Stroke* 24:670-675, 1993.

71. Malatino LS, et al: Cerebral blood flow velocity after hyperventilation-induced vasoconstriction in hypertensive patients, *Stroke* 23:1728-1732, 1992.

72. Marinkovic SV, et al: Perforating branches of the middle cerebral artery, *Stroke* 16:1022-1029, 1985.

73. Markwalder TM, et al: Dependency of blood flow velocity in the middle cerebral artery on the end-tidal carbon dioxide partial pressure: a transcranial Doppler study, *J Cereb Blood Flow Metab* 4:368-372, 1984.

74. Massaro AR, et al: Characterization of arteriovenous malformation feeding vessels by carbon dioxide reactivity, *AJNR AMJ Neuroradiol* 15:55-61, 1994.

75. Matsuda M, Shiino A, Handa J: Sequential changes of cerebral blood flow after aneurysmal subarachnoid hemorrhage, *Acta Neurochir (Wien)* 105:98-106, 1990.

76. Mattle HP, et al: Transient cerebral circulatory arrest coincides with fainting in cough syncope, *Cerebrovasc Dis* 4:232, 1994 (abstract).

77. Mchedlishvili G: Physiological mechanisms controlling cerebral blood flow, *Stroke* 11:240-248, 1980.

78. Mchedlishvili GI, Mitagvaria NP, Ormotsadze LG: Vascular mechanisms controlling a constant blood supply to the brain ("autoregulation"), *Stroke* 4:742-750, 1973.

79. Miller JD, Smith RR, Holaday HR: Carbon dioxide reactivity in the evaluation of cerebral ischemia, *Neurosurgery* 30: 518-521, 1992.

80. Muller HR: Evaluation of vasomotor reactivity by transcranial Doppler and acetazolamide test before and after extracranial-intracranial bypass, *Stroke* 23:1840, 1992.

81. Muller HR, et al: Response of middle cerebral artery volume flow to orthostasis, *Cerebrovasc Dis* 1:82-89, 1991.

82. Naylor AR, et al: Parametric imaging of cerebral vascular reserve, *Eur J Nucl Med* 18:259-264, 1991.

83. Nelson RJ, et al: Transcranial Doppler ultrasound studies of cerebral autoregulation and subarachnoid hemorrhage in the rabbit, *J Neurosurg* 73:601-610, 1990.

84. Norrving B, Nilsson B, Risberg J: rCBF in patients with carotid occlusion: resting and hypercapneic flow related to collateral pattern, *Stroke* 13:155-162, 1982.

85. Paulson OB, Strandgaard S, Edvinsson L: Cerebral autoregulation, *Cerebrovasc Brain Metab Rev* 2:161-192, 1990.

86. Paulson OB, et al: Effect of captopril on the cerebral circulation in chronic heart failure, *Eur J Clin Invest* 16:124-132, 1986.

87. Petersen P, et al: Cerebral blood flow before and after cardioversion of atrial fibrillation, *J Cereb Blood Flow Metab* 9:422-425, 1989.

88. Piepgras A, et al: A simple test to assess cerebrovascular reserve capacity using transcranial Doppler sonography and acetazolamide, *Stroke* 21:1306-1311, 1990.

89. Powers WJ, Tempel LW, Grubb RL: Influence of cerebral hemodynamics on stroke risk: one year follow-up of 30 medically treated patients, *Ann Neurol* 25:325-330, 1989.

90. Powers WJ, et al: The effect of hemodynamically significant carotid artery disease on the hemodynamic status of the cerebral circulation, *Ann Intern Med* 106:27-35, 1987.

91. Provinciali L, Ceravolo MG, Minicotti P: A transcranial Doppler study of vasomotor reactivity in symptomatic carotid occlusion, *Cerebrovasc Dis* 3:27-32, 1993.

92. Rajagopalan B, et al: Changes in cerebral blood flow in patients with severe congestive heart failure before and after captopril treatment, *Am J Med* 76(supplement 5B):86-89, 1984.

93. Ringelstein EB, Otis SM: *Physiological testing of vasomotor reserve.* In Newell DW, Aaslid R, editors: *Transcranial Doppler,* New York, 1992, Raven Press.

94. Ringelstein EB, et al: Noninvasive assessment of CO_2-induced cerebral vasomotor response in normal individuals and patients with internal carotid artery occlusions, *Stroke* 19:963-969, 1988.

95. Ross DJ, et al: Regional metabolic supply dependency in chronic congestive heart failure, *J Intensive Care Med* 8:87-90, 1993.

96. Rubba P, et al: Cerebral blood flow velocity and systemic vascular resistance after acute reduction of low-density lipoprotein in familial hypercholesterolemia, *Stroke* 24:1154-1161, 1993.

97. Russell D, et al: Cerebral vasoreactivity and blood flow before and 3 months after carotid endarterectomy, *Stroke* 21:1029-1032, 1990.

98. Saha M, et al: The impact of cardiac index on cerebral hemodynamics, *Stroke* 24:1686-1690, 1993.

99. Saver JL, Feldmann E: *Basic transcranial examination: technique and anatomy.* In Babikian VL, Wechsler LR, editors: *Transcranial Doppler ultrasonography,* St Louis, 1993, Mosby–Year Book.

100. Schöning M, Walter J, Scheel P: Estimation of cerebral blood flow through color duplex sonography of the carotid and vertebral arteries in healthy adults, *Stroke* 25:17-22, 1994.

101. Schwarze JJ, et al: Intracranial arterial resistance during carotid endarterectomy evaluated by transcranial Doppler ultrasound, *Ann Neurol* 34:289, 1993 (abstract).

102. Seiler RW, Nirkko A: Effect of nimodipine on cerebrovascular response to CO_2 in asymptomatic individuals and patients with subarachnoid hemorrhage: a transcranial Doppler ultrasound study, *Neurosurgery* 27:247-251, 1990.

103. Shigemori M, et al: Intracranial haemodynamics in diffuse and focal brain injuries: evaluation with transcranial Doppler ultrasound, *Acta Neurochir (Wien)* 107:5-10, 1990.

104. Shinoda J, et al: Acetazolamide reactivity on cerebral blood flow in patients with subarachnoid hemorrhage, *Acta Neurochir (Wien)* 109:102-108, 1991.

105. Sorteberg W, et al: Blood velocity and regional blood flow in defined cerebral arterial systems, *Acta Neurochir (Wien)* 97:47-52, 1989.

106. Sorteberg W, et al: Effect of acetazolamide on cerebral artery blood velocity and regional cerebral blood flow in normal subjects, *Acta Neurochir (Wien)* 97:139-145, 1989.

107. Steiger HJ, et al: Transcranial Doppler monitoring in head injury: relations between type of injury, flow velocities, vasoreactivity, and outcome, *Neurosurgery* 34:79-86, 1994.

108. Stromberg DD, Fox J: Pressures in the pial arterial microcirculation of the cat during changes in systemic arterial blood pressure, *Circ Res* 31:229-239, 1972.

109. Sugimori H, et al: Cerebral hemodynamics in hypertensive patients compared with normotensive volunteers, *Stroke* 25:1384-1389, 1994.

110. Sullivan HG, et al: The rCBF response to diamox in normal subjects and cerebrovascular disease patients, *J Neurosurg* 67:525-534, 1987.

111. Tranmer BI, et al: Loss of cerebral autoregulation during cardiac output variations in focal cerebral ischemia, *J Neurosurg* 77:253-259, 1992.

112. Trimble BA, et al: Transcranial Doppler during cardiopulmonary resuscitation, *Neurology* 40:144, 1990 (abstract).

113. Van Durme JP: Tachyarrhythmias and transient cerebral ischemic attacks, *Am Heart J* 89:538-540, 1975.

114. Vinall PE, Simeone FA: Cerebral autoregulation: An *in vivo* study, *Stroke* 12:640-642, 1981.

115. Vorstrup S, Brun B, Lassen NA: Evaluation of the cerebral vasodilatory capacity by the acetazolamide test before EC-IC bypass surgery in patients with occlusion of the internal carotid artery, *Stroke* 17:1291-1298, 1986.

116. Wahlgren NG, et al: Sympathetic nerve stimulation in humans increases middle cerebral artery blood flow velocity, *Cerebrovasc Dis* 2:359-364, 1992.

117. Wei EP, et al: Determinants of response of pial arteries to norepinephrine and sympathetic nerve stimulation, *Stroke* 6:654-658, 1975.

118. Wood JH: *Cerebral blood flow,* New York, 1987, McGraw-Hill.

119. Yamashita I, et al: The effect of EC-IC bypass surgery on resting cerebral blood flow and cerebrovascular reserve capacity studied with stable Xe-CT and acetazolamide test, *Neuroradiology* 33:217-222, 1991.

120. Yonas H, et al: Increased stroke risk predicted by compromised cerebral blood flow reactivity, *J Neurosurg* 79:483-489, 1993.

121. Zanette EM, et al: Transcranial Doppler ultrasonography and single photon emission tomography following cerebral infarction, *Cerebrovasc Dis* 3:37-374, 1993.

122. Zierler BK, et al: Accuracy of duplex scanning for measurement of arterial volume flow, *J Vasc Surg* 16:520-526, 1992.

Transcranial Doppler Monitoring of Vasospasm after Subarachnoid Hemorrhage

Michael A. Sloan

Delayed narrowing or vasoconstriction of intracerebral arteries, or vasospasm (VSP), is detectable on cerebral angiography in 21% to 70% of patients who suffer subarachnoid hemorrhage (SAH) due to a ruptured berry aneurysm.[128,150,159,167] Vasospasm may also occur following lobar hemorrhage with extension to the subarachnoid space[147] or SAH of unknown cause.[6,125] Angiographic VSP following aneurysmal SAH tends to occur between days 2 and 17 after SAH, with maximal severity between days 7 and 12. Rarely, VSP may last for 3 to 4 weeks or even longer.[159,167] Recent data from the International Cooperative Study in the Timing of Aneurysm Surgery (CASTOS) study suggest that the overall rate of focal neurologic deficits attributable to VSP ("clinical VSP") is 24% by 14 days.[159] Vasospasm-related ischemic neurologic deficits are the major cause of morbidity and mortality in survivors of aneurysmal SAH.[75,76,159,166,168] Given these adverse outcomes, early, reliable diagnosis and timely institution of treatment may well mitigate the devastating consequences of this disorder.

In 1982, Aaslid and associates[1] described the method of transcranial Doppler sonography (TCD) and immediately demonstrated its ability to noninvasively detect flow velocity (FV) acceleration attributable to VSP.[2,3] It is felt that TCD is of established value in the detection and monitoring of VSP following SAH.* However, the reliability of TCD in clinical management has recently been questioned.[85,113]

This chapter has five objectives: First, the pathoanatomy and pathophysiology of VSP are reviewed to provide a basis for understanding the phenomena that can be evaluated by TCD in this setting. Second, general aspects of the investigation of VSP by TCD are discussed. Third, the sensitivity and specificity of TCD, as well as reasons for inaccurate test results, are presented. Fourth, strategies to improve the accuracy of TCD are explored. Finally, general guidelines that illustrate the value of TCD in clinical management of SAH patients are provided.

*References 26, 28, 50, 86, 92, 94, 95, 110, 139, 143.

VASOSPASM: PATHOPHYSIOLOGIC CONSIDERATIONS

Current understanding of the mechanism(s), pathogenesis, and evaluation of VSP following SAH have recently been reviewed.[41,74,98,152] Diverse experimental[34,41,74,98,164] and clinical[7,43,80,116] studies have convincingly shown that the amount of and duration of vessel exposure to blood in the subarachnoid space on computed tomographic (CT) scans determines the occurrence of VSP. Two major theories explain the mechanism(s) of VSP.[152] The structural theory rests on the observation that VSP leads to smooth-muscle cell damage and/or myonecrosis and induces a change in smooth-muscle cell phenotype. Subsequent migration of these cells (myofibroblasts) into the tunica intima is followed by their proliferation. The spasmogen theory suggests that VSP is prolonged vasoconstriction caused by or associated with prolonged exposure to a variety of chemical mediators, such as blood breakdown products (hemoglobin,[98] oxyhemoglobin,[98] and bilirubin), eicosanoids, free radicals, inflammation, vasoconstrictor neuropeptides, and disturbed endothelial function.[41,74,98,152] These theories are based upon experiments performed in a wide variety of animal species, using differing SAH models with various in vitro and in vivo conditions and assessments at different time points after SAH by various methodologies. Despite these caveats, many findings are consistent.[152] The structural and spasmogen theories are in all likelihood interdependent, thus resulting in multifactorial biochemical mechanism(s) for the production of VSP.[152] Moreover, recent experimental observations suggest that the vasoconstriction may be responsive to vasodilator agents at various time points after SAH.[83,164]

ANGIOGRAPHIC ASSESSMENT OF VASOSPASM

The technical and scientific aspects of the angiographic assessment of VSP have recently been reviewed.[128,150,152] There is an excellent correlation between angiographic residual lumen diameters (RLDs) and morphometric measurements from a variety of experimental animal models. The incidence of angiographic VSP is highly variable,[105,128,159,167] and the accuracy of angiographic determination is generally limited to the vessels of the circle of Willis and their first- and second-order branches.[128] Angiographic VSP may spread to involve more proximal portions of the arterial tree or the other vessels. In general, severe (more than 50% narrowing) diffuse VSP in an arterial territory favors the development of clinical VSP.[42,43,80,128,143,150] Because the reliability of measurements may vary, depending upon whether standard biplane or digital intraarterial techniques are used, it is important for investigators to define carefully both the technique and method of angiographic measurements.[150]

CEREBRAL BLOOD FLOW, METABOLISM, AND AUTOREGULATION FOLLOWING SUBARACHNOID HEMORRHAGE

Cerebral blood flow (CBF), as assessed by a variety of techniques,[150] is reduced after SAH.[55,70,102] Although CBF may be decreased soon after SAH, it often declines progressively during the first 2 to 3 weeks after onset,[102,104,106] whether or not an aneurysm is present,[104] and begins to improve in the third week.[102] Lower CBF values are frequently found in patients with Hunt and Hess grades III or IV.[102,106,118] A strong correlation exists between severe VSP (more than 50% diameter reduction) and a clinically important reduction in regional cerebral blood flow (rCBF).[55,70,79,118,142] Patients exhibit decreased alertness and mild neurologic deficits, severe (often irreversible) deficits, and irreversible deficits at CBF values of 20 to 30 ml/100 g per minute, less than 20 ml/100 g per minute, and less than 15 ml/100 g per minute, respectively.[121,174] Patients with less decline in CBF[104] or improvement in CBF postoperatively[106] tend to have a more favorable outcome.

A significant increase in intracranial pressure (IICP) that reduces cerebral perfusion pressure (CPP) to less than 40 mm Hg is associated with significant compromise of CBF,[54,163] increased cerebral blood volume (CBV),[54] disruption of oxidative metabolism,[54] and increasing clinical grade.[53,61] There can be a biphasic course of IICP, with an early phase in the minutes to hours after aneurysm rupture[25,53,129] and a later phase during the VSP period.[163] Severe VSP is often accompanied by brain infarction[121,142] or swelling, edema, and persistent IICP.[163]

Normal autoregulatory mechanisms may be altered after SAH,[30,39,112,162] whether or not VSP is present.[39] The autoregulatory impairment may be global or regional and often directly correlates with clinical grade[30,162] or the presence of severe or diffuse VSP.[39,162] The presence of IICP sufficient to reduce CPP to less than 40 mm Hg may also impair autoregulation.[54]

VASOSPASM: CLINICAL ASPECTS

The clinical features associated with VSP* and their prognostic significance have been documented.† Neurologic changes may develop insidiously over hours to days, progress rapidly over minutes to hours, or rarely appear as an ictus. Some degree of obtundation is almost universal, irrespective of VSP site.[11] Typical syndromes consistent with middle cerebral artery (MCA),[11,42,65,80] anterior cerebral artery (ACA),[11,42,43] posterior cerebral artery (PCA),[11,42,80,101] and vertebrobasilar‡ territory ischemia have been described. Symptoms and signs may

---

*References 11, 12, 36, 42, 43, 63, 80, 101, 105, 114.
†References 43, 79, 80, 159, 166, 168.
‡References 11, 12, 36, 63, 101, 105, 168.

fluctuate, vary between specific vascular territories, and have a marked dependence on blood pressure, intravascular volume status, and posture.[11,154] A number of other factors have also been associated with clinical VSP, including intraventricular blood,[7] poor clinical grade,[65,160] acute hydrocephalus,[25,161] older age,[160] pre-existing hypertension,[160] hyperglycemia on admission,[84] treatment with fluid restriction or antifibrinolytic agents,[7] and impaired CBF response to hypotension.[119] The occurrence of, severity of, and outcome from clinically important VSP ultimately depends upon the intensity of the stimulus (blood and its by-products), individual differences in responses to spasmogens and their structural concomitants, and the success of therapeutic interventions.[152]

TRANSCRANIAL DOPPLER SONOGRAPHY INVESTIGATION OF VASOSPASM
General aspects

Transcranial Doppler sonography has been extensively used to monitor noninvasively patients with aneurysmal SAH.* The time course of FV acceleration related to arterial narrowing from VSP parallels the development of angiographic VSP. Several studies indicate that pathologically elevated FVs may rarely occur in the MCA,[9,24,116,169] intracranial internal carotid artery (IICA),[24] PCA,[149,173] vertebral artery (VA),[149,153] and basilar artery (BA)[149,153] on day 3 or sooner after SAH onset.[172a] However, other studies did not find elevated MCA-FVs before day 3.[60,157] The reasons for these different results are unclear. Flow velocities in the MCA increase roughly in proportion to the degree of arterial narrowing present.[2,143] Early investigators showed that the time course of MCA-FV acceleration due to VSP correlated well with clinical grade, CT localization of subarachnoid clot, and angiographic data.[57-59,116,134] With increasing degrees of VSP, musical murmurs with pure tonal qualities may be heard near the IICA bifurcation in systole and diastole, presumably reflecting periodic formation of vortices.[2] Velocities are often asymmetrically increased, with higher FVs on the side of aneurysmal rupture,[67,134] although on some occasions the contralateral side may have higher FVs.

Correlation of flow velocity with residual lumen diameter

The relation between FVs and VSP severity has been investigated for all intracerebral vessels, either by comparison with RLD (biplane angiography)* or stenosis grade.[24,153,173] Statistically significant inverse† or direct[39,153,173] correlations between FVs and RLD or stenosis grade, respectively, have demonstrated for the proximal MCA,‡ IICA,[58] PCA,[58,92,94,95,173] VA,[153] and BA.[153] In one study, the relation for the IICA was not confirmed.[24] In general, there is often a considerable spread of the data.[24,58,143,153,173] This may be explained in part by variable resting vessel diameters in the population under study.[110,167] The lack of correlation between FVs and RLD[94,143] or stenosis grade[173] in the ACA may be due to congenital anatomic variations (atretic A1 segments with normal velocities)[94] or the frequent presence of an aberrant anatomic course with resultant suboptimal angle of insonation.[173] Some investigators have also proposed that the ACA frequently serves as a collateral channel.[110]

Relation between CBF and MCA-FVs

Under circumstances where arterial P_{CO_2} content, CPP, and brain metabolism are held constant, a proportional relation presumably exists between FV and rCBF, provided that the defined perfusion territory (amount of brain tissue) and luminal area are unchanged.[82,155] In two studies, Aaslid and colleagues induced small, stepwise changes in blood pressure in healthy subjects[4] or changes in perfusion with carotid compression[5] and found an excellent correlation between calculated changes in FV and CBF based on signal power.[4,5] In studies of patients undergoing carotid endarterectomy[93,111] or aneurysm clipping,[111] changes in MCA-FV correlated with ICA flow, although in one study[93] the relationship between blood flow and FV was nonlinear. In a recent small study, Giller and associates[47] showed that the mean diameter change in the large cerebral arteries (IICA, MCA, VA) was less than 4% and as large as 21% to 29% in smaller arteries (ACA, M2 portion of MCA) to end-tidal CO_2 and blood pressure changes during craniotomy.

An additional layer of complexity exists in the less easily controlled and highly variable situation in the clinical setting. Using a computer model simulating the effects of proximal MCA stem and diffuse MCA territory VSP, Pucher and associates[122,123] illustrated the difficulties in equating rCBF with MCA-FV. In the setting of VSP, the location, length, and extent of vessel narrowing and the status of autoregulatory capacity are often unknown. As a result of MCA-VSP, there may be an unpredictable and variable combination of elevated or decreased FV and of unchanged or decreased volume flow since FV values may represent two different sides of the velocity profile and levels of cerebral perfusion.[123] In the clinical setting, the effects of blood pressure, hematocrit,[18,19] P_{CO_2},[62,110] and ICP[54,163] must also be considered. For these reasons, changes in FVs are not

---

*References 1, 38, 58, 92, 94, 95, 110, 143.
†References 1-3, 8, 9, 13, 21-25, 27-29, 31, 32, 37, 38, 44, 50, 52, 53, 56, 60, 66, 69, 81, 85, 86, 89, 92, 94, 95, 103, 109, 110, 116, 120, 126, 127, 130, 134-140, 143-146, 153, 157, 158, 165, 169, 171-173.

‡References 1, 24, 38, 58, 94, 110, 143.

necessarily a reliable index of changes in rCBF in patients with VSP.

The lack of correlation between FVs, clinical grade, and neurologic deficits in some studies[28,85,139,140] has prompted investigations using TCD and rCBF techniques, such as single photon emission computed tomography (SPECT),[90] xenon-enhanced CT,[139] and xenon clearance,[26,32,139] to clarify the meaning of specific FV values in particular situations. The two techniques are complementary in that TCD permits assessment for the presence and severity of arterial narrowing and rCBF techniques evaluate the adequacy of cerebral perfusion in affected vascular territories. In one study,[32] vessels with high FVs had decreased rCBF in the supplied cortical areas. In another study,[139] the time course of rCBF reduction usually followed the elevation in FVs detected by TCD. Moreover, extreme FV accelerations were accompanied by rCBF values of approximately 20 ml/100 g per minute.

Evaluation of autoregulatory capacity

Several methods to assess cerebrovascular responsiveness have been developed,* such as the response to hypercapnia or hypocapnia,[47,62,137] acetazolamide infusion,[139] hypotension,[47,93] and the transient hyperemic response in MCA-FVs following transient carotid compression.[46] Hassler and Chioff showed a progressive loss of vasodilatory capacity to hypercapnia with increasing VSP severity with an essentially normal vasoconstrictive response to hypocapnia, even with severe VSP.[62] Nimodipine does not appear to affect the ability of the cerebral vasculature to respond to changes in Pco_2.[137]

Clinical–TCD correlations

In general, mean MCA-FVs up to 120 cm/s correlate with mild angiographic VSP (usually less than 25% diameter narrowing), and mean MCA-FVs between 120 cm/s and 200 cm/s correlate with moderate angiographic VSP (25% to 50% diameter narrowing), whereas FVs greater than 200 cm/s imply severe angiographic VSP (greater than 50% diameter narrowing).[110] Mean MCA-FVs of 140 cm/s or higher have been associated with delayed ischemic neurologic deficits.[60] In addition, the rate of rise of MCA-FVs can predict the site of VSP-induced cerebral ischemia.[58] A rapid early rise in FVs (more than 25% increase per day[37] in the preoperative phase[68]) and values greater than 200 cm/s often occur up to 2 days before onset of clinical VSP and infarction in the MCA territory.[134] In some cases, there is no difference in FVs whether or not blood is seen on the initial CT, but a greater degree of rise in FV is observed when blood is present on the CT scan.[67]

Recent studies suggest that the preceding correlations are imperfect. Grade IV and V patients tend to have the lowest FVs.[81,85,139] In several studies, there were no significant differences between the time course of FVs and individual Hunt and Hess grades[28,60,85] or between FVs and Hunt and Hess grades on admission.[140] In one study, normal CBF was measured in patients with so-called critical MCA-FVs.[103] In another study, there was no specific MCA-FV value that was a reliable indicator of the patient who would become symptomatic.[37] In addition, there may be no significant difference between FVs in patients with or without neurologic deficits[85] or a correlation between maximal FVs and severity of neurologic deficits.[140] These discrepant results might reflect improved ischemic tolerance due to concurrent nimodipine treatment,[60] presence of adequate collateral pathways,[150,156] technical limitations,[40,49,143] imprecise description of the nature of neurologic deficit,[85] and lack of clear definitions for VSP by angiography or TCD.[85] Moreover, clinically important VSP may have occurred in vessels that may not have been routinely insonated or reported, such as the MCA-M2 or MCA convexity branches,[109,143] IICA,[37,69,143,146,150] ACA,[3,49,86,94,171] PCA,[21,92,94,95] VA,[36,145] and BA.[31,50,144,153]

Other factors affecting FV determinations

A large number of anatomic and physiologic factors may, either in isolation or in concert, affect FV determinations in patients with VSP after SAH (box).[150]

Technical factors are of great importance, especially operator skill and experience. Patients are often agitated and poorly cooperative, and gentle sedation and rest before proceeding to perform the study optimize results. Suboptimal transtemporal windows may occur in as many as 38% of patients.[40,49] As experience is gained, the likelihood of a limited TCD study due to a suboptimal window[40,49] or missing an abnormally increased FV[150] should lessen.

A variety of anatomic factors may obscure detection of elevated FVs. Variations in the configuration of the circle of Willis are well known. The resting diameters of large cerebral arteries, such as the proximal MCA, are subject to substantial variation between individuals.[110,167] Aberrant vessel course may increase the Doppler angle and lead to considerable error in FV measurements, even lack of signal detection, when using conventional TCD technique.

As suggested by the computer simulation of MCA-VSP,[122,123] the site(s) and severity of VSP may limit its detection by TCD. As the severity of the vasospastic process surpasses the critical degree of stenosis, FVs decrease, often with progressive weakening of the signal,[110] which becomes barely audible.[33] In some instances, FVs may fluctuate from day to day, depending

*References 44-47, 62, 93, 100, 137, 141.

Factors that influence flow velocity values related to vasospasm following subarachnoid hemorrhage

Technical factors

Operator skill and experience
Adequacy of ultrasonic windows (especially transtemporal)
Patient cooperation
Adequacy of Doppler angle

Anatomic factors

Variations in configuration of circle of Willis
Resting arterial diameters
Aberrant vessel course
Site(s), extent, and severity of vasospasm
Coexisting proximal hemodynamically significant lesion(s)
    Extracranial common carotid artery/internal carotid artery high-grade stenosis/occlusion
    Intracranial internal carotid artery stenosis/vasospasm
Clip artifacts

Physiologic factors – increased intracranial pressure

Mass effect – regional/diffuse
Hydrocephalus

Physiologic factors – systemic
Cardiovascular
    Blood pressure
    Cardiac output
    Volume status
    Arrhythmias (atrial fibrillation, premature ventricular contractions)
Metabolic/rheologic
    PCO_2 variations
    Viscosity (hematocrit, fibrinogen)
    Temperature

Effects of therapeutic interventions

"Triple-H" therapy (hypertension, hypervolemia, hemodilution)
Calcium channel blockers (nimodipine, nicardipine)
Transluminal angioplasty
Vasodilators – papaverine

Combination

upon VSP severity and the contribution of other factors that influence FV determinations (see box). It can be difficult to consistently capture a weak signal on successive days, which may lead to a diagnostic and clinical dilemma. The absence of a signal may indicate vascular occlusion.[78,105] On occasion, signals may weaken, disappear, and then reappear when VSP resolves. In addition, patients with proximal and distal or diffuse VSP in an arterial territory may also have low FVs.[143,150] In the

patient with decreasing MCA-FVs, VSP may be subsiding or spreading to more proximal portions of the arterial tree, thus altering perfusion pressure more distally.[23,24,127,150] Patients with a coexisting proximal hemodynamic lesion, such as IICA-VSP, [23,24,150] high-grade extracranial internal carotid stenosis,[91,143] or occlusion,[131] may have dampened MCA signals. Finally, convexity VSP may occur in up to 7.5% of patients with anterior circulation aneurysms,[109] thus leading to dampened, high-resistance waveforms and lower mean MCA-FVs.

The presence of IICP, either regional or generalized, may be associated with significant compromise in CBF and CPP. In one study,[81] a resistance index of Pourcelot (RI) value greater than 0.6 was associated with ICP above 20 mm Hg and MCA-FVs less than or equal to 150 cm/s, and an RI of less than 0.5 was associated with ICP below 20 mm Hg and MCA-FVs greater than 120 cm/s, with changes in MCA-FV clearly reflecting the degree of and evolution of the vasospastic process. Sander and Klingelhöfer[129] and Byrd and colleagues[25] have documented changes in MCA Doppler waveforms during[25] and following[129] rebleeding from an aneurysm. As the ICP and RI increased, mean MCA-FVs decreased, and vice versa during resolution of IICP. Sloan reported increased FVs in the right PCA and BA, as well as decreases in PI and RI in the IICAs, left VA, and BA, following a right frontotemporal lobectomy for a large right MCA and PCA infarction complicating SAH due to a giant right ICA bifurcation aneurysm.[150]

A variety of cardiovascular, metabolic, and rheologic conditions may also influence FV determinations.[44,62,127] The impact of blood pressure and volume status fluctuations on FVs may depend upon the magnitude of the parameter change, the site and severity of VSP, and the presence and extent of autoregulation.[44] There is an inverse correlation between hematocrit and FV values, particularly when hematocrit is less than 30%,[18,19] although the effects of changes in blood viscosity[170] and hematocrit level[18,170] remain to be determined in relation to varying degrees of VSP.

Finally, recent studies suggest that "triple-H" therapy[107,115] or dobutamine[88] improves blood pressure, cardiac performance, CBF, and clinical outcome in patients with symptomatic VSP. Recent studies suggest that MCA-FVs may increase in the intracranial arteries as a response to various treatments, although the magnitude and significance of these findings remain to be more fully characterized.[88] Nimodipine therapy does not appear to prevent angiographic VSP,[10] but it may lessen the severity with resultant decrease in FVs.[59,60,116,135] When nimodipine is discontinued, FVs may rise as a result of recurrent arterial narrowing,[59] which has been associating with worsened clinical status.[101,116] In the Nicardipine in SAH trial,[56] use of nicardipine was associated with a significantly reduced occurrence of moderate or severe angiographic VSP, the proportion of individuals with mean MCA-FVs greater than 120 cm/s, and the proportion of individuals with mean MCA-FVs greater than 200 cm/s. Neurointerventional procedures, such as transluminal balloon angioplasty* and papaverine† have been shown to improve vascular patency and clinical outcome, with immediate and sustained reduction in FVs in the vessel undergoing balloon angioplasty.[87,108] Then again, elevated FVs following neurointerventional procedures may also suggest the presence of postischemic hyperemia or the coexistence of persistent or recurrent VSP and hyperemia.[48] Correlation with clinical findings and CBF techniques should help distinguish between these possibilities.

SENSITIVITY AND SPECIFICITY FOR DETECTION OF VASOSPASM

Investigators have focused primarily on the detection of angiographic MCA-VSP‡ and ACA-VSP,[50,86] although it has been demonstrated that TCD can detect angiographic VSP in the IICA,[24,146,147] PCA,[21,173] VA,[145,153] and BA[144,153] as well. Cerebral angiography, whether standard biplane or digital intraarterial,§ remains the gold standard against which TCD has been compared in order to define true positive (TP), true negative (TN), false positive (FP), and false negative (FN) TCD results. It has recently been recognized that true positives for occlusion (TPo)[171,173] and false positives for occlusion (FPo)[21,86,171,173] may occur. In the case of FPos, the TCD result may be classified this way regardless of whether VSP is present in varying degrees in a patent artery. From a clinical perspective, no meaningful conclusion can be drawn regarding the status of such a vessel. However, the most conservative approach to defining the accuracy of TCD in this situation is to include FPos in the analysis.[21,149,171,173] Available data on the sensitivity and specificity of TCD for detection of VSP are summarized in Table 15-1. The positive and negative predictive value data should be cautiously interpreted, particularly when the prior probability of disease or the number of evaluable vessels is low.

Middle cerebral artery

Inspection of Table 15-1 indicates that the prevalence of and definitions for angiographic MCA-VSP, as well as the diagnostic FV criteria for MCA-VSP, varies widely between studies. In one recent study performed prima-

rily in the nimodipine era,[22,24] the FV criterion of 120 cm/s retained high specificity but had a surprising 39% sensitivity for MCA-VSP. It should be noted that for 19 of 24 (79.2%) of the FN-TCD studies, the operator detected a mean MCA-FV of at least 120 cm/s on a different day than the TCD-angiogram correlation, particularly if vessels were evaluated four or more times. The maximum possible sensitivity of TCD for MCA-VSP in this study might have been 80%, a value comparable with results from the prenimodipine era.‖ These latter data suggest that sensitivity of TCD for MCA-VSP may be significantly affected by the timing of correlative angiography and, to some extent, by the number and results of TCD studies performed. Moreover, the findings of the latter may influence the performance of the former.[24]

Anterior cerebral artery

As for the MCA, prevalence of disease and diagnostic FV criteria (relative or absolute) varied widely.[50,86,171,173] Recent studies[86,171,173] indicate that TCD has low sensitivity for angiographic ACA-VSP. When the FPos were excluded[171,173] or the diagnostic FV criterion was raised to 130 cm/s [148,173] or 140 cm/s,[86] a specificity of 96%[148,173] to 100%[86] was obtained.

Other vessels

In one study with a moderate prevalence of IICA-VSP,[24,146] TCD had low sensitivity but excellent specificity. In a recent study with a low prevalence of PCA-VSP,[21,173] TCD had fair sensitivity and moderate specificity. As with the ACA, elimination of FPos substantially improved specificity. In a study with a low prevalence of VA-VSP,[145,153] TCD had low to moderate sensitivity and good to excellent specificity. In a study with moderate prevalence of BA-VSP,[144,153] sensitivity and specificity were good. Based upon considerations similar to the MCA, the maximal possible sensitivity of TCD for VA-VSP might be 66.7% and 85% for BA-VSP.[153] More studies are needed to confirm or refute these results.

FALSE POSITIVES AND FALSE NEGATIVES

A number of causes for both FP and FN TCD studies have been demonstrated.[23,24,149,153,173] Each vessel has at least one known cause for FPs and FNs, with varying proportions of respective causes between vessels.

False positives

Increased collateral flow (CF) in a vessel is associated with the presence of moderate to severe stenosis (more than 50% diameter reduction) in anatomically related or physiologically linked vessels. In the study of Wozniak

---

*References 36, 63, 64, 67, 87, 96, 97, 108, 175.
†References 27a, 72, 77, 83, 97, 99, 133.
‡References 28, 50, 86, 92, 94, 139, 143.
§References 21, 22, 24, 144, 146, 173.

‖References 28, 50, 86, 92, 139, 143.

Table 15-1. Sensitivity and specificity of transcranial Doppler for detection of vasospasm following subarachnoid hemorrhage

Study	N	Prevalence of disease (%)	Positive test (mean flow velocity)	Sensitivity	Specificity	Predictive value Positive	Predictive value Negative
Middle cerebral artery (MCA)							
Grolimund[50]	93 patients	20	120 cm/s	78	85	57	80
Compton[28]	20 patients	30	100 cm/s	68	96	87	87
Lindegaard[94]	51 patients	31[a]	110 cm/s	85	98	95	94[b]
	112 MCAs		100 cm/s	94[c]	90	81	97[b]
Sekhar[139]	21 patients	38[d]	155 cm/s	75	100	85	85
Lennihan[86]	41 patients	10.6	120 cm/s	86	86	42[b]	98[b]
	66 MCAs		140 cm/s	86	98	83[b]	98[b]
Sloan[143]	34 patients	85[e]	120 cm/s	59	100	100	30
	52 MCAs	46[e]	120 cm/s	84	89	87	90
Burch[22,24]	87 MCAs	44	120 cm/s	39	94	83	66
		44[f]	120 cm/s	80	94	91[b]	87[b]
Anterior cerebral artery (ACA)							
Grolimund[50]	93 patients	15	50% increase in FV	71	100	100	95
Lennihan[86]	66 ACAs[g]	22.7	120 cm/s	13	96	49[b]	79[b]
			140 cm/s	13	100	100[b]	80[b]
Wozniak[171,173]	87 ACAs	68	120 cm/s	18	65	52	27
	73 ACAs[h]	66	120 cm/s	15	96	88	37
Intracranial internal carotid artery (IICA)							
Burch,[24] Sloan[146]	90 IICAs	49	90 cm/s	25	91	76	58
Vertebral artery (VA)							
Sloan[145,153]	64 VAs	25	60 cm/s	44	88	54	82
Basilar artery (BA)							
Sloan[144,153]	42 BAs	31	60 cm/s	77	79	62	89
Posterior cerebral artery (PCA)							
Burch[21], Wozniak[173]	84 PCAs	32	90 cm/s	48	69	42	74
	77 PCAs[h]	30	90 cm/s	48	78	48	78

[a]Vasospasm defined as MCA diameter less than or equal to 2.1 mm.
[b]Calculated values.
[c]Reported values.
[d]Vasospasm diagnosed on basis of clinical deficits and appropriate reduction in regional cerebral blood flow.
[e]Vasospasm defined by criteria adapted from Fisher, et al.[42,43]
[f]Calculations based upon the assumption that angiographic vasospasm was present on the day of the highest MCA-FV.
[g]Calculations based upon exclusion of 9 false positives for occlusion (see text for definition).
[h]Calculations based upon exclusion of false positives for occlusion and true positives for occlusion.

and colleagues,[173] only 1 in 13 (8%) FVs for ACA-VSP was attributed to CF. Moreover, there was no clear relationship between asymmetric FVs and the presence of angiographic ACA-VSP. Adjacent vessel VSP, a "technical" category, is the unintended insonation of VSP in a nearby vessel. It has been observed for MCA (insonation of terminal IICA),[143] VA (insonation of BA-VSP),[153] and PCA (insonation of BA or superior cerebellar artery).[173] Hyperemia and/or hyperperfusion reflects the presence of abnormally high FVs in a nonvasospastic vessel on day 2 or earlier after SAH. This finding has been demonstrated in the VA,[149,153] BA,[149,153] IICA,[24,149] MCA,[24,149] and PCA[149,173] all in the same patient. Another or an unknown cause is present when no known anatomic or physiologic condition can explain the elevated FVs. This finding has been observed in all vessels except the ACA. More data are needed to determine the cause of FP results in these cases.

False positives for occlusion (ACA and PCA)[149,173] can occur for the following reasons: (1) Anatomic factors, such as tortuous or aberrant vessel course into a different two-dimensional or three-dimensional plane than the ultrasonic beam, may preclude an optimal angle

Table 15-2. Proposed criteria for optimal diagnosis of vasospasm after subarachnoid hemorrhage by transcranial Doppler sonography

Vessel	Number of vessels	Possible vasospasm	Probable vasospasm	Presumed definite vasospasm
Intracranial internal carotid artery[24,146]	90	80 (89)	110 (98)	130 (100)
Middle cerebral artery[22,24]	87	100 (88)	110 (94)	130 (96)
Anterior cerebral artery*[171,173]	87	110 (92)	120 (96)	130 (100)
	73			
Vertebral artery[145,153]	64	55 (78)	60 (86)	80 (100)
Basilar artery[141]	41	60 (82)	80 (96)	90 (100)
Basilar artery[153]	42	60 (79)	80 (93)	95 (100)
Posterior cerebral artery*[21,173]	84	80 (69)	90 (78)	110 (93)
	77			

*Optimal diagnostic criteria are based on exclusion of false positives for occlusion and true positives for occlusion.
Flow velocities in cm/s.
Numbers in parentheses refer to specificities at each respective flow velocity criterion for each vessel.
Criteria for possible, probable, and presumed definite were arbitrarily chosen.

of insonation and lead to lack of vessel detection; (2) a proximal hemodynamically significant lesion (50% or greater diameter reduction) may lead to a decrease in cerebral perfusion[55,70,79,117] with resultant dampening of FVs, thus making it difficult to detect the vessel; and (3) operator error or inexperience may be invoked if there is no anatomic or technical difficulty that would explain the lack of ability to insonate the vessel.

False negatives

Anatomic factors, such as tortuous or aberrant vessel course, may preclude an optimal angle of insonation with resultant underestimation of FVs. This cause is especially prominent for the IICA (100%), PCA (80%), VA (78%), and ACA (51%).[23] For the PCA,[173] a fetal origin may compound the problem. A proximal hemodynamic lesion (50% or greater diameter reduction) may cause a decrease in cerebral perfusion[55,70,79,117] with resultant dampening of FVs in a vasospastic vessel distal to the lesion. This phenomenon has occasionally been observed,[23,24,67,143,150,173] particularly for the MCA[24] and ACA.[23,173] Operator error or inexperience may be invoked if there is no anatomic reason or technical difficulty that would explain the lack of VSP detection. This cause has been found to be especially prominent for MCA-VSP,[23,24] although its role may be overemphasized because of the effect of the timing of angiography.[24] It has also been documented for ACA-VSP,[23,173] PCA-VSP,[23,173] and BA-VSP.[23,153] In the majority of cases, the VSP missed by the sonographer was 50% or less diameter stenosis, a degree of narrowing deemed insufficient to cause a hemodynamic disturbance and possibly lead to neurologic deterioration. Nevertheless, these results emphasize the need for ongoing quality assurance activities to ensure optimal TCD technique, particularly when new sonographers are being trained.

IMPROVING VASOSPASM DETECTION BY TRANSCRANIAL DOPPLER SONOGRAPHY

Precision in the diagnosis of VSP by TCD may be enhanced in several ways. First, one may optimize traditional handheld TCD technique by considering the variations in anatomic configuration and trajectory for each vessel. At each insonation site, the sonographer should carefully vary the probe position and direction in order to anticipate the possibility that the vessel under study may have an atypical three-dimensional course. Prior knowledge of the anatomic reasons for FP and FN studies will help the sonographer to think three-dimensionally as the study is being performed and thus minimize error.

Second, one may set the diagnostic criterion at a higher level to maximize specificity to minimize or eliminate false positives,[86,148] with some sacrifice in sensitivity. The finding of a wide range of FVs for any grade of VSP severity[24,143,153,173] suggests the need for the sonographer to consider VSP as being present at a given FV with varying degrees of confidence. Such an approach is supported by the general finding of a significant relation between FVs and severity of stenosis. Table 15-2 summarizes one set of criteria for optimal diagnosis of VSP after SAH in all major cerebral arteries. Table 15-3 illustrates how often the proposed possible, probable, and presumed definite categories of sonographic VSP have been reported for each vessel.*

A third way to improve the accuracy of TCD is to use FV ratios. Aaslid and colleagues[3] and Lindegaard and associates[92,94,95] developed the V_{MCA}/V_{ICA} ratio — or the ratio of MCA-FVs (V_{MCA}) to the ipsilateral distal extracranial ICA FVs (EICA-FV) by way of the submandibular approach (V_{ICA}) — to analyze the decrease

*References 8, 60, 116, 136, 151, 172.

Table 15-3. Reported prevalence of sonographic vasospasm by transcranial Doppler

Study	Number of patients	Number of vessels	Possible n (%)	Probable n (%)	Presumed definite n (%)
Intracranial internal carotid artery					
Wozniak[172]	239	467	271 (58%)	137 (29%)	71 (16%)[a]
Middle cerebral artery					
Seiler[136]	118[b]	—	80%	73%	52%
Pasqualin[116]	68[b]	—	37 (54%)	33 (49%)	21 (31%)
Harders[60]	100[b]	—	86%	77%	63%
Alexander[8]	93	—	—	39.3%[c]	—
Wozniak[172]	239	463	319 (69%)	294 (64%)	215 (46%)[d]
Anterior cerebral artery					
Wozniak[172]	239	435	178 (41%)	132 (30%)	95 (22%)[e]
Vertebral artery					
Sloan[151]	239	447	291 (65%)	264 (59%)	127 (28%)[f]
Basilar artery					
Sloan[151]	239	232	174 (75%)	111 (48%)	82 (35%)[g]
Posterior cerebral artery					
Sloan[151]	239	449	276 (62%)	238 (53%)	144 (32%)

[a]Possible VSP = ≥ 80 cm/s, probable VSP = ≥ 110 cm/s, presumed definite VSP ≥ 130 cm/s.
[b]Estimated values.
[c]Based on MCA-FV ≥ 120 cm/s, Lindegaard ratio ≥ 3.
[d]Possible VSP = ≥ 100 cm/s, probable VSP = ≥ 110 cm/s, presumed definite VSP = ≥ 130 cm/s.
[e]Possible VSP = ≥ 110 cm/s, probable VSP = ≥ 120 cm/s, presumed definite VSP = ≥ 130 cm/s.
[f]Possible VSP = ≥ 55 cm/s, probable VSP = ≥ 60 cm/s, presumed definite VSP = ≥ 80 cm/s.
[g]Possible VSP = ≥ 60 cm/s, probable VSP = ≥ 80 cm/s, presumed definite VSP = ≥ 90 cm/s.
[h]Possible VSP = ≥ 80 cm/s, probable VSP = ≥ 90 cm/s, presumed definite VSP = ≥ 110 cm/s.

in EICA-FVs that sometimes occurs with VSP or IICP. A V_{MCA}/V_{ICA} less than 3 reportedly is rarely found in patients with VSP, whereas a value greater than 6 appears to distinguish severe from moderate MCA-VSP.[138] The Lindegaard ratio changes very little when MCA-FVs and cerebral blood flow increase as a result of acute hypercarbia.[14] The presence of hyperemia and/or hyperperfusion may be suspected in patients with elevated MCA-FVs and a V_{MCA}/V_{ICA} less than 3, particularly in the early days following SAH. Moreover, a state of elevated MCA-FV of any degree and normal to elevated cerebral blood flow—that is, "high Vmca hyperemia"—may lead to FP TCD studies in patients with closed-head injury. Increasing the V_{MCA}/V_{ICA} ratio to at least 4 may be more predictive of ischemic VSP.[71] These latter observations may well be relevant to the detection of VSP following SAH by TCD. It is not known how the utility of V_{MCA}/V_{ICA} is affected by the presence of proximal hemodynamically significant lesions and IICP.[150] More data are needed to clarify the relationship between elevated MCA-FVs, Lindegaard ratios, cerebral blood flow, and ischemic VSP following SAH. Finally, studies are presently underway to develop a

"posterior circulation velocity index," or "Vba/Vva," in order to help distinguish between BA-VSP, hyperemia, and collateral effects.

A fourth way to optimize the diagnostic precision of TCD is to actually image the vessels. Non-contrast-enhanced* and contrast-enhanced[17,124] transcranial color-coded sonography (TCCS) and transcranial imaging (TCI) are promising techniques to delineate vessel course, determine vessel lumen size, and optimize the angle of insonation. The comparative efficacy of these techniques for detection of VSP in general and specific vessels in particular remains to be demonstrated.

Finally, the apparent lack of correlation between FVs, CBF, and neurologic status[37,85,103] has prompted investigations using both TCD and CBF techniques such as xenon/CT-CBF,[139] SPECT,[29,51,89,90] and xenon clearance.[18,32,139] In patients with MCA territory deficits and indeterminate conventional TCD studies by the transtemporal approach, CBF studies may be more sensitive for the detection of hemispheric hypoperfusion attributable to VSP.[28,29,32,89] Thus, in some situations, evalua-

*References 13, 16, 17, 35, 73, 132.

tion with TCD and CBF studies should be considered as complementary noninvasive alternatives to angiography.

VALUE OF TRANSCRANIAL DOPPLER SONOGRAPHY IN CLINICAL MANAGEMENT

Transcranial Doppler findings may be predictive of outcome after SAH. An average rate of rise in FVs of more than 20 cm per second per day between days 3 and 7 after SAH,[60] a rapid early rise in FVs (more than 25% per day),[37,68,116] a mean maximal absolute rise in MCA-FVs or ACA-FVs of 65 ± 5 cm/s over a 24-hour period,[52] and a higher V_{MCA}/V_{ICA} (6 ± 0.3)[52] have been found in SAH patients who develop a delayed ischemic neurologic deficit. An increase of MCA-FVs of more than 50 cm/s predicts the presence of more than 20% arterial constriction on a subsequent angiogram; both parameters are associated with clinical VSP.[120] Higher maximal mean MCA-FVs,[130] such as mean FV values equal to or greater than 180 to 200 cm/s, often occur up to 2 days before MCA territory infarction[26,52,58,134] and have been associated with a poor clinical outcome.[68,130] Increased pulsatility index and poor cerebrovascular reactivity to acetazolamide have also been associated with incipient cerebral ischemia and poor prognosis.[158] Several of these findings are illustrated in Figure 15-1.

The presence and temporal profile of VSP in all basal cerebral arteries can be detected and serially monitored by TCD. All available vessels should be evaluated. The pattern of FV elevation may indicate the need to follow the patient carefully for evidence of deficits related to specific vessels with abnormal FVs. For example, Figure 15-2 illustrates the importance of elevated FVs in the right VA and BA in a patient with clinical VSP in the vertebrobasilar territory. The sonographer and clinician must carefully consider the patient's clinical findings, the FV values from all vessels in relation to their likelihood of reflecting VSP, the limitations of TCD technique, and, in some cases, correlation with CBF and neuroimaging data. Analysis of all available data may then permit optimal interpretation and use of TCD results.

The frequency with which TCD should be performed may be guided by the patient's clinical presentation, knowledge of risk factors for VSP, knowledge of clinical and sonographic predictors of outcome, and early clinical course. It is useful to obtain a baseline TCD upon admission and perform studies daily or every other day in order to look for a rapid rate of rise in FVs and detect the occasional case of early hyperemia and/or hyperperfusion. If the baseline study shows elevated FVs, daily TCD studies should be performed and prophylactic hypervolemia should be given. If a rapid rate of rise in FVs and detect the occasional case of early hyperemia and or hyperperfusion. If the baseline study shows elevated FVs, daily TCD studies should be performed and prophylactic hypervolemia should be given. If a

rapid rate of rise in FVs occurs or if such a patient deteriorates, then triple-H therapy should be instituted. If the baseline study shows elevated FVs and the V_{MCA}/V_{ICA} is less than 3, patients should also be monitored daily to every other day and perhaps have correlative rCBF studies in order to distinguish hyperemia from VSP in problematic cases. Testing of autoregulatory capacity may be helpful. Serial TCD studies should be performed at least every other day for a period of 2 to 3 weeks or longer, depending upon the patient's status. Asymptomatic patients with unimpressive TCD findings may be evaluated every 2 to 3 days during the period at risk.

The patient who is deteriorating may have a variety of TCD findings. The patient who has persistently elevated FVs and does not improve, has a normal or nondiagnostic TCD study, or continues to deteriorate despite aggressive medical therapy should be considered a candidate for urgent neurointerventional procedures, either balloon angioplasty,* intraarterial papaverine,[27a,72,77,97] or a combination[72,97] of the two, based upon consideration of vessel anatomy[96] or need for a specific catheter type.[64] These procedures should ideally be performed within a few hours of recognition that the deterioration is nonresponsive to aggressive medical treatment. Vasospastic vessels that are felt to be responsible for symptoms, whether or not associated with the highest FVs, should be treated first. Effectiveness of treatment is demonstrated by normalization of FVs in the treated vessel(s). The magnitude or duration of the therapeutic effect may be quite variable.[27a,97,99,153a] For example, VSP has recurred within 24 to 48 hours in some patients treated with papaverine.[97,99,153a] Daily TCD studies should be performed following treatment to identify and distinguish patients who develop recurrent VSP and require retreatment.[27a,48,66] The finding of increased pulsatility or resistivity and decreased peak systolic and diastolic FVs may complement clinical and neuroimaging data and suggest the presence of localized or generalized IICP or hydrocephalus, thus necessitating appropriate diagnostic evaluation and treatment.

Finally, the use of TCD may facilitate the optimal timing of aneurysm surgery, as well as intraoperative and postoperative management.[150] It may be prudent to delay surgery until the period of reactive VSP is resolving. Nevertheless, immediate postoperative angioplasty may lead to a good outcome in desperate situations,[87] such as the patient with severe VSP before surgery. At the time of surgery, TCD can detect altered flow patterns in the aneurysm,[59] assess autoregulation,[44] and evaluate clip placement and detect iatrogenic stenosis or occlusion[27] in selected cases. This may facilitate operative technique and minimize the risk of

*References 12, 36, 63, 64, 66, 87, 97, 108, 175.

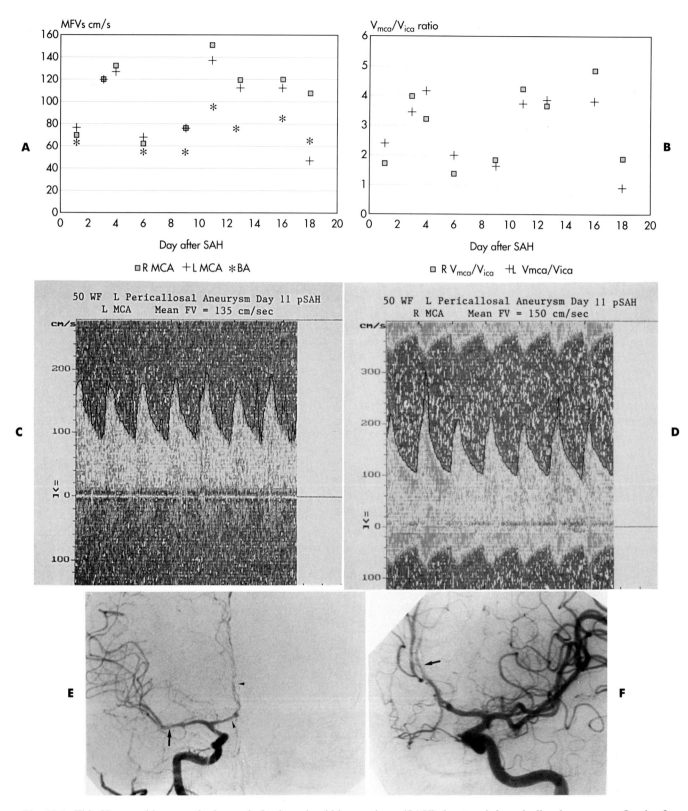

Fig. 15-1. This 50-year-old woman had a grade I subarachnoid hemorrhage (SAH) due to a left pericallosal aneurysm. On day 2, she received nimodipine and underwent an uneventful aneurysm clipping. On day 3, she was lethargic, and mild bilateral MCA-VSP was diagnosed, based on the presence of both (**A**) flow velocity and (**B**) V_{MCA}/V_{ICA} ratio criteria and borderline elevated right ACA flow velocities. Despite treatment with intravascular hydration, vasopressors, and mannitol, she developed right more than left hemiparesis and aphasia over the next 1 to 2 days. On day 6, clinical improvement was accompanied by decline in flow velocities (**A**). Over the next 4 days, she spoke slowly in short phrases and was without weakness; vasopressors were tapered and discontinued. On day 11, (**C**), left MCA, and (**D**), right MCA, and BA flow velocities and (**B**) V_{MCA}/V_{ICA} ratios increased. Over the next several days, she developed recurrent right arm weakness and also had moderate to severe impairment in memory, linguistic organization, work fluency, processing, problem solving, impulsivity, distractibility, and euphoria. Cerebral angiography on day 17 revealed severe VSP in the right MCA (**E**, *arrow*), right ACA (**E**, *arrowhead*) and A2 segment of the left ACA (**F**, *arrow*) and moderate to severe BA-VSP. Nimodipine was discontinued after day 21. She was discharged on day 27 to a cognitive rehabilitation center. (*MCA,* Middle cerebral artery; *VSP,* vasospasm; V_{MCA}, MCA flow velocities; V_{ICA}, distal extracranial ICA flow velocities by way of the submandibular approach; *ACA,* anterior cerebral artery; *BA,* basilar artery.)

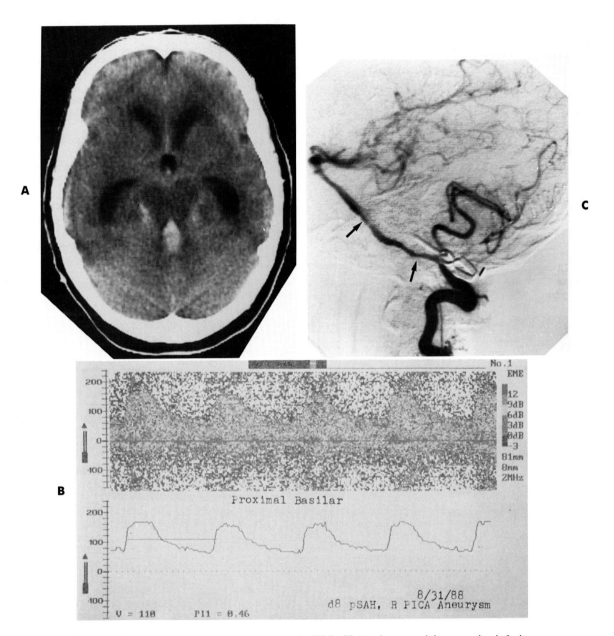

Fig. 15-2. This 69-year-old woman had a grade IV SAH (**A**) due to a right posterior inferior cerebellar artery aneurysm, with depressed level of consciousness and quadriparesis. After treatment with dexamethasone (Decadron), mannitol, and an intraventricular catheter for hydrocephalus, she underwent emergency aneurysm clipping on day 1. Over the next several days, she became more alert and purposeful and had somewhat improved motor function. On day 5, she had impaired vertical gaze, right lower facial weakness and right more than left hemiparesis. Transcranial Doppler (**B**) revealed elevated mean flow velocities in the right VA (104 cm/s) and BA (84 cm/s). Over the next 2 to 3 days, she improved slightly. On day 8, she was drowsy and had impaired horizontal and vertical gaze, hypometric saccades, bifacial weakness, and worsening quadriparesis. Mean flow velocities (**B**) were higher in the right VA (111 cm/s) and BA (110 cm/s). **C,** Cerebral angiography revealed severe VSP in the right VA and BA. Two months later, she was transferred to a chronic care facility in a vegetative state. (*SAH,* subarachnoid hemorrhage; *VA,* vertebral artery; *BA,* basilar artery; *VSP,* vasospasm.)

complications. Transfer from the intensive care unit and mobilization of postoperative patients may be guided by the timing of resolution of elevated FVs in pertinent vessels.

REFERENCES

1. Aaslid R, Markwalder T, Nornes H: Noninvasive transcranial Doppler ultrasound recording of flow velocities in basal cerebral arteries, *J Neurosurg* 57:769-774, 1982.
2. Aaslid R, Nornes H: Musical murmurs in human cerebral arteries after subarachnoid hemorrhage, *J Neurosurg* 60:32-36, 1984.
3. Aaslid R, Huber P, Nornes H: A transcranial Doppler method in the evaluation of cerebrovascular spasm, *Neuroradiology* 28:11-16, 1986.
4. Aaslid R, et al: Cerebral autoregulation dynamics in humans, *Stroke* 20:45-52, 1989.
5. Aaslid R, et al: Assessment of cerebral autoregulation dynamics from simultaneous arterial and venous transcranial Doppler recordings in humans, *Stroke* 22:1148-1154, 1991.
6. Acosta JA, et al: Detection of vasospasm following nonaneurysmal subarachnoid hemorrhage by transcranial Doppler, *J Neuroimaging* 4:63, 1994.
7. Adams HP, et al: Predicting cerebral ischemia after aneurysmal subarachnoid hemorrhage: Influences of clinical condition, CT results, and antifibrinolytic therapy: report of the Cooperative Aneurysm Study, *Neurology* 37:1586-1591, 1987.
8. Alexander M, Martin NA: Cerebral hyperemia in subarachnoid hemorrhage and trauma, *Stroke* 24:520, 1993.
9. Alexander MJ, et al: Determinants of cerebral vasospasm in unruptured aneurysms, *Stroke* 24:518, 1993.
10. Allen GS, et al: Cerebral arterial spasm: a controlled trial of nimodipine in patients with subarachnoid hemorrhage, *N Engl J Med* 308:619-624, 1983.
11. Barker FG, Heros RC: Clinical aspects of vasospasm, *Neurosurg Clin N Am* 1:277-288, 1990.
12. Barnwell SL, et al: Transluminal angioplasty of intracerebral vessels for delayed cerebral arterial spasm: reversal of neurological deficits after delayed treatment, *Neurosurgery* 25:424-429, 1989.
13. Becker G, et al: Diagnosis and monitoring of subarachnoid hemorrhage by transcranial color-coded real-time sonography, *Neursurgery* 28:814-820, 1991.
14. Benalcazar HE, Martin NA, Thomas-Lukes K, Rinsky BS: How do transcranial Doppler velocities and the Lindegaard ratio change in hyperemia? A quantitative analysis, *Stroke* 25:238,1994.
15. Black PM: Hydrocephalus and vasospasm after subarachnoid hemorrhage from ruptured intracranial aneurysm, *Neurosurgery* 18:12-16, 1986.
16. Bogdahn U, et al: Transcranial color-coded real-time sonography in adults, *Stroke* 21:1680-1688, 1990.
17. Bogdahn U, et al: Contrast-enhanced transcranial color-coded real-time sonography: results of a phase II study, *Stroke* 24:676-684, 1993.
18. Brass LM, Prohovnik I, Mohr JP: Multivariate analysis improves the correlation between middle cerebral artery blood velocity and cerebral blood flow, *J Cardiovasc Technol* 9:58-59, 1990.
19. Brass LM, et al: Transcranial Doppler measurements of the middle cerebral artery: effect of hematocrit, *Stroke* 19:1966-1969, 1988.
20. Brouwers PJAM et al: Amount of blood on computed tomography as an independent predictor after aneurysm rupture, *Stroke* 24:809-814, 1993.
21. Burch CM, et al: Sensitivity and specificity of transcranial Doppler in the detection of posterior cerebral artery vasospasm, *J Neuroimaging* 2:57, 1992.

22. Burch CM, et al: Re-evaluation of transcranial Doppler criteria for the diagnosis of middle cerebral artery vasospasm, *Stroke* 24:517, 1993.
23. Burch CM, et al: Causes of false negative transcranial Doppler (TCD) examinations in subarachnoid hemorrhage, *Stroke* 24:519, 1993.
24. Burch CM, et al: Detection of intracranial internal carotid artery and middle cerebral artery vasospasm following subarachnoid hemorrhage, *J Neuroimaging* (in press).
25. Byrd SM, et al: Influences of intracranial pressure on transcranial Doppler spectral waveforms during rupture of an intracranial aneurysm, *Stroke* 24:519, 1993.
26. Caplan LR, et al: Transcranial Doppler ultrasound: present status, *Neurology* 40:696-700, 1990.
27. Chyatte D, Kisiel D, Brass LM: Intraoperative transcranial Doppler monitoring during aneurysm clipping, *J Cardiovasc Technol* 9:106, 1990.
27a. Clousten JE, et al: Intraarterial papaverine infusion for cerebral vasospasm following subarachnoid hemorrhage, *Am J Neuroradiol* 16:27-38, 1995.
28. Compton JS, Redmond S, Symon L: Cerebral blood velocity in subarachnoid hemorrhage: a transcranial Doppler study, *J Neurol Neurosurg Psychiatry* 50:1499-1503, 1987.
29. Davis SM, et al: Correlations between cerebral arterial velocities, blood flow, and delayed ischemia after subarachnoid hemorrhage, *Stroke* 23:492-497, 1992.
30. Dernback PD, et al: Altered cerebral autoregulations and CO_2 reactivity after aneurysmal subarachnoid hemorrhage, *Neurosurgery* 22:822-826, 1988.
31. DeWitt LD, Wechsler L: Transcranial Doppler, *Stroke* 19:915-921, 1988.
32. Doberstein C, et al: Assessment of cerebral blood flow using transcranial Doppler ultrasonography and the intravenous xenon-133 technique, *J Cardiovasc Technol* 9:60-61, 1990.
33. Douville CM, et al: Detection of vasospasm following subarachnoid hemorrhage using transcranial Doppler, *J Vasc Technol* 14:111-115, 1990.
34. Duff TA, et al: Erythrocytes are essential for development of cerebral vasculopathy resulting from subarachnoid hemorrhage in cats, *Stroke* 19:68-72, 1988.
35. Eicke BM, Tegeler CH, Dalley G, Myers LG: Angle correction in transcranial Doppler sonography, *J Neuroimaging* 4:29-33, 1994.
36. Eskridge JM, Newell DW, Pendleton GA: Transluminal angioplasty for treatment of vasospasm, *Neurosurg Clin N Am* 1:387-399, 1990.
37. Fahmy MA, Smith RR: Identification of presymptomatic vasospasm by transcranial Doppler sonography, *Stroke* 23:156, 1992.
38. Farrar K, Ferguson G: Cerebral blood flow and arterial caliber following subarachnoid hemorrhage, *J Cardiovasc Technol* 9:88-89, 1990.
39. Fein JM: Focal autoregulatory disturbances in middle cerebral artery vasospasm, *Stroke* 4:333-334, 1973.
40. Feinberg WM, et al: Clinical characteristics of patients with inadequate temporal windows, *J Cardiovasc Technol* 9:55-56, 1990.
41. Findlay JM, Macdonald RL, Weir BKA: Current concepts of pathophysiology and management of cerebral vasospasm following aneurysmal subarachnoid hemorrhage, *Cerebrovasc Brain Metab Rev* 3:336-361, 1991.
42. Fisher CM, Kistler JP, Davis JM: Relation of cerebral vasospasm to subarachnoid hemorrhage visualized by computerized tomographic scanning, *Neurosurgery* 6:1-9, 1980.
43. Fisher CM, Roberson GM, Ojemann RG: Cerebral vasospasm with ruptured saccular aneurysm—the clinical manifestations, *Neurosurgery* 1:245-248, 1977.

44. Giller CA: Transcranial Doppler monitoring of cerebral blood velocity during craniotomy, *Neurosurgery* 25:769-776, 1989.

45. Giller CA: The frequency-dependent behavior of cerebral autoregulation, *Neurosurgery* 27:362-368, 1990.

46. Giller CA: A bedside test for cerebral autoregulation using transcranial Doppler ultrasound, *Acta Neurochir (Wien)* 108:7-14, 1991.

47. Giller CA, et al: Cerebral arterial diameters during changes in blood pressure and carbon dioxide during craniotomy, *Neurosurgery* 32:737-742, 1993.

48. Giller CA, Purdy P, Giller A, et al: Elevated transcranial Doppler ultrasound velocities following therapeutic arterial dilation, *Stroke* 26:123-127, 1995.

49. Gomez CR, Gomez SM, Hall IS: The elusive transtemporal window: a demographic and technical study, *J Cardiovasc Technol* 8:176-177, 1989.

50. Grolimund P, et al: Evaluation of cerebrovascular disease by combined extracranial and transcranial Doppler sonography: experience in 1,039 patients, *Stroke* 18:1018-1024, 1987.

51. Grosset DG, et al: Prediction of symptomatic vasospasm after subarachnoid hemorrhage by rapidly increasing transcranial Doppler velocity and cerebral blood flow changes, *Stroke* 23:674-679, 1992.

52. Grosset DG, et al: Use of transcranial Doppler sonography to predict development of a delayed ischemic deficit after subarachnoid hemorrhage, *J Neurosurg* 78:183-187, 1993.

53. Grote E, Hassler W: The critical first minutes after subarachnoid hemorrhage, *Neurosurgery* 22:654-661, 1988.

54. Grubb RL, et al: Effects of increased intracranial pressure on cerebral blood volume, blood flow, and oxygen utilization in monkeys, *J Neurosurg* 43:385-398, 1975.

55. Grubb RL, et al: Effects of subarachnoid hemorrhage on cerebral blood volume, blood flow, and oxygen utilization in humans, *J Neurosurg* 46:446-453, 1977.

56. Haley EC, Kassell NF, Torner JC, and the participants: A randomized trial of nicardipine in subarachnoid hemorrhage: angiographic and transcranial Doppler ultrasound results, *J Neurosurg* 78:548-553, 1993.

57. Harders A: *Monitoring hemodynamic changes related to vasospasm in the circle of Willis after aneurysm surgery.* In Aaslid R, editor: *Transcranial Doppler ultrasonography,* Vienna, 1986, Springer-Verlag.

58. Harders AG: *Neurosurgical applications of transcranial Doppler sonography,* Vienna, 1987, Springer-Verlag.

59. Harders AG, Gilsbach JM: Time course of blood velocity changes related to vasospasm in the circle of Willis measured by transcranial Doppler ultrasound, *J Neurosurg* 66:718-728, 1987.

60. Harders AG, Gilsbach JM, Hornyak ME: *Incidence of vasospasm in transcranial Doppler sonography and its clinical significance: a prospective study in 100 consecutive patients who were given intravenous nimodipine and who underwent early aneurysm surgery.* In Wilkins RH, editor: *Cerebral vasospasm,* New York, 1988, Raven Press.

61. Hase U, et al: Intracranial pressure and pressure volume relation in patients with subarachnoid haemorrhage (SAH), *Acta Neurochir (Wien)* 44:69-80, 1978.

62. Hassler W, Chioff F: CO_2 reactivity of cerebral vasospasm after aneurysmal subarachnoid haemorrhage, *Acta Neurochir (Wien)* 98:167-175, 1989.

63. Higashida RT, et al: Transluminal angioplasty for treatment of intracranial arterial vasospasm, *J Neurosurg* 71:648-653, 1989.

64. Higashida RT, et al: New microballoon device for transluminal angioplasty of intracranial arterial vasospasm, *Am J Neuroradiol* 11:233-238, 1990.

65. Hijdra A, et al: Aneurysmal subarachnoid hemorrhage: compli-

cations and outcome in a hospital population, *Stroke* 18:1061-1067, 1987.

66. Hurst RW, et al: Role of transcranial Doppler in neuroradiological treatment of intracranial vasospasm, *Stroke* 24:299-303, 1993.

67. Hutchison K, Weir B: Transcranial Doppler studies in aneurysm patients, *Can J Neurol Sci* 16:411-416, 1989.

68. Iacopino DG, et al: Flow velocity increase revealed by transcranial Doppler examination in patients operated for intracranial aneurysms: physiopathological and clinical considerations, *Stroke* 23:462, 1992.

69. Iacopino DG, et al: Transorbital Doppler: an approach that increases transcranial Doppler sensitivity in the detection of SAH vasospasm, *Stroke* 24:519, 1993.

70. Ishii R: Regional cerebral blood flow in patients with ruptured intracranial aneurysms, *J Neurosurg* 50:587-594, 1979.

71. Jackson M, Thomas-Lukes K, McBride DQ, Martin NA: The use of transcranial Doppler to distinguish vasospasm from hyperemia in head injury patients, *Stroke* 25:756, 1994.

72. Kaku Y, et al: Superselective intra-arterial infusion of papaverine for the treatment of cerebral vasospasm after subarachnoid hemorrhage, *J Neurosurg* 77:842-847, 1992.

73. Kaps M, et al: Imaging of the intracranial vertebrobasilar system using color-coded ultrasound, *Stroke* 23:1577-1582, 1992.

74. Kassell NF, et al: Cerebral vasospasm following aneurysmal subarachnoid hemorrhage, *Stroke* 16:562-572, 1985.

75. Kassell NF, et al: The International Cooperative Study on the Timing of Aneurysm Surgery, part I: overall management results, *J Neurosurg* 73:18-36, 1990.

76. Kassell NF, et al: The International Cooperative Study on the Timing of Aneurysm Surgery, part II: surgical results, *J Neurosurg* 73:37-47, 1990.

77. Kassell NF, et al: Treatment of cerebral vasospasm with intra-arterial papaverine, *J Neurosurg* 77:848-852, 1992.

78. Katsiotas PA, Taptas JN: Embolism and spasm following subarachnoid hemorrhage, *Acta Radiol* 7:140-144, 1968.

79. Kelly PF, et al: Cerebral perfusion, vascular spasm, and outcome in patients with ruptured intracranial aneurysms, *J Neurosurg* 47:44-49, 1977.

80. Kistler JP, et al: The relation of cerebral vasospasm to the extent and location of subarachnoid blood visualized by CT scan: a prospective study, *Neurology* 33:424-436, 1983.

81. Klingelhöfer J, et al: Cerebral vasospasm evaluated by transcranial Doppler ultrasonography at different intracranial pressures, *J Neurosurg* 75:752-758, 1991.

82. Kontos HA: Validity of cerebral arterial blood flow calculations from velocity measurements, *Stroke* 20:1-3, 1989.

83. Kuwayama A, et al: Papaverine hydrochloride and experimental hemorrhagic cerebral arterial spasm, *Stroke* 3:27-33, 1972.

84. Lanzino G, et al: Blood glucose levels predict outcome in patients with subarachnoid hemorrhage and vasospasm: analysis of 635 patients enrolled in the nicardipine study, *Stroke* 24:169, 1993.

85. Laumer R, et al: Cerebral hemodynamics in subarachnoid hemorrhage evaluated by transcranial Doppler sonography, part I: reliability of flow velocities in clinical management, *Neurosurgery* 33:1-9, 1993.

86. Lennihan L, et al: Transcranial Doppler detection of anterior cerebral artery vasospasm, *J Neurol Neurosurg Psychiatry* 56:906-909, 1993.

87. LeRoux PD, et al: Severe symptomatic vasospasm: the role of immediate postoperative angioplasty, *J Neurosurg* 80:224-229, 1994.

88. Levy ML, et al: Cardiac performance enhancement from dobutamine in patients refractory to hypervolemic therapy for cerebral vasospasm, *J Neurosurg* 79:494-499, 1993.

89. Lewis DH, et al: Brain SPECT and transcranial Doppler ultrasound in vasospasm-induced delayed cerebral ischemia after

subarachnoid hemorrhage, *J Stroke Cerebrovasc Ds* 2:12-21, 1992.

90. Lewis DH, et al: Brain SPECT and the effect of cerebral angioplasty in delayed ischemia due to vasospasm, *J Nucl Med* 33:1789-1796, 1992.

91. Lindegaard K-F, et al: Assessment of intracranial hemodynamics in carotid artery disease by transcranial Doppler ultrasound, *J Neurosurg* 63:890-898, 1985.

92. Lindegaard K-F, et al: A non-invasive Doppler ultrasound method for the evaluation of patients with subarachnoid hemorrhage, *Acta Radiol* 369 (suppl):96-98, 1987.

93. Lindegaard K-F, et al: Variations in middle cerebral artery blood flow investigated with noninvasive transcranial blood velocity measurements, *Stroke* 18:1025-1030, 1987.

94. Lindegaard K-F, et al: Cerebral vasospasm after subarachnoid haemorrhage investigated by means of transcranial Doppler ultrasound, *Acta Neurochir (Wien)* 42 (suppl):81-84, 1988.

95. Lindegaard K-F, et al: Cerebral vasospasm diagnosis by means of angiography and blood velocity measurements, *Acta Neurochir (Wien)* 100:12-24, 1989.

96. Linskey ME, et al: Fatal rupture of the intracranial carotid artery during transluminal angioplasty for vasospasm induced by subarachnoid hemorrhage, *J Neurosurg* 74:842-847, 1991.

97. Livingston K, Hopkins LN: Intraarterial papaverine as an adjunct to transluminal angioplasty for vasospasm induced by subarachnoid hemorrhage, *Am J Neuroradiol* 14:346-347, 1993.

98. Macdonald RL, Weir BKA: A review of hemoglobin and the pathogenesis of cerebral vasospasm, *Stroke* 22:971-982, 1991.

99. Marks MP, Steinberg GK, Lane B: Intraarterial papaverine for the treatment of vasospasm, *Am J Neuroradiol* 14:822-826, 1993.

100. Markwalder TM, et al: Dependency of blood flow velocity in the middle cerebral artery on end-tidal carbon dioxide partial pressure: a transcranial Doppler ultrasound study, *J Cereb Blood Flow Metab* 4:368-372, 1984.

101. Mathiesen T, Lindquist C: Delayed brainstem ischemia following rupture of a basilar artery aneurysm and its reversal by nimodipine, *Acta Neurol Scand* 82:150-152, 1990.

102. Matsuda M, Shiino A, Handa J: Sequential changes of cerebral blood flow after aneurysmal subarachnoid haemorrhage, *Acta Neurochir (Wien)* 105:98-106, 1990.

103. Meixensberger J, et al: Blood flow velocity and cerebral blood flow after subarachnoid hemorrhage, *Stroke* 23:476, 1992.

104. Meyer CHA, et al: Progressive change in cerebral blood flow during the first three weeks after subarachnoid hemorrhage, *Neurosurgery* 12:58-76, 1983.

105. Millikan CH: Cerebral vasospasm and ruptured intracranial aneurysm, *Arch Neurol* 32:433-449, 1975.

106. Mountz JM, et al: Pre- and post-operative cerebral blood flow changes in subarachnoid haemorrhage, *Acta Neurochir (Wien)* 109:30-33, 1991.

107. Muizelaar JP, Becker DP: Induced hypertension for the treatment of cerebral ischemia after subarachnoid hemorrhage, *Surg Neurol* 25:317-325, 1986.

108. Newell DW, Winn HR: Transcranial Doppler in cerebral vasospasm, *Neurosurg Clin N Am* 1:319-328, 1990.

109. Newell DW, et al: Angioplasty for the treatment of symptomatic vasospasm following subarachnoid hemorrhage, *J Neurosurg* 71:654-660, 1989.

110. Newell DW, et al: Distribution of angiographic vasospasm after subarachnoid hemorrhage: implications for diagnosis by TCD, *Neurosurgery* 27:574-577, 1990.

111. Newell DW, et al: Comparison of flow and velocity during dynamic autoregulation testing in humans, *Stroke* 25:793-797, 1994.

112. Nornes H, Knutzen HB, Wikeby P: Cerebral arterial blood flow and aneurysm surgery, part 2: induced hypotension and auto-

113. Norris J: Does transcranial Doppler have any clinical value? *Neurology* 40:329-331, 1990.

114. Ohno K, et al: Symptomatic cerebral vasospasm of unusually late onset after aneurysm rupture, *Acta Neurochir (Wien)* 108:163-166, 1991.

115. Origitano TC, et al: Sustained increased cerebral blood flow with prophylactic hypertensive hypervolemic hemodilution ("Triple-H" therapy) after subarachnoid hemorrhage, *Neurosurgery* 27:729-740, 1990.

116. Pasqualin A, et al: *Transcranial Doppler findings in the early stage of subarachnoid hemorrhage: relation to the amount of cisternal blood deposition and modality of treatment.* In Wilkins RH, editor: *Cerebral vasospasm,* New York, 1988, Raven Press.

117. Petruk KC, et al: Cerebral blood flow following induced subarachnoid hemorrhage in the monkey, *J Neurosurg* 37:316-324, 1972.

118. Petruk KC, et al: Clinical grade, regional cerebral blood flow, and angiographical spasm in the monkey after subarachnoid and subdural hemorrhage, *Stroke* 4:431-445, 1973.

119. Pickard JD, et al: *Autoregulation of cerebral blood flow and the prediction of late morbidity and mortality after cerebral aneurysm surgery.* In Wilkins RH, editor: *Cerebral vasospasm,* Baltimore, 1980, Williams & Wilkins.

120. Piepgras A, Hagen T, Schmiadek P: Reliable prediction of grade of angiographic vasospasm by transcranial Doppler sonography, *Stroke* 25:260, 1994.

121. Powers WJ, et al: Regional cerebral blood flow and metabolism in reversible ischemia due to vasospasm, *J Neurosurg* 62:539-546, 1985.

122. Pucher RK, Auer LM: Effects of vasospasm in the middle cerebral artery territory on flow velocity and volume flow: a computer simulation, *Acta Neurochir (Wien)* 93:123-128, 1988.

123. Pucher RK, Mokry M, Auer LM: *Numerical simulation of vasospasm in the middle cerebral artery territory.* In Wilkins RH, editor: *Cerebral vasospasm,* New York, 1988, Raven Press.

124. Ries F, et al: A transpulmonary contrast medium enhances the transcranial Doppler signal in humans, *Stroke* 24:1903-1909, 1993.

125. Rinkel GJE, van Gijn J, Wijdicks EFM: Subarachnoid hemorrhage without detectable cause: a review of the causes, *Stroke* 24:1403-1409, 1993.

126. Romner B, et al: Transcranial Doppler sonography 12 hours after subarachnoid hemorrhage, *J Neurosurg* 70:732-736, 1989.

127. Romner B, et al: Correlation of transcranial Doppler sonography findings with timing of aneurysm surgery, *J Neurosurg* 73:72-76, 1990.

128. Sanchez R, Pile-Spellman J: Radiologic features of cerebral vasospasm, *Neurosurg Clin N Am* 1:289-306, 1990.

129. Sander D, Klingelhöfer J: Changes of cerebral hemodynamics during rebleeding subsequent to subarachnoid hemorrhage with vasospasm, *Neurol Res* 14:352-354, 1992.

130. Sander D, Klingelhöfer J: Cerebral vasospasm following post traumatic subarachnoid hemorrhage evaluated by transcranial Doppler ultrasonography, *J Neurol Sci* 119:1-7, 1993.

131. Schneider PA, et al: Effect of internal carotid artery occlusion on intracranial hemodynamics: transcranial Doppler evaluation and clinical correlations, *Stroke* 19:589-593, 1988.

132. Schoning M, Buchholz R, Walter J: Comparative study of transcranial color duplex sonography and transcranial Doppler sonography in adults, *J Neurosurg* 78:776-784, 1993.

133. Segawa H, et al: *Efficacy of intracisternal papaverine on symptomatic vasospasm.* In Wilkins RH, editor: *Cerebral vasospasm,* New York, 1988, Raven Press.

134. Seiler RW, et al: Cerebral vasospasm evaluated by transcranial ultrasound correlated with clinical grade and CT-visualized

113. regulatory capacity, *J Neurosurg* 17:819-827, 1977.

subarachnoid hemorrhage, *J Neurosurg* 64:594-600, 1986.

135. Seiler RW, Grolimund P, Zurbruegg HR: Evaluation of the calcium-antagonist nimodipine for the prevention of vasospasm after aneurysmal subarachnoid haemorrhage: a prospective transcranial Doppler ultrasound study, *Acta Neurochir (Wien)* 85:7-16, 1987.

136. Seiler RW, et al: Outcome of aneurysmal subarachnoid hemorrhage in a hospital population: a prospective study including early operation, intravenous nimodipine, and transcranial Doppler ultrasound, *Neurosurgery* 23:598-604, 1988.

137. Seiler RW, Nirkko AC: Effect of nimodipine on cerebrovascular response to CO_2 in asymptomatic individuals and patients with subarachnoid hemorrhage: a transcranial Doppler ultrasound study, *Neurosurgery* 27:247-251, 1990.

138. Seiler RW, Newell DW: *Subarachnoid hemorrhage and vasospasm.* In Newell DW, Aaslid R, editors: *Transcranial Doppler,* New York, 1992, Raven Press.

139. Sekhar LN, et al: Value of transcranial Doppler examination in the diagnosis of cerebral vasospasm after subarachnoid hemorrhage, *Neurosurgery* 22:813-821, 1988.

140. Shigemori M, et al: *Evaluation of intracranial hemodynamics in subarachnoid hemorrhage by use of three dimensional transcranial Doppler (3D-TCD) ultrasound.* Proceedings of the fourth international symposium on intracranial hemodynamics: Transcranial Doppler and Cerebral Blood Flow, Orlando, Florida, February 11-14, 1990.

141. Shinoda J, et al: Acetazolamide reactivity on cerebral blood flow in patients with subarachnoid haemorrhage, *Acta Neurochir (Wien)* 109:102-108, 1991.

142. Simeone FA, Trepper P: Cerebral vasospasm with infarction, *Stroke* 3:449-455, 1972.

143. Sloan MA, et al: Sensitivity and specificity of transcranial Doppler ultrasonography in the diagnosis of vasospasm following subarachnoid hemorrhage, *Neurology* 39:1514-1518, 1989.

144. Sloan MA, et al: Sensitivity and specificity of transcranial Doppler in the detection of basilar artery vasospasm, *Stroke* 23:469, 1992.

145. Sloan MA, et al: Sensitivity and specificity of transcranial Doppler in the detection of vertebral artery vasospasm, *Stroke* 23:469, 1992.

146. Sloan MA, et al: Sensitivity and specificity of transcranial Doppler in the detection of internal carotid siphon vasospasm, *J Neuroimaging* 2:57, 1992.

147. Sloan MA, Kittner SJ, Rigamonti D: Detection of vasospasm complicating lobar hematoma by transcranial Doppler sonography, *J Neuroimaging* 2:213-215, 1992.

148. Sloan MA, et al: Optimal diagnosis of vasospasm following subarachnoid hemorrhage by transcranial Doppler sonography (TCD), *Stroke* 24:518, 1993.

149. Sloan MA, et al: Causes of false positive transcranial Doppler (TCD) examinations in subarachnoid hemorrhage, *Stroke* 29:519, 1993.

150. Sloan MA: *Detection of vasospasm following subarachnoid hemorrhage.* In Babikian VL, Wechsler LR, editors: *Transcranial Doppler ultrasonography,* St Louis, 1993, BC Decker/Mosby–Year Book.

151. Sloan MA, et al: Prevalence of posterior circulation vasospasm: a transcranial Doppler study, *Stroke* 25:743, 1994.

152. Sloan MA: *Cerebral vasoconstriction: physiology, pathophysiology, and occurrence in selected cerebrovascular disorders.* In Caplan LR, editor: *Brain ischemia: basic concepts and their clinical relevance* London, 1994, Springer-Verlag.

153. Sloan MA, et al: Transcranial Doppler detection of vertebrobasilar vasospasm following subarachnoid hemorrhage, *Stroke* 25: 2187-2197, 1994.

153a. Sloan M, et al: Hemodynamic effects of intraarterial papaverine

for vasospasm following subarachnoid hemorrhage, *Cerebovasc Dis* 4(suppl 3):9, 1994.

154. Solomon RA, Post KD, McMurty JC III: Depression of circulating blood volume in patients after subarachnoid hemorrhage: implications for the management of symptomatic vasospasm, *Neurosurgery* 15:354-361, 1984.

155. Sorteberg W, et al: Blood velocity and regional blood flow in defined cerebral arterial systems, *Acta Neurochir (Wien)* 97:47-52, 1989.

156. Symon L, Bell BA, Kendall BE: *The relationship between vasospasm and cerebral ischemia and infarction.* In Wilkins RH, editor: *Cerebral vasospasm,* Baltimore, 1980, Williams & Wilkins.

157. Todaro C, et al: How early does the cerebral vasospasm begin after subarachnoid hemorrhage? *Stroke* 24:518, 1993.

158. Tomita Y, et al: Transcranial Doppler blood flow mapping in vasospasm after subarachnoid hemorrhage: prediction of cerebral ischemia and outcome of patients, *J Cardiovasc Technol* 9:286-287, 1990.

159. Torner JC, Kassell NF, Haley EC: The timing of surgery and vasospasm, *Neurosurg Clin N Am* 1:335-347, 1990.

160. Torner JC, Kassell NF: Predictors of asymptomatic and symptomatic vasospasm, *Stroke* 25:257, 1994.

161. Van Gijn J, et al: Hydrocephalus and vasospasm after aneurysmal hemorrhage, *J Neurosurg* 63:355-362, 1985.

162. Voldby B, Enevoldsen EM, Jensen FT: Cerebrovascular reactivity in patients with ruptured intracranial aneurysms, *J Neurosurg* 62:59-67, 1985.

163. Voldby B, Enevoldsen EM: Intracranial pressure changes following aneurysm surgery, part I: clinical and angiographic correlations, *J Neurosurg* 56:186-196, 1988.

164. Vorkapic P, Bevan RD, Bevan JA: Longitudinal time course of reversible and irreversible components of chronic cerebrovasospasm of the rabbit basilar artery, *J Neurosurg* 74:951-955, 1991.

165. Wechsler LR, Ropper AH, Kistler JP: Transcranial Doppler in cerebrovascular disease, *Stroke* 17:905-912, 1986.

166. Weir B, et al: Relative prognostic significance in vasospasm following subarachnoid hemorrhage, *Can J Neurol Sci* 2:109-114, 1975.

167. Weir B, et al: Time course of vasospasm in man, *J Neurosurg* 48:173-178, 1978.

168. Weir BKA: *The effect of vasospasm on morbidity and mortality after subarachnoid hemorrhage from ruptured aneurysm.* In Wilkins RH, editor: *Cerebral vasospasm,* Baltimore, 1980, Williams & Wilkins.

169. Williams AR, Chehrazi BB, Lemons VR: Elevated transcranial Doppler (TCD) measured flow velocities after severe head injury (SHI), *Stroke* 24:520, 1993.

170. Wood JH, Kee DB: Hemorheology of the cerebral circulation in stroke, *Stroke* 16:765-772, 1985.

171. Wozniak MA, et al: Sensitivity and specificity of transcranial Doppler for the diagnosis of anterior cerebral artery vasospasm, *J Neuroimaging* 3:75, 1993.

172. Wozniak MA, et al: Prevalence of anterior circulation vasospasm: a transcranial Doppler study, *Stroke* 25:744, 1994.

172a. Wozniak M, et al: Distribution of pathologically elevated flow velocities occurring on days 1-3 following subarachnoid hemorrhage, *Cerebrovasc Dis* 4(suppl 3):9, 1994.

173. Wozniak MA, et al: Detection of vasospasm by transcranial Doppler: the challenges of the anterior cerebral and posterior cerebral arteries. Submitted to *J Neuroimaging.*

174. Yonas H, et al: Determination of irreversible ischemia by xenon-enhanced computed tomographic monitoring of cerebral blood flow in patients with symptomatic vasospasm, *Neurosurgery* 24:368-372, 1989.

175. Zubkov YN, Nikiforov BM, Shustin VA: Balloon catheter technique for dilation of constricted cerebral arteries after aneurysmal SAH, *Acta Neurochir (Wien)* 70:65-79, 1984.

16

Cerebrovascular Diseases

E. Bernd Ringelstein

Not surprisingly, transacranial Doppler sonography (TCD) was first applied to patients exhibiting intracranial arterial vasospasm due to subarachnoid hemorrhage (SAH).[1] Soon after, reports were published that demonstrated the usefulness of TCD in the detection of stenoses and occlusions of the middle cerebral artery (MCA) or the internal carotid artery siphon.[43,54] It is the use of TCD in the study of occlusive disease in the anterior and posterior cerebral arteries, together with its diagnostic capacity and possible methodologic refinements, that is the subject of this chapter. The broad spectrum of diseases in which TCD is of significant clinical value are also considered, as are various aspects of the pathophysiology of stroke and cerebrovascular occlusive disease (CVOD).

In the anterior cerebral circulation, three different predilection sites for atherothrombosis,* embolism and dissection,[40] or thrombosis due to sickle cell disease[4] have been identified, namely, (1) the M1 segment of the MCA and (2) the basilar artery, which are similar sites with a predilection to occlusive disease; (3) the top of the basilar artery and the P1 segments of the posterior cerebral arteries, (4) the superior cerebellar arteries, and (5) the posterior inferior cerebellar arteries[17,45] have a predilection to occlusion.

*References 10, 13, 17, 23, 56, 57.

Previous studies of acute stroke patients have consistently shown that the cause of cerebral infarction often remains unidentified, even after arteriographic investigation. The limitation has been ascribed to the delay involved in such investigation. This is not the case with TCD and other ultrasound techniques, which combine noninvasive qualities with an ability to examine the cerebral vasculature instantaneously. The TCD's capacity to evaluate stroke etiology has improved to such an extent that, when combined with transoesophageal echocardiography and magnetic resonance imaging (MRI) of cerebral small vessel disease, it is close to perfect.

Because they are addressed elsewhere in this book, topics such as microembolus detection, analysis of the configuration of the circle of Willis, and cardiac influences on cerebral blood flow velocities are not detailed in this chapter.

DIAGNOSIS AND FOLLOW-UP
OF INTRACRANIAL OCCLUSIVE DISEASE
Anterior circulation

Stenosis and occlusion of the middle cerebral artery. Although in situ (autochthonous) occlusive disease of the MCA and carotid siphon is responsible for only a small percentage of ischemic strokes,[23,35] a timely diagnosis of MCA or carotid siphon stenosis may be

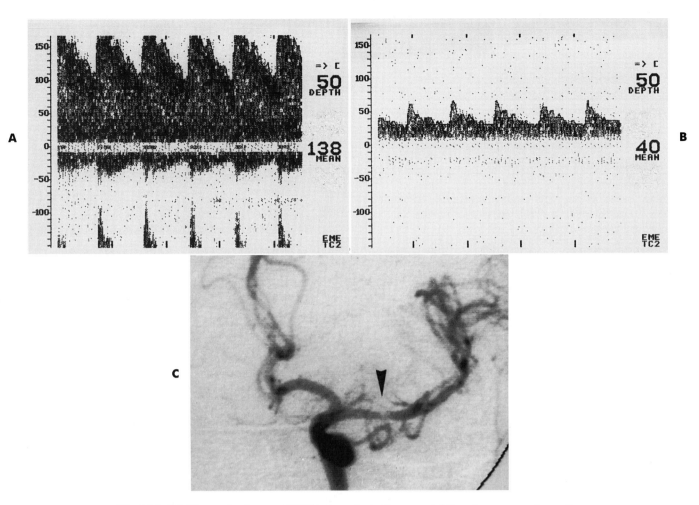

Fig. 16-1. Middle cerebral artery (MCA) stenosis. **A,** Transcranial Doppler sonography on the left side shows a markedly increased flow velocity (mean 138 cm/s) within the M1 segment of the MCA. Turbulent flow and vessel wall covibration phenomena are indicated by spectral broadening and increased low-frequency components during systole (transtemporal insonation). **B,** Normal flow signal (mean velocity 40 cm/s) of the contralateral MCA at the same insonation depth, presented for comparison. **C,** Angiogram indicated MCA stenosis (*arrow*). (From Ley-Pozo J, Ringelstein EB: Noninvasive detection of occlusive disease of the carotid siphon and middle cerebral artery, *Ann Neurol* 28:640-647, 1990.)

crucial in the prevention of a catastrophic stroke, once transient ischemic attacks (TIAs) or crescendo TIAs have been experienced. Asian populations, especially the Japanese, suffer from this type of cerebrovascular disease two to three times more frequently than Europeans.[12] In the past, most MCA or siphon stenoses were not diagnosed before completion of the stroke, if at all, because clinicians were reluctant to perform potentially harmful cerebral arteriography on the stroke-threatened patient with progressive symptoms. The validation of TCD as a reliable tool for intracranial exploration has radically changed this situation. Patients presenting with repetitive TIAs or crescendolike transient hemispheric stroke symptoms are not only checked for extracranial internal carotid artery stenosis or ICA dissection but also

receive TCD examinations to check the patency of large intracranial arteries before other diagnostic steps are performed.[32,41]

The tentative diagnosis of intracranial artery stenosis can be made according to typical TCD findings. An MCA stenosis produces (1) increased flow velocity, (2) "turbulence" (i.e., disturbed flow) immediately distal to the stenosis, (3) low-frequency noise produced by nonharmonic covibrations of the vessel wall, and, in rare instances, (4) musical murmurs due to harmonic covibrations producing pure tones[2,33] (Fig. 16-1). Side-to-side differences in flow velocity are also helpful in making the diagnosis (box).

In patients with intracranial atherosclerotic stenoses sensu strictu, the anatomic extension of flow abnormali-

According to Ley-Pozo J, Ringelstein EB: Noninvasive detection of occlusive disease of the carotid siphon and middle cerebral artery, *Ann Neurol* 28:640-647, 1990.
*Not distinguishable from very distal carotid siphon stenosis.
†Most authors consider a 20 cm/s side-to-side difference in flow velocities pathologic but nonspecific.

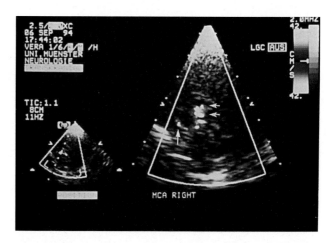

Fig. 16-2. Transcranial color-coded Duplex scanning. The intracranial vascular tree is visible in an axial view (*top*, lateral; *bottom*, medial). The color spots indicate the C1 segment of the carotid siphon (*white arrow*), and the proximal MCA is seen as a red spot. A tight MCA stenosis (*double arrow*) can also be seen.

ties should always be "circumscribed," that is, restricted to certain insonation depths. The site of the highest flow velocities corresponds to the stenotic channel itself. The corresponding echo may be very faint and may be "overheard" or "overlooked" because of the intrusive low-frequency downstream noise. Approximately 5 mm upstream and 10 to 15 mm downstream from the lesion—beyond the site of the greatest flow velocities—flow abnormalities are less pronounced or absent.

It is difficult to quantify MCA stenosis, largely because angiography has shown itself to be unreliable in that it is able to visualize the main stem of the MCA in only one plane, the anterior-posterior. As a rule of thumb, stenoses that reduce the cross-sectional area of the MCA by up to 50% (an approximate 30% reduction in diameter) cannot be detected by TCD. In clinical practice, however, this is not a significant shortcoming because lesions of that size are hardly ever symptomatic. The following general principles may be useful in the quantification of intracranial stenoses: A "circumscribed" increase of flow velocity, exceeding the corresponding site of the contralateral artery by 30 cm/s and unassociated with turbulence or low-frequency noise, indicates a moderate stenosis with a lumen reduction of approximately 60% to 70%. It corresponds to a diameter narrowing of approximately 40% to 50%. High-grade stenoses causing 80% or more reduction in diameter (corresponding to at least 70% loss of cross-sectional area) produce all of the abnormalities listed in the box. Very high-grade stenoses (at least 90%) create flow

velocities of 200 cm/s or more and even musical murmurs.[2] An illustrative example of a high-grade MCA stenosis is shown in Figure 16-1.

Similar observations may be made in stenoses of the MCA M2 segment, although these cannot be reliably detected by TCD. Two or three first-grade MCA branches may exist, and they cannot be unequivocally identified by TCD examination. Stenoses of the M2 segment are very rare, representing less than 10% of all MCA lesions. Furthermore, more distal stenoses of the MCA branches cannot be detected at all, mainly because their flow direction is almost perpendicular to the ultrasound beam. A study of a high-grade M2 stenosis has been published by Ringelstein and associates.[50]

Color-coded transcranial Doppler (CC-TCD) does not significantly improve TCD's diagnostic capacity in this field, although it does facilitate easier and faster anatomic orientation within the skull and cerebral vascular tree[8] (Fig. 16-2; see also Plate 62).

One difficulty for both TCD and CC-TCD is the lack of an adequate ultrasound window in the temporal bone in 15% to 20% of older patients and in women in particular. This problem should, however, be overcome by the routine introduction of echocontrast agents into clinical practice (Fig. 16-3).

In the hands of an experienced vascular technician, a well-trained nurse, or a physician, TCD (including CC-TCD) is sufficiently reliable for clinical purposes and is thus of considerable practical value. In my experience, positive TCD findings that appear false are likely to indicate inaccurate "negative" results from poor-quality arteriograms, when all ultrasound criteria listed in the preceding paragraphs are fulfilled. Studies designed to evaluate TCD's potential for detecting intracranial

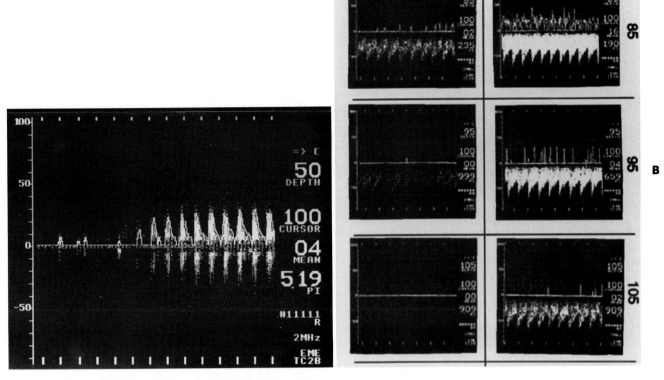

Fig. 16-3. Effect of the echocontrast agent SHU508A. **A,** The middle cerebral artery of an elderly woman is insonated; no signal is detected. After injection of SHU508A, a strong middle cerebral artery echo appears and is sustained for several minutes. **B,** *Left column:* In an elderly, short-necked, obese patient with brainstem stroke, the vertebrobasilar system could be traced suboccipitally only up to an insonation depth of 95 mm (note very faint vertebral or basilar artery flow signal). *Right column:* After intravenous injection of SHU508A, the entire vertebrobasilar axis could be traced up to an insonation depth of 105 mm, thus excluding basilar artery thrombosis or stenosis. (Modified from Dorr JM, Doherty CC, Ringelstein EB, Schlief R: A new ultrasound contrast medium as a diagnostic aid in patients with insufficient transcranial Doppler sonography [TCD] signals, *Journal of Clinical Ultrasound* [in press].)

occlusive disease in the anterior cerebral circulation reflect its high sensitivity and specificity.* Details of the largest series investigated, which used arteriograms as its gold standard, are given in Tables 16-1 and 16-2. From a clinical standpoint, a 6-month TCD follow-up of MCA stenoses is useful because it helps the clinician make decisions regarding anticoagulation. The latter can be discontinued without any harm to the patient when complete occlusion or MCA recanalization (Fig. 16-4) can be demonstrated.

The diagnosis of an acute ("embolic") MCA occlusion is often triggered by the clinical discovery of abrupt hemiplegia, forced deviation, dysphasia, or neglect. In rare cases of local, in situ atherothrombotic ("chronic") MCA occlusion, the lesion may remain asymptomatic, but only if it has been collateralized by a moyamoyalike network of tortuous, dilated, lenticulostriate arteries. The presence of these collaterals cannot be diagnosed

*References 15, 24, 25, 33, 36, 38, 40, 50, 60.

Table 16-1. Comparison of transcranial Doppler and arteriographic findings corresponding to the carotid siphon (*N* = 139 visualized arteries)

	Transcranial Doppler sonography			
Arteriography	**Normal**	**Stenosis**	**Occlusion**	**Total**
Normal	111	4	0	115
Stenosis	1	16	0	17
Occlusion	1	0	6	7
TOTAL	113	20	6	139

Kappa = 0.86; 95% confidence interval = 0.72-0.996.
Quality features of TCD: sensitivity for stenosis/occlusion 94.1/85.7; specificity for stenosis/occlusion 96.7/100; positive predictive value for stenosis/occlusion 80/100; negative predictive value for stenosis/occlusion 99.2/99.3; diagnostic accuracy for stenosis/occlusion 96.4/99.3.
From Ley-Pozo J, Ringelstein EB: Noninvasive detection of occlusive disease of the carotid siphon and middle cerebral artery, *Ann Neurol* 28:640-647, 1990.

Table 16-2. Comparison of transcranial Doppler sonographic and arteriographic findings corresponding to the middle cerebral artery (M1 segment) (N = 169 visualized arteries)

Arteriography	Transcranial Doppler sonography			
	Normal	Stenosis	Occlusion	Total
Normal	142	1	1	144
Stenosis	2	12	0	14
Occlusion	0	1	10	11
TOTAL	144	14	11	169

Kappa = 0.91; 95% confidence interval = 0.79-1.
Quality features of TCD: sensitivity for stenosis/occlusion 85.7/90.9; specificity for stenosis/occlusion 98.7/99.4; positive predictive value for stenosis/occlusion 85.7/90.9; negative predictive value for stenosis/occlusion 98.7/99.4; diagnostic accuracy for stenosis/occlusion 97.6/98.8.
From Ley-Pozo J, Ringelstein EB: Noninvasive detection of occlusive disease of the carotid siphon and middle cerebral artery, *Ann Neurol* 28:640-647, 1990.

with certainty by TCD, but they should be suspected if "multiple stenoses" are found close to depths of insonation corresponding to the MCA or the carotid siphon.[59] (See discussion of stenotic mimicry later in this chapter.) The definitive diagnosis of pseudo-moyamoya, however, is made by cerebral arteriography.

The vast majority of MCA occlusions are embolic, with either arterial or cardiac sources for emboli in the acute stage of a stroke; TCD findings are unaffected by the source of emboli. In the diagnosis of acute MCA occlusion, it is important to remember that an occlusion produces no MCA signal at all. Nevertheless, this "negative" finding can equally be caused by factors such as artifact, inadequacy of the investigator's technique, or variations in the patient's skull. Consequently, "positive" observations must also be made in order to establish the diagnosis. One such positive finding is the presence of an anterior cerebral artery (ACA) signal; another is a posterior cerebral artery (PCA) signal.[5,20,44,47] Increased flow velocity in an ACA or PCA indicates the recruitment of leptomeningeal anastomoses toward the ischemic MCA territory and may further support the diagnosis of an acute MCA occlusion.[11,60] The diagnosis of clinically relevant recruitment of leptomeningeal collaterals can be made where flow velocity in a basal cerebral artery increases in absolute terms, or when it exceeds that of its contralateral counterpart by 20 cm/s or more.

Frequent TCD follow-up studies of MCA occlusion can show spontaneous or therapeutically induced clot lysis and vessel recanalization.[26]

Spontaneous lysis occurs frequently and rapidly,[22] 65% of embolic MCA occlusions being completely recanalized within 3 days. The recanalization curve has a steep initial upstroke, with asymptomatic flattening after a few days (Fig. 16-5) and the recanalization rate reaching more than 80% in 3 weeks.[46] The clinical importance of early recanalization is self-evident. The presence of existing collateral channels distal to the circle of Willis (i.e., the leptomeningeal collateral network), together with early revascularization of the MCA, helps maintain blood flow and reduce the infarct's size, thus significantly improving the patient's poststroke prognosis.[50]

Occlusions of major MCA branches cannot be diagnosed by TCD because these lesions produce exclusively "negative" findings. Stenosis of the M2 segment, as mentioned previously, can occasionally be diagnosed by TCD because of the "positive" findings they produce.

I am aware of only one instance in which TCD data led to the false-positive diagnoses of MCA occlusion. This was in the case of a hemiplegic patient who had a marked displacement of the MCA from a large parenchymal hematoma. The patient's actual condition was not ascertained by a computed tomography (CT) scan performed prior to the TCD examination.

Other stenoses of the anterior basal cerebral arteries are rare (except for the carotid siphon). An example of the stenosis of the A1 segment of the anterior cerebral artery is shown in Fig. 16-6, *B* and *C*.

Stenosis and occlusion of the carotid siphon. The clinical and ultrasonographic features of siphon stenoses are similar to those of MCA stenoses (Fig. 16-6, *A* and *B*). Acute siphon occlusion by cardiac embolus, autochthonous thrombosis, or carotid dissection may remain asymptomatic or lead to only a minor stroke. More frequently, however, an embolus blocks the inner ICA bifurcation and leads to an infarct in the MCA distribution. Depending on the configuration of the anterior portion of the circle of Willis, the infarct can extend into the adjacent ACA territory. Acute brain infarcts of two major and adjacent territories will be lethal because of excessive brain swelling with subsequent herniation.

It is possible today to use extracranial Doppler sonography to make the diagnosis of a distal ICA occlusion. Typical findings include markedly reduced flow velocities in the proximal ICA and the common carotid artery. The flow signal is characterized by reverberating systolic low flow within a blind stump and by the absence of any flow during diastole.[43] The same reverberating flow signal can be observed with TCD during submandibular insonation of the distal but still "extradural" ICA (Figs. 16-7, *A* on p. 180 and 16-8, *A* on p. 181).

In patients with intact circles of Willis in whom the clot occludes the lumen of the distal ICA, flow in the ipsilateral ACA frequently becomes retrograde, indicating the presence of collateral flow. When the clot also blocks the proximal MCA, however, the combined

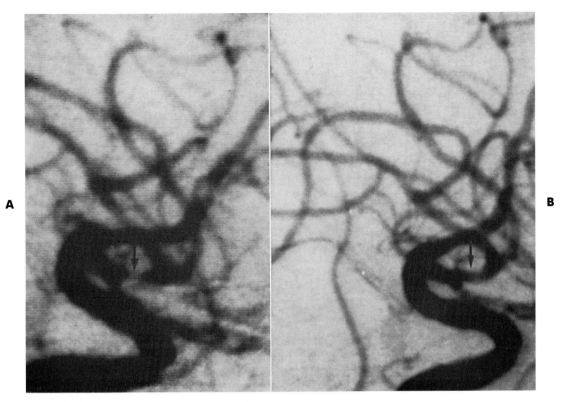

Fig. 16-4. Recanalization of middle cerebral artery (MCA) severe stenosis after 2 years of anticoagulation. The patient first presented with crescendo transient ischemic attacks. **A,** The original angiogram shows a subtotal MCA stenosis (*arrow*). Note the unusual projection, obtained because the lesion could not be visualized on regular anteroposterior views. The diagnosis was made by transcranial Doppler (TCD). **B,** The atherothrombotic plaque regressed while the patient was anticoagulated with warfarin. TCD was repeated every 3 months, and repeat angiography was performed when the TCD findings became normal. The flat plaque seen on the angiogram (*arrow*) did not cause detectable flow abnormalities.

findings of distal ICA occlusion (reverberating flow) and proximal MCA occlusion (lack of MCA flow) are observed.

In patients with moyamoya disease and complete siphon occlusion, the aforementioned blind stump of the ICA is associated with multiple, additional, high-grade stenotic signals in the vicinity of the carotid siphon, representing the collateral network (rete mirabile), which gives the disease its name, *moyamoya* or "fog," referring to the misty appearance of the collateral network on cerebral artenography.[59]

The diagnosis of siphon stenosis (Fig. 16-6, *A* and *B*) is made difficult by the unpredictable topography of both the carotid siphon and the osseous openings within the orbits and also by the variability of the lesion's pathology, which can include atherosclerosis and dissection. In addition, the proximity of the carotid siphon to other vascular channels that produce compensatory high flow and initiate stenosis further complicates the diagnosis.

Most problematic in this respect is the diagnosis of high-grade siphon stenosis when the ipsilateral posterior communicating artery (PCoA) functions as a collateral channel. The hyperperfused PCoA findings can be misdiagnosed as corresponding to siphon stenosis. Similar false conclusions might be drawn in patients with small, cavernous sinus–to–carotid artery fistulae, when key symptoms such as proptosis or oculomotor abnormalities are absent.[53] This shortcoming is partially compensated for by the accessibility of the siphon from both the transtemporal and transorbital pathways. The diagnosis can be verified by compressing the common carotid artery in the neck while the suspected siphon stenosis, actually the PCoA, is insonated. Flow stops in true siphon stenosis but increases in collateralizing channels ("stenotic mimicry").

Carotid artery dissections. The TCD diagnosis of carotid artery dissection should not be a major challenge to the examiner because findings, although not particularly specific, do exhibit clear, general characteristics. A stenotic lesion that is detected during TCD testing with the submandibular approach and located more than 2 cm distal to the carotid bifurcation almost certainly

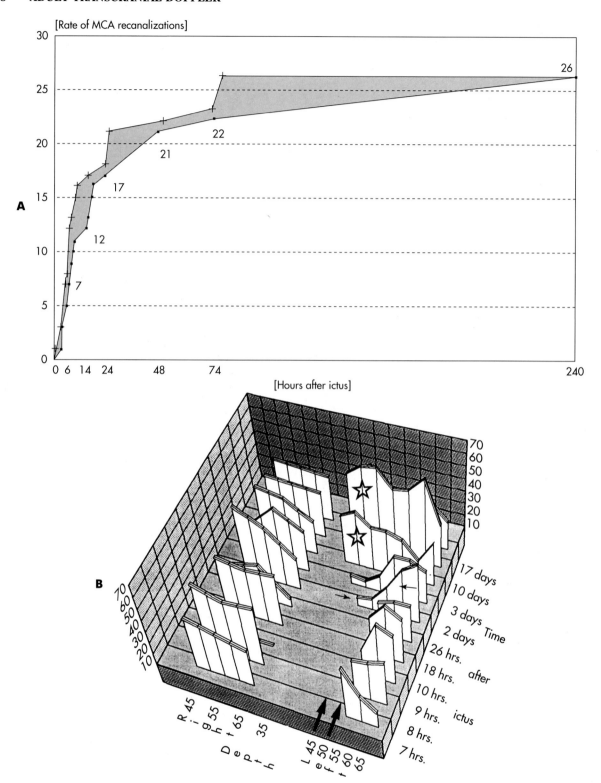

Fig. 16-5. Recanalization of the embolically occluded middle cerebral artery. **A,** In a series of 34 acute stroke patients with proven embolic middle cerebral artery (MCA) occlusion, repeat transcranial Doppler (TCD) investigations revealed an exponential, asymptotic recanalization curve. The left edge of the hatched zone indicates the time when the MCA was still occluded, and the right edge indicates the time when TCD revealed partial or total recanalization. **B,** Three-dimensional graph of MCA flow velocities in an acute stroke patient with MCA occlusion (*abscissa,* insonation depths of the right and left MCAs; *ordinate,* mean flow velocity in cm/s; *Z axis,* time; *0,* witnessed time of ictus). On the left side, flow signals could be obtained from the C1 segment of the carotid siphon but not the middle cerebral artery (*arrows*). Recanalization occurred at 26 hours poststroke (*horizontal arrowhead*) and led to hyperperfusion with abnormally high MCA flow velocities (*asterisk*). (**A** from Ringelstein EB, Biniek R, Weiller C, et al: Type and extent of hemispheric brain infarctions and clinical outcome in early and delayed middle cerebral artery recanalization, *Neurology* 42:289-298, 1992; **B** modified from same source.)

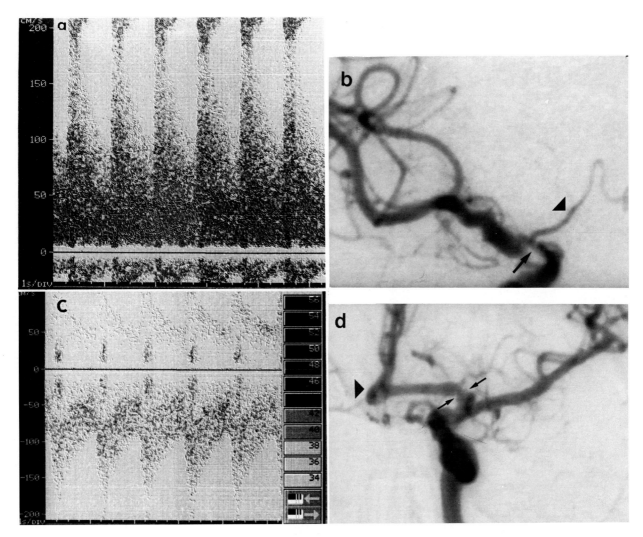

Fig. 16-6. Internal carotid artery (ICA) siphon and contralateral anterior cerebral artery (ACA) stenosis. **A,** Transtemporal transcranial Doppler (TCD) reveals very high flow velocities (mean 120 cm/s) at an insonation depth of 65 or 60 mm, leading to the diagnosis of tight left ICA C1 stenosis. **B,** Arteriogram shows a high-grade C1 stenosis (*arrow*) immediately proximal to the origin of the anterior choroidal artery (*arrowhead*). **C,** High flow velocities and bidirectional low-frequency echoes (*arrowheads*) on the right (downward flow signal represents the anterior cerebral artery; a faint upward flow signal represents the proximal middle cerebral artery). **D,** Arteriography reveals a stenosis close to the origin of the right ACA (*arrows*). Both pericallosal arteries (*arrowhead*) are fed by this A1 segment.

consists of carotid artery dissection (Fig. 16-8). In rare cases, however, these TCD findings may be caused by atherosclerotic lesions in this segment of the carotid artery. A young patient with an acute distal carotid artery occlusion but no vascular risk factors should be examined for dissection. The latter typically manifests as a reverberating flow signal corresponding to a blind ICA stump with to-and-fro movement of the blood column (Fig. 16-9, *A*).

The diagnosis of acute ICA dissection is therapeutically important. For patients who present with nonstroke symptoms (such as ptosis, miosis, anterior lateralized neck pain, pulsating tinnitus, or caudal cranial nerve palsy), it leads the clinician to begin immediate anticoagulation therapy before a frank stroke occurs. Thereafter, if the dissection results in complete ICA occlusion, daily TCD follow-up studies quickly shed light upon the nature of the underlying vascular lesion. The TCD findings may change every day and eventually show complete recanalization of the ICA in most cases.[40] Moreover, follow-up ultrasound findings can provide a basis regarding the duration of anticoagulation.

Pseudo-aneurysms are difficult to access by TCD and normally cannot be diagnosed by conventional techniques. Color-coded extracranial and transcranial duplex sonography might be helpful in such cases, although

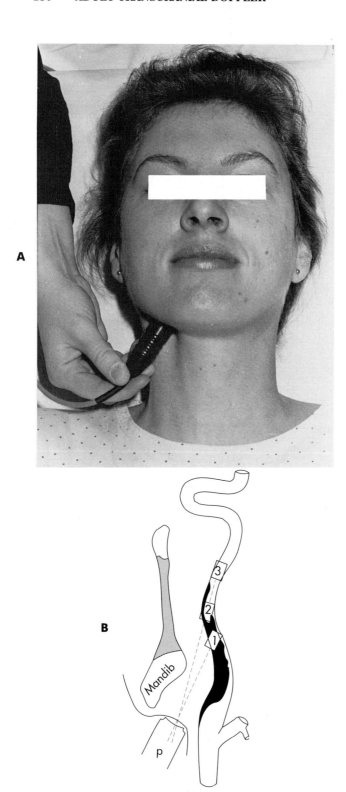

Fig. 16-7. A and **B,** Submandibular approach to the very distal, retromandibular but still extracranial internal carotid artery. (*Mandib,* Mandible; *P,* probe; *1, 2, 3,* sample volumes at various insonation depths.) (Modified from Müllges W, Ringelstein EB, Leibold M: Non-invasive diagnosis of internal carotid artery dissections, *J Neurol Neurosurg Psychiatry* 55:98-104, 1992.)

their accuracy has not been ascertained. We obtain repeat angiograms once the dissection has resolved ultrasonographically, in order to check for residual pseudo-aneurysms of the distal carotid artery. These aneurysms may subsequently present as pulsating tumors and may rupture or act as a source of emboli. Progressive aneurysms should be treated surgically.[40]

Posterior circulation

Ultrasound access to the vertebral arteries is limited. Color-coded duplex sonography could considerably improve ultrasound diagnosis of extracranial vertebral artery occlusive disease.[3] The assessment of intracranial occlusive disease affecting the distal vertebral, basilar, posterior cerebral, or even cerebellar arteries remains difficult.

The distal vertebral artery is a predilection site for stenosis and for embolically active atherothrombotic plaques. The insonation depth to assess the distal vertebral artery begins at about 50 mm. The ultrasound beam hits the caudal basilar artery at around 85 to 100 mm, and the top of the basilar artery can be evaluated at an insonation depth somewhere between 100 and 125 mm (see Chapter 12).

The entire length of the vertebrobasilar axis should be scrutinized for stenoses and occlusions as these lesions are of major clinical importance. Although they are rare, distal vertebral artery lesions can be life-threatening once they have become symptomatic, shedding emboli into the basilar trunk. Occlusion of the mouth of the posterior inferior cerebellar artery may lead to cerebellar infarction with subsequent compression of the brainstem.

An atheroma of the intracranial vertebrobasilar artery may cause a branch occlusion and lacunar brainstem infarction.[19] Superimposed thrombi may extend to the ostia of additional perforating branches, leading to progressive brainstem strokes.[18] A major superimposed thrombus can lead to distal vertebral artery stenosis or complete occlusion, frequently blocking the posterior inferior cerebellar artery and leading to cerebellar infarction. Alternatively—and even more deteriously—the thrombus may shed emboli into distal cerebellar arteries or the basilar artery.

A combination of extracranial and transcranial Doppler sonographic techniques can be used to diagnose most of these lesions.[45] The potential therapeutic consequences of such diagnoses are evident; large-vessel disease in the posterior circulation may require anticoagulation or therapeutic lysis, whereas small-vessel disease does not. In clinical practice, the ultrasonic proof of a patent vertebrobasilar avenue is of obvious significance in the diagnostic workup of patients presenting to the emergency ward with acute coma or a focal brainstem deficit.

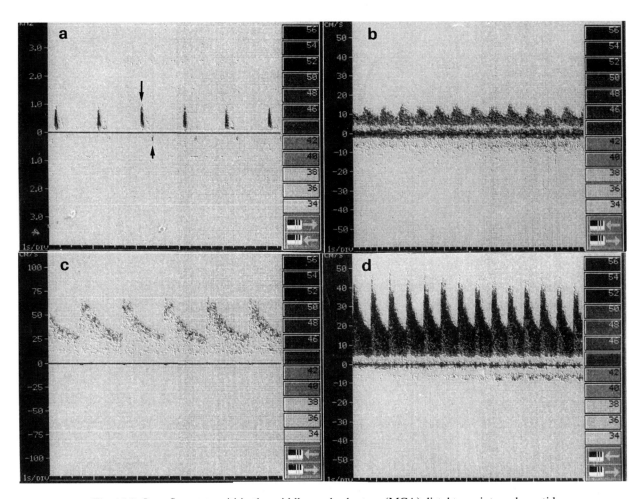

Fig. 16-8. Low-flow state within the middle cerebral artery (MCA) distal to an internal carotid artery (ICA) occlusion. **A,** Submandibular transcranial Doppler (TCD) insonation of the distal carotid artery revealed reverberating flow *(arrows)* within the blind stump of the distally occluded left internal carotid artery. Note the small amplitude of the signal and the absence of flow during diastole. This 43-year-old patient had suffered an ICA dissection and a severe stroke. **B,** Markedly decreased flow velocities in the left middle cerebral artery (mean flow velocity approximately 10 cm/s). The MCA was exclusively supplied from the retrogradely perfused ophthalmic artery. The left anterior cerebral and posterior communicating arteries were absent, leading to a diagnosis of "isolated middle cerebral artery." **C** and **D,** Normal MCA and ICA flow velocities on the contralateral side for comparison.

The extracranial diagnosis of basilar artery and distal vertebral artery occlusions is made by observing unilateral or bilateral reverberating flow signals in the blind arterial loop(s).[51] Stenosis, by contrast, can only be diagnosed by TCD, using the occipital approach. It is possible to identify any stenosis of clinical significance (i.e., one with a lumen reduction of 50% or more). Figure 16-9 shows examples of an asymptomatic collateralized extracranial vertebral artery occlusion, a clinically relevant mid-basilar artery stenosis, and an additional distal basilar tandem stenosis. Any circumscribed acceleration of blood flow, particularly if associated with disturbed flow ("turbulence"), low-frequency noise (reflecting arterial wall covibrations), or even musical murmurs, is highly indicative of a stenosing lesion. The differential diagnosis should consider the possibility of vasospasm due to subarachnoid hemorrhage or spasm due to basilar migraine. Additional clues to accurate diagnosis include history, neck stiffness, headache, and findings in cerebral blood flow measurements of the suspected stenosis. Further indicators of vasospasm include the great length of the involved segment, a finding unusual for atherothrombotic stenosis, and the gradual reduction of turbulent flow, with normalization of velocities within days. In patients with spasm, findings corresponding to the "stenotic" lesion also fluctuate on a daily basis. If a precise diagnosis is needed quickly, particularly in patients with progressive symptoms, vertebrobasilar arteriography should be performed immediately. Arteriography, however, is not immediately

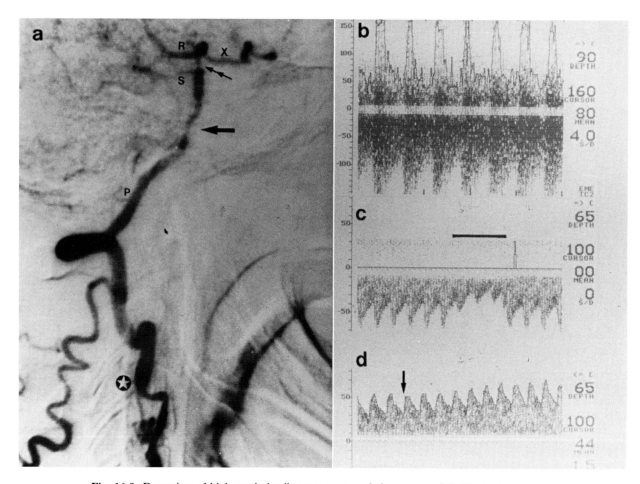

Fig. 16-9. Detection of high-grade basilar artery stenosis by means of TCD. **A,** Angiogram, performed after ultrasound diagnosis, revealed (1) collateralized extracranial vertebral artery occlusion (*asterisk*); (2) subtotal, extended stenosis of the vertebrobasilar junction and the basilar trunk (*arrow*); (3) tandem stenosis of the distal basilar artery (*double arrow*); and (4) nonfilling of right posterior cerebral artery (PCA). (*R,* stump of PCA; *X,* Posterior communicating artery; *S,* superior cerebellar artery; *P,* posterior inferior cerebellar artery.) **B,** Transforaminal insonation of the basilar artery revealed a high-flow velocity signal (mean velocity of approximately 120 cm/s; normal range, 41 ± 10 cm/s). This led to the presumptive diagnosis of high-grade basilar trunk stenosis or collateralized basilar trunk occlusion. **C,** The P2 segment of the PCA on the left could be insonated transtemporally. Compression of the left common carotid artery (*black bar*) proved the predominant dependency of this artery from the carotid distribution. **D,** The identity of the P2 segment was confirmed by the striking increase of flow velocity when the patient opened his eyes (*arrow*). This led to the differential diagnosis of embryonal type of left PCA blood supply or partial occlusion of the top-of-basilar artery. The patient had recurrent vertebrobasilar transient ischemic attacks that progressed to a hemiparesis without visual field defects. TCD findings prompted arteriography. (From Ringelstein EB: Ultrasound evaluation of the posterior cerebral circulation. In Hofferberth B, Brune GG, Sitzer G, Weger HD, editors: *Vascular brain stem diseases,* Basel, 1990, Karger.)

necessary if the vertebrobasilar arterial pathway can be insonated throughout its length and is found to be normal. Diagnoses other than vertebrobasilar occlusive disease are more probable.

Because posterior fossa leptomeningeal collateral pathways can mimic vertebrobasilar stenoses, thus confusing the examiner, TCD is not an appropriate instrument for the diagnosis of basilar artery occlusion. If the basilar occlusion is proximal to or at the mid-basilar portion, extracranial Doppler findings in the vertebral arteries are frequently diagnostically abnormal. More distal occlusions, however, can easily be missed by ultrasound examination of any type. A countercheck on the distal basilar artery through the transtemporal window is, therefore, strongly recommended. Normal perfusion of the basilar bifurcation can be deduced if flow velocities in the P1 segments of the posterior cerebral arteries are normal. Compression tests may be necessary to confirm that these segments are not fed by the internal carotid arteries.

The distal vertebral artery is a predilection site for both atherothrombosis and vertebrobasilar dissection. During vigorous head turning, the transverse processes of the atlas could injure the intima of the vertebral arteries, causing a dissection of these vessels. The examiner should use clinical clues to make the diagnosis because this condition resembles both distal vertebral artery occlusion and stenosis. The diagnosis of dissection should be triggered by the patient's young age and lack of vascular risk factors, leading to vertebral arteriography in the disease's early stages. A precise and early diagnosis of the condition is key to initiate anticoagulation therapy. The prognosis can be good.[40]

Occlusion or stenosis of the posterior cerebral artery is relatively rare. If a PCA occlusion is diagnosed, the examiner should look carefully for intracardiac or vertebral sources of embolism. In the even rarer case of P1 segment stenosis, anticoagulation is the preferred form of therapy at the present time.

Another rare but distinct vascular condition of the posterior fossa is the megadolichobasilar artery.[39] It cannot be diagnosed by extracranial ultrasound, but some intracranial features, although not diagnostic, are characteristic. Flow velocities are low throughout the trunk of the basilar artery.[6] At increasing insonation depths, flow directions may change, depending on the curvature of these extremely elongated vessels. Ultrasound findings, in conjunction with a history of transient or severe brainstem stroke, should prompt diagnostic CT or MRI imaging (Fig. 16-10).

SECONDARY EFFECTS OF EXTRACRANIAL OCCLUSIVE DISEASE ON INTRACRANIAL TRANSCRANIAL DOPPLER FINDINGS
The role of the Circle of Willis

Low-flow phenomena distal to stenosing lesions include the downstream signal's reduced pulsatility, preserved diastolic blood flow, and, generally, reduced mean flow velocity. Severe stenoses and occlusions of the ICA or the common carotid artery may affect cerebral perfusion pressure, thus reducing MCA flow velocity and regional cerebral blood flow (rCBF) in parallel.[27,28] In most cases this does not lead to tissue damage, but in some patients with carotid occlusion or very tight stenosis, low-flow infarcts may occur in the centrum semiovale, which is the terminal supply area of the deep perforators. In even rarer instances, low-flow infarcts occur in the cortical watershed areas.[29,48,49] The severity of the cervical carotid stenosis should not be taken as a reliable indicator of intracranial hemodynamic change in the distal hemisphere[9,42,48] because the circle of Willis may fully compensate for the pressure drop resultant from these lesions. The insufficiency of the circle of

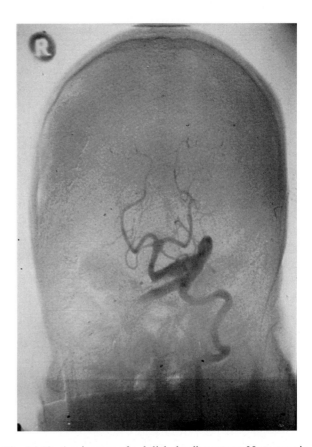

Fig. 16-10. Angiogram of a dolichobasilar artery. Note ectasia, elongation, and curvature of distal vertebral and basilar arteries.

Willis is reliably indicated by strong retrograde flow through the ophthalmic artery.[55] Analysis of the circle of Willis may be performed by TCD in combination with carotid compression maneuvers.[49]

Vasomotor reactivity

Measurement of intracranial vasomotor reserve provided a reliable estimate of the hemodynamic compromise distal to extracranial occlusive disease. The observation of intracranial severe hemodynamic impairment indicates an increased risk of subsequent stroke[30] or ischemic ophthalmopathy.[14,48] Pulsatility indices[21,37] correlate well with the actual intracranial hemodynamic state when large numbers of patients are studied[52] but are of little or no predictive value in individual cases.

Other abnormal flow phenomena

A to-and-fro movement of the blood arterial is found in arterial segments that connect major extracranial and intracranial arterial trunks (Fig. 16-11). A typical example of this phenomenon is the pendulumlike flow in the basilar artery, the main collateral pathway between

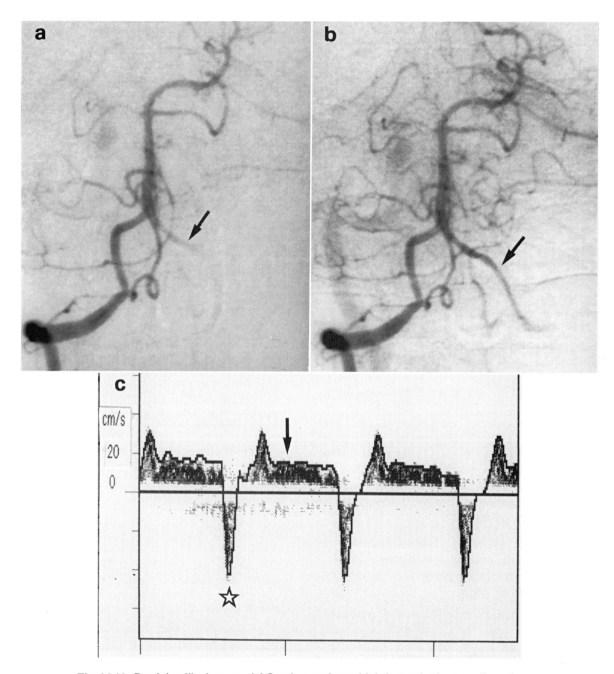

Fig. 16-11. Pendulumlike intracranial flow in a patient with left vertebral artery dissection. **A** and **B,** Right vertebral arteriogram shows retrograde opacification of the left vertebral artery (*arrow*). The left vertebral artery was occluded at the level of the atlas loop (not shown). **C,** In the distal vertebral artery (*left*), blood flow was pendulumlike with a sharp retrograde flow (*asterisk*). The blood supply came from two sources: the right vertebral artery during early systole (*asterisk*) and cervical collateral pathways during late systole and diastole (*arrow*) (*abscissa:* 1 second/division).

the anterior and posterior circulation, which can be seen in patients with severe subclavian steal (Fig. 16-12).[31] Identical flow phenomena can also be seen in other collateral flow channels, such as the Willisian communicating arteries or the major pial arteries. In patients with moyamoya disease, this flow phenomenon is observed even in enlarged deep perforating arteries such as the posterior choroidal artery. Unlike the pendulumlike, "reverberating" flow found in blind loops during systole (Fig. 16-8, *A*), the to-and-fro phenomenon that exists in arteries connecting two vascular beds occurs throughout the full cardiac cycle (Figs. 16-11 and 16-12). In very rare

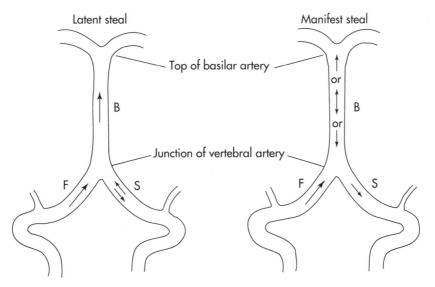

Fig. 16-12. Pendulumlike flow in the basilar artery. To-and-fro-movement of the blood column within the stealing vertebral artery in moderate (*left*) and severe (*right*) subclavian steal. Pendulumlike flow may be registered in the distal stealing vertebral artery (*left*) or even the basilar artery (*right*). Note that this flow phenomenon is completely different from the reverberating flow shown in Fig. 16-8, *A.* (*F.* Contralateral feeding vertebral artery; *S,* homolateral stealing vertebral artery; *B,* basilar trunk.)

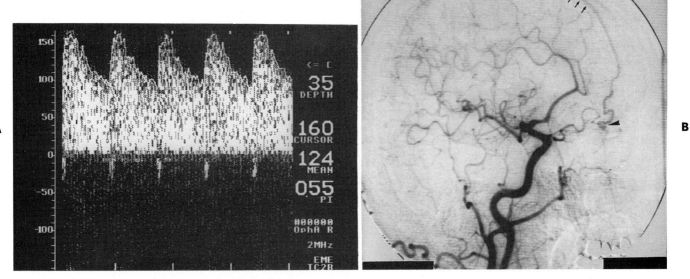

Fig. 16-13. High-flow velocity findings in the ophthalmic artery mimicking stenosis. **A,** At an insonation depth of 35 mm, a very high mean flow velocity of 124 cm/s was found in the right ophthalmic artery. The patient had a history of intermittent headaches. Because flow abnormalities were found at various depths, the diagnosis of a shunt was made. **B,** Carotid arteriography shows a dural fistula fed by the ophthalmic artery (*arrowhead*) and leading to arterialization of the superior sagittal sinus (*arrows*). (From Sommer C, Müllges W, Ringelstein EB: Noninvasive assessment of intracranial fistulas and other small arteriovenous malformations, *Neurosurgery* 30:522-528, 1992.)

cases, "alternating flow" may also be seen in residual primitive arteries such as the hypoglossal (arteria hypoglossica primitiva) or trigeminal (arteria trigemina primitiva), primitive arteries that connect the ICA with the basilar artery.

HIGH-FLOW VELOCITY PHENOMENA OTHER THAN STENOSIS AND SPASM
Hyperfusion and stenotic mimicry

Several nonspecific cerebral insults can lead to vasoparalysis and to increased flow velocities in the pial arteries, a phenomenon called *hyperperfusion.* Ischemia caused by arterial occlusion, cardiac arrest, hypoxia, vasospasm, spreading depression in migraine, head trauma, and inflammation in patients with meningitis, encephalitis, and cerebritis have all been associated with hyperperfusion. Figure 16-5, *B,* is an illustrative example of hyperperfusion in the MCA distribution after lysis of an occluding embolus. Hyperperfusion may last for several days and can lead to the mistaken diagnosis of stenosis. It is mentioned in this chapter because it is a frequent cause of stenotic mimicry, leading to false-positive diagnoses. It is a pathologic but nonspecific finding and, unlike atherosclerotic lesions and vasospasm, is observed throughout the entire length of the artery under study. Depending on its etiology, it may be restricted to one arterial territory (e.g., to a recanalized MCA) or widespread to most of the cerebral vascular tree (e.g., following cardiac arrest).

In most migraine sufferers, hyperperfusion is found throughout the hemisphere corresponding to focal ischemic signs and with throbbing hemicrania. As a rule, hyperperfusion does not produce flow velocities as excessively high as those associated with high-grade stenoses. If flow velocities exceed the normal values (i.e., mean value plus 2 standard deviations) for a given arterial segment or if a side-to-side difference of 20 cm/s or more is observed, hyperperfusion should be diagnosed. Hyperperfused arteries may also have a low-frequency sound caused by arterial wall covibrations.

Cryptogenic AVMs

Highly circumscribed stenotic mimicry may also be due to arteriovenous fistulae and cryptogenic arteriovenous malformations (cAVMs), which may cause focal epilepsy, headache, papilledema, oculomotor palsies, subarachnoid hemorrhage, and focal or generalized neurologic symptoms or signs caused by congestive encephalopathy. The latter is often the case when the pathological supply to cerebral veins or sinuses forms and leads to congestion of brain areas remote from the dural fistula itself. Carotid artery–to–cavernous sinus fistulae have already been mentioned as a possible alternative diagnosis to that of siphon stenosis. Other feeders of fistulae may be located within the orbits, where they mimic stenosis of the ophthalmic artery (Fig. 16-13), and within the silvian fissure, where they mimic stenosis of the MCA's M2 segment. By visualizing congestive brain edema or congested veins and sinuses, MRI may be helpful and can pinpoint small AVMs. If the MRI findings are normal, however, a selective cerebral angiogram is necessary to establish an accurate diagnosis. As mentioned previously, carotid compression tests can also be helpful in distinguishing between true atherosclerotic stenoses and stenotic mimicry.

CONCLUSIONS

In the hands of experienced investigators, TCD has proved to be a highly reliable and clinically valuable diagnostic tool. This is especially true in patients exhibiting symptoms of acute or subacute cerebrovascular disease associated with in situ thrombosis or embolic occlusion of large pial arteries, carotid or vertebrobasilar dissection, fibromuscular dysplasia, atheromatous stenoses, and intracranial low-flow phenomena caused by extracranial occlusive disease. It can also identify collateral pathways and estimate their perfusion capacities and aid in the detection of cerebral congestion due to fistulae and small AVMs.

REFERENCES

1. Aaslid R, Markwalder TM, Nornes H: Noninvasive transcranial Doppler ultrasound recording of flow velocities in basal cerebral arteries, *J Neurosurg* 57:769-774, 1982.
2. Aaslid R, Nornes H: Musical murmurs in human cerebral arteries after subarachnoid hemorrhage, *J Neurosurg* 60:32-36, 1984.
3. Ackerstaff RGA, Grosveld WJHM, Eikelboom BC, Ludwig JW: Ultrasonic Duplex scanning of the prevertebral segment of the vertebral artery in patients with cerebral atherosclerosis, *Eur J Vasc Surg* 2:387-393, 1988.
4. Adams RJ, McKie V, Nichols F, et al: The use of transcranial ultrasonography to predict stroke in sickle cell disease, *N Engl J Med* 326:605-610, 1992.
5. Arnolds BJ, von Reutern GM: Transcranial Doppler sonography. Examination technique and normal reference values, *Ultrasound Med Biol* 12:115-123, 1986.
6. Babikian VL: The effects of dolichoectasia on transcranial Doppler measurements, *J Neuroimaging* 2:19-24, 1992.
7. Bartels E, Flügel KA: Quantitative measurements of blood flow velocity in basal cerebral arteries with Transcranial Duplex colour-flow imaging: a comparative study with conventional transcranial Doppler sonography, *J Neuroimaging* 4:77-81, 1994.
8. Becker G, Lindner A, Bogdahn U: Imaging of the vertebrobasilar system by transcranial colour-coded real-time sonography, *J Ultrasound Med* 12:495-501, 1993.
9. Bishop CCR, Powell S, Insall M, et al: Effect of internal carotid artery occlusion on middle cerebral artery blood flow at rest and in response to hypercapnia, *Lancet* 1:710-712, 1986.
10. Bogousslavsky J, Barnett HJM, Fox AJ: Atherosclerotic disease of the middle cerebral artery, *Stroke* 17:1112-1120, 1986.
11. Brass L, Duterte DL, Mohr JP: Anterior cerebral artery velocity changes in disease of the middle cerebral artery stem, *Stroke* 20:1737-1740, 1989.
12. Caplan LR, Gorelick PB, Hier DB: Race, sex and occlusive cerebrovascular disease: a review, *Stroke* 17:648-655, 1986.

13. Caplan LR, et al: Occlusive disease of the middle cerebral artery, *Neurology* 35:975-982, 1985.
14. Copetto JR, Wand M, Bear L, Sciarra R: Neovascular glaucoma and carotid artery obstructive disease, *Am J Ophthalmol* 99:567-570, 1985.
15. De Bray JM, et al: Transcranial Doppler evaluation of middle cerebral artery stenosis, *J Ultrasound Med* 7:611-616, 1988.
16. Dorr JM, Doherty CC, Ringelstein EB, Schlief R: A new ultrasound contrast medium as a diagnostic aid in patients with insufficient transcranial Doppler sonography (TCD) signals, *Journal of Clinical Ultrasound,* 1995 (in press).
17. Fisher CM: Atherosclerosis of the carotid and vertebral arteries: extracranial and intracranial, *J Neuropathol Exp Neurol* 24:455-476, 1965.
18. Fisher CM: Bilateral occlusions of basilar artery branches, *J Neurol Neurosurg Psychiatry* 40:1182-1189, 1977.
19. Fisher CM, Caplan LR: Basilar artery branch occlusion: a cause of pontine infarction, *Neurology* 21:900-905, 1971.
20. Gillard JH, Kirkham FJ, Lem SD: Anatomical validation of middle cerebral artery position as identified by transcranial pulsed Doppler ultrasound, *J Neurol Neurosurg Psychiatry* 49:1025-1029, 1986.
21. Giller CA, Hodges K, Batjer HH: Transcranial Doppler pulsatility in vasodilation and stenosis, *J Neurosurg* 72:901-906, 1990.
22. Gomez CR, et al: Transcranial Doppler findings in acute spontaneous recanalization of middle cerebral artery embolism, *J Neuroimaging* 1:63-67, 1991.
23. Hass WK, Fields WS, North RR, et al: Joint study of extracranial arterial occlusion II: arteriography, technique, sites, and complications, *JAMA* 203:961-968, 1968.
24. Hennerici M, Rautenberg W, Schwartz A: Transcranial Doppler ultrasound for the assessment of intracranial arterial flow velocity, part 2: evaluation of intracranial arterial disease, *Surg Neurol* 27:523-532, 1987.
25. Kaps M: Transcranial Doppler ultrasound findings in middle cerebral artery occlusion, *Stroke* 21:532-537, 1990.
26. Karnik R, Stelzer P, Slany J: Transcranial Doppler sonography monitoring of local intra-arterial thrombolysis in acute occlusion of the middle cerebral artery, *Stroke* 23:284-287, 1992.
27. Kelley RE, Namon RA, Juang SH, et al: Transcranial Doppler ultrasonography of the middle cerebral artery in the hemodynamic assessment of internal carotid artery stenosis, *Arch Neurol* 47:960-964, 1990.
28. Kirkham FJ, Padayachee TS, Parsons S, et al: Transcranial measurement of blood velocities in the basal cerebral arteries using pulsed Doppler ultrasound: velocity as an index of flow, *Ultrasound Med Biol* 12:15-21, 1986.
29. Kleiser B, Krapf H, Widder B: Carbon dioxide reactivity and patterns of cerebral infarction in patients with carotid artery occlusion, *J Neurol* 238:392-394, 1991.
30. Kleiser B, Widder B: Course of carotid artery occlusions with impaired cerebrovascular reactivity, *Stroke* 23:171-174, 1992.
31. Klingelhöfer J, Conrad B, Benecke R, Frank B: Transcranial Doppler ultrasonography of carotid-basilar collateral circulation in subclavian steal, *Stroke* 19:1036-1042, 1988.
32. Kushner MJ, Zanette EM, Bastianello S, et al: Transcranial Doppler in acute hemispheric brain infarction, *Neurology* 41:109-113, 1991.
33. Ley-Pozo J, Ringelstein EB: Noninvasive detection of occlusive disease of the carotid siphon and middle cerebral artery, *Ann Neurol* 28:640-647, 1990.
34. Ley-Pozo J, Willmes K, Ringelstein EB: Relationship between pulsatility indices of Doppler flow signals and CO_2-reactivity within the middle cerebral artery in extracranial occlusive disease, *Ultrasound Med Biol* 16:763-772, 1990.
35. Lhermitte F, Gautier JC, Derouesne C, Guiraud B: Ischemic accidents in the middle cerebral artery territory, *Arch Neurol* 19:248-256, 1968.
36. Lindegaard KF, Bakke SJ, Aaslid R, Nornes H: Doppler diagnosis of intracranial artery occlusive disorders, *J Neurol Neurosurg Psychiatry* 49:510-518, 1986.
37. Lindegaard KF, Bakke SJ, Grolimund P, et al: Assessment of intracranial hemodynamics in carotid artery disease by transcranial Doppler ultrasound, *J Neurosurg* 63:890-898, 1985.
38. Mattle H, Grolimund P, Huber P, et al: Transcranial Doppler sonographic findings in middle cerebral artery disease, *Arch Neurol* 45:289-295, 1988.
39. Moseley F, Holland M: Ectasia of the basilar artery: the breadth of the clinical spectrum and the diagnostic value of computed tomography, *Neuroradiology* 18:83-91, 1979.
40. Müllges W, Ringelstein EB, Leibold M: Non-invasive diagnosis of internal carotid artery dissections, *J Neurol Neurosurg Psychiatry* 55:98-104, 1992.
41. Niederkorn K, Myers LG, Nunn CL: Three dimensional transcranial Doppler blood flow mapping in patients with cerebrovascular disorders, *Stroke* 19:1335-1344, 1988.
42. Powers WJ, Press GA, Grubb RL, et al: The effect of hemodynamically significant carotid artery disease on the hemodynamic status of the cerebral circulation, *Ann Intern Med* 6:27-35, 1987.
43. Ringelstein EB: *Continuous-wave Doppler sonography of the extracranial brain-supplying arteries.* In Weinberger J, editor: *Noninvasive assessment of the cerebral circulation in cerebrovascular disease* (Frontiers of Clinical Neuroscience Series), New York, 1989, Alan R Liss.
44. Ringelstein EB: *A practical guide to transcranial Doppler sonography.* In Weinberger J, editor: *Non-invasive assessment of the cerebral circulation in cerebrovascular disease* (Frontiers of Clinical Neuroscience Series), New York, 1989, Alan R Liss.
45. Ringelstein EB: *Ultrasound evaluation of the posterior cerebral circulation.* In Hofferberth B, Brune GG, Sitzer G, Weger HD, editors: *Vascular brain stem diseases,* Basel, 1990, Karger.
46. Ringelstein EB, Biniek R, Weiller C, et al: Type and extent of hemispheric brain infarctions and clinical outcome in early and delayed middle cerebral artery recanalization, *Neurology* 42:289-298, 1992.
47. Ringelstein EB, Otis SM, Spaar-Kahlscheuer B, Niggemeyer E: Transcranial Doppler sonography: anatomical landmarks and normal velocity values, *Ultrasound Med Biol* 16:745-761, 1990.
48. Ringelstein EB, Sievers C, Ecker S, et al: Noninvasive assessment of CO_2-induced cerebral vasomotor response in normal individuals and patients with internal carotid artery occlusions, *Stroke* 19:963-969, 1988.
49. Ringelstein EB, Weiller C, Weckesser M, Weckesser S: Cerebral vasomotor reactivity is significantly reduced in low-flow as compared to thromboembolic infarctions: the key role of the circle of Willis, *J Neurol Sci* 121:103-109, 1994.
50. Ringelstein EB, Zeumer H, Korbmacher G, Wulfinghoff F: Transkranielle Dopplersonographie der hirnversorgenden Arterien: atraumatische Diagnostik von Stenosen und Verschlüssen des Karotissiphons und der A. cerebri media, *Nervenarzt* 56:296-306, 1985.
51. Ringelstein EB, Zeumer H, Poeck K: Non-invasive diagnosis of intracranial lesions in the vertebrobasilar system: a comparison of Doppler sonographic and angiographic findings, *Stroke* 15:848-855, 1985.
52. Schneider PA, Rossman ME, Bornstein EF, et al: Effect of internal carotid artery occlusion on intracranial hemodynamics: transcranial Doppler evaluation and clinical correlation, *Stroke* 19:589-593, 1988.
53. Sommer C, Müllges W, Ringelstein EB: Noninvasive assessment of intracranial fistulas and other small arteriovenous malformations, *Neurosurgery* 30:522-528, 1992.

54. Spencer MP, Whisler D: Transorbital Doppler diagnosis of intracranial arterial stenosis, *Stroke* 17:916-921, 1986.

55. Tatemichi TK, Chamorro A, Petty GW, et al: Hemodynamic role of ophthalmic artery collateral in internal carotid artery occlusion, *Neurology* 40:461-464, 1990.

56. Toole JF: Middle cerebral artery stenosis: a neglected problem? *Surg Neurol* 27:44-46, 1987.

57. Wechsler LR, Kistler JP, Davis KR, Kaminski MJ: The prognosis of carotid siphon stenosis, *Stroke* 17:714-718, 1986.

58. Wechsler LR, Ropper LH, Kistler JP: Transcranial Doppler in cerebrovascular disease, *Stroke* 17:905-912, 1986.

59. Weiller C, Müllges W, Leibold M, et al: Infarctions and non-invasive diagnosis in Moyamoya disease: two case reports, *Neurosurg Rev* 14:75-77, 1991.

60. Zanette EM, Fieschi C, Bozzao L, et al: Comparison of cerebral angiography and transcranial Doppler sonography in acute stroke, *Stroke* 20:899-903, 1989.

Trauma and Brain Death

David W. Newell

Transcranial Doppler ultrasonography (TCD) can provide information that is useful in the management of closed head injury in patients in the neurosurgical intensive care unit (box).

EPIDEMIOLOGY AND PATHOPHYSIOLOGY OF CLOSED HEAD INJURY

Trauma is the third most common cause of death in the United States and the leading cause of death in Americans younger than 40 years old. About 420,000 head injuries occur in the United States each year, for an annual frequency rate of 200 per 100,000.[40] Head injuries, therefore, are much more common than brain tumors or cerebral aneurysms, and head-injured patients constitute a large portion of patients receiving care in the neurosurgical intensive care unit. The development of new intensive management methods for head injury has been aided by improved understanding of pathophysiology obtained with neuroimaging techniques, cerebral blood flow examinations, and newer monitoring devices such as the TCD. These intensive-monitoring management techniques have helped clinicians to accomplish one of the main goals of head injury management: preventing secondary deterioration resulting from decreased cerebral perfusion.

For practical purposes, brain injury can be divided into two components: primary injury, which is caused at the time of impact by physical forces that produce mechanical damage and disruption of axons and neural circuits; and secondary injury, which comprises damage following the primary injury as the brain is subjected to further insults. Secondary injuries include hemorrhages, which cause further tissue damage, and decreased cerebral perfusion, which results from decreased arterial pressure or intracranial pressure (ICP). Increased ICP can result from secondary hemorrhages, swelling, edema, or vascular instability due to interruption of the normal vascular control mechanisms. Impaired cerebrovascular control can be caused by cerebral blood volume increases, which can cause secondary increases in ICP and aggravate ischemic injury.[49]

Successful intensive care management provides brain-injured patients with optimal conditions for brain recovery (i.e., conditions that meet the metabolic requirements of the injured brain and those that prevent further, secondary injury). In head-injury management, TCD can be used to detect some of the circulatory abnormalities and to guide intensive care unit therapy directed toward preserving cerebral blood circulation.

TRANSCRANIAL DOPPLER DETECTION OF BLOOD FLOW CHANGES AFTER HEAD INJURY

The recording of blood flow velocity in basal cerebral arteries makes use of several physical principles to detect

Uses for transcranial Doppler ultrasonography

- Records blood flow velocity from cerebral arteries, aiding noninvasive diagnosis
- Permits closer examination of pathophysiology of circulatory disturbances after head injury
- Provides continuous measurement of velocity changes in head-injured patients in an easily accessible format; adds to understanding of pathophysiology of disordered cerebrovascular control
- Enables determination of cerebral autoregulation and CO_2 reactivity in head-injured patients
- Alerts clinicians to presence of posttraumatic vasospasm and vascular dissection, permitting early use of measures to prevent cerebral infarction
- Quickly detects markedly increased intracranial pressure
- Confirms brain death in comatose patients
- Reliably determines arrest of cerebral circulation, which can shorten observation time for organ retrieval in patients with brain death
- May allow noninvasive estimation of intracranial pressure in head-injured patients

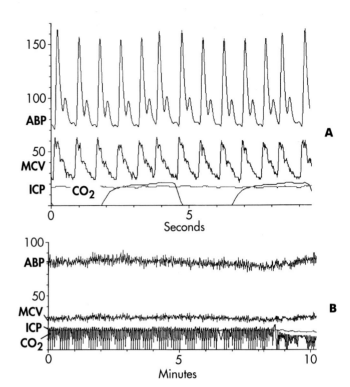

Fig. 17-1. Multimodality recording of middle cerebral artery velocity, arterial blood pressure, end-tidal CO_2, and intracranial pressure. **A,** Short recording interval permitting waveform analysis; **B,** longer recording interval allowing trend analysis, which can be used to examine relative flow changes under certain conditions and interactions among the recorded parameters. *ABP,* arterial blood pressure; *MCV,* middle cerebral velocity.

changes in these vessels and the cerebral circulation.[4,29] The following two principles are used diagnostically in monitoring flow and velocity.

Principle 1. Under conditions of constant flow and insonation angle, changes in velocity are inversely proportional to changes in cross-sectional area of the insonated vessel. Because of this principle, TCD can detect stenosis due to fixed or reversible lesions of the intracranial arteries (e.g., vascular spasm).

Principle 2. When the diameter of the vessel being monitored is constant and the insonation angle does not change, changes in velocity are directly proportional to changes in volume flow through the vessel.[1,64] This principle can be applied to detect relative changes in blood flow through the inflow artery, which can be used to calculate vascular reactivity in distal regulating arteries.

Transcranial Doppler can also detect intracranial artery emboli and aid in measuring changes in mean velocity and in the pulsatility index. The latter parameter can reflect progressive increases in resistance of the cerebral circulation, indicating very high ICP.[24]

Continuous monitoring of middle cerebral artery (MCA) velocity waveforms can reveal changes in cerebral blood flow that occur in response to different circumstances in the neurosurgical intensive care unit.[10,31,43,44,46] Blood flow changes resulting from various waves in ICP can be assessed with such monitoring. Assessment of MCA responses to induced or spontaneous blood pressure changes may aid in the evaluation of

autoregulatory mechanisms. It is also possible to assess relative blood-flow changes resulting from alterations in CO_2 concentration or different medications. Figure 17-1 illustrates continuous recording of MCA velocity, arterial blood pressure, ICP, and end-tidal CO_2.

A waves

First described by Lundberg,[32] A waves correspond to spontaneous increases in ICP associated with states of reduced intracranial compliance. Also termed *plateau waves,* these waves are associated with sudden marked increases in ICP to levels of 60 to 80 mm Hg. They may persist for 5 to 20 minutes and then spontaneously subside. It is thought that A waves represent a disorder of cerebral circulatory control resulting from a positive-feedback cycle established between vasodilatation and increases in ICP.[32,48,56] Previous measurements of cerebral blood flow and volume have indicated increased volume and decreased flow during the peak of the wave. Transcranial Doppler monitoring has revealed markedly decreased MCA velocity and increased pulsatility index during the wave's peak.[33,54] In many patients, markedly increased velocity is present after the wave, probably indicating hyperemia in response to cerebral ischemia.

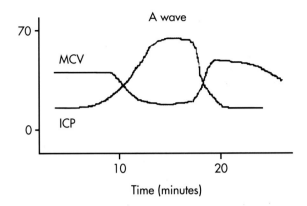

Fig. 17-2. Typical relationship between ICP and middle cerebral artery velocity during a Lundberg A, or plateau, wave. *ICP,* intracranial pressure; *MCV,* middle cerebral velocity.

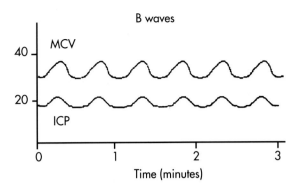

Fig. 17-3. Typical recording of ICP B waves. Note the in-phase relationship between middle cerebral artery velocity and ICP. *ICP,* intracranial pressure; *MCV,* middle cerebral velocity.

Figure 17-2 illustrates the relationship between ICP and MCA velocity during a typical wave. A waves are significant because (1) they represent a state of reduced intracranial compliance and (2) their continued presence or an increase in their frequency may indicate impending herniation.[32]

B waves

Lundberg also described B waves, waves in the ICP tracing approximately 10 to 20 mm Hg in amplitude that repeat at a frequency of 0.5 to 2 per minute.[32] Simultaneous TCD monitoring of MCA velocity and ICP during B waves in head-injured patients has revealed much about their cause and significance. Fluctuations in MCA velocity always occur simultaneously and in phase with ICP B waves in head-injured patients.[43] It has also been found that the ICP B waves' amplitude is related to the amplitude of the middle cerebral velocity wave and the ICP at the time of recording. These findings indicate that the B wave corresponds to an amplification of changes in cerebral blood volume produced by intermittent vasodilatation and vasoconstriction at regular intervals. Figure 17-3 illustrates the relationship between MCA velocity and ICP during typical B waves.

Similar waves were found in a high percentage of normal volunteers, indicating the B waves probably result from physiologic phenomena—specifically, from the amplification of vasomotor waves associated with reduced intracranial compliance.[6] During TCD testing, marked fluctuations in intracranial velocity at this frequency are often seen. These fluctuations may be a source of error in accurate velocity determinations; for this reason, the examiner must record average measurements of the mean velocity during the waves.

Carbon dioxide reactivity

The ability of the brain's distal regulating vessels to dilate and constrict in response to changes in CO_2 is

termed *CO_2 reactivity*.[38] It can be measured in both MCA distributions accurately with TCD.[7,20] Carbon dioxide reactivity can be impaired or abolished in head-injured patients. A marked decrease in reactivity after head injury is also associated with poor prognosis.* The TCD measurements of reactivity have several advantages over the older method of xenon-labeled blood flow: They are noninvasive, do not use radioisotopes, and are much easier to perform.

Autoregulation

Autoregulation is the ability of the cerebral circulation to maintain constant blood flow under conditions of changing cerebral perfusion pressure.[27,50] This important compensatory mechanism can rapidly adjust cerebral blood flow in response to altered ICP or arterial blood pressure. Autoregulation can be impaired or abolished in head-injured patients, significantly affecting management.[36,37] In cases of impaired autoregulation, hypotension must be prevented because cerebral ischemia can develop relatively quickly compared to patients with normal autoregulation. It is also important to prevent marked increases in arterial blood pressure; such increases contribute to cerebral swelling, edema, and secondary hemorrhage.[63]

Autoregulation plays a significant role in mediating cerebrovascular responses to various therapies used to control ICP. Muizelaar and associates showed that mannitol is more effective in decreasing ICP in patients with intact autoregulation than in those with impaired autoregulation.[37] In patients who have intact autoregulation, when arterial hypertension is induced, ICP may decrease; in patients without autoregulation, induced arterial hypertension causes increased ICP.[36]

Transcranial Doppler can be used to measure cerebral autoregulation.[3,5,19,41,42] Middle cerebral artery velocity responses to static[29] or rapid dynamic changes in

*References 11, 12, 16, 17, 22, 26, 44, 58, 59.

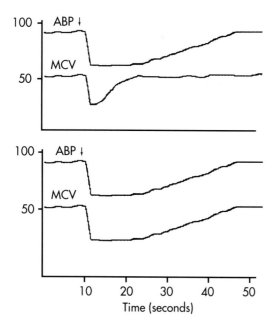

Fig. 17-4. Typical responses to a rapid autoregulatory stimulus induced by transient reduction in arterial blood pressure *(ABP)*. These are filtered tracings of arterial blood pressure and middle cerebral velocity *(MCV)*. Upper tracing indicates a normal MCV response to a step change in blood pressure with a rapid return to baseline within 10 seconds. In the lower tracing, an abnormal response of MCV is seen in response to a step change in arterial blood pressure. The phenomenon is seen in patients with impaired autoregulation following head injury. *Arrow* denotes onset of blood pressure decrease.

blood pressure[5,42] correlate well with changes in flow and can be used to determine the effectiveness of the autoregulatory response. In addition, TCD can be used to observe MCA velocity response to transient reductions of cerebral perfusion pressure induced by carotid compression.[19] Figure 17-4 illustrates the response of MCA velocity to a rapid change in arterial blood pressure in intact and absent autoregulation.

Response to medication

Mannitol increases cerebral blood flow,[37,39] especially (and to a greater degree) in patients with disturbed autoregulatory mechanisms. This effect is clearly detected in the TCD measurements of MCA velocity measurements.[46]

Barbiturates. The administration of barbiturates can decrease ICP in head-injured patients. However, the response varies for several reasons, including lack of vascular reactivity and decreased cerebral metabolism.[47] Transcranial Doppler can help assess the vascular response to barbiturates and correlate it with the degree of ICP reduction so that a given dose can be seen to achieve a specific effect.[44] In addition, the reduction in MCA velocity achieved with barbiturates can be correlated with TCD measurements of CO_2 reactivity.[44]

These data may be valuable in determining which patients may benefit from barbiturate therapy.

VASOSPASM

Cerebral vasospasm remains an important cause of neurologic deterioration in patients in whom subarachnoid hemorrhage occurs after rupture of an intracranial aneurysm. Transcranial Doppler can be used to detect and monitor the course of the vasospasm and to direct therapy in these patients.[2,21,30,60,61] Vasospasm can also occur after head injury and is associated with traumatic subarachnoid hemorrhage. It is likely that a similar mechanism—namely, hemoglobin induced arterial spasm and arteriopathy—causes both conditions.

Posttraumatic vasospasm has clearly been shown to be responsible for clinical deterioration and infarction in some patients with closed head injury.[28,34] Figure 17-5 shows the radiographic studies of a patient found to have severe posttraumatic vasospasm, illustrating the usefulness of TCD in such cases.

Like vasospasm in patients with subarachnoid hemorrhage, asymptomatic vasospasm is more common than vasospasm causing delayed ischemic neurologic deficits. Weber and colleagues, using TCD, found a 40% incidence of vasospasm in a group of severely head-injured patients.[66] Martin and associates reported a 27% incidence in another group of patients with head injury; severe vasospasm was confirmed with cerebral angiography.[34]

The concurrent existence of cerebral hyperemia is a special consideration when obtaining TCD measurement of vasospasm in head-injured patients. Hyperemia increases blood flow velocities in the basal intracranial arteries and may yield false-positive indications of vasospasm when the criteria for vasospasm in subarachnoid hemorrhage are used. For this reason, blood flow velocity recordings are frequently obtained from the most distal portion of the extracranial internal carotid artery (V_{ICA}) before it enters the skull base. Ratios of the intracranial MCA velocities (V_{MCA}) to the extracranial velocities expressed as V_{MCA}/V_{ICA}, should be used to correct for hyperemia when TCD is used to detect posttraumatic vasospasm. A V_{MCA}/V_{ICA} ratio greater than 3 indicates vasospasm, and a ratio greater than 6 denotes severe vasospasm.[30,61]

VASCULAR DISSECTION

An important complication of head injury is dissection of the carotid arteries, both extracranially and at the skull base, producing devastating delayed cerebral infarction. One diagnostic clue is the presence of intracranial arterial emboli. Our laboratory found a 60% incidence of such emboli on the side of the dissection in 15 patients (unpublished data) (Table 17-1). Most of these dissections were traumatic. Figure 17-6 shows the

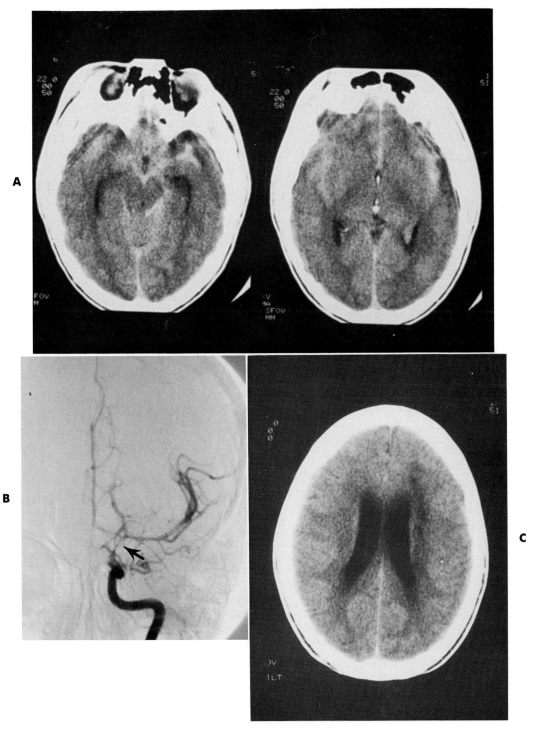

Fig. 17-5. Radiographic studies of a patient who sustained a cerebral infarction resulting from posttraumatic vasospasm. **A,** Initial computed tomography scan on admission reveals blood in the subarachnoid cisternae. **B,** Cerebral angiography indicates severe left distal internal carotid artery and proximal middle cerebral artery vasospasm *(arrow).* **C,** Computed tomography scan shows delayed infarction resulting from left-sided spasm.

Table 17-1. Middle cerebral artery embolus monitoring in patients with carotid artery dissection

Patient characteristics	Number
Average age (years)	31
Gender (M/F)	7/8
Cause of dissection	
Traumatic	10
Spontaneous	4
Undetermined	1
Diagnostic test	
Angiography	14
Computed tomography	1
MCA emboli	
Present	9 (60%)
Absent	6 (40%)

radiographic and TCD findings in a patient with traumatic carotid dissection.

PROGNOSIS OF HEAD INJURY AS DETERMINED WITH TRANSCRANIAL DOPPLER CRITERIA

Low velocities in the intracranial arteries after head injury can result from diminished cerebral blood flow due to severely reduced cerebral metabolism or from high ICP. An inverse correlation has been demonstrated between the severity of head injury and mean MCA velocity.[9] Poor prognosis is indicated when the flow velocity determined on admission is low. Chan and colleagues reported that a low cerebral blood flow velocity (less than 28 cm/s in both MCAs) is a predictor of early death.[9]

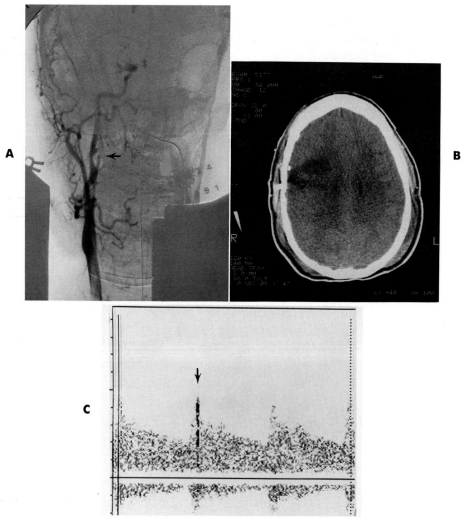

Fig. 17-6. A, Angiography demonstrating internal carotid dissection in a patient with head and spine injuries. **B,** Computed tomography scan reveals brain infarction distal to the dissection. **C,** Spectral tracing of the middle cerebral artery waveform with intraarterial microembolus *(arrow)* was obtained with transcranial Doppler.

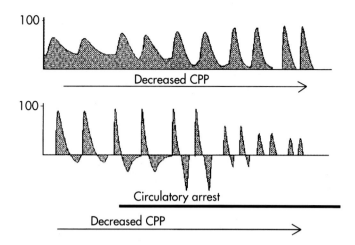

Fig. 17-7. Progressive change in the waveform morphology of the middle cerebral velocity, with progressive increase in resistance to flow in the cerebral circulation leading to cerebral circulatory arrest. Note the initial decrease in diastolic velocity leading to an increased pulsatility index. With further obstruction of flow, an alternating flow pattern becomes evident, with subsequent progression to short systolic spikes and then to no signal at all. The final stages correlate with cerebral circulatory arrest. *CPP,* cerebral perfusion pressure. (From Hassler W, Steinmetz H, Pirschel J: Transcranial Doppler study of intracranial circulatory arrest, *J Neurosurg* 71:195-201, 1989.)

TRANSCRANIAL DOPPLER FINDINGS WITH INCREASED INTRACRANIAL PRESSURE

Two parameters of the TCD velocity tracing can be evaluated for a determination of ICP: mean velocity and pulsatility index. Under normal circumstances, mean velocity remains stable, with ICP increasing until the lower limit of autoregulation is reached. Then there is progressive reduction in mean velocity corresponding to progressive reduction in cerebral blood flow. A marked increase in the pulsatility index is an even earlier indicator of increased ICP. As the pulsatility index increases, there is progressive reduction of diastolic velocity but no initial change in mean velocity. With further increases in ICP, mean velocity is reduced simultaneously with a further increase in the pulsatility index. These changes probably occur as a result of progressive increases in the resistance of the cerebrovascular bed.

At very high ICPs, which produce cerebral circulatory arrest, the MCA velocity waveform progresses through a predictable sequence: A progressive reduction in diastolic velocity to zero is followed by an alternating flow pattern with a reduced diastolic component (Fig. 17-7). Further obstruction of flow causes development of an alternate flow that is antegrade in systole and retrograde in diastole. Further progression leads to small systolic peaks and then to a complete absence of the waveform. These TCD changes have been correlated with previously described angiographic findings showing a lack of opacification of the cerebral arterial tree.[24] Both cerebral angiography and radionuclide isotope scanning show that an alternating flow pattern on TCD corresponds to arrest of the cerebral circulation.

Changes in pulsatility index and mean velocity alone, however, are not specific for increased ICP. High resistance in the cerebrovascular bed, producing increased pulsatility and decreased velocity, is also seen with intense vasoconstriction resulting from vigorous hyperventilation, low cerebral metabolism, and cerebrovasoconstrictive drugs such as barbiturates. This is why isolated mean velocity and pulsatility index measurements do not predict ICP reliably. The pulsatility index can also be markedly affected by cardiac factors. However, in patients who are carefully observed and demonstrate no concomitant cardiac changes, alterations in arterial CO_2 content, or changes in other factors that produce vasoconstriction, progressive increases in the pulsatility index can indicate an incipient increase in ICP.

Transcranial Doppler can be used to estimate increased ICP and to provide information about cerebral perfusion in critically ill patients in spite of the limitations mentioned earlier. Intracranial pressure monitoring, which has become routine in neurosurgical intensive care, can provide information about cerebral perfusion pressure and warn of impending herniation. Direct monitoring of ICP, however, is an indirect method of evaluating cerebral perfusion. Recording of blood flow velocity in the basal intracranial arteries can yield information about cerebral perfusion, as long as the limitations discussed are considered. Evaluation of mean velocity and pulsatility index can be valuable in clinical

Table 17-2. Transcranial Doppler studies comparing sonographic results to clinical and blood flow findings in suspected brain death

Author	Clinical	Blood flow study	Method of comparison	Comments
Ropper et al.[55]	Yes	No	EEG	3 False positives
Kirkham et al.[25]	Yes	No	EEG	Pediatric population
Bode et al.[8]	Yes	No		Pediatric population
Velthoven et al.[65]	Yes	Yes	Angiography/EEG	
Newell et al.[45]	Yes	Yes	Radioisotope	1 False positive
Hassler et al.[24]	Yes	Yes	Angiography	
Powers et al.[52]	Yes	Yes	Radioisotope	
Petty et al.[51]	Yes	No	EEG	Comparison group of non–brain-dead comatose patients
Messer et al.[35]	Yes	No		Pediatric population
Shiogai et al.[62]	Yes	No	EEG/SSEP	
Zurynski et al.[68]	Yes	Yes	Angiography	Basilar artery included
Yokota et al.[67]	Yes	Yes	Angiography	
Rozsa et al.[57]	Yes	No		
Ducrocq et al.[14]	Yes	Yes	Angiography/EEG	
Davalos et al.[13]	Yes	No	EEG	Barbiturates present
Feri et al.[18]	Yes	No	EEG	

EEG, Electroencephalogram; *SSEP*, somatosensory evoked potential.

situations in which ICP is in question. In our intensive care unit, it has been observed that marked side-to-side differences in velocity and pulsatility are occasionally seen in patients with large, unilateral mass lesions. Intracranial pressure monitoring may not always accurately reflect the perfusion pressure in both hemispheres; ICP is usually measured unilaterally. Examination of patients with TCD can also be useful when there is concern about the validity of ICP measurements from transducer readings. Occasionally, ICP transducers give falsely high or low readings as a result of technical problems. Under these circumstances, TCD has been found useful in determining whether the circulatory pattern is normal or abnormal; such information can corroborate or refute ICP readings.

It was recently noted that the effectiveness of cerebral autoregulation appears to be correlated with the intrinsic cerebrovascular tone. Both cerebrovascular tone pressure and critical closing pressure of the cerebral circulation can be obtained from an analysis of the MCA velocity and arterial pressure waveforms. In the future, it may be possible to predict ICP reliably from these parameters with the use of TCD and arterial blood pressure recordings.

BRAIN DEATH

Transcranial Doppler is considered the confirming test in the diagnosis of brain death. It can reliably detect arrest of the intracranial circulation, which often occurs in brain death. The true diagnosis of brain death is made on a clinical basis; blood flow studies such as cerebral angiography, radioisotope scanning, and TCD serve only to confirm the diagnosis. According to the president's commission on guidelines for determination of brain death in the United States,[53] confirmatory tests can be used in patients who fulfill the clinical criteria for brain death to shorten the observation period preceding organ harvest or the discontinuation of mechanical ventilation.

Several studies have examined the role of TCD in the determination of brain death.* These studies have compared (1) clinical findings and (2) the results of blood flow studies with sonographic waveforms in patients in whom brain death occurs. Table 17-2 lists some of these studies. Note that most of these studies have indicated sensitivities and specificities of the TCD technique approaching 100%. However, several caveats apply to TCD and all other confirming tests of cerebral blood flow. First, false positives occur in rare circumstances; for instance, in pathologic conditions producing transient cerebral circulatory arrest. This finding has been documented in patients with subarachnoid hemorrhage caused by marked increase in ICP.[15,23] However, cerebral circulatory arrest in this case may be transient and may reverse in minutes. Cerebral blood flow is restored, and Doppler waveforms return to normal. When TCD is used to confirm arrest, it must be repeated, or arrest must be documented for a sufficient period (30 minutes, under normothermic conditions) to

*References 8, 12, 14, 24, 45, 51, 55, 57, 62, 65, 67, 68.

show incompatibility with survival. False-positive TCD results are also seen in patients who have sustained cerebral circulatory arrest but still have residual brainstem function.[45] This minimal activity can sustain respiratory effort or minimal cranial nerve function for a short time. False-negative TCD results have been reported in unusual situations in which abnormally low diastolic pressure is present (e.g., in patients with intraaortic balloon pumps). In addition, false-negative results have been reported in patients with clinical brain death, such as cases in which massive destruction of the brainstem occurs as a result of posterior fossa lesions, abolishing brainstem function and fulfilling the criteria for brain death. Transcranial Doppler waveforms may indicate preserved blood flow in patients who are clinically dead but have preserved supratentorial blood flow and therefore persistent electroencephalographic (EEG) activity.

These examples of false-positive and false-negative results do not indicate the failure of the TCD technique itself but emphasize why results of confirmatory tests do not always concur with the clinical diagnosis of brain death. Despite these shortcomings, TCD is extremely valuable in documenting cerebral circulatory arrest in patients suspected of being brain dead. This is especially true in patients in whom clinical diagnosis is made difficult or suspect because of extensive trauma and cranial nerve damage. Transcranial Doppler may also be used to establish arrest of the cerebral circulation after trauma in patients who have been given paralytic agents that complicate clinical evaluation. In these cases TCD examination can help avoid unneeded surgery.

CONCLUSIONS

Transcranial Doppler is increasingly accepted in neurosurgical intensive care as a valuable tool in the assessment of cerebral circulation under various circumstances. It has proved useful in further defining pathophysiology with alterations of cerebrovascular control after head injury and provides guidance in the management of such cases. In the early diagnosis of various complications associated with head injury such as vasospasm and carotid dissection, TCD can be clinically useful. It can also alert clinicians to the presence of markedly increased ICP, although at this writing TCD waveforms alone are not specific enough to predict moderate ICP increases. An experienced interpreter can identify Doppler waveforms indicating the arrest of cerebral circulation, a useful finding in the diagnosis of brain death. Transcranial Doppler can also be used in cases of suspected brain death to shorten the observation period before organ harvest. The decision to discontinue ventilatory support and nursing care can be based on the confirmatory findings of TCD.

REFERENCES

1. Aaslid R: *Cerebral hemodynamics.* In Newell DW, Aaslid R, editors: *Transcranial Doppler,* New York, 1992, Raven Press.
2. Aaslid R, Huber R, Nornes H: Evaluation of cerebrovascular spasm with transcranial Doppler ultrasound, *J Neurosurg* 60:37-41, 1984.
3. Aaslid R, Lindegaard K-F, Sorteberg W, et al: Cerebral autoregulation dynamics in humans, *Stroke* 20:45-52, 1989.
4. Aaslid R, Markwalder T-M, Nornes H: Noninvasive transcranial Doppler ultrasound recording of flow velocity in basal cerebral arteries, *J Neurosurg* 57:769-774, 1982.
5. Aaslid R, Newell DW, Stooss R, et al: Assessment of cerebral autoregulation dynamics from simultaneous arterial and venous transcranial Doppler recordings in humans, *Stroke* 22:1148-1154, 1991.
6. Auer LM, Sayama I: Intracranial pressure oscillations (B-waves) caused by oscillations in cerebrovascular volume, *Acta Neurochir (Wien)* 68:93-100, 1983.
7. Bishop CC, Powell S, Rutt D, et al: Transcranial Doppler measurement of middle cerebral artery blood flow velocity: validation study, *Stroke* 17:913-915, 1986.
8. Bode H, Sauer M, Pringsheim W: Diagnosis of brain death by transcranial Doppler sonography, *Arch Dis Child* 63:1474-1478, 1988.
9. Chan K-H, Miller JD, Dearden NM: Intracranial blood flow velocity after head injury: relationship to severity of injury, time, neurological status and outcome, *J Neurol Neurosurg Psychiatry* 55:787-791, 1992.
10. Chan K-H, Miller JD, Dearden NM, et al: The effect of changes in cerebral perfusion pressure upon middle cerebral artery blood flow velocity and jugular bulb venous oxygen saturation after severe brain injury, *J Neurosurg* 77:55-61, 1992.
11. Cold GE: Measurement of CO_2 reactivity and barbiturate reactivity in patients with severe head injury, *Acta Neurochir (Wien)* 98:153-163, 1989.
12. Cold GE, Jensen FT, Malmros R: The cerbrovascular CO_2 reactivity during the acute phase of brain injury, *Acta Anaesthesiol Scand* 21:222-231, 1977.
13. Davalos A, Rodriguez-Rago A, Maté G, et al: Value of the transcranial Doppler examination in the diagnosis of brain death, *Med Clin (Barc)* 100:249-252, 1993.
14. Ducrocq X, Pincemaille B, Braun M, et al: Value of transcranial Doppler ultrasonography in patients with suspected brain death, *Ann Fr Anesth Reanim* 11:415-423, 1992.
15. Eng CC, Lam A, Byrd S, et al: The diagnosis and management of a perianesthetic cerebral aneurysmal rupture aided with transcranial Doppler ultrasonography, *Anesthesiology* 78:191-194, 1993.
16. Envoldsen E: CBF in head injury, *Acta Neurochir Suppl (Wien)* 36:133-136, 1986.
17. Envoldsen EM, Jensen FT: Autoregulation and CO_2 responses of cerebral blood flow in patients with acute severe head injury, *J Neurosurg* 48:689-703, 1978.
18. Feri M, Ralli L, Felici M: Transcranial Doppler in the diagnosis of brain death, *Minerva Anestesiol* 59:11-18, 1993.
19. Giller CA: A bedside test for cerebral autoregulation using transcranial Doppler ultrasound, *Acta Neurochir (Wien)* 108:7-14, 1991.
20. Giller CA, Bowman G, Dyer H, et al: Cerebral artery diameters during changes in blood pressure and carbon dioxide during craniotomy, *Neurosurgery* 32:737-742, 1993.
21. Grosset DG, Straiton J, McDonald I, et al: Use of transcranial Doppler sonography to predict development of a delayed ischemic deficit after subarachnoid hemorrhage, *J Neurosurg* 78:183-187, 1993.

22. Grosset DG, Strebel S, Straiton J, et al: *Impaired carbon dioxide reactivity predicts poor outcome in severe head injury: a transcranial Doppler study.* In Avezaat CJJ, van Eijndhoven JHM, Maas AIR, et al, editors: *Intracranial pressure 8,* Berlin and Heidelberg, 1993, Springer Verlag.

23. Grote E, Hassler W: The critical first minutes after subarachnoid hemorrhage, *Neurosurgery* 22:654-661, 1988.

24. Hassler W, Steinmetz H, Pirschel J: Transcranial Doppler study of intracranial circulatory arrest, *J Neurosurg* 71:195-201, 1989.

25. Kirkham FJ, Levin SD, Padayachee TS, et al: Transcranial pulsed Doppler ultrasound findings in brain stem death, *J Neurol Neurosurg Psychiatry* 50:1504-1513, 1987.

26. Langfitt TW, Obrist WD: Cerebral blood flow and metabolism after intracranial trauma, *Prog Neurol Surg* 10:14-48, 1981.

27. Lassen NA: Cerebral blood flow and oxygen consumption in man, *Physiol Rev* 39:183-237, 1959.

28. Lewis DH, Eskridge JM, Newell DW, et al: Single-photon emission computed tomography, transcranial Doppler ultrasound, and cerebral angioplasty for posttraumatic vasospasm, *J Neuroimaging* 3:252-254, 1993.

29. Lindegaard K-F, Lundar T, Wiberg J, et al: Variations in middle cerebral artery blood flow investigated with noninvasive transcranial blood velocity measurements, *Stroke* 18:1025-1030, 1987.

30. Lindegaard K-F, Nornes H, Bakke SJ, et al: Cerebral vasospasm diagnosis by means of angiography and blood velocity measurements, *Acta Neurochir (Wien)* 100:12-24, 1989.

31. Lundar T, Lindegaard K-F, Nornes H: Continuous recording of middle cerebral artery blood velocity in clinical neurosurgery, *Acta Neurochir (Wien)* 102:85-90, 1990.

32. Lundberg N: Continuous recording and control of ventricular fluid pressure in neurosurgical practice, *Acta Psychiatr Scand (Suppl)* 149:1-193, 1960.

33. Lundberg N, Cronqvist S, Kjallquist A: Clinical investigation on interrelations between intracranial pressure and intracranial hemodynamics, *Prog Brain Res* 30:70-75, 1968.

34. Martin N, Doberstein C, Zane C, et al: Post traumatic vasospasm: transcranial Doppler ultrasound, cerebral blood flow and angiographic findings, *J Neurosurg* 77:575-583, 1992.

35. Messer J, Burtscher A, Haddad J, et al: Contribution of transcranial Doppler sonography to the diagnosis of brain death in children, *Arch Fr Pediatr* 47:647-651, 1990.

36. Muizelaar JP: *Cerebral blood flow, cerebral blood volume, and cerebral metabolism after severe head injury.* In Becker DP, Gudeman SK, editors: *Textbook of head injury,* Philadelphia, 1989, WB Saunders.

37. Muizelaar JP, Lutz HA III, Becker DP, et al: Effect of mannitol on ICP and CBF and correlation with pressure autoregulation in severely head-injured patients, *J Neurosurg* 61:700-706, 1984.

38. Muizelaar JP, van der Poel H, Li Z, et al: Pial arteriolar vessel diameter and CO_2 reactivity during prolonged hyperventilation in the rabbit, *J Neurosurg* 69:923-927, 1988.

39. Muizelaar JP, Wei EP, Kontos HA, et al: Mannitol causes compensatory cerebral vasoconstriction and vasodilation in response to blood viscosity changes, *J Neurosurg* 59:822-828, 1983.

40. Narayan RK: *Emergency room management of the head-injured patient.* In Becker DP, Gudeman SK, editors: *Textbook of head injury,* Philadelphia, 1989, WB Saunders.

41. Nelson RJ, Czosnyka M, Pickard JD, et al: Experimental aspects of cerebrospinal hemodynamics: the relationship between blood flow velocity waveform and cerebral autoregulation, *Neurosurgery* 31:705-710, 1992.

42. Newell DW, Aaslid R, Lam A, et al: Comparison of flow and velocity during dynamic autoregulation testing in humans, *Stroke* 25:793-797, 1994.

43. Newell DW, Aaslid R, Stooss R, et al: The relationship of blood flow velocity fluctuations to intracranial pressure B waves, *J Neurosurg* 76:415-421, 1992.

44. Newell DW, Aaslid R, Stooss R, et al: Experience using continuous transcranial Doppler monitoring in head injured patients, *Neurosurgery* (in press).

45. Newell DW, Grady S, Sirotta P, et al: Evaluation of brain death using transcranial Doppler, *Neurosurgery* 24:509-513, 1989.

46. Newell DW, Seiler RW, Aaslid R: *Head injury and cerebral circulatory arrest.* In Newell DW, Aaslid R, editors: *Transcranial Doppler,* New York, 1992, Raven Press.

47. Nordstrom C-H, Messeter K, Sunbärg G, et al: Cerebral blood flow, vasoreactivity, and oxygen consumption during barbiturate therapy in severe traumatic brain lesions, *J Neurosurg* 68:424-431, 1988.

48. Nornes H, Magnes B, Aaslid R: *Observations of intracranial pressure plateau waves.* In Lundberg N, Ponten U, Brock M, editors: *Intracranial pressure 2,* New York, 1975, Springer Verlag.

49. Obrist WD, Langfitt TW, Jaggi JL, et al: Cerebral blood flow and metabolism in comatose patients with acute head injury: relationship to intracranial hypertension, *J Neurosurg* 61:241-253, 1984.

50. Paulson OB, Strandgaard S, Edvinsson L: Cerebral autoregulation, *Cerebrovasc Brain Metab Rev* 2:161-192, 1990.

51. Petty GW, Mohr JP, Pedley TA, et al: The role of transcranial Doppler in confirming brain death: sensitivity, specificity, and suggestions for performance and interpretation, *Neurology* 40:300-303, 1990.

52. Powers AD, Gradeber MC, Smith RR: Transcranial Doppler ultrasonography in the determination of brain death, *Neurosurgery* 24:884-889, 1989.

53. President's Commission: Guidelines for the determination of brain death, *JAMA* 246:2184-2187, 1981.

54. Risberg J, Lundberg N, Ingvar DH: Regional cerebral blood volume during acute transient rises of the intracranial pressure (plateau waves), *J Neurosurg* 31:303-310, 1969.

55. Ropper AH, Kehne SM, Wechsler L: Transcranial Doppler in brain death, *Neurology* 37:1733-1735, 1987.

56. Rosner MJ, Becker DP: Origin and evolution of plateau waves: experimental observations and a theoretical model, *J Neurosurg* 60:312-324, 1984.

57. Rozsa L, Szabo S, Gombi R, et al: Intracranial pressure increase and changes in cerebrovascular circulation, associated with brain death, studied by transcranial Doppler sonography, *Orv Hetil* 132:2785-2788, 1991.

58. Sander D, Klingelhofer J: Correlation between CO_2 reactivity, ICP and outcome in severe cerebral disease, *J Cardiovasc Tech* 9:261-262, 1990.

59. Schalen W, Messeter R, Nordstrom CH: Cerebral vasoreactivity and the prediction of outcome in severe traumatic brain lesions, *Acta Anaesthesiol Scand* 35:113-122, 1991.

60. Seiler RW, Grolimund P, Aaslid R, et al: Cerebral vasospasm evaluated by transcranial ultrasound correlated with clinical grade and CT-visualized subarachnoid hemorrhage, *J Neurosurg* 64:594-600, 1986.

61. Seiler RW, Newell DW: *Subarachnoid hemorrhage and vasospasm.* In Newell DW, Aaslid R, editors: *Transcranial Doppler,* New York, 1992, Raven Press.

62. Shiogai T, Sato E, Tokitsu M, et al: Transcranial Doppler monitoring in severe brain damage: relationships between intracranial haemodynamics, brain dysfunction and outcome, *Neurol Res* 12:205-213, 1990.

63. Simard JM, Bellefleur M: Systemic arterial hypertension in head trauma, *Am J Cardiol* 63:32-35, 1989.

64. Sorteberg W: *Cerebral blood velocity and cerebral blood flow.* In Newell DW, Aaslid R, editors: *Transcranial Doppler,* New York, 1992, Raven Press.

65. Velthoven VV, Calliauw L: Diagnosis of brain death: transcranial Doppler sonography as an additional method, *Acta Neurochir (Wien)* 95:57-60, 1988.

66. Weber M, Grolimund P, Seiler RW: Evaluation of post-traumatic cerebral blood flow velocities by transcranial Doppler ultrasonography, *Neurosurgery* 27:106-112, 1990.

67. Yokota H, Nakazawa S, Shimura T, et al: Hypothalamic and pituitary function in brain death, *Neurol Med Chir (Tokyo)* 31:881-886, 1991.

68. Zurynski Y, Dorsch N, Pearson I, et al: Transcranial Doppler ultrasound in brain death: experience in 140 patients, *Neurol Res* 13:248-252, 1991.

18

Transcranial Doppler Ultrasonography Monitoring during Cognitive Testing

Jürgen Klingelhöfer
Dirk Sander

In 1928, J. F. Fulton reported for the first time the close coupling between neuronal activity and regional cerebral blood flow (rCBF). Fulton described an increased blood flow murmur over a patient's occipital angioma while the patient was reading.[17] Today, the primary methods for in vivo evaluation of rCBF are the xenon-133 inhalation and injection techniques, single photon emission computed tomography (SPECT), and positron emission tomography (PET). These methods are used to assess rCBF and metabolic activity during different functional activities, such as talking, reading, or performing other cognitive tasks.[19,22,38,42,45,53] The results indicate a spatial distribution of rCBF that is task-specific. Thinking, for example, is associated with an increase in rCBF in the superior prefrontal cortex,[47] whereas auditory discrimination tends to produce a selective increase in the right hemispheric rCBF. The comparable increase produced by speaking is most prominent in the left hemisphere.[38,49] It should be borne in mind, however, that factors other than the aforementioned kinds of functional activity—factors such as handedness, gender, anxiety, and motivation—have an impact on cognitive performance and rCBF in normal subjects.[19,20,43,44,46]

Although the methods of rCBF measurement already alluded to have the advantage of high spatial resolution, their temporal resolution is not sufficiently fast to detect those changes of cerebral perfusion that occur within seconds and correspond to rapid alterations of the functional state. Such methods, then, cannot provide adequate data on the dynamics of rCBF adjustment. If we can arrive at a better understanding of the temporal course of local cerebral perfusion in its qualitative and quantitative details, we should eventually be able to answer unsolved questions about coupling mechanisms linking neuronal activity, regional cerebral perfusion, and metabolism.[23,33]

Coupling may be explained by the dependence of rCBF on brain tissue metabolism. Because rCBF is regulated by changes in the diameters of small-resistance vessels while the diameters of the large basal arteries remain constant, changes in brain perfusion should produce comparable changes in the blood flow velocity of the large cerebral arteries.[1,2,4,6,52]

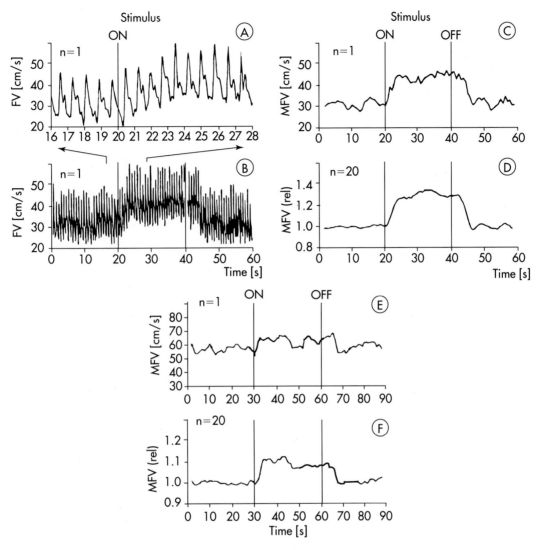

Fig. 18-1. General experimental procedure. **A,** Envelope of Doppler frequency spectra in the right posterior cerebral artery during stimulation. **B,** Same recording as **A** at a different time resolution. **C,** Mean flow velocity *(MFV)* response of the same recording as in **A** and **B**. The MFV was calculated from the envelope curve using a computer-assisted integration procedure. **D,** Average MFV responses under the same conditions as in **A** and **B** derived from 20 single trials (relative values). The reference point for averaging was the stimulus onset. **E,** The right middle cerebral artery MFV response during the performance of a complex spatial task. **F,** Average MFV responses under the same conditions as in **E,** derived from 20 single trials (relative values). The reference point for averaging was the stimulation onset.

The introduction of transcranial Doppler sonography (TCD) by Aaslid and colleagues in 1982 made it possible to make continuous measurements of blood flow velocity (FV) in the large basal arteries.[3] The high temporal resolution of TCD has provided data on cerebral hemodynamics in relation to neuronal functional change. For example, by monitoring the posterior cerebral artery (PCA) (an artery that has the exclusive supply of the visual cortex) during visual stimulation, it has been possible to study functionally evoked velocity responses (Fig. 18-1).[1,12] By assessing the range of stimulus presentation and its perception, as well as the

applied methodologic procedures, it has become possible to investigate the influence of different sensory modalities on cerebral hemodynamics during the performance of complex tasks.

The following pages present an overview of recently performed TCD studies, subdivided according to the stimuli applied during testing. The Sensory Stimulation section deals with investigations into the activation of only one sensory modality (visual, auditory, or vibratory stimulation). Under Stimulation with Associative Tasks, we summarize studies characterized by the activation of additional cerebral centers in the performance of complex tasks such as viewing pictures, reading, and tactile discrimination.

SENSORY STIMULATION
Light, color, and checkerboard-pattern reversal stimulation

Using TCD, Aaslid studied the visually evoked FV response in 10 normal patients by means of simple on-off light stimulus.[1] By calculating the envelope curve of the velocity spectrum and filtering it with a cutoff frequency of 0.4 Hz, Aaslid was able to analyze blood flow changes in the PCA, middle cerebral artery (MCA), and superior cerebellar artery (SCA). He found an average FV increase of 16.4% in the PCAs and 3.3% in the MCAs. The FV values in the SCAs showed no significant change in response to the stimulus.

Conrad and Klingelhöfer made a detailed analysis of the effects of white screen and checkerboard-pattern stimulation on local cerebral perfusion.[12] Using the original TCD envelope curve, they calculated, by means of a computer-assisted integration procedure, the mean flow velocity (MFV) during one cardiac cycle. During the test, 10 normal patients were asked to look at a small light in the center of a white or checkered screen. White screen stimulation resulted in sudden increases in FV values (Fig. 18-2), although habituation occurred within 30 to 40 seconds and was accompanied by a nearly continuous but gradual decrease of MFV. The 10 Hz dynamic checkerboard stimulus caused a steeper increase of MFV at the onset, an increase that attained a plateau situated 30.9% ± 7.2% higher than the baseline (Fig. 18-2). At the termination of the 10 Hz checkerboard stimulus, a second, smaller increase of FV was noted in 40% of subjects, a phenomenon the investigators termed "off-reaction." During the poststimulus period, the MFV decreased below the level of the prestimulus period in 60% of the patients. This finding was called "undershooting reaction." Conrad and Klingelhöfer suggested that the results from the checkerboard stimulation may have been caused by an increase in the visual field's contrast borders. The difference in the response of MFV to the white and the checkered screen stimuli is similar to that observed in patients concentrating on a picture's center as opposed to performing free scanning. This is because velocity habituation occurs when the visual cortex receives no new information. It thus appears that MFV changes so rapidly to meet altered stimulus conditions that even neuronal "off effects" are observable when the stimulus is terminated. The delay in the decrease of MFV after stimulus cessation may have been due to neuronal activity outlasting the stimulus.[7] Conrad and Klingelhöfer attributed the "undershooting reaction" that was observed in the poststimulus phase to excessive blood supply during visual stimulation, resulting in poststimulus counterregulation. The adaptation of MFV to the resting condition would then imply the existence of an oscillating regulatory mechanism.

Gomez and colleagues recorded changes of the PCA MFV during total darkness; intermittent light stimulation of 5, 10, 20, 30, and 60 Hz; and continuous illumination.[18] They expected a progressive increase in PCA MFV as a result of temporal summation of the stimuli. The highest increases, however, were recorded at 10 Hz (21% ± 5%) and 20 Hz (19% ± 5%) and were significantly different from those obtained at other frequencies. Frequencies greater than 20 Hz caused velocity changes that were almost the same as those found during continuous illumination. From the pattern they observed, Gomez and associates concluded that optimal stimulation frequency creates an overall balance of excitation of both "on" and "off" neuronal populations. According to these observations, the optimal frequency of intermittent visual stimulation required to induce measurable changes in PCA velocity responses is in the range of 10 to 20 Hz.

Harders and colleagues analyzed changes of the PCA MFV during illumination of the right and/or left visual fields in 24 right-handed subjects.[21] They demonstrated that the increase in velocity in the right PCA during activation of the left visual field was significantly higher than that of the left PCA during activation of the right visual field. Activation of both visual fields produced similar increases in the two PCAs. Harders and associates interpreted this higher MFV response in the right PCA as being indicative of the dominance of the right visual field in right-handed persons.

Simultaneous, bilateral TCD recordings of the PCAs were recently performed to confirm the greater increase of the right PCA MFV during half and full stimulation of the visual field.[54] The method was also used in a study of 16 normal subjects to investigate the influence of stimulus size and duration (50, 100, and 150 ms) on the FV response. The FV increase was found to correlate positively with the size of the stimulus, although the increase was only by average factors of 1.4 and 1.8, while the stimulus size increased by factors of 22 and 553, respectively (Fig. 18-3). This relatively slight FV response was attributed to the substantially lower receptor cell density in the periphery of the retina and to the disproportionate representation of central retinal fields on the visual cortex.

Njemanze and associates carried out experiments to determine the relationship between cerebral lateralization and color perception.[39] Their experiments involved the repeated measurement of MFV in eight normal subjects under conditions of darkness (eyes closed in a dark room), light (eyes open in ambient room light), and after exposure to a variety of color stimuli. Although light stimulation gave rise to generally equal MFV

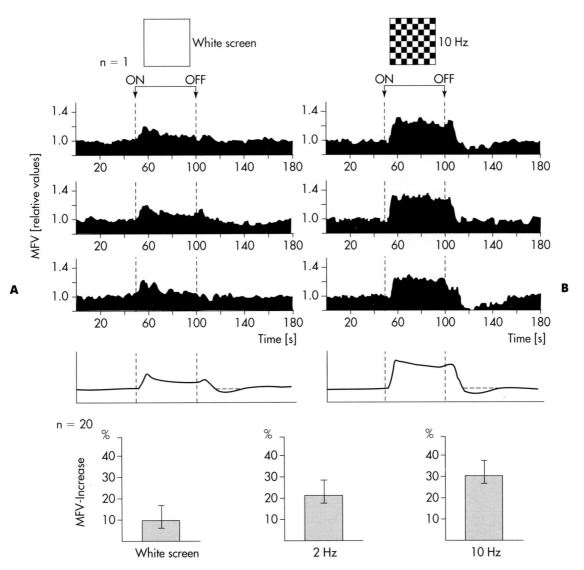

Fig. 18-2. Qualitative and quantitative effects of white screen and checkerboard stimulation on right posterior cerebral artery flow patterns. **A,** Normalized mean flow velocity *(MFV)* response of three representative subjects (single trials) during white screen stimulation *(left column)* and 10 Hz checkerboard stimulation *(right column)*. The schematic drawing at the bottom illustrates the general behavior of MFV changes. **B,** Percentage increase of MFV during white screen as well as 2 Hz and 10 Hz checkerboard stimulation relative to the corresponding resting phase (10 subjects, two trials). The subjects were asked to look at a central point of the screen. The values represent means ± SEM.

increases in the two PCAs, darkness and color produced significantly greater MFV values in the right PCA. The right PCA MFV was always higher than that of the left during the presentation of color stimuli. Furthermore, it was found that primary psychological colors (blue, yellow, red, and green) induced greater MFV lateralization than did a blue-green mixture. Njemanze and colleagues therefore concluded that the right visual cortex is selectively sensitive to certain wavelengths.

Preliminary investigations have also been performed to evaluate the PCA MFV response to visual stimuli in

patients with occipital lesions. Maravic and associates studied the effect of on-off light stimuli, red color slides, and visual imagery in 12 patients with PCA infarctions and complete homonymous hemianopsia, quadrantanopsia, or multiple defects in both visual fields.[34] In patients with complete homonymous hemianopsia, no velocity response could be gauged on the affected side. Patients with quadrantanopsia showed perceptible decreases of the PCA MFV response after exposure to on-off light and color slide stimuli, but not after exposure to complex scenes. Maravic and colleagues postulated a

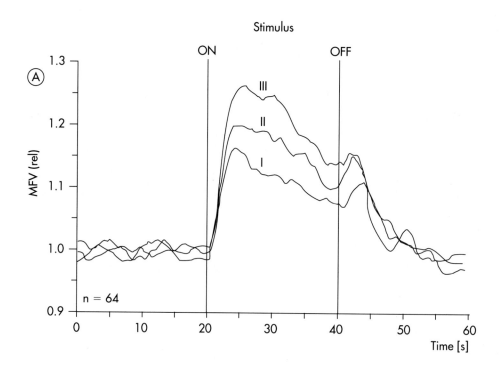

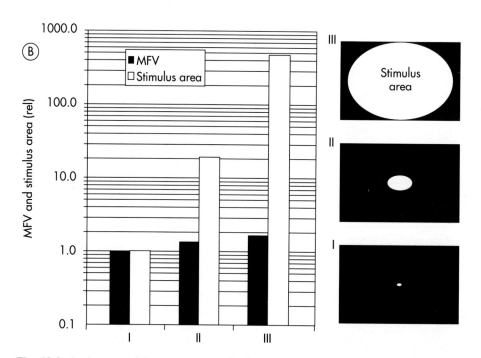

Fig. 18-3. A, Average right posterior cerebral artery mean flow velocity *(MFV)* responses during stimulation with different large stimuli *(I, II, III)* (16 subjects, four trials). The reference point for averaging was the stimulus onset. The subjects were asked to look at a central point of the screen. **B,** Relationship between MFV responses and the three stimulus sizes. The MFV values and the stimulus sizes are normalized to 1 by using the smallest stimulus size.

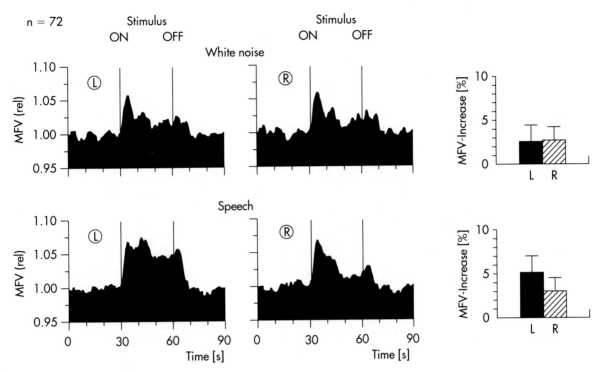

Fig. 18-4. Average mean flow velocity *(MFV)* responses in the left *(L)* and right *(R)* middle cerebral arteries during auditory stimulation (24 subjects, three trials). The reference point for averaging was the stimulus onset. Percentage increases of MFV for the four modalities are presented by the bar graphs.

proportional relationship between the visually induced FV response and the extent of activated visual cortex. In a similar study of seven patients with ischemic lesions of the visual cortex, a markedly reduced FV response was found on the affected side.[50] The amplitude of FV response was dependent on the degree of infarction.

Carvajal-Lizano and Thie studied the PCA MFV changes during the interictal periods of 25 migraineurs.[10] They manually recorded the MFV every 4 seconds using stroboscopic stimulation at frequencies of 2 and 10 Hz. Vasoreactivity was always more pronounced in migraine sufferers than in healthy, age-matched controls, suggesting abnormalities of visual vasoreactivity in these patients. The diagnostic value of these observations has yet to be determined.

Auditory stimulation

Bruneau and associates studied the relationship of MCA FV dynamics to auditory stimulation in 34 children, 12 of whom were autistic, 12 normal, and 10 mentally retarded.[8] Auditory stimuli (200 ms bursts of a 750 Hz tone at an intensity of 80 dB) were simultaneously administered to both ears by means of earphones. Measurements of the maximal systolic and diastolic FVs and MFV were made while the children were at rest and during the first 5 seconds of stimulus administration. In normal children, the left MCA MFV

increased by an average of 5.3% over baseline values, although no comparable change was observed in the right MCA. A similar but less asymmetric pattern was found in the mentally retarded children, in whom left and right MCA MFVs rose by 8% and 4.5%, respectively. Results in autistic children, however, differed significantly, showing decreased FV levels in both MCAs. This suggests an abnormality in the metabolic changes triggered by auditory stimulation, an abnormality possibly related to the known impaired development of cerebral lateralization in these children.

Klingelhöfer and colleagues subjected 24 healthy, right-handed individuals to speech or white noise that was administered to both ears simultaneously (Fig. 18-4).[27] They obtained continuous and simultaneous measurements of the FVs in each subject's left and right MCAs. White noise stimulation caused only minor velocity increases, which were virtually the same on both sides (right, 2.5% ± 1.5%; left, 2.5% ± 1.9%). Speech, by contrast, produced a significantly greater MFV increase in the left (2.7 ± 2.2%) than in the right MCA (0.5% ± 2.3%). Klingelhöfer and associates suggested that the small FV increase during white noise stimulation corresponds to the activation of the primary auditory regions of the two temporal lobes.[31] They also proposed that the left MCA's MFV response to speech stimulation indicates the dominance of the left hemisphere in language processing in right-handed subjects. These results are in accord with rCBF findings and cerebral glucose metabolism measurements.[9,29,38,41]

Vibratory stimulation

Kelley and colleagues studied the relationship between vibratory stimulation and FV in 20 exclusively right-handed subjects.[26] They measured blood pressure and pulse before and after the study and performed a series of alternate recordings from the MCAs using a switchbox. Compared to baseline values, FVs did not significantly increase during stimulation. Kelley and associates concluded that the type of vibratory apparatus used produced too slight a stimulus to elicit significant FV changes and that their observations may reflect the limited sensitivity of TCD.

STIMULATION WITH ASSOCIATIVE TASKS
Complex pictures

Conrad and Klingelhöfer monitored the MFV of study subjects as they looked at five different pictures of increasing complexity.[12] The average MFV increased with growing picture complexity, reaching a maximum increase of 38.8% ± 6.5% over baseline values. Fixing the subject's attention on the central point of a complex picture elicited an increase of only 19.1% ± 4.2% and generally indicated stronger FV habituation than did the results of stimulation with a white screen. Based on these findings, Conrad and Klingelhöfer suggested that the act of perceiving visual stimuli causes distinct MFV changes in occipital areas involved in visual information processing. This was thought to indicate that visual analysis uses independent processing systems or that the increased number of eye movements necessary to scan complex pictures increases the variation of oculomotor projection.[32] The study's results agree with quantitative observations produced by rCBF and PET studies.[30,36,42]

Sitzer and associates studied 10 healthy subjects in an attempt to determine the influence of end-tidal $paCO_2$ on visually induced PCA FV changes.[50] As the subjects watched a color video movie, hypercapnia was found to reduce the maximal response amplitude from an average of 30% in normocapnia to 15% in mild hypercapnia and 8% in severe hypercapnia. Sitzer and colleagues also noted an average reduction of 20% in the maximal response amplitude during hypocapnia. They suggested that their results are consistent with the notion of a nonlinear relationship between the end-tidal $paCO_2$ and stimulus-induced FV changes.

Searching task

Twelve normal subjects, some of whom had been assigned a searching task, were asked to look at a series of complex pictures while they underwent simultaneous and bilateral PCA FV monitoring.[54] The initial increase

in MFV was steeper in subjects performing the search than in those merely looking at the pictures (Fig. 18-5). After the searchers identified their targets, their MFVs remained high for a few seconds before dropping markedly. The frequency of eye movements was higher when the subjects were searching than when they were merely viewing the same picture. Eye movement frequency was also reduced after the target had been identified.

Reading aloud

Droste and associates asked 70 subjects to read four-syllable nouns aloud, a task involving visual, motor, and cognitive components.[15] The right MCA was insonated first in 36 subjects, the left in the other 34. Little difference was observed between the two sides, the left MCA MFV increasing by an average of 10.6% and the right by 9.9%. In another study, Droste and colleagues asked subjects to select from a series of written nouns those that began with a certain letter.[15] The right MCA FV increased by an average of 1.8% and the left by 3.8%, again showing little difference between the two sides. Droste and co-workers suggested that the bilateral increase of MFVs was a consequence of increased cortical metabolism in cerebral territories supplied by the MCAs. The lack of significant differentiation between the two sides was explained by factors of motivation and habituation. It was noted that the side examined first had higher MFV values, a finding the authors ascribed to the subjects' higher motivation and excitement during the first measurements. Although one might expect to find a higher left MCA MFV in right-handed subjects, handedness did not appear to affect the test's results.

Word association

Markus and Boland asked 18 healthy subjects to perform a word association test by producing words with a semantic connection to the one with which they were presented.[35] A subject given the word *apple*, for example, might produce words like *fruit*, *tree*, or *food*. Subjects had to perform the task without speaking. Twelve subjects were right-handed, three were left-handed, and three were ambidextrous. Half of the subjects had their right MCAs studied first, and the other half, their left MCAs. In right-handed subjects, the left MCA MFV increased by an average of 4% compared to baseline values, while no significant changes were recorded on the right side. In left-handed subjects, similar differences were observed between the two sides, the MFV increasing by an average of 7.7% on the right and by only 0.4% on the left. Markus and Boland explained the higher left MCA MFV response in right-handed subjects and the opposite in left-handed subjects in terms of hemispheric dominance. They also hypothesized that the lack of cerebral later-

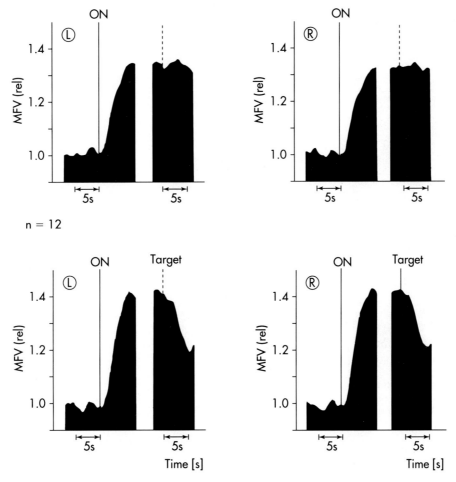

Fig. 18-5. Average mean flow velocity *(MFV)* responses in the left *(L)* and right *(R)* posterior cerebral arteries of subjects who were free viewing a complex picture with *(lower part)* and without *(upper part)* a searching task (12 subjects, one trial). The reference point for averaging was the stimulus onset *(left column,* ON) and a trigger for target identification *(right column,* target).

alization in ambidextrous subjects may reflect a bilateral language-processing ability.

Complex spatial tasks

In a test requiring sensory, motor, and cognitive-spatial functions, Kelley and associates instructed 20 right-handed subjects to handle mah-jongg tiles while blindfolded.[26] The subjects were then asked to place each tile in one of three boxes according to the symbol printed on it. The tiles had to be sorted with one hand, half of the subjects beginning with their left, the others with their right. Because the TCD device did not allow for simultaneous measurements, serial alternating recordings of the MCA were made with a switchbox. Subjects sorting with the right hand demonstrated an average MFV increase over baseline values of 4.9% in the right MCA and 5.9% in the left. In subjects using the left hand, the right MCA MFV increased by an average of 7.4% while that of the left MCA rose by only 1.4%.

Such MFV increases in the MCA opposite to the active hand reflect the contralateral representation of motor activity. Kelley and colleagues suggested that the relatively high right MCA MFV values when the right hand was in use indicate the right hemisphere's dominant role in spatial cognition.

In another study, the MCA MFV was monitored by means of bilateral recordings in 24 normal, right-handed subjects as they compared a series of wooden figures visually and by touching them, one hand at a time[27] (Fig. 18-6). When the task was performed with the left hand, the right MCA MFV increased by 9.2% ± 3% over baseline values while the left MCA MFV rose by only 4.5% ± 2.2%. When the right hand was used, left MCA MFV increased by 7.4% ± 2.8%, while the right MCA MFV rose by 6.2% ± 3%. Both studies produced significant differences between the two sides. Considerably higher increases of MFV were recorded in the hemisphere contralateral to the performing hand. In

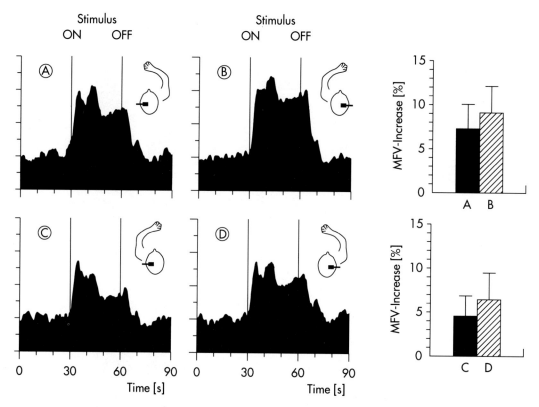

Fig. 18-6. Average mean flow velocity *(MFV)* responses in the middle cerebral arteries during the performance of a complex spatial task with the contralateral (**A** and **B**) or ipsilateral (**C** and **D**) hand (24 subjects, four trials). The reference point for averaging was the stimulus onset. The percentage increases of MFV for the four modalities are presented by the bar graphs.

addition, under the same experimental conditions, the right MCA MFV increase was higher than that on the left (Fig. 18-6). Klingelhöfer and associates proposed that the task required activation of the visual, sensory, and motor cortical areas. They suggested that the processing of the visual task involved both hemispheres to the same extent, whereas sensory input and control of the operational hand involved respective contralateral hemispheres. Increases in the left MCA MFV were thought to be comparable to those observed during simple finger activity. Increases in right MCA MFV during contralateral or ipsilateral hand activity, however, were ascribed to the right hemisphere's dominance in the performance of spatial tasks.[5,11,19,51]

Kelley and co-workers studied the MFV and the peak systolic velocity of 21 healthy subjects as they played a joystick-controlled video game.[25] Each subject was instructed to hold the joystick mount with the left hand and use the right to move the joystick, which directed a ball on the screen. The anterior cerebral artery (ACA), MCA, and PCA were insonated during the game, and blood pressure, pulse rate, and anxiety levels were measured at the beginning and end of the study. In addition, the end-tidal $paCO_2$ was recorded every 30

seconds. Playing the video game caused the following MFV increases over baseline: right ACA, 6.1%; left ACA, 2.1%; right MCA, 13.6%; left MCA, 8.3%; right PCA, 11.8%; left PCA, 15.6%. Blood pressure, pulse rate, and anxiety scores remained nearly unchanged, and $paCO_2$ levels were constant. Noting the higher MFVs in the right MCA and ACA, Kelley and associates suggested that attention and visual-spatial orientation, largely right-hemispheric functions, had a greater impact than motor activity on the right MCA MFV.

Face recognition

From a series of 80 faces, 68 subjects were asked to pick out those that appeared more than once.[15] The average increase of MFV in the right MCA (5.1%) was noticeably higher than that in the left MCA (2.6%), a result that was not significantly affected by handedness. The higher right MCA FV responses were thought to reflect increased cortical activity of the right hemisphere, which is associated with the performance of spatial tasks.

Memory test

O'Dell and associates monitored the MCA MFV in 24 healthy subjects who were asked to perform memory

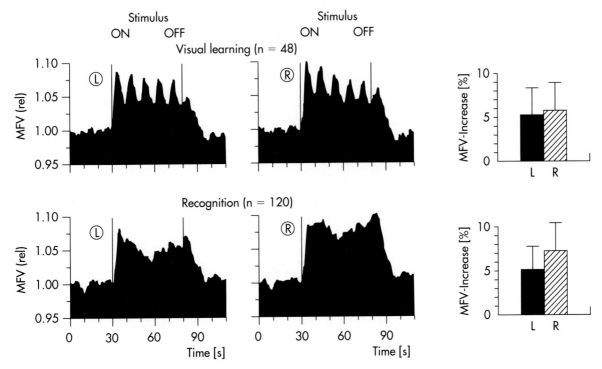

Fig. 18-7. Average mean flow velocity *(MFV)* responses in the left *(L)* and right *(R)* middle cerebral arteries during a memory test with a series of 50 drawings. During visual learning (24 subjects, two trials), five drawings per trial were shown (10 seconds per single drawing). During recognition (24 subjects, five trials), 10 drawings per trial were shown (5 seconds per single drawing). The reference point for averaging was the stimulus onset. The percentage increases of MFV for the four modalities are presented by the bar graphs.

tasks.[40] The tasks consisted of remembering letters, generating and maintaining images, and answering general knowledge questions. Although MFVs increased significantly during task performance, a subject's gender and the type of memory task had no measurable effect on the increase.

In a study performed by Klingelhöfer and co-workers, 24 normal, right-handed subjects memorized 10 drawings and were then asked to pick them out of a selection of 50. Bilateral, simultaneous MCA FV recordings were obtained throughout the course of the test[27] (Fig. 18-7). During the test's memorization stage, the MFV increased 5.8% ± 3.1% above baseline values in the right MCA and 5.3% ± 2.9% in the left MCA. During the second stage of the test, recognition of a presented picture produced velocity increases of 7.4% ± 3% and 5% ± 2.6% in the right and left MCAs, respectively. Comparing the velocity responses of the two stages of testing, Klingelhöfer and colleagues found a right MCA MFV increase of 1.6% ± 2.6% during picture recognition; there was no significant change in the left MCA MFV (Fig. 18-7). They suggested that their findings are consistent with different patterns of cortical activity for learning and memorization.[13,48] Moreover, higher increases in right MCA velocity during the recognition

stage were considered to indicate greater right-hemispheric activity during visual memory recall.[13,40]

DYNAMIC ASPECTS

One major advantage of TCD over other techniques used for the measurement of cerebral perfusion is its excellent time resolution. This is a crucial factor, given the rapidity of FV changes. Aaslid determined through an on-off light stimulation test on 10 subjects that only 2.3 seconds elapse between exposure to the light stimulus and the buildup of 50% of the full FV response, a response that begins to adapt slightly after about 10 seconds.[1] Similar observations were made by Conrad and Klingelhöfer,[12] who used a 10 Hz checkerboard pattern for visual stimulation. In two sets of trials on 10 subjects, 50% and 90% of the FV maximum was reached after, respectively, 2 ± 0.8 and 4.2 ± 1.7 seconds. In 95% of the recordings, a reduction in MFV 5 ± 2.1 seconds after stimulus cessation was detected.

Similarly rapid regulating mechanisms have been detected in other analyses of MCA velocity dynamics. A test involving the performance of a complex spatial task (the visual and tactile comparison of wooden figures) was performed left-handed by 24 subjects who had bilateral, simultaneous recordings of both MCAs: Only

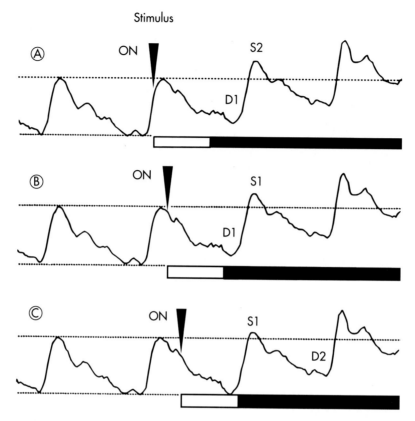

Fig. 18-8. Illustration of the principal procedure using a pulse-dependent triggering of visual stimuli. The relationship between stimulus onset *(ON)* and the subsequent diastolic *(D1)*/peak systolic *(S1)* flow velocity is adjustable through the use of a quartz-controlled, two-level, pulse-triggered timer. The optimal time for stimulus onset **(B)** is attained when the individual reaction time ends shortly before the onset of subsequent diastolic flow velocity. The stimulus onset was chosen too early in **A** and too late in **C**.

2.6 ± 0.6 seconds elapsed between stimulation onset and 50% of full MFV response in the right MCA, and 2.3 ± 0.5 seconds passed before similar results were observed in the left MCA. After stimulus cessation, the MFV took an average of only 4.1 seconds (right MCA) and 4.2 seconds (left MCA) to begin its decline, reaching normal levels in both MCAs about 11 seconds after the stimulus had been terminated. The time scale of the FV response is similar to that of rCBF measured in animal experiments.[14,16,37]

Until recently, the temporal resolution of FV changes was linked to the length of the cardiac cycle, and it was therefore difficult for researchers to detect the shortest latency periods between stimulus onset and FV response. It has finally become possible to extend the existing rate of temporal resolution resulting from the heart rate by using a pulse-dependent triggering of the visual stimuli. In a recent investigation (Fig. 18-8), color slides of complex pictures were used to stimulate 12 healthy subjects.[28] Electromagnetic shutters and a quartz-controlled, pulse-triggered timer ensured a defined temporal limit to the stimuli. In these experiments, stimulus onset was triggered pulse-dependently in order to establish precisely the beginning of FV reactive changes. The electronic timer was set in such a way that the FV increase occurred in the subsequent diastole (Fig. 18-8). Using this method, it was possible to determine that the shortest latency periods between stimulus onset and FV increase varied from 520 to 1080 ms for each individual; the average shortest latency period of the whole population was $717.3 \text{ ms} \pm 190 \text{ ms}$. Measurements from animal experiments show similar latency periods between visual stimulation and the reactive increase of cerebral blood volume in the region of the visual cortex. The discovery of latency periods lasting less than 1 second shows that the control of cerebral vascular resistance—and the coupling between changes in neuronal activity and rCBF—must be regulated by rapidly acting mechanisms.[23]

ADDITIONAL FACTORS INFLUENCING FLOW VELOCITY RESPONSES

The influence of factors such as blood pressure, heart rate, and $paCO_2$, which could account for some of the observed velocity responses, has been analyzed in only a few investigations. In one of these, Kelley and co-

Table 18-1. Comparison of different transcranial Doppler studies with respect to side-to-side differences

Applied stimulus	Examined vessels	Significant hemispheric difference	Study
Half-field stimulation	PCA (P2)	Y	Harders et al.[21]
		Y	Wittich et al.[54]
Full-field stimulation	PCA (P2)	N	Harders et al.[21]
		Y	Wittich et al.[54]
Psychological color perception	PCA (P2)	Y	Njemanze et al.[39]
Auditory stimulation (750 Hz tone bursts, normal children)	MCA	Y	Bruneau et al.[8]
White noise	MCA	N	Klingelhöfer et al.[28]
Speech	MCA	Y	Klingelhöfer et al.[28]
Reading aloud	MCA	N	Droste et al.[15]
Word associations	MCA	Y	Markus and Boland[35]
Complex spatial task	MCA	Y	Kelley et al.[26]
		Y	Klingelhöfer et al.[27]
Memory test	MCA	Y	Droste et al.[15]
		Y	Klingelhöfer et al.[27]
		N	O'Dell et al.[40]

PCA, Posterior cerebral artery; *MCA*, middle cerebral artery.

workers studied these three factors before and after the stimulation phase, finding no significant changes.[25] Changes of these factors during the stimulation phase itself, however, have not been adequately studied.

To examine the relationship between respiration, arterial blood pressure, heart rate, and MCA FV responses during stimulation, we established a test in which six subjects performed a complex spatial task (the visual and tactile comparison of wooden figures). We monitored the subjects' end-tidal CO_2 concentration, systemic arterial blood pressure, and TCD indices. The factors studied showed only minor changes during the stimulation period, the heart rate increasing by 3% ± 2.6% and the arterial blood pressure rising by 2.2% ± 1.8% over baseline values. End-tidal CO_2 concentration decreased by 1% ± 0.9% as a result of slightly increased breathing frequency. The MFV increase during stimulation did, however, correlate slightly with changes in heart rate ($r = 0.27$) and blood pressure ($r = 0.35$), and we could not, therefore, completely exclude the possibility that the observed changes in these two factors did boost the MFV increase. Then again, the observed CO_2 reduction during stimulation probably decreased MFV slightly, and it can therefore be assumed that these three factors almost nullify each other in tests involving large groups of subjects.

These observations, along with recorded differences in right and left MCA MFV, indicate that perfusion changes reflect functional neuronal activity and are not caused by variations in cardiovascular or respiratory factors. This view is also supported by other authors, including Kelley and colleagues, who recorded task-specific perfusion patterns in the basal arteries during brain activity.[25] In response to visual stimulation, Aaslid observed significant average increases of MFV in the PCA (16.4%) and MCA (3.3%) only, the SCA registering an average increase of only 1.2%.[1] Jorgensen and associates showed that despite significant increases in blood pressure, the observed velocity increases in the contralateral MCA during hand contraction disappeared when the arm was placed under local anesthesia.[24] These findings suggest that vegetative reactions, which should influence the hemodynamics of all vessels in the same way, induce only slight MCA FV changes.

Another apparently significant factor is the sequence of MCA recording. Until recently, the simultaneous insonation of both MCAs was not possible for technical reasons, and most of the previous studies, therefore, have had to divide subjects into two groups, measuring the right MCA before the left or vice versa.[8,15,26,35] It has been reported that MFV values in the MCA measured first tend to be higher than those measured from the subsequently examined side.[15] This has been ascribed to various factors, such as habituation and the study subject's loss of motivation, factors that might play a significant role in the early stages of a study but whose influence dwindles as the test progresses.

These factors are of only slight significance during visual stimulation because of the reactive velocity increase in the PCA. They can be important, however, in the comparative analysis of differences between the two sides in subjects performing hemisphere-specific tasks. The influence of these factors may explain discrepant results found in studies with hemisphere-specific tasks (Table 18-1). To eliminate the interaction between side and order in such studies, then, recordings should be made bilaterally and simultaneously. In addition, a stimulus-triggered averaging method should be utilized in order to better distinguish FV increases resulting from neuronal activity and those from more random FV changes in the resting phase.

CONCLUSION

Functionally evoked changes of TCD parameters demonstrate that reactive perfusion patterns are specific to the type of stimuli. The high temporal resolution of TCD makes it possible to observe hemodynamic adjustments that occur in units of seconds. This makes TCD a powerful tool in the detection of rapid regulatory mechanisms related to changes in functional neuronal activity. Bilateral recording, combined with averaging techniques, helps to identify the effect of additional systemic factors that influence the FV response, especially in situations of hemisphere-specific perfusion differences. The development and standardization of tasks that produce these perfusion patterns may offer the possibility of a noninvasive means to study further the hemispheric dominance of language.

REFERENCES

1. Aaslid R: Visually evoked dynamic blood flow response of the human cerebral circulation, *Stroke* 18:771-775, 1987.
2. Aaslid R, Lindegaard K-F, Sorteberg W, et al: Cerebral autoregulation dynamics in humans, *Stroke* 20:45-52, 1989.
3. Aaslid R, Markwalder TM, Nornes H: Noninvasive transcranial Doppler ultrasound recording of flow velocity in basal cerebral arteries, *J Neurosurg* 57:769-774, 1982.
4. Aaslid R, Newell DW, Stooss R, et al: Assessment of cerebral autoregulation dynamics by simultaneous arterial and venous transcranial Doppler, *Stroke* 22:1148-1154, 1991.
5. Benton AL: *Spatial thinking in neurological patients: historical aspects.* In Potegal M, editor: *Spatial abilities: development and physiological foundations,* New York, 1982, Academic Press.
6. Bishop CCR, Powell S, Rutt D, et al: Transcranial Doppler measurement of middle cerebral artery blood flow velocity: a validation study, *Stroke* 17:913-915, 1986.
7. Brown JL: *Afterimages.* In Graham CH, editor: *Vision and visual perception,* New York, 1965, Wiley.
8. Bruneau N, Dourneau M-C, Garreau B, et al: Blood flow response to auditory stimulations in normal, mentally retarded, and autistic children: a preliminary transcranial Doppler ultrasonographic study of the middle cerebral arteries, *Biol Psychiatry* 32:691-699, 1992.
9. Carmon A, Lavy S, Gordon H, et al: *Hemispheric differences in rCBF during verbal and nonverbal tasks.* In Ingvar DH, Lassen DH, editors: *Brain work,* Copenhagen, Munksgaard, 1975.
10. Carvajal-Lizano M, Thie A: Vasoreactivity to visual stimuli in migraine, *J Neurol* 239(suppl 3):524, 1992.
11. Cohen H, Levy JJ: Cerebral and sex differences in the categorization of haptic information, *Cortex* 22:253-259, 1986.
12. Conrad B, Klingelhöfer J: Dynamics of regional cerebral blood flow for various visual stimuli, *Exp Brain Res* 77:437-441, 1989.
13. Deutsch G, Papanicolaou AC, Eisenberg HM, et al: CBF gradient changes elicited by visual stimulation and visual memory tasks, *Neuropsychologia* 24:283-287, 1986.
14. Dirnagl U, Lindauer U, Villringer A: Role of nitric oxide in the

coupling of cerebral blood flow to neuronal activation in rats, *Neurosci Lett* 149:43-46, 1993.
15. Droste DW, Harders AG, Rastogi E: A transcranial Doppler study of blood flow velocity in the middle cerebral arteries performed at rest and during mental activities, *Stroke* 20:1005-1011, 1989.
16. Frostig RD, Lieke EE, Tso DY, et al: Cortical functional architecture and local coupling between neuronal activity and the microcirculation revealed by *in vivo* high-resolution optical imaging of intrinsic signals, *Proc Natl Acad Sci U S A* 87:6082-6086, 1990.
17. Fulton JF: Observations upon the vascularity of the human occipital lobe during visual activity, *Brain* 51:310-320, 1928.
18. Gomez SM, Gomez CR, Hall IS: Transcranial Doppler ultrasonographic assessment of intermittent light stimulation at different frequencies, *Stroke* 21:1746-1748, 1990.
19. Gur RC, Gur RE, Obrist WD, et al: Sex and handedness differences in cerebral blood flow during rest and cognitive activity, *Science* 217:659-661, 1982.
20. Gur RC, Gur RE, Skolnick BE: Effects of task difficulty on regional cerebral blood flow: relationships with anxiety and performance, *Psychophysiology* 25:392-399, 1988.
21. Harders AG, Laborde G, Droste W, et al: Brain activity and blood flow velocity changes: a transcranial Doppler study, *Int J Neurosci* 47:91-102, 1989.
22. Ingvar DH, Schwartz MS: Blood flow patterns induced in the dominant hemisphere by speech and reading, *Brain* 97:273-288, 1974.
23. Jadecola C: Regulation of the cerebral microcirculation during neuronal activity: is nitric oxide the missing link? *Trends Neurosci* 16:206-214, 1993.
24. Jorgensen LG, Perko G, Payne G, et al: Effect of limb anesthesia on middle cerebral artery response to handgrip, *Am J Physiol* 264, H553-H559, 1993.
25. Kelley RE, Chang JY, Scheinman NJ, et al: Transcranial Doppler assessment of cerebral flow velocity during cognitive tasks, *Stroke* 23:9-14, 1992.
26. Kelley RE, Chang JY, Suzuki S, et al: Selective increase in the right hemisphere transcranial Doppler velocity during a spatial task, *Cortex* 29:45-52, 1993.
27. Klingelhöfer J, Matzander G, Sander D, et al: Bilateral changes of middle cerebral artery blood flow velocities in various hemisphere-specific brain activities, *J Neurol* 241:264-265, 1994.
28. Klingelhöfer J, Wittich I, Sander D, et al: Latencies of visually evoked perfusion changes in the posterior cerebral artery territory, *J Neurol* 239:23, 1992.
29. Larsen B, Skinhoj E, Endo H: *Localisation of basic speech functions as revealed by rCBF measurements in normal subjects and patients with aphasia.* In Meyer JS, Lechner H, Reivich M, et al, editors: *Cerebral vascular disease,* Amsterdam, 1977, Exerpta Medica.
30. Lassen NA, Ingvar DH, Skinhoj E: Brain function and blood flow, *Sci Am* 239:50-59, 1978.
31. Le Scao Y, Baulieu JL, Robier A, et al: Increment of brain temporal perfusion during auditory stimulation, *Eur J Nucl Med* 18:981-983, 1991.
32. Livingstone MS, Hubel DH: Psychological evidence for separate channels for the perception of form, colour, movement, and depth, *J Neurosci* 7:3416-3468, 1987.
33. Lou HC, Edvinsson L, MacKenzie ET: The concept of coupling blood flow to brain function: revision required? *Ann Neurol* 22:289-297, 1987.
34. von Maravic M, Kessler CH, Böhning A, et al: Visual stimuli and posterior cerebral artery blood flow, *J Neurol* 239:24, 1992.
35. Markus HS, Boland M: "Cognitive activity" monitored by non-invasive measurement of cerebral blood flow velocity and its application to the investigation of cerebral dominance, *Cortex* 28:575-581, 1992.
36. Meyer JS, Hayman LA, Amano T, et al: Mapping of local blood

flow of human brain by CT scanning during stable xenon inhalation, *Stroke* 12:426-436, 1981.

37. Ngai AC, Ko KR, Morii S, et al: Effect of sciatic nerve stimulation on pial arterioles in rats, *Am J Physiol* 254:H133-H139, 1988.

38. Nishizawa Y, Olsen TS, Larsen B, et al: Left-right cortical asymmetries of regional cerebral blood flow during listening to words, *J Neurophysiol* 48:458-466, 1982.

39. Njemanze PC, Gomez CR, Horenstein S: Cerebral lateralization and color perception: a transcranial Doppler study, *Cortex* 28:69-75, 1992.

40. O'Dell DM, Roberts AE, McKinney WM: Transcranial Doppler monitoring of middle cerebral artery blood flow velocities during three memory tasks, *J Neuroimaging* 2:186-189, 1992.

41. Petersen SE, Fox PT, Posner MI, et al: Positron emission tomographic studies of the cortical anatomy of single-word processing, *Nature* 331:585-589, 1988.

42. Phelps ME, Mazziota JC, Huang SC: Study of cerebral function with positron computed tomography, *J Cereb Blood Flow Metab* 2:113-162, 1982.

43. Reiman EM, Fusselman MJ, Fox PT, et al: Neuroanatomical correlates of anticipatory anxiety, *Science* 243:1071-1073, 1989.

44. Risberg J, Halsey JH, Wills EL, et al: Hemispheric specialization in normal man studied by bilateral measurements of the regional cerebral blood flow: a study with the 133-Xe inhalation technique, *Brain* 98:511-524, 1975.

45. Risberg J, Ingvar DH: Patterns of activation in the grey matter of the dominant hemisphere during memorizing and reasoning, *Brain* 96:737-756, 1973.

46. Rodriguez G, Cogomo P, Gris A, et al: Regional cerebral blood flow and anxiety: a correlation study in neurologically normal patients, *J Cereb Blood Flow Metab* 9:410-416, 1989.

47. Roland PE, Friberg L: Localization of cortical areas activated by thinking, *J Neurophysiol* 53:1219-1243, 1985.

48. Roland PE, Gulyás B, Seitz RJ, et al: Functional anatomy of storage, recall, and recognition of a visual pattern in man, *Neuroreport* 1:53-56, 1990.

49. Roland PE, Skinhoj E, Lassen NA: Focal activations of human cerebral cortex during auditory discrimination, *J Neurophysiol* 45:1139-1151, 1981.

50. Sitzer M, Diehl RR, Hennerici M: Visually evoked cerebral blood flow responses: normal and pathological conditions, *J Neuroimaging* 2:65-70, 1992.

51. Skolnick BE, Gur RC, Stern MB, et al: Reliability of regional cerebral blood flow activation to cognitive tasks in elderly normal subjects, *J Cereb Blood Flow Metab* 13:448-453, 1993.

52. Sorteberg W, Lindegaard K-F, Rootwelt K, et al: Blood velocity and regional blood flow in defined cerebral artery systems, *Acta Neurochir (Wien)* 97:47-52, 1989.

53. Squire LR, Ojeman JG, Miezin FM, et al: Activation of the hippocampus in normal humans: a functional anatomical study of memory, *Proc Natl Acad Sci U S A* 89:1837-1841, 1992.

54. Wittich I, Klingelhöfer J, Matzander G, et al: Influence of visual stimuli on the dynamics of reactive perfusion changes in the posterior cerebral artery territory, *J Neurol* 239:9, 1992.

Transcranial Color Doppler Imaging

Ulrich Bogdahn
Georg Becker

Significant improvements have recently been made in transcranial color-coded real-time sonography (TCCS), also known as transcranial duplex sonography. In addition to its ability to reveal vascular and parenchymal anatomy, this modified technique also detects a wide variety of cerebrovascular pathologies such as cerebral infarcts and hematomas, arteriosclerotic vascular changes, arteriovenous malformations (AVMs), and aneurysms. It also permits the imaging of parenchymal abnormalities in patients with central nervous system tumors or degenerative disorders such as monopolar depression; it can identify and monitor disturbances of cerebrospinal fluid circulation. The use of transpulmonary stable ultrasound contrast agents improves both signal quality and image intensity, permitting a considerably broader spectrum of applications. While complementing magnetic resonance imaging (MRI) and computerized tomography (CT) findings and providing new diagnostic information on parenchymal lesions, TCCS permits the identification of large intracranial vessels within the B-mode image considerably faster than conventional pulsed transcranial sonography (TCD). This results in briefer examinations while simultaneously improving standardization and reproducibility. This technique also provides real-time localization of vascular and parenchymal pathology by color imaging superimposed on the black-and-white B-mode image.

ULTRASOUND ANATOMY OF THE ADULT BRAIN

Besides detecting blood flow in the basal cerebral arteries and their branches, TCCS provides two-dimensional views of brain parenchyma, the echogenicity and echotexture of which are similar in adults to those reported in pediatric and intraoperative neurosonology studies.* The brain parenchyma, including almost all supratentorial and infratentorial brain nuclei and fiber tracts, is homogeneously hypoechogenic with areas of interspersed hyperechogenic pixels. Hyperechogenic areas that can be identified within this hypoechogenic matrix include the red nucleus, the fiber tracts and nuclei of the brainstem raphe, and the aqueduct within the butterfly-shaped mesencephalic brainstem. At the diencephalic level, the hyperechogenic posterior limb of the internal capsule separates the hypoechogenic thalamus from the hypoechogenic lenticular nuclei. Dorsal portions of the thalamus are interspersed with hyperechogenic pixels, probably caused by thalamoperforating arteries. At the level of the anterior horns of the lateral ventricles, the head of the caudate nucleus exhibits

*References 6, 16, 20, 22, 47, 49, 51, 55.

increased echogenicity, especially in elderly subjects. The sylvian fissure may be seen as a hyperechogenic, pulsating line separating the temporal lobe from the parietal lobe and diencephalon. The hyperechogenic falx cerebri is visible between the two hemispheres, and sulci are identifiable as hyperechogenic ribbons on the surface of the brain and cerebellum.

The supratentorial ventricular system, comprised of both lateral ventricles in addition to the third ventricle, serves as a central structure for orientation. The ventricles are anechoic and are surrounded by a thin, hyperechogenic margin that represents the impedance step between cerebrospinal fluid and parenchyma. The choroid plexus may be discerned as pulsating, hyperechogenic structures within the cerebral ventricles. The hyperechogenic septum pellucidum can be identified between the frontal horns. Although age-adjusted normative values are not yet available, in patients with ventricular enlargement, TCCS findings concerning the diameters of the third ventricle and frontal horns closely correspond to those of CT.[9] According to CT data and our own preliminary experiences, 0.7 cm is the upper limit of normal for the width of the third ventricle and 1.9 cm for the lateral ventricles[35,45] measured at the level of the frontal horns.

The basal cerebral, superior cerebellar, retrothalamic, and quadrigeminal cisternae exhibit distinctly increased echogenicity. It is difficult to separate the quadrigeminal cisterna from the homogeneously hyperechogenic pineal gland, located dorsal to the third ventricle. The hyperechogenic opercular cisterna separates the frontal lobe from the temporal lobe, and the major branches of the basal cerebral arteries can be distinguished as pulsating tubes within the basal cerebral cisternae.

Arterial system

The principal advantage of transcranial duplex imaging rests in its ability to permit angle-corrected determination of Doppler flow velocities. Studies made by Schöning and co-workers[5,46,53] reveal that in children under 10 years of age the maximum flow velocities ($\pm$ SD) were 79.9 $\pm$ 17.7 cm/s in the anterior cerebral artery (ACA), 92.2 $\pm$ 13 cm/s in the middle cerebral artery (MCA), and 63.9 $\pm$ 13.6 cm/s in the posterior cerebral artery (PCA). Children over age 10 and adolescents up to 18 years of age had respective maximum flow velocities of 69.4 $\pm$ 13.8 and 39.9 $\pm$ 10.5 cm/s in the ACA, 83.2 $\pm$ 11.9 and 50.8 $\pm$ 9 cm/s in the MCA, and 55.6 $\pm$ 10.1 and 33.1 $\pm$ 6.3 cm/s in the PCA. The time-averaged maximum velocity decreased significantly with age, whereas resistance and pulsatility indices remained stable throughout childhood and adulthood. Schöning and his colleagues also compared TCCS with conventional TCD and reported a good

correlation of comparable parameters, improved recording quality and interexaminer reproducibility, and a higher detection rate for anatomically difficult locations.[54] Moreover, angle-corrected Doppler flow velocities were found to be approximately 10% to 15% higher than those recorded with TCD. Several groups have reported improved detection of the vertebrobasilar system lesions by TCCS and have stressed the additional advantage of angle correction.[8,40,57] Angle-corrected peak systolic and end-diastolic flow velocities were 50/24 cm/s in the vertebral artery, 59/28 cm/s in the basilar artery, and 56/30 cm/s in the posterior inferior cerebellar artery. Although previous TCD studies had suggested that the basilar artery could be identified at a depth of 80 to 90 mm, TCCS studies reveal that it may be detected at a depth of 70 to 75 mm.[8,40,57]

Signal intensity is a crucial parameter in transcranial Doppler imaging. An improvement in the signal-to-noise ratio therefore might improve the potential of transcranial ultrasound examinations. Schwarz and co-workers demonstrated a 20 to 25 dB increase in intensity after the intravenous administration of a new transpulmonary stable ultrasound contrast agent, SHU508A, which is composed of galactose microbubbles.[58] This contrast agent has been recently tested in the context of phase 2 and 3 clinical trials in various fields of ultrasound imaging.[53] Its only contraindication is galactose hypersensitivity. Results for TCCS applications are very encouraging because peripheral branches of the basal arteries, the cerebellar arteries, and the basal venous system can be visualized.[19] In patients for whom conventional TCD examination is unyielding because of poor acoustic bone windows, at least the proximal branches of the large intracranial arteries may be evaluated. A number of arterial abnormalities (discussed later in this chapter) and lesions at the distal portion of the basilar artery (see Plates 63 to 66) may be examined under highly improved conditions.

Venous system

Although Aaslid and co-workers used a conventional TCD when describing blood flow in the straight sinus in 1991,[2] TCD testing has, until recently, generally been restricted to the examination of large basal arteries. The delineation of the basal cerebral venous system by TCCS[19] and improved imaging following the injection of SHU508A have disclosed new information. In all seven patients we studied recently, the inferior sagittal and straight sinuses, the internal cerebral vein, and the vein of Galen could be identified and further assessed by Doppler sampling. The confluens sinuum and the transverse and sigmoid sinuses were not consistently identified.[34] Doppler recordings from the straight sinus revealed an angle-corrected average peak systolic flow velocity of 19.8 cm/s and end-diastolic velocity of 18.5

cm/s.[7] The Doppler frequency spectra showed slight pulsatility. In a second study, a population of 10 individuals was evaluated after the administration of SHU508A: Angle-corrected peak systolic and end-diastolic velocities for the straight sinus were 20.2 cm/s and 17.9 cm/s respectively; flow in the confluens sinuum (systolic 12 cm/s, diastolic 10.3 cm/s, N = 3) (see Plates 67 and 68) and the inferior sagittal sinus (systolic 20.2 cm/s, diastolic 15 cm/s, N = 1) was quantified in only a few cases. Clearly, a larger study is necessary to establish definitive data.

Experience regarding transcranial ultrasound examination of patients with cerebral venous thrombosis remains limited. In two patients with superior sagittal sinus thrombosis, flow velocities in the straight sinus (88 and 92 cm/s) and the great vein of Galen (84 and 92 cm/s) were elevated to approximately 4 times the norm, indicating increased collateral venous flow. TCCS may therefore, in the future, allow monitoring of cerebral venous thrombosis.[7]

CAVERNOUS HEMANGIOMAS

Cavernomas are often detected either fortuitously by MRI or during emergency surgery for intracerebral hemorrhage. As a result, no ultrasound data exist concerning their preoperative diagnosis. In order to explore the potential of contrast-enhanced TCCS in delineating these vascular malformations, we studied 10 patients with cavernomas diagnosed on the basis of a clinical history of intracranial hemorrhage and of typical MRI and intraoperative findings. Nine lesions were identified as hyperechogenic areas, the dimensions and locations of which corresponded to the MRI findings. Cavernomas could not be detected on unenhanced TCCS testing, but flow within the lesions was detected after the administration of 8 ml of SHU508A at a concentration of 400 mg/ml (see Plates 69 to 72). Doppler sampling of the cavernomas revealed mean peak systolic flow velocities of approximately 10 to 15 cm/s and diastolic flow of a venous pattern, a hemodynamic pattern that was confirmed intraoperatively. Due to the multidirectional flow in these lesions, angle correction was not performed.[16]

We suspect that when contrast agents become available for routine clinical use, contrast-enhanced TCCS may be especially helpful intraoperatively as well as during postoperative follow-up and may become a valuable tool for detecting the source of atypical parenchymal hemorrhage in the emergency room.

ANEURYSMS AND ARTERIOVENOUS MALFORMATIONS

The role of TCCS in the screening and follow-up of patients with AVMs is not clear. Several reports illustrate the potential of unenhanced TCCS in delin-eating the entire vascular tree of AVMs, thereby improving anatomic orientation.[5,13,15] Although the sensitivity of the method is as yet unknown, it seems that as long as a patient has an ultrasonic temporal bone window, an AVM can probably be detected. In B-mode images, the lesions appear as hyperechogenic structures interspersed with zones of low density. Color Doppler displays flow within AVMs, while feeding and draining vessels, along with collateral supply, can be identified anatomically. Doppler sampling frequently displays turbulent and multidirectional flow, with velocities in the main feeders reaching or exceeding levels as high as 180 cm/s. Depending on the location of the Doppler sample, however, its spectrum is more or less modulated by the pulse amplitude.

The administration of ultrasound contrast agents may aid in the delineation of the entire AVM and the identification of malformations not detected by unenhanced TCCS (see Plates 73 to 76). Similarly, contrast enhancement may permit diagnosis of aneurysms already detected by unenhanced TCCS with improved resolution and identification of smaller, undetected, aneurysms (see Plates 77 to 79). It is conceivable that contrast administration will assist in the differential diagnosis of intracranial hemorrhages, detecting the source of hemorrhage for emergency clot evacuation.[17] Moreover, TCCS may have a role in the postoperative and postinterventional follow-up of AVM patients, allowing an unlimited number of repeat examinations.

SONOGRAPHIC FINDINGS IN INTRACRANIAL HEMORRHAGES

Intracerebral hemorrhage accounts for approximately 10% of all strokes.[46] Although hypertensive microvascular angiopathy is usually considered the most common cause of hemorrhage in the basal ganglia, thalamus, and pons, nonhypertensive causes such as AVMs, intracranial tumors, amyloid angiopathy, and venous thrombosis are frequently identified in patients with lobar hemorrhage.

An acute intracerebral hematoma appears on ultrasound images as a homogeneously hyperechogenic lesion, sharply delineated from the adjacent parenchyma (see Plates 80 to 82).[12,21,28,34,59] The high contrast between hemorrhage and parenchyma during this stage allows an unequivocal diagnosis by means of TCCS in all patients. The clot is often surrounded by a thin, hyperechogenic "halo," indicating compression of the adjacent tissue.[12] Over time, the initially homogeneous lesion becomes interspersed with hypoechogenic areas so that in the subacute state, the clot appears as a lesion with a hypoechogenic center surrounded by a hyperechogenic margin.[12,28,59] It has been suggested that decreased echogenicity may be due to the lysis of red blood cells in the center of the hematoma.[28] Echogenicity decreases over a period of 1 to 4 weeks, and the margin becomes blurred; complete resolution of the hematoma seems to occur after a minimum of 2 to 5 weeks.

Intraventricular hematomas appear as hyperechogenic masses within the ventricles. Although TCCS may fail to detect small amounts of blood within the occipital horn,[10,59] in patients with extensive hemorrhage a hyperechogenic castlike pattern may be observed. Intraventricular blood usually resolves within 5 weeks. Complications such as cerebrospinal fluid circulation disturbances, compression of adjacent structures, or midline shift, which arise after intraventricular or intracerebral hemorrhages, are detectable by TCCS.

In patients with acute hemiparesis of unknown etiology, TCCS helps to differentiate cerebral infarction from intracerebral hemorrhage.[12] In contrast to intracerebral hematomas, infarcted brain tissue displays no change in echogenicity and echotexture. The diagnosis of ischemic stroke is primarily based, therefore, on the demonstration of vascular pathology, such as occlusion of cerebral arteries, with color-coded B-mode imaging and Doppler analysis and on the finding of reduced brain pulsation in ischemic parenchyma. In the chronic stage of cerebral infarction, however, increased echogenicity can be observed in the affected brain territory.

Because the basal cisternae normally have an echogenicity similar to that of blood, making the differentiation between cerebrospinal fluid and blood difficult, TCCS is not well suited to the detection of subarachnoid hemorrhage.[9] Extensive subarachnoid hematomas are associated with widening of the basal cisternae and sylvian fissure and can lead to acute hydrocephalus.

SONOGRAPHIC FINDINGS IN BRAIN TUMORS

Transcranial sonography has been utilized to detect brain tumors since the early 1960s and, in the pre-CT era, was credited with surprisingly high accuracy of tumor identification.[9,30,31] Although CT and MRI have replaced sonography in the diagnosis of brain tumors in adults, ultrasound has become—because of its fine resolution, portability, ease of use, and relative cost-effectiveness—an established diagnostic method in pediatric and intraoperative neuroimaging.* The detailed information regarding the ultrasound pattern of brain tumors that was obtained from these fields has been combined with modern transcranial Duplex techniques and applied to the study of adult brain tumors.[13]

Although adult brain tumors vary histologically, they tend to exhibit the same increased echogenicity. The hyperechogenic matrix is often interspersed with more or less extensive hypoechogenic areas, the size and distribution of which can affect the tumor's sonographic image. The latter can range from the homogeneously hyperechogenic to the hypodense surrounded by a thin, hyperechogenic margin. Comparison of ultrasound findings with those of histopathology shows that the echogenicity of brain tumors may be related to tumoral cell density or to the composition of their extracellular constituents.[29] Specifically, hyperechogenic areas correspond to solid tumor tissue, and hypodense areas within the hyperdense matrix represent necrotic or cystic tumor regions (see Plates 83 to 89).[11,29,33,41,44] Cysts are anechoic and distinctly circumscribed, whereas meningiomas, lymphomas, ependymomas, and solid astrocytomas appear as predominantly hyperechogenic lesions. Glioblastomas, high-grade gliomas, and metastatic lesions frequently exhibit nonhomogeneous echotexture, and cystic astrocytomas are almost always hypoechogenic with a hyperechogenic portion near the borderzone. Regardless of their histologic grade and biologic behavior, approximately 5% of cerebral brain tumors are isoechogenic when compared with normal brain tissue and are therefore not detectable by TCCS, even when the bone window is adequate.[13] Nevertheless, a study comparing TCCS, CT, and histologic findings suggests that TCCS has superior sensitivity and higher resolution than CT in differentiating tumor components such as necrotic, cystic, and solid areas and in identifying peritumoral tissue.[11]

Brain tumors are occasionally surrounded by a thin, hypoechogenic peritumoral halo, suspected of being secondary to compression of adjacent tissue and consequent changes in tissue impedance.[13] Although there is some difference of opinion regarding the echogenicity of edema in areas surrounding brain tumors—some investigators reporting an increase,[44,49] others a decrease[22,33]—most agree that edema is isoechogenic relative to normal brain parenchyma and is therefore undetectable by TCCS.[13,29,42] Our preliminary findings suggest that increased echogenicity always implies a solid tumor or gliosis.[11,29,41,42]

Brain tumor extension can be precisely delineated by TCCS, and the findings are similar to results obtained from intraoperative ultrasound studies.[29,33,41] Comparative studies of CT and TCCS reveal the latter's advantages in estimating tumor size, particularly with regard to tumors of low attenuation on CT.[11,41] The isoechogenicity of brain edema and TCCS's excellence in determining tissue components may serve to explain the method's accuracy in the delineation of solid tumor extent, although it should also be emphasized that TCCS, like all neuroimaging methods, fails to depict the far peripheral tumor zone, where it diffusely infiltrates normal tissue.

Postoperative insonation, through either the intact skull or through the craniotomy defect, allows unequivo-

*References 24, 29, 33, 36, 41, 42, 43, 63.

cal identification of residual tumor tissue or tumor regrowth.[25,39,52,62,64] The resection defect is displayed as an echogenic area, and its cavity is separated from adjacent brain parenchyma by a thin, echogenic margin. The tumor-free resection line appears as a slightly hyperechogenic margin less than 0.5 cm in thickness, and residual tumor tissue is detected as a hyperechogenic area adjacent to the resection cavity. Postoperative TCCS examinations are delayed for 1 to 2 weeks after surgery because artifacts may interfere with the ability to detect residual tumor tissue. Air trapped in the resection cavity, for example, causes a distinct increase in echogenicity that prevents tumor identification within the resection site. Additionally, bleeding along the resection line or in the area adjacent to it may also confuse the interpretation of early postoperative TCCS studies. The increased echogenicity of blood, unlike that of remaining tumor tissue, gradually decreases within the first 2 postoperative weeks.[12,59]

Ultrasound is highly effective not only in the identification of residual tumor tissue but also in the detection of tumor recurrence.* Comparing CT, MRI, and TCCS postoperative data in a series of 69 children, Dittrich and co-workers demonstrated that ultrasound and MRI are almost equally sensitive, both surpassing CT in these two areas.[25] Moreover, De Slegte and co-workers presented data from postoperative sonographic follow-up examinations suggesting that ultrasound provides valuable information about tumor response to chemotherapy and radiation. Their observation of residual tumor exhibiting increased tumor matrix irregularity indicated tumor necrosis following adjuvant therapy.[62] Our preliminary experiences comparing CT, TCCS, and histologic findings suggest that TCCS is more sensitive than postoperative CT in the identification of residual tumor tissue and is generally quicker in detecting tumor recurrence (see Plates 83 to 89).

TUMOR VASCULARIZATION

The potential of TCCS in the detection of primary intracranial tumor vascularization was recently studied in a series of 28 patients whose primary central nervous system tumors were examined before and after administration of SHU508A.[18] Conventional CT and MRI examinations were obtained prior to TCCS testing. All lesions appeared hyperechogenic in B-mode, a finding that correlated well with the CT and MRI data. Color flow signals associated with these hyperechogenic lesions were detected only rarely prior to SHU508A administration. However, after contrast administration, most low-grade and all high-grade tumors had color flow signals. Although high-grade malignant tumors always displayed atypical arterial and venous Doppler spectra

*References 11, 25, 33, 39, 42, 52, 62, 64.

with an irregular distribution of Doppler shift and signal intensities (see Plates 90 to 92), only some of the low-grade tumors produced these atypical patterns, and then only inconsistently. Contrast-enhanced TCCS was found to be superior to intraarterial digital subtraction angiography in displaying tumor-related pathologic flow, thereby indicating TCCS's high sensitivity to tumor vascularization. Increased vascular proliferation as seen in histologic examination always correlated with atypical flow phenomena in high-grade lesions. These results suggest that TCCS data on tumor vascularization may provide new prognostic information on the biology of individual tumors. It is conceivable that in the future TCCS may be used prior to surgery in the detection and characterization of brain tumors, during treatment in the monitoring of tumor progression or recurrence, and following radiation in distinguishing radionecrosis from recurrence.

SONOGRAPHIC FINDINGS IN HYDROCEPHALUS

Distinguishing between high- and low-pressure hydrocephalus is a frequent clinical problem in neurology. Brain CT and MRI permit a morphologic diagnosis of ventriculomegaly but, except for the finding of transependymal cerebrospinal fluid reabsorption, cannot assist in estimating intraventricular pressure. Neurosonography, however, has proved valuable in the diagnosis of hydrocephalus in infants.[26,60] A study correlating TCCS and CT findings in patients with low- and high-pressure hydrocephalus revealed that TCCS permits quantification of the ventricular enlargement and an approximate estimation of the intracranial pressure (ICP).[9] The TCCS data on the width of the third ventricle closely correlate with CT findings, although a slightly poorer correlation has been noted regarding the width of the lateral ventricles' frontal horns. This discrepancy is due to differences in the scanning planes employed by the two methods, in that sonographic depiction of lateral ventricles from the temporal bone window requires a tilting of the TCCS scanning plane, which results in slightly different readings from those produced by CT's strictly axial planes.

Because the ability of brain structures to undulate is affected by increased ICP, dynamic neurosonographic examinations may be used to estimate ICP levels by examining such undulation. The septum pellucidum's undulatory ability may be recorded by TCCS by continuously rotating the head at an angle of 20° from the vertical body axis while holding the transducer at the temporal acoustic bone window. Because of the different degrees of inertia exhibited by the cerebrospinal fluid and brain parenchyma, the angular acceleration results in a movement of the ventricular compartment relative to the parenchyma. This relative movement is transferred to the septum pellucidum when it is loosely attached to its fixation points, as in low-pressure hydrocephalus. By contrast, high-pressure hydrocephalus stretches the septum pellucidum and increases its tension (see Plates 93 and 94), the raised ICP resulting in reduction or loss of undulation. Experience with these dynamic neurosonographic studies shows that ICP values lower than 18 cm H_2O are always accompanied by septum pellucidum undulation, whereas ICP values above 21 cm H_2O always occur with septum pellucidum stiffness.[9] Because the test is probably limited by several factors, it may provide only a gross estimation of ICP.

Raised ICP also has effects on cerebral blood flow that can be recorded by TCD.[1,37] When ICP exceeds the diastolic blood pressure, there is both a relative reduction in end-diastolic flow velocity and increases of the pulsatility index and the ratio between peak systolic and end-diastolic velocities. Doppler waveforms, however, can also be affected by several other factors, such as CO_2 pressure or red blood cell count. Thus TCCS allows only a gross bimodal estimation of the ICP, loss of septum pellucidum undulation identifying ICP values above 20 cm H_2O and an increase in the pulsatility index indicating ICP values near or above the diastolic blood pressure.

PERSPECTIVES ON TRANSCRANIAL COLOR-CODED REAL-TIME SONOGRAPHY AS A PARENCHYMAL NEUROIMAGING MODALITY

Unlike CT and MRI, ultrasound imaging is based on the interactions of ultrasound waves with tissue. Therefore, TCCS could provide unique insights into normal and abnormal physiology and may yet unveil new pathogenetic considerations. Its uniqueness is illustrated by findings in patients with unipolar depression who were found to have reduced echogenicity of the brainstem raphe.[14] Because differences in the raphe's echogenicity were not detected in either healthy adults or in patients with a bipolar disorder, it is assumed that the reduction accompanying unipolar depression may reflect a degree of structural disruption of the raphe, normally a sonographically homogeneous area. The raphe contains cell groups of serotoninergic nuclei interwoven with crossing tegmental and median forebrain bundle fibers and is therefore rich in noradrenergic, cholinergic, and serotoninergic pathways. Interestingly, there is considerable evidence suggesting that the raphe may be involved in the pathogenesis of affective disorders,* an observation first clearly demonstrated clinically by TCCS.

REFERENCES

1. Aaslid R, Lundar T, Lindegaard KF: *Estimation of cerebral perfusion pressure from arterial blood pressure and transcranial*

Doppler recordings. In Miller JD, Teasdale GM, Rowan JO, editors: *Intracranial pressure 6,* Berlin, 1986, Springer Verlag.
2. Aaslid R, Newell DW, Stoss R, et al: Assessment of cerebral autoregulation dynamics from simultaneous arerial and venous transcranial Doppler recordings in humans, *Stroke* 22:1148-1154, 1991.
3. Ball WA, Whybrow PC: Biology of depression and mania, *Curr Opin Psychiatry* 6:27-34, 1993.
4. Bartels E, Flügel KA: Quantitative measurement of blood flow velocity in basal cerebral arteries with transcranial duplex flow imaging, *J Neuroimaging* 4:77-81, 1994.
5. Bartels E, Rodiek SO, Flügel KA: Evaluation of arterio-venous malformations with transcranial color-Doppler imaging, Innsbruck, 1993, Euroson.
6. Becker G, Bogdahn U: *Transcranial color-coded real-time sonography in adults.* In Babikian V, Wechsler L, editors: *Transcranial doppler ultrasonography,* St Louis, 1993, Mosby–Year Book.
7. Becker G, Bogdahn U, Gehlberg C, et al: Examination of intracerebral venous system by transcranial color-coded real-time sonography: normal values of venous blood flow velocities and sonographic findings in cortical vein thrombosis, *J Neuroimaging* 5:87-94, 1995.
8. Becker G, Bogdahn U, Lindner A: Imaging of the vertebro-basilar system by transcranial color-coded real-time sonography, *J Ultrasound Med* 12:395-401, 1993.
9. Becker G, Bogdahn U, Straßburg H-M, et al: Identification of ventricular enlargement and estimation of ventricular pressure by transcranial color-coded real-time sonography, *J Neuroimaging* 4:17-22,
10. Becker G, Greiner K, Kaune B, et al: Diagnosis and monitoring of subarachnoid hemorrhage by transcranial color-coded real-time sonography, *Neurosurgery* 28:814-820, 1991.
11. Becker G, Krone A, Koulis D, et al: Reliability of transcranial color-coded real-time sonography in the assessment of brain tumors: correlation between ultrasound, computerized tomography and biopsy findings, *Neuroradiology* 36:585-590, 1994.
12. Becker G, Lindner A, Winkler J, et al: Differentiation between ischemic and hemorrhagic stroke by transcranial color-coded real-time sonography, *J Neuroimaging* 3:41-47, 1993.
13. Becker G, Perez J, Krone A, et al: Transcranial color-coded real-time sonography in the evaluation of intracranial neoplasms and arteriovenous malformations, *Neurosurgery* 31:420-428, 1992.
14. Becker G, Struck M, Bogdahn U, Becker T: Echogenicity of the brainstem raphe in patients with major depression, *Psychiat Res Neuroimaging* 55:75-84, 1994.
15. Becker G, Winkler J, Hoffmann E, Bogdahn U: Imaging of cerebral arteriovenous malformations by transcranial colour-coded real-time sonography, *Neuroradiology* 32:280-288, 1990.
16. Berland LL, Bryan CR, Sekar BC, Moss CN: Sonographic examination of the adult brain, *J Clin Ultrasound* 16:337-345, 1988.
17. Bogdahn U, Becker G, Fröhlich T: Contrast enhanced transcranial color coded real time sonography of cerebrovascular disease, *Echocardiography* 10:678, 1993.
18. Bogdahn U, Becker G, Frölich T, et al: Contrast-enhanced transcranial color-coded real-time sonography allows detection of primary central nervous system tumor vascularisation, *Radiology* 192:141-148, 1994.
19. Bogdahn U, Becker G, Schlief R, et al: Contrast-enhanced transcranial color-coded real-time sonography, *Stroke* 24:676-684, 1993.
20. Bogdahn U, Becker G, Winkler J, et al: Transcranial color-coded real-time sonography of adults, *Stroke* 21:1680-1688, 1990.
21. Bowermann RA, Donn SM, Silver TM, Jaffe MH: Nature history of neonatal periventricular/intraventricular hemorrhage and its complications: sonographic observations, *AJNR Am J Neuroradiol* 5:527-538, 1984.

*References 3, 22, 36, 45, 47, 58.

22. Chandler WF, Knake JE, McGillicuddy JE, et al: Intraoperative use of ultrasound in neurosurgery, *J Neurosurg* 57:157-163, 1982.

23. Chan-Palay V, Asan E: Quantification of catecholamine neurons in the locus coeruleus in human brains of normal young and older adults and in depression, *J Comp Neurol* 287:357-372, 1989.

24. Chuang S, Harwood-Nash D: Tumors and cysts, *Neuroradiology* 28:463-475, 1986.

25. Dittrich M, Gutjahr P, Dinkel E, et al: Postoperative sonographische Verlaufsuntersuchungen im Kindesalter, *Klin Padiatr* 199:403-410, 1987.

26. Dittrich M, Straßburg H-M, Dinkel E, Hackelöhr B-J: *Zerebrale Ultraschalldiagnostik in Pädiatrie und Geburtshilfe,* Berlin, 1985, Springer Verlag.

27. Dussik KT: Über die Möglichkeit hochfrequente mechanische Schwingungen als diagnostisches Hilfsmittel zu verwenden, *Zschr Ges Neurol Psychiatr* 174:465-482, 1942.

28. Enzmann DR, Britt RH, Loyons BE, et al: Natural history of experimental intracerebral hemorrhage: sonography, computed tomography and neuropathology, *AJNR Am J Neuroradiol* 2:517-526, 1981.

29. Enzmann DR, Wheat R, Marshall WH, et al: Tumors of the central nervous system studied by computed tomography and ultrasound, *Radiology* 154:393-399, 1985.

30. French LA, Wild JJ, Neal D: The experimental application of ultrasonic to the localisation of brain tumors, *J Neurosurg* 8:198-203, 1951.

31. Freund HJ, Somer JC, Kendel KH, et al: Electronic sector scanning in the diagnosis of cerebrovascular diseases and space-occupying processes, *Neurology* 23:1147-1159, 1973.

32. Furuhata H: Noninvasive measurement of the intracranial circulation by transcranial Doppler sonography, Tokyo *Jikeikei Medical Journal* 104:971-992, 1989.

33. Gooding GA, Boggan JE, Weinstein PR: Characterisation of intracranial neoplasms by CT and intraoperative sonography, *AJNR Am J Neuroradiol* 5:517-520, 1984.

34. Grant EG: Sonography of the premature brain: intraventricular hemorrhage and periventricular leukomalacia, *Neuroradiology* 28:476-490, 1986.

35. Gyldensted C, Kosteljanetz M: Measurements of the normal ventricular system with computer tomography of the brain: a preliminary study on 44 adults, *Neuroradiology* 10:205-213, 1976.

36. Han BK, Babock DS, Oestreich AE: Sonography of brain tumors in infants, *AJN* 143:31-36, 1984.

37. Hassler W, Steinmetz H, Gawlowski J: Transcranial Doppler ultrasonography in raised intracranial pressure and intracranial circulatory arrest, *J Neurosurg* 68:745-751, 1988.

38. Hillegaart V: Functional topography of brain seritonergic pathways in rat, *Acta Physiol Scand Suppl* 598:1-54, 1991.

39. Hoffman RB, Laudau B: Ultrasound B-scan imaging of intracranial lesion through a bone flap defect, *J Clin Ultrasound* 4:125-127, 1975.

40. Kaps M, Seidel G, Bauer T, Behrmann B: Imaging of the intracranial vertebrobasilar system using color-coded ultrasound, *Stroke* 23:1577-1582, 1993.

41. Knake JE, Chandler WF, Gabrielsen TO, et al: Intraoperative sonographic delineation of low-grade brain neoplasms defined poorly by computed tomography, *Radiology* 151:735-739, 1984.

42. LeRoux PD, Berger MS, Ojemann GA, et al: Correlation of intraoperative ultrasound tumor volumes and margins with pre-operative cmputerized tomography scans, *J Neurosurg* 71:691-698, 1989.

43. Martin PJ, Evans DJ, Naylor AR: Transcranial color coded sonography of the basal circulation, *Stroke* 25:390-396, 1994.

44. McGahan JP, Ellis WG, Budenz RW, et al: Brain gliomas: Sonographic characterisation, *Radiology* 159:485-492, 1986.

45. Meese W, Kluge W, Grumme T, Hopfenmüller W: CT evaluation of the CSF spaces of healthy persons, *Neuroradiology* 19:131-136, 1980.

46. Mohr JP, Caplan LR, Melski JW, et al: The Harvard cooperative stroke register: a prospective register, *Neurology* 28:754-762, 1978.

47. Naidrich TP, Yousefzadeh DK, Gusnard DA: Sonography of the neonatal head, *Neuroradiology* 28:408-427, 1986.

48. Paulus W, Jellinger K: The neuropathologic basis of different clinical subgroups of Parkinson's disease, *J Neuropathol Exp Neurol* 50:743-755, 1991.

49. Quencer RM, Montalvo BM: Intraoperative cranial sonography, *Neuroradiology* 28:528-550, 1986.

50. Rizvi TA, Ennis M, Shipley MT: Reciprocal connections between medial preoptic area and the midbrain periaqueductal gray in rat: a WGA-HRP and PHA-L study, *J Comp Neurol* 315:1-15, 1992.

51. Rubin JM, Mirfakhraee M, Duda EE, et al: Intraoperative ultrasound examination of the brain, *Radiology* 137:831-832, 1980.

52. Rubinstein JB, Pasto ME, Rifkin MD, Goldberg BB: Real-time neurosonography of brain through calvarial defects with computed tomography correlation, *J Ultrasound Med* 137:831-832, 1980.

53. Schlief R: Diagnostic potential of intravenous contrast enhancement in various areas of cardiovascular Doppler ultrasound: efficacy results of a multinational clinical trial with the galactose-based agent SHU508A, *Echocardiography* 10:665-682, 1993.

54. Schöning M, Buchholz R, Walter J: Comparative study of transcranial color duplex sonography and transcranial Doppler sonography in adults, *J Neurosurg* 78:776-784, 1993.

55. Schöning M, Grunert D, Stier B: Transkranielle real-time Sonographie bei Kindern und Jugendlichen. Ultraschallanatomie des Gehirns, *Ultraschall Med* 9:286-292, 1988.

56. Schöning M, Staab M, Walter J, Niemann G: Transcranial color duplex sonography in childhood and adolescence, *Stroke* 24:1305-1309, 1993.

57. Schöning M, Walter J: Evaluation of the vertebro-basilar-posterior system by transcranial color Duplex sonography in adults, *Stroke* 23:1280-1286, 1992.

58. Schwarz KQ, Bechar H, Schimpfky C, et al: A study of the magnitude of Doppler enhancement with SHU 508 A in multiple vascular regions, *Radiology* (in press).

59. Seidel G, Kaps M, Dorndorf W: Transcranial color-coded duplex sonography in intracerebral hematomas in adults, *Stroke* 24:1519-1527, 1993.

60. Shackelford GD: Neurosonography of hydrocephalus in infants, *Neuroradiology* 28:452-462, 1986.

61. Simpson PE, Weiss JM: Altered activity of the locus coeruleus in animal model of depression, *Neuropsychopharmacology* 1:287-295, 1988.

62. De Slegte RGM, Valk J, Kaiser MC: Sonography of the postoperative brain: a report on 2 years of experiences, *Neuroradiology* 28:591-598, 1986.

63. Straßburg H-M, Sauer M, Weber S, Gilsbach J: Ultrasonographic diagnosis of brain tumor in infancy, *Pediatr Radiol* 14:284-287, 1984.

64. Winkler P, Helmke K: Ultrasonic diagnosis and follow-up of malignant brain tumors in childhood, *Pediatr Radiol* 15:215-219, 1985.

Echocontrast Agents in Transcranial Doppler Sonography

Fernand Ries

Neuroimaging methods have improved significantly during the last two decades. Unlike computed tomography, magnetic resonance imaging, and positron emission tomography, ultrasonography offers the advantage of being noninvasive, although it is often considered unreliable as a screening method. This is especially true when the ultrasound investigation relies on the Doppler method unsustained by visual imaging, as is the case in the duplex system. Transcranial Doppler sonography (TCD) is, however, a reliable, noninvasive means of investigating the intracranial cerebrovascular circulation.[2] Recent developments in transcranial color-coded duplex imaging (TCCD) promise further steps in the noninvasive hemodynamic and morphologic investigation of the cerebrovascular circulation.[7]

As well as being well suited to the evaluation of occlusive disease of the basal cerebral arteries, TCD is utilized to evaluate patients with cerebral vascular malformations, increased intracranial pressure, microangiopathy, and brain death. It is also useful in patient monitoring during therapeutic or radiologic interventions and during surgery. However, technical considerations such as restricted emission power and the presence of artifacts produced by higher gain settings can limit its use. In addition, in more than 15% of patients over 60 years of age, a technically satisfactory study cannot be made. This is due to hyperostosis of the skull bone, which is found mainly in elderly female patients and which becomes a limiting factor in attempting to use the transtemporal window.[39] This limitation is related to an insufficient signal-to-noise ratio, caused by the skull's absorption or reflection of 60% to 80% of the emitted ultrasound energy.[16] In some patients, no reflected signal is received at all. In the case of a minimally reflected ultrasound signal, the required high-energy emission leads to increased scattering of the ultrasound beam. This produces a large sample volume of limited spatial resolution or, in extreme cases, two different ultrasound foci.

One possible way to solve this problem is to improve the electronic processing of the signal. Reduced backscattering of the emitted signal, however, can be overcome only by improving the acoustic characteristics of reflected ultrasound waves. This may be achieved with the use of echocontrast agents.

THE SIGNAL ENHANCEMENT PRINCIPLE

The principles of ultrasound signal enhancement have been known for some time, and the behavior of gas bubbles has already been studied under in vitro conditions.[20,22] The echocontrast effect is due to the difference in the acoustic impedance of two reflecting media. Acoustic impedance, the resistance that ultrasound encounters as it passes through different tissues, is the product of tissue density and ultrasound velocity; it is expressed in rayl (R). The greatest difference in acoustic impedance occurs at the borderzone of air and soft or solid tissue,[20] where blood has a value of 1.62 R and gas of 0.004 R. Signal enhancement is due to the fact that oscillating air bubbles absorb a part of the emitted ultrasound energy and reradiate it, thereby increasing the ultrasound signal.

Due to high interfacial tension, gas bubbles have a tendency to shrink and disappear in only a few seconds. An air bubble's dissolution may be delayed by means of plasma proteins, such as albumin, which act as membranes at the gas-liquid interface, thus reducing surface tension. As a result, bubbles take much longer to dissolve, although their capacity for oscillation is reduced. The resonant oscillation of gas bubbles in an ultrasound field can produce cavitation effects. Oscillation properties and, consequently, the risk of cavitation increase with the similarity of the oscillatory frequency to that of the ultrasound emission.[41]

Other technical considerations related to the use of echocontrast agents include the bubble-eliminating function of the pulmonary reticuloendothelial system and the likelihood of bubbles being destroyed by high intraarterial pressure. Further difficulties are raised by possible rheologic differences between the contrast medium and red blood cells, the boluslike behavior of the injected contrast agent, and difficulties in adjusting such technical settings as wall filter, gain, and sample volume.

METHODS OF SIGNAL ENHANCEMENT

Contrast agents used as signal-enhancing media have to be stable compounds that are relatively easy to manufacture. They should have the characteristics of intravascular blood pool agents and exhibit increased echogenicity, thus allowing the visualization of the bloodstream. They should also cause no relevant side effects to the patient, and the contrast effect should be both reproducible and quantifiable. As a result of all these requirements, contrast enhancement of the venous system, the right heart, and body cavities was achieved first, and contrast agents that are able to pass through the lungs, aiding in the imaging of the left heart and cerebral or peripheral arterial vessels, have been devised only recently.[29]

In the past, as well as industrially manufactured contrast media, investigators have used contrast agents of their own making. "Handmade" agents may be produced simply by shaking a syringe partially filled with a liquid until bubbles form. Various liquids have been studied for this purpose, including saline or glucose solutions, colloids like oxypolygelin, or gas-generating agents such as H_2O_2.[22]

The second generation of echocontrast agents is industrially prepared. They include the microbubble foam (perfluoro-octyl-bromide, PFOB),[1] sonicated albumin (Albunex),[11,18] x-ray contrast medium sonicated by high-energy ultrasound emission, nitrogen-filled liposomes,[37] and air microbubbles bound to saccharide carrier microparticles (Echovist, Levovist).[30] Contrast agents utilizing air-filled microballoons consisting of polyglutamate polymers have also been tested recently.[9,32,38]

Handmade agents are cheap and easily available, but their effects are usually investigator-dependent and nonreproducible. Their signal-enhancement properties cannot be quantified, and they are insufficiently stable. They may cause side effects such as thromboembolic events due to macrobubble formation or impurities. They may also contain elements that could produce allergic reactions.[21]

A significant problem associated with industrially manufactured contrast agents relates to their reduced stability during passage through the heart and lungs, where most carriers tend to be crushed by the high intraarterial pressure. Several solutions have been proposed to circumvent this problem. One agent that is stable for several heart cycles uses saccharide crystals containing air-filled channels. When agitated in an aqueous solution, the crystals disintegrate. The resulting gas bubbles, each about 2 to 10 μm in diameter, are stabilized at the air-liquid contact zone by an interfacial membrane of denatured proteins. The bubbles have a coating of palmitic acid that protects them from destruction by the lungs' reticuloendothelial system. The saccharide crystals dissolve completely and are metabolized by the liver.

ECHOCONTRAST STUDIES IN NEUROSONOLOGY
Experimental results

The first studies and clinically relevant observations concerning echocontrast agents were obtained during echocardiographic testing.[12,15] Initially TCD was used to investigate the application problems of industrially manufactured contrast agents in a pilot study of anesthetized pigs.[25] The contrast medium used in that study consisted of galactose microparticles (SHU454, Echovist, Schering AG, Berlin); it was shown to enhance the TCD signal following intracardiac and intraarterial injection. Signal enhancement was dose-dependent, and

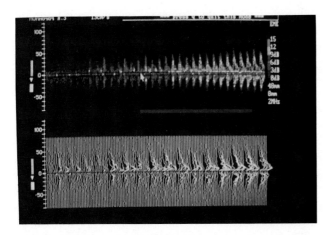

Fig. 20-1. Middle cerebral artery M1 segment signal enhancement by galactose-based air microbubbles (concentration of 300 mg MP per ml) in a 68-year-old female patient. *Upper display:* Following contrast agent injection, the originally missing native Doppler signal reaches a stable intensity level after about 26 heart cycles. *Lower display:* Amplitude to frequency display of the enhanced frequency spectrum. The color-coded dB scale for evaluation of signal increase is presented at the display's right margin.

Table 20-1. Time course of signal increase: time evolution of signal increase with averaged values and standard deviation for different concentrations; signal increase is related to first documentation, peak increase, and maximal duration of enhancement

Concentration (mg MP/ml)	First signal (s)	t peak (s)	t max (s)
200			
x̄ (±SD)	25,3 (5,9)	41,3 (17,1)	118 (69,8)
Median	25	35	90
Range	15-39	17-76	30-247
300			
x̄ (±SD)	27,6 (7,8)	55,5 (27,7)	237 (112,3)
Median	27	46	196
Range	12-45	19-143	60-477
400			
x̄ (±SD)	30,6 (12,3)	66,1 (31,8)	293 (122)
Median	30	62	265
Range	7-68	25-154	73-600

S, Seconds; *MP,* Microparticles; *t peak,* time to peak increase; *t max,* maximal duration of increase.

its duration and peak intensity were greatly influenced by the suspension's stability. Intravenous injection did not lead to a signal increase because the insufficient stability of air microbubbles during the transpulmonary passage led to their rapid dissolution during the first heart cycles. Intravenous administration of the contrast agent thus proved unsuitable for transcranial insonation.

Changes in the pharmaceutical design of the drug have led to improved stability without significant deficiencies in other relevant areas (SHU508A, Levovist, Schering AG, Berlin). The new galactose microparticles are roughly spherical and average 3.2 μm in size, 99% of the particles being less than 8 μm and 50% less than 2 μm. The carrier comes in the form of a dry, granular substance that, when dissolved in sterile water, binds air microbubbles and forms a milky suspension.

Clinical studies

Published studies of phase 2 and 3 trials in humans have addressed questions about the quality of signal enhancement during transcranial insonation and have explored ways of quantifying enhancement and assessing its diagnostic reliability.[6,24,26,27] These studies involved patients scheduled for TCD examination according to previously established criteria. The purpose of ultrasound testing was to detect cerebrovascular malformations and intracranial lesions causing arterial stenosis or occlusion and to monitor cerebrovascular spasm following subarachnoid hemorrhage. The studies also sought to assess the hemodynamic effects of extracranial carotid stenoses or occlusions.

A phase 2 study performed at our center involved 20 patients who were selected on the basis of a poor (N = 5) or absent (N = 15) native TCD signal obtained through the temporal bone window. Computerized tomography studies indicated that 19 of the 20 patients had abnormally thick temporal bones.

The TCD examinations were performed with a Transscan instrument (Eden Medizin Elektronik, Überlingen, Germany) equipped with a pulsed, 2 MHz ultrasound probe fixed with a system of rods and joints. A color-coded image of blood flow velocity and flow direction was obtained, and the reflected signal's amplitude was assessed.[23] Evaluation of the signal increase was based on the color-coded decibel (dB) scale (Fig. 20-1). The effect of contrast agent concentration on the duration of signal enhancement was studied. A tracing was considered to be continuously enhanced until it was seen to drop to an amplitude less than 3 dB above the original signal or, if the unenhanced native signal had been completely undetectable, when it dropped to less than 3 dB. A distinction was made between inhomogeneous, brief, maximal, spot increases (dBmax) occurring in certain phases of the pulse curve cycle, and the basal increase (dBbas) present throughout the whole cardiac cycle that defined the contours of the pulse curve (Tables 20-1 and 20-2).

The effect of contrast agent concentration was also assessed. Various concentrations of Levovist (200-, 300-, or 400-mg microparticles [MP] per ml solution) were used to insonate the left middle cerebral artery (MCA).

The concentration showing the best signal-enhancing effect was then used to insonate the right MCA. A subgroup of 60 injections showed signal enhancement free from high-frequency artifacts (Fig. 20-1). These pulse curves were used to further evaluate pharmacodynamic effects (Figs. 20-2 and 20-3).

The following criteria were evaluated:
• Time interval to first signal increase
• Time to peak intensity (values for dBmax and dBbas)
• Duration of the signal increase (values for dBmax and dBbas)
• Pharmacodynamic effects during signal increase and washout phase
• Peak intensity of dBmax and dBbas values
• Evaluation of flow pattern changes
• Diagnostic reliability
• Clinically manifest side effects

Adverse events and eventual minor side effects were documented during the examination and the 24 hours subsequent to contrast medium administration. The likelihood of these side effects being caused by the contrast injection was then rated as probable, possible, or improbable.

The successful documentation of an enhanced Doppler signal in at least one transtemporal insonation was possible in all study patients. In 5 of 37 (14%) vessels, however, a diagnostically useful signal increase sufficient in terms of duration and quality could not be obtained.

The first acoustic signal increase appeared an average of 21 seconds after contrast injection. The first enhanced pulse curves were seen 25 to 30 (mean 28) seconds after injection, the interval increasing slightly at higher contrast concentrations. This relatively long delay was attributed to the time spent to detect a vessel with a nonexistent native signal. The time interval from the beginning of injection to the peak of signal increase was dose-dependent for both dBmax and dBbas values. The average duration of signal increase was conspicuously high for all contrast agent concentrations, even when extensive, individual variations in duration were taken into account. In some cases, a longer-lasting signal was detected for up to 8 minutes. In 13 of 94 (14%) injections, the end of signal increase overlapped with a faint native signal not detected prior to contrast injection. Contrary to the preliminary hypotheses, signal

Table 20-2. Extent of signal increase: extent of signal increase with averaged values and standard deviation for the basal (dBbas) and maximal (dBmax) increase for different concentrations; signal increase is related to peak increase and maximal duration of signal enhancement

Concentration (mg MP/ml)	Peak SI Basal (dB)	Maximal (dB)	Last SI Basal (dB)	Maximal (dB)
200				
x̄ (±SD)	9,1 (5,0)	17,5 (6,0)	4,9 (2,1)	9,0 (5,0)
Median	8	17	5	11
Range	2-20	8-32	2-9	2-16
300				
x̄ (±SD)	12 (5,4)	20,7 (5,5)	4,6 (2,6)	9,3 (4,7)
Median	11	21	5	8
Range	5-28	13-37	0-11	2-23
400				
x̄ (±SD)	13,1 (5,6)	22,7 (5,9)	4,9 (3,2)	8,8 (5,6)
Median	12	23	5	8
Range	5-30	10-42	0-17	0-26

MP, Microparticles; *SI*, signal increase.

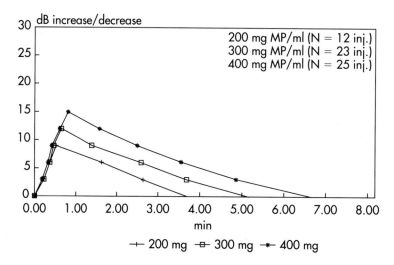

Fig. 20-2. Time course and extent of basal signal enhancement. Characteristics of signal increase and decrease at different concentrations (total of 60 injections).

increase and decrease were roughly linear, and there was no plateau during the contrast's washout phase (Figs. 20-2 and 20-3). The average dBbas-dBmax increase for the different concentrations was also dose-dependent (Table 20-2), with a significantly higher increase produced by the 200 mg to 300 mg MP per ml concentrations. The 300 mg to 400 mg MP per ml concentrations produced no corresponding increase.

The quantification of signal enhancement did not necessarily correspond to the diagnostic reliability, which was shown to be dose-dependent. Although these Doppler investigations revealed normal studies in 7 of 20 (35%) patients with known pathologic findings, they also led to the diagnosis of intracranial stenoses in 2 of 20 (10%) patients and microangiopathy in 11 of 20 (55%) others.

In a subsequent phase 3 study, we examined 32 patients with inadequate temporal bone windows. Aiming at a complete investigation of the basal cerebral arteries, this study used the previously established optimal concentration of 200 mg MP per ml for insufficient native signals and 300 mg MP per ml for absent native signals in a total of 115 injections. The study's primary focus was on diagnostic reliability.

The optimal concentration of contrast agent was shown to be 300 mg MP per ml, although the 400 mg MP per ml concentration yielded better results in investigations requiring the insonation of deeper brain areas. Reliable diagnoses were made in 27 of 32 (84%) patients. In four patients, the signal increase was insufficient, and in one, due to a displaced injection catheter, it was absent altogether. The concentrations used for optimal diagnostic evaluation were 200 mg MP per ml in 1 case, 300 mg MP per ml in 13 cases, and 400 mg MP per ml in 17 cases. Dose-dependent peak

intensities and duration of signal increase were similar to the phase 2 study results.

The distal branches of the basal cerebral arteries, especially the M1 segment of the MCA, were far better situated for contrast-enhanced imaging than those areas of the circle of Willis and the anterior cerebral artery that were located more proximally. The time-dependent nature of the signal increase was evident when signal enhancement lasted more than 3 minutes. In such cases, diagnostically reliable signals were produced mainly at insonation depths of 40 to 55 mm. In both studies it proved difficult to evaluate changes in flow pattern because an inadequate or absent native signal was required as an inclusion criterion.

There were no side effects severe enough to warrant interruption of the study or to provide medical therapy. In 12 of the phase 2 study's 97 injections (12.4%), patients experienced minimal side effects such as dysesthesia (N = 2, 2%), a general feeling of warmth (N = 3, 3%), or pain at the injection site (N = 7, 7%). Such side effects were observed in 9 of 20 (45%) patients. Side effects occurred in only one (5%) patient injected with the 200 mg MP per ml concentration, in 5 (14%) patients injected with the 300 mg MP per ml concentration, and in 6 (15%) injected with the 400 mg MP per ml concentration. In the phase 3 study, there were even fewer side effects, and they were limited to transient local pain at the injection site in 7 of 32 patients (22%). One patient experienced a feeling of cold and paresthesia in the lower extremities.

DISCUSSION

Ultrasound signal-enhancing techniques based on reflecting contrast agents are becoming increasingly important diagnostic tools, especially when restrictions

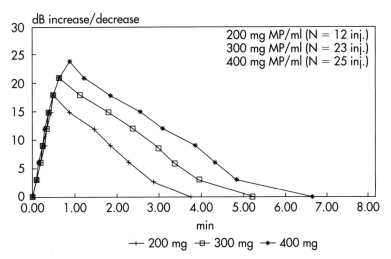

Fig. 20-3. Time course and extent of maximal signal enhancement. Characteristics of signal increase and decrease at different concentrations (total of 60 injections).

on invasive diagnostic techniques are taken into consideration.

Contrast-enhancing techniques were first used in B-mode echocardiography[12,15] and have since been introduced to vascular ultrasonographic testing. They have recently been utilized to measure tissue perfusion[5,13] and to characterize tumors. The Doppler mode, which is based on the frequency shift caused by moving particles, is superior to the B-mode in its ability to detect individual air microbubbles. This is mainly due to the higher noise level of the B-mode's echo intensity. The B-mode's signal sensitivity threshold is about 50 dB, a level surpassed by the Doppler mode, which is still sensitive at a threshold of 85 to 90 dB.[30]

Many questions about TCD signal enhancement and its application possibilities have already been answered in animal studies utilizing carrier-bound air microbubbles.[25] However, if contrast media are to be used for intracranial imaging in humans, a stable transpulmonary suspension has to be developed. The spatial resolution of TCCD imaging, the most promising TCD technique, may be improved through the use of such stable contrast media.[6] In addition, the diagnostic reliability of signal-enhancing techniques has to be further assessed. Research should focus on ways of quantifying signal increase, of differentiating artifacts from embolic material, and of delineating those pharmacokinetic properties that may influence diagnostic evaluation. It should also be noted that signal increase characteristics may depend on the time elapsing between the intravenous injection and the appearance of air microbubbles in cerebral arteries. A decreased cardiac ejection fraction or ventricular insufficiency may prolong this silent period, whereas an intracardiac shunt, such as a patent foramen ovale, might reduce it to less than the minimal time required for heart-lung passage. A pharmacodynamic evaluation should therefore take into account factors like microbubble recirculation, clustering, and the increased destabilization of critically low concentrations of injected suspensions.

A computerized Doppler technique is currently being developed in order to limit reliance on purely visual and nonstandardized evaluations of signal enhancement.[31,34] The effective increase in ultrasound intensity has to be calculated based on the understanding that an insufficient or absent native signal may correspond to a comparatively marked signal increase. Further analysis needs to be done on the relevance accorded to a maximal increase during only part of each cardiac cycle, as opposed to a basal increase allowing complete hemodynamic assessment. This analysis should look at the frequency spectra of both physiologic and nonphysiologic blood flow patterns, noting changes that might indicate eventual alterations in hemodynamics and microcirculation. In vivo investigations of animals subjected to this procedure, however, have revealed no fluctuations in arteriolar diameter or in capillary characteristics.[14]

As well as contrast-enhanced transcranial insonation, extracranial duplex testing can also be significantly improved by signal enhancement. This was evidenced by a recent color duplex study on the quantification of high-grade internal carotid artery stenosis.[36]

The detection of vascular malformations by TCCD[4] and its characterization of intracranial tumors according to their vascularization type[3] might also be made more diagnostically reliable with the use of echocontrast media. The combination of color-coded imaging and echocontrast agents is expected to make ultrasound a viable means of evaluating smaller peripheral vessels as well as the venous system. For example, in a study of TCCD signal enhancement,[6] 10 patients formerly diagnosed with angiomas, cavernous sinus fistulae, cavernomas, aneurysms, glioblastomas, and encephalitis were injected with Levovist. In most patients, contrast agent administration made it possible to produce color-coded images of the large intracranial basal vessels' peripheral branches as well as of the deep cerebral veins and the inferior sagittal sinus. In addition, the entire vertebrobasilar system, including the cerebellar arteries, could be traced through a transforaminal approach.

Any perspective on the development of echocontrast agents in neurosonology should take various contrast media into account. One of these is sonicated albumin, which is composed of albumin-coated air microbubbles that have the same signal-enhancing properties for transcranial insonation as the saccharide-based contrast agent described previously. However, contrary to theoretical expectations,[10] clinical studies show a briefer and more turbulent signal increase for sonicated albumin than for the saccharide-based agent.[28] This may be due to an instability of sonicated albumin microbubbles during cardiopulmonary passage; this instability may affect the microbubble size and the suspension's homogeneity.[35] If the carrier specifications could be improved, sonicated albumin could prove to be useful in transcranial ultrasound enhancement. However, the saccharide-based agent is, so far, the only one to have demonstrated lasting stability during cardiopulmonary passage. Another contrast medium, perflubron, may prove to offer similar enhancing properties. Its blood flow enhancement is marked and demonstrates a shear rate dependency that is responsible for a backscattering of flowing blood.[1] The fact that perflubron may also be used as a contrast medium in computed tomography and magnetic resonance tomography opens up new possibilities for simultaneous neuroimaging methods.

There is little significant evidence at present suggesting against the use of saccharide-based contrast media. Side effects observed in our studies were exclusively related to injection problems or consisted of reversible sensations of short duration, such as a feeling of warmth. As the highest concentration of 400 mg MP per ml seems to be responsible for most side effects and yields only a minimal improvement in diagnostic ability, the 300 mg MP per ml concentration is recommended for patients with inadequate native signals.

No relevant complications were reported in a review of other contrast media.[8] The condition known as *decompression sickness,* however, has to be further explored. Decompression sickness may be related to an impairment of the blood-brain barrier secondary to the passage of bubbles smaller than 20 μm in size. In an animal experiment featuring the injection of 15 μm microbubbles directly into the carotid artery, albumin-binding dye was observed in the neocortex as long as 3 hours after injection. This could be interpreted as a dysfunction of the blood-brain barrier.[19] In our pilot study, however, in which we performed neuropathologic exams on animal brains after contrast injection, we were unable to produce similar findings.[23]

Flow quantification is not possible with Doppler measurements alone. A very precise assessment of the vessel diameter and of the angle-corrected flow velocity is required. This has been achieved with transcranial insonation only recently. A computer-based Doppler technique, combined with the use of contrast agents, has made such flow quantification theoretically possible.[33] Another approach to this problem measures flow based on the dilution characteristics of injected contrast agents. This was attempted in an in vitro study using sonicated albumin.[17] Taking time-intensity curves as a basis for a mathematical dilution formula, various flow rates could be reliably quantified. This presents the possibility of a new approach to flow quantification by means of Doppler measurements. It is important, however, that pitfalls be avoided in the transfer of in vitro model results to in vivo systems. The last consideration is of particular concern, given that the relative insensitivity of commercially available ultrasound devices, largely a result of the "electronic threshold," makes proper flow quantification nearly impossible.[40]

Although the need for the enhancement of TCD signals occurs mostly in elderly patients, the growing number of applications for TCD and TCCD suggests the development of a new realm of extracranial and transcranial ultrasound imaging for all age groups.

REFERENCES

1. Andre MP, Steinbach G, Mattrey RF: Enhancement of the echogenicity of flowing blood by the contrast agent perflubron, *Invest Radiol* 28:502-506, 1993.
2. Arnolds B, von Reutern GM: Transcranial Doppler sonography: examination technique and normal reference values, *Ultrasound Med Biol* 12:115-123, 1986.
3. Becker G, Demuth K, Krone A, et al: Imaging of intracranial neoplasms and arteriovenous malformations by transcranial color-coded real-time sonography, *Neurosurgery* 31:420-428, 1992.
4. Becker G, Winkler J, Hoffmann E, Bogdahn U: Imaging of cerebral arterio-venous malformations by transcranial color-coded real-time sonography, *Neuroradiology* 32:280-288, 1990.
5. Bleeker H, Shung K: On the application of ultrasonic contrast agents for blood flowmet and assessment of cardiac perfusion, *J Ultrasound Med Biol* 9:461-471, 1990.
6. Bogdahn U, Becker G, Schlief R, et al: Contrast-enhanced transcranial colour-coded real time sonography: results of a phase-2 study, *Stroke* 24:676-684, 1993.
7. Bogdahn U, Becker G, Winkler J, et al: Transcranial color-coded real-time sonography in adults, *Stroke* 21:1680-1688, 1990.
8. Bommer WJ, Shah PM, Allen H, et al: The safety of contrast echocardiography: report of the Committee on Contrast Echocardiography for the American Society of Echocardiography, *J Am Coll Cardiol* 3:6-12, 1984.
9. de Jong N, Hoff L, Skotland T, Bom N: Absorption and scatter of encapsulated gas filled microspheres: theoretical considerations and some measurements, *Ultrasonics* 10:95-103, 1992.
10. de Jong N, Ten Cate FJ: Principles and recent developments in ultrasound contrast agents, *Ultrasonics* 29:324-330, 1991.
11. Feinstein SB, Cheirif J, Ten Cate FJ, et al: Safety and efficacy of a new transpulmonary ultrasound contrast agent: initial multi-center clinical results, *J Am Coll Cardiol* 16:316-324, 1990.
12. Feinstein SB, Shah PM: Advances in contrast two-dimensional echocardiography, *Cardiovasc Clin* 17:95-102, 1986.
13. Fobbe F, Siegert J, Fritzsch T: Color-coded duplex sonography and ultrasound contrast media: detection of renal perfusion defects in experimental animals, *Rofo Fortschr Geb Rontgenstr Neuen Bildgeb Verfahr* 154:242-245, 1991.
14. Fritzsch T, Maaß B, Müller B, et al: *Composition and tolerance of galactose-based echo contrast media.* In Katayama H, Brash RC, editors: *New dimensions of contrast media,* Tokyo, 1991, Excerpta Medica.
15. Gramiak R, Shah PM: Echocardiography of the aortic root, *Invest Radiol* 3:356-366, 1968.
16. Grolimund P: *Transmission of ultrasound through the temporal bone.* In Aaslid R, editor: *Transcranial Doppler sonography,* Vienna and New York, 1986, Springer Verlag.
17. Heidenreich PA, Wiencek JG, Zaroff JG, et al: In vitro calculation of flow by use of contrast ultrasonography, *J Am Soc Echocardiogr* 6:51-61, 1993.
18. Hellebust H, Christiansen C, Skotland T: Biochemical characterization of air-filled albumin microspheres, *Biotechnol Appl Biochem* 18:227-237, 1993.
19. Hills BA, James PB: Microbubble damage to the blood-brain barrier: relevance to decompression sickness, *Undersea Biomed Res* 18:111-116, 1991.
20. Meltzer RS, Tickner GE, Sahines TP, Popp RL: The source of ultrasound contrast effect, *J Clin Ultrasound* 8:121-127, 1980.
21. Nanda NC: *Echocontrast enhancers: how safe are they?* In Nanda NC, R Schlief, editors: *Advances in echo imaging using contrast enhancement,* Dordrecht, 1993, Kluwer.
22. Ophir J, Parker KJ: Contrast agents in diagnostic ultrasound, *Ultrasound Med Biol* 15:319-333, 1989.
23. Ries F: *Three-dimensional transcranial Doppler scanning.* In Bernstein EF, editor: *Vascular diagnosis,* ed 4, St Louis, 1993, Mosby–Year Book.
24. Ries F, Honisch C, Lambertz M, Schlief R: A transpulmonary contrast medium enhances the transcranial Doppler signal in humans, *Stroke* 24:1903-1909, 1993.
25. Ries F, Kaal K, Schultheiss R, et al: Air microbubbles as a contrast medium in transcranial Doppler sonography, *J Neuroimaging* 1:173-178, 1991.
26. Ries F, Lambertz M, Hartmann J, et al: Applications and

perspectives of a transpulmonary contrast agent in cerebrovascular imaging, *Stroke* 23:512, 1993 (abstract).

27. Rosenkranz K, Zendel W, Langer R, et al: Contrast-enhanced transcranial Doppler using a new transpulmonary echo contrast agent based on saccharide microparticles, *Radiology* 187:439-443, 1993.

28. Russell D, Brucher R, Dahl A, Jacobsen J: Contrast enhanced Doppler examination of internal and middle cerebral arteries, *Stroke* 23:513, 1993 (abstract).

29. Schlief R: Ultrasound contrast agents, *Curr Opin Radiol* 3:198-207, 1991.

30. Schlief R, Schürmann R, Balzer T, et al: Saccharide-based contrast agents and their application in vascular Doppler ultrasound, *Adv Echo-Contrast* 3:60-76, 1994.

31. Schlief R, Schwarz KQ, Ries F, et al: Dopplerintensitometrie: eine neue Methode zur quantitativen Analyse von Blutflußvolumen mit Echokontrastmitteln, *Ultraschall Med* 7:199, 1992 (abstract).

32. Schneider M, Bussat P, Barrau MB, et al: Polymeric microballoons as ultrasound contrast agents: physical and ultrasonic properties compared with sonicated albumin, *Invest Radiol* 27:134-139, 1992.

33. Schwarz KG, Bezante GP, Chen XC, Schlief R: Quantitative echo contrast concentration measurement by Doppler sonography, *Ultrasound Med Biol* 19:289-297, 1993.

34. Schwarz KG, Bezante GP, Chen XC, et al: Volumetric arterial flow quantification using echo contrast. An in-vitro comparison of three ultrasonic intensity methods: radio-frequency, video and Doppler, *Ultrasound Med Biol* 19:447-460, 1993.

35. Shapiro JR, Reisner SA, Lichtenberg GS, Meltzer RS: Intravenous contrast echocardiography with use of sonicated albumin in humans: systolic disappearance of left ventricular contrast after transpulmonary transmission, *J Am Coll Cardiol* 16:1603-1607, 1990.

36. Sitzer M, Fürst G, Siebler M, Steinmetz H: Usefulness of intravenous contrast medium in the characterization of high-grade internal carotid stenosis with color Doppler-assisted duplex imaging, *Stroke* 25:385-389, 1994.

37. Unger EC, Lund PJ, Shen DK, et al: Nitrogen-filled liposomes as a vascular US contrast agent: preliminary evaluation, *Radiology* 185:453-456, 1992.

38. Wheatley MA, Schrope B, Shen P: Contrast agents for diagnostic ultrasound: development and evaluation of polymer-coated microbubbles, *Biomaterials* 11:713-717, 1990.

39. Widder B: *Transkranielle Dopplersonographie bei zerebrovaskulären Erkrankungen,* Berlin, 1987, Springer Verlag.

40. Wiencek JG, Feinstein SB, Walker R, Aronson S: Pitfalls in quantitative contrast echocardiography: the steps to quantitation of perfusion, *J Am Soc Echocardiogr* 6:395-416, 1993.

41. Williams AR: Basic principles restated: cardiological applications of ultrasound, *Adv Echo-Contrast* 2:6-7, 1992.

SECTION FOUR

Embolus Detection with Doppler Ultrasonography

Background and Principles

Rainer Brucher
David Russell

Although cerebral embolism is one of the most common mechanisms of a stroke, at present we do not have methods that can be used routinely in the clinical setting to detect emboli. This often results in diagnostic uncertainty and delays in the initiation of appropriate treatment to prevent further emboli from entering the cerebral circulation.

Doppler ultrasound may theoretically be used to detect emboli. This method is usually used to measure blood flow velocities because movement of red blood cells causes a detectable Doppler frequency shift. Normally, the Doppler signal is a complex combination of all frequency shifts in that the red blood cells at various radii from the center of the vessel are moving at different velocities. The process of determining the individual frequency shifts from this complex Doppler signal is called *spectral analysis,* which is usually accomplished with a mathematical algorithm called the fast fourier transform (FFT).

THE INTENSITY OF THE DOPPLER SIGNAL

The Doppler spectrum also contains information regarding the intensity or amount of sound that is reflected back to the transducer. This is proportional to the number of red blood cells and indicates the amount of blood in the sample volume. The intensity of the reflected sound at a particular frequency depends on the number of red blood cells moving at a particular velocity. The signal power of each velocity component can be coded in a color or gray scale on a computer display using the spectrum analysis technique.

An embolus moving through the sample volume increases the amount of ultrasound being reflected back to the transducer because the amount of sound being reflected depends to a large extent on the size and acoustic impedance of particles in the blood (Fig. 21-1). We now consider in more detail the factors that determine the intensity of the Doppler signal.

The intensity of the Doppler signal or the amount of sound reflected back to the transducer mainly depends on two principles: reflection and scattering (Fig. 21-2). If the interface or object is larger in diameter than the wavelength of the ultrasound, then reflection occurs, whereas scattering takes place if the particle is smaller than the ultrasound wavelength. Particles with diameters that approximate the ultrasound wavelength show both characteristics.

Large interfaces are called *specular reflectors;* when sound is directed at an angle, the angle of reflection is equal to the angle of incidence. However, to obtain

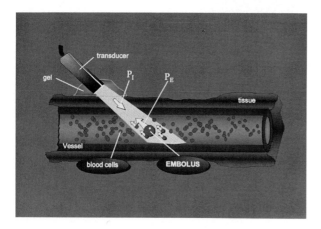

Fig. 21-1. Insonation of an artery as an embolus passes through. The embolus causes the reflection of an increased amount of Doppler power (P_E). (P_I, power of the incident Doppler beam.)

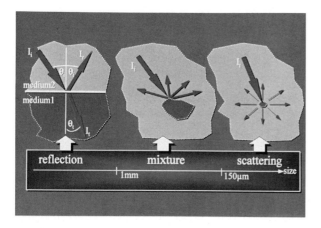

Fig. 21-2. Principles for reflection when ultrasound (2 MHz) travels through one medium (medium 2) and meets another (medium 1). The amount of scattering and reflection at the interface depends on the size of medium 2 (horizontal axis). (I_i, Incident ultrasound intensity; I_r, reflected intensity; I_t, transmitted intensity; Θ_i, angle of insonation; Θ_t, transmission angle.)

maximal detection of the reflected signal, the transducer must be oriented so that the incident sound beam strikes the interface perpendicularly. The amount of sound that is reflected at an interface depends on the acoustic impedance change from one medium to the next. Acoustic impedance (Z) is a measure of the resistance to sound passing through a medium and is the product of density (Σ) times velocity (c); that is $Z = \Sigma c$. It is similar to electrical resistance, which is the degree of difficulty experienced by an electron in traversing a specific type of material. High-density materials have high velocities and therefore high acoustic impedances. Similarly, low-density materials, such as gases, have low acoustic impedances. If the acoustic impedance of an embolus in the bloodstream is the same as that for blood, the sound is readily transmitted from blood to embolus. If there is

an acoustic impedance difference, however, more sound is reflected at the interface. The reflection coefficient (α_R) is expressed as follows:

$$\alpha_R = \left(\frac{(Z_2 - Z_1)}{(Z_2 + Z_1)}\right)^2$$

where α_R = reflection coefficient, Z_1 = acoustic impedance of medium 1, and Z_2 = acoustic impedance of medium 2.

Multiplying this relation by 100 gives the percentage reflection. Note that it does not matter which impedance is the larger or smaller for the two materials. The difference between the two impedances, when squared, gives the same number. Thus, the same percentage of reflection occurs at an interface, whether going from a high acoustic impedance to a lower acoustic impedance or vice versa. If the acoustic impedance difference is small, the intensity of the reflected wave is small. If the acoustic impedance difference is large, as with blood ($Z_1 = 1.6$ kg/m^2/second $\times 10^{-6}$) compared to air ($Z_2 = 0.0004$ kg/m^2/second $\times 10^{-6}$), a large fraction of the ultrasound is reflected at a blood-air interface:

$$\% \text{ Reflection} = \left(\frac{(Z_1 - Z_2)}{(Z_1 + Z_2)}\right)^2 \times 100\%$$
$$= \left(\frac{(1.6 \times 10^6) - (0.0004 \times 10^6)}{(1.6 \times 10^6) + (0.0004 \times 10^6)}\right)^2 \times 100$$
$$= 99.9\%$$

Scattering is another interaction between ultrasound and tissue that is of importance in the consideration of the intensity of the Doppler signal due to emboli. This wave behavior is also called *nonspecular reflection*. Scattering occurs because the interfaces are much smaller than one wavelength of the incident ultrasound. Each individual interface then acts as a new, separate sound source, and sound is reflected in all directions (Fig. 21-2). This is the case in the measurement of blood flow velocities. In this situation the primary target is the red blood cell with a size of 7 to 10 μm. The wavelength (λ) of the ultrasound can be calculated and depends on the velocity (c) of sound in the medium and on the frequency (f) of the ultrasound being used: $c = f \lambda$. Because the velocity of sound is constant for a particular medium (average of soft tissue = 1.540 m/s), increasing the frequency will cause the wavelength to decrease. For example, the wavelength for 10 MHz ultrasound in soft tissue is approximately 0.15 mm, whereas for 2 MHz ultrasound it is 0.77 mm. Increasing the ultrasound frequency may therefore, at least in theory, facilitate detection of emboli because the emboli may then behave as specular rather than nonspecular reflectors. In other words, the intensity of the ultrasound returning to the Doppler transducer will be determined more by reflection and less by scattering.

When scattering is present, the intensity of the Doppler signal depends on transmitted frequency (fourth power) and the diameter of the object (sixth power), in addition to the density and compressibility (similar to acoustic impedance) of the object (second power).

When 2 MHz transmitted frequency is being used for embolus detection, the intensity of the reflected signal is dependent on scattering for particles less than 150 μm in size, whereas reflection is present for particles more than 1 mm in diameter. A combination of scattering and reflection is present for particles between 150 μm and 1 mm (Fig. 21-2).

DURATION, SPECTRAL BROADENING, AND SAMPLE VOLUME

The duration of the intensity increase caused by an embolus (i.e., the number of spectral lines showing a power increase) depends on the time taken for the embolus to travel through the sample volume (transit time). This will understandably depend on both the velocity of the embolus and the size of the sample volume.

Spectral broadening of the embolic signal is at least partly due to changes in insonation angle as the embolus passes through the sample volume. Each FFT lasts 10 ms, and in this period 128 frequency samples are measured. Movement of the embolus causes changes in the insonation angle, resulting in different Doppler shift measurements, that is, the measurement of several different frequencies during one 10 ms sampling period (i.e., spectral broadening).

The amount of ultrasound reflected by an embolus is also dependent on the intensity of the ultrasound beam that insonates the embolus. The intensity of the transmitted ultrasound in the sample volume is not, however, uniform. The borders of the sample volume have less intensity than the middle. The reflected power due to the embolus therefore gradually increases, reaching a maximum when the embolus passes the center of the sample volume. This effect can be minimized by using a relatively large sample volume so that the incident intensity remains relatively constant for one spectral line (t = 10 ms).

EXPERIMENTAL STUDIES

Because gases cause a large reflection of ultrasound, it is not surprising that the first clinical reports of emboli detection using Doppler ultrasound have implicated these substances. Doppler signals thought to be due to air or other gases have been reported in decompression sickness,[1] open-heart surgery,[2-5] hip arthroplasty,[6] and carotid endarterectomy.[7] Other studies have suggested the detection of emboli composed of elements other than gas. Kelly and colleagues described Doppler signals

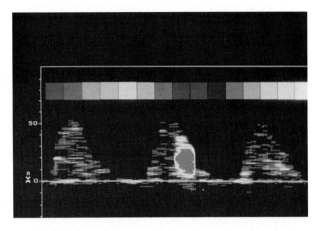

Fig. 21-3. Doppler signal caused by a whole-blood embolus in the rabbit aorta. The embolus caused a Doppler signal *(orange)* with intensity 15 dB greater than that of the surrounding blood *(blue)*. Each shade from left to right on color scale *(top)* represents increase in signal intensity of 3 dB. Blood flow velocities are shown in centimeters per second on the vertical axis; time base is 2.5 seconds.

in the femoral veins of patients following fractures of the tibia or femur that the authors proposed to be due to fat emboli.[8] Similar findings were reported by Herndon and associates during total hip replacement.[9] Spencer and co-workers performed transcranial Doppler examinations of the middle cerebral artery in patients undergoing carotid endarterectomy and found Doppler signals that suggested the presence of not only air emboli but also emboli composed of solid elements that they called "formed-element emboli."[10]

In clinical studies, however, it is extremely difficult to prove the origin of Doppler signals and especially to determine whether this method can detect not only gas emboli but also emboli composed of solid materials.

In an attempt to clarify these questions, an animal model was developed that could be used to detect arterial emboli composed of materials that are often involved in cerebral embolism.[11] The artery used was the rabbit aorta, which is similar in diameter to that of the middle cerebral artery in humans. Emboli introduced into the rabbit aorta via the left renal artery consisted of clotted whole blood, platelets, atheromatous material, fat, or air. The ultrasound examination was carried out continuously during the studies, using a multifrequency transcranial Doppler apparatus with a 2-MHz probe and a sample volume of 15 mm at a depth of 15 mm. The intensity of the Doppler spectrum was measured and displayed as a 15-shade color scale, each shade representing a 3-dB difference. All emboli introduced were clearly detected because they caused a Doppler signal at least 15 dB greater than that of the surrounding blood (Fig. 21-3; see also Plate 95). A more detailed analysis of the Doppler signals showed a significant positive correlation between the maximum intensity of the Doppler signals caused by emboli and embolus size.[12] This was the case for each embolus type studied.

In summary, emboli have the following Doppler characteristics:

1. They cause short (less than 0.1 second) increases in the Doppler signal power.
2. They are unidirectional within the Doppler spectrum.
3. Their duration in the spectrum depends on their velocity and on the size of the sample volume.
4. They may cause spectral broadening in the Doppler spectrum.
5. The intensity of the Doppler signal is dependent on the size of the embolus for each embolus type.
6. They sound like whistles or chirps.

Artifacts, by contrast, cause signal intensity increases that are simultaneous in both Doppler shift directions, that is, around the zero line.

REFERENCES

1. Spencer MP, Campbell SD, Sealey JL, et al: Experiments on decompression bubbles in the circulation using ultrasonic and electromagnetic flowmeters, *J Occup Med* 2(5):238-244, 1969.
2. Spencer MP, Lawrence GH, Thomas GI, Sauvage LR: The use of ultrasonics in the determination of arterial aeroembolism during open heart surgery, *Ann Thorac Surg* 8:489-497, 1969.
3. Padayachee TS, Parsons S, Theobald R, et al: The detection of microemboli in the middle cerebral artery during cardiopulmonary bypass. A transcranial Dopler ultrasound investigation using membrane and bubble oxygenators, *Ann Thorac Surg* 44:298-302, 1987.
4. Pugsley W: The use of Doppler ultrasound in the assessment of microemboli during cardiac surgery, *Perfusion* 4:115-122, 1989.
5. Pugsley W, Klinger L, Paschalis C, et al: Microemboli and cerebral impairment during cardiac surgery, *Vasc Surg* 24:34-43, 1990.
6. Svartling N: Detection of embolized material in the right atrium during cementation in hip arthroplasty, *Acta Anaesthesiol Scand* 23:203-208, 1988.
7. Padayachee TS, Gosling RG, Bishop CC, et al: Monitoring middle cerebral artery blood velcity, *Br Surg* 73:98-100, 1986.
8. Kelly GL, Dodi G, Eisman B: Ultrasound detection of fat emboli, *Surg Forum* 23:459-461, 1972.
9. Herndon JH, Bechtol CO, Dallas P, Crickenberger DP: Use of ultrasound to detect fat emboli during total hip replacement, *Acta Orthop Scand* 46:108-118, 1975.
10. Spencer MP, Thomas GI, Nicholls SC, Sauvage LR: Detection of middle cerebral artery emboli during carotid endarterectomy using transcranial Doppler ultrasonography, *Stroke* 21:415-423, 1990.
11. Russell D, Madden KP, Clark WM, et al: Detection of arterial emboli using Doppler ultrasound in rabbits, *Stroke* 22:253-258, 1991.
12. Russell D, Brucher R, Madden KP, et al: The intensity of the Doppler signal caused by arterial emboli depends on embolus size. In Oka M, von Reutern G-M, Furuhata H, Kodaira K, editors: *Recent advances in neurosonology: proceedings of the fourth meeting of the Neurosonology Research Group of the World Federation of Neurology, Hiroshima,* 6-8 June, 1991, Amsterdam, 1992, Excerpta Medica.

Methods and Clinical Potential

David Russell
Rainer Brucher

It is possible to detect emboli traveling through the cerebral circulation by using Doppler ultrasound. This requires examination of the common or internal carotid artery in the neck or transcranial Doppler examination of the major intracranial arteries. Bilateral Doppler examinations may be used to detect emboli entering both sides of the brain. In addition, two Doppler probes positioned over different vessels can be used to follow the path of an embolus through various cerebral vessels, for example, the internal carotid and the middle cerebral arteries.

The major intracranial arteries, especially the middle cerebral artery, are generally used for cerebral embolus detection. This is because probe fixation is easier over the temporal bone of the skull, and it is best achieved using flat monitoring probes. Good probe fixation is very important because embolus detection is best when there is a good Doppler signal compared to background noise and a constant power and insonation angle.

INSTRUMENTATION

The Doppler instrumentation used for emboli detection should have a high dynamic range (i.e., in excess of 50 dB), and the receiver should enable measurement of the signal power increase caused by emboli, which may be more than 40 dB. Gain or automatic gain control may further extend the dynamic range, and this is mandatory for gaseous embolus detection because these usually overload the Doppler instrumentation.

The amplitude of the transmitted ultrasound has to be adjustable so that the blood flow velocity curve can be readily differentiated from background noise. The axial length of the sample volume should be adaptable in relation to the size of the vessel, so that homogeneous insonation of the latter may be obtained. There should be a way of analyzing the increase in power caused by an embolus in both the time and the spectral domains. The exact resolution in time with regard to the entrance of an embolus into the sample volume can be accomplished only by analysis of the power increase in the time domain. This form of analysis is necessary for multigate Doppler examinations as described later. Analyses in the spectral domain offer greater detail regarding an embolic event, and emboli that are moving simultaneously through the sample volume with different velocities can be detected. Fast Fourier transformation (FFT) with medium resolution of the Doppler frequency should be of sufficient speed to allow an instant picture of blood flow velocities. Spectral broadening caused by curved paths or by the transit time of the embolus through the sample volume is therefore reduced. Furthermore, an overlapping in time of each FFT up to 60% should be possible. This improves power estimations in the frequency domain and subsequently sensitivity for embolus detection.

Storage of the Doppler data facilitates "off-line" assessment of possible embolic signals but is usually not possible using the Doppler instrumentation's hard disk, which is quickly overloaded. The examination may be recorded, however, using high-quality videotapes or digital audio tapes (DAT). Replaying the audiosignal recording through the Doppler instrument allows both auditory and visual reassessment of possible embolic signals as often as required. A DAT recorder with high-quality digital storage and stereo channels for forward and backward flow is recommended.

Automatic detection

The possibility of detecting cerebral emboli automatically would represent a considerable advance with regard to the clinical application of this method. There is discussion as to which Doppler characteristics of emboli should be used in the clinical situation. Most workers recognize emboli on the basis of their sound as they pass through the sample volume and as a color change in the Doppler spectrum, which is color coded for Doppler power intensity. However, this has the weakness of observer bias, which would be eliminated by an automatic assessment.

Analysis of the Doppler power increase caused by emboli has shown that the following parameters may be used for automatic embolus detection: enhanced power and peak power.[3] Enhanced power (Fig. 22-1) is the total power increase caused by the embolus relative to the mean Doppler power of the background signal. The mean Doppler power is due to the red blood cells in the sample volume, that is, normal sample volume without embolus. Assuming that the diameter of the vessel remains constant, then the sample volume will contain a relatively constant number of red blood cells. The mean Doppler power of the background signal should therefore be relatively constant. The relative comparison of total power increase and mean power eliminates attenuation effects because both parameters are equally affected. The peak power is the maximum power increase caused by the embolus (Fig. 22-1).

Neuronal networks can also be developed for automatic embolus detection.[11] The latter is based on artificial intelligence, where neuronal processing in the brain is simulated. Networks can be programmed to detect patterns in the Doppler spectrum caused by emboli by exposing the network system to many different types of emboli because this is a learning process based on experience.

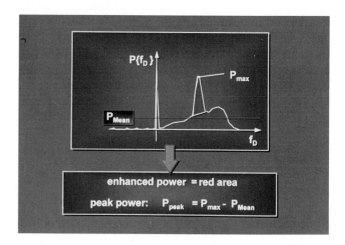

Fig. 22-1. Power increase (enhanced power) caused by an embolus (one spectral line). Doppler frequencies are shown on the horizontal axis (f_D) and the power distribution on the vertical axis [($P(f_D)$)]. Positive Doppler shifts are on the right side of the horizontal axis. (*Pmax*, Maximum power increase caused by embolus; *Pmean*, mean Doppler power of the background Doppler signal.)

Artifacts

Artifacts, too, may cause power increases in the Doppler spectrum. They are usually due to electrical interference, to fast movements of the probe, which may occur when the patient talks or chews, or possibly to bumping of the probe. This results in rapid relative movements of the probe toward and away from the head, causing Doppler shifts, and occurs within 1 ms and therefore faster than the duration of one FFT, which usually lasts 10 ms. The power increase due to artifacts is therefore seen simultaneously in both the forward and reverse flow of the Doppler spectrum (Fig. 22-2). Large, solid emboli or air emboli may cause overloading of the Doppler spectrum, which may appear similar to artifacts. It is therefore important for artifact rejection that the Doppler has a good dynamic range up to 50 dB.

Multigate Doppler may also help in differentiating emboli from artifacts. In this method, two sample volumes are positioned at a distance from each other of at least 5 mm in the same vessel. The delay between the appearance of an embolus in the two Doppler signals is then measured. It is only in the time domain that resolution is good enough to allow calculation of this delay. Artifacts, by contrast, cause simultaneous Doppler shifts and therefore appear in both sample volumes at the same time.

CLINICAL APPLICATION

The potential for cerebral embolus detection in the clinical situation is considerable. The ability to detect cerebral emboli may be of help in resolving the

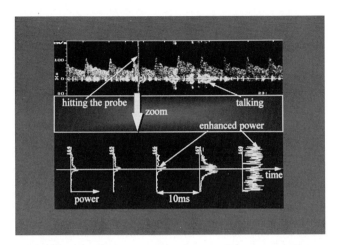

Fig. 22-2. Doppler recording from a middle cerebral artery with artifacts due to hitting the probe and talking *(top)*. Detailed examination (5 spectral lines) of artifact caused by hitting the probe is shown at the bottom. This shows that the artifact caused a power increase in both the positive (above the horizontal line representing the time axis) and negative (below the time axis) flow directions. Doppler signal power is shown to the right of each spectral line. Vertical axis *(top)* is blood flow velocity in cm/s. The interval between each spectral line is 10 ms.

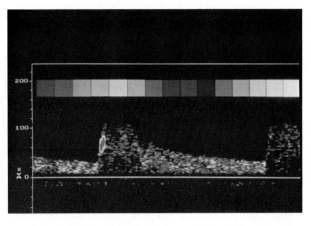

Fig. 22-3. Detection of a middle cerebral artery embolus *(orange)* in a patient with a prosthetic heart valve. Each shade from left to right on the color scale *(top)* represents an increase in signal intensity of 3 dB. Blood velocities are shown in centimeters per second on the vertical axis and the time base is 1.25 seconds.

controversy regarding transient ischemic attacks (TIAs) because it remains a matter of opinion as to what proportion of patients experience TIAs due to embolic versus hemodynamic events.

It is very difficult, however, to obtain Doppler monitoring during symptoms such as TIAs, which occur sporadically and seldom. Doppler examination during cerebral ischemic symptoms requires the development of small, portable Doppler systems that allow ambulatory bilateral monitoring of the cerebral circulation over long periods.

Clinical experience with cerebral embolus detection has so far been limited to patient groups or clinical situations that carry an increased risk for embolic stroke. In these situations a surprisingly high incidence and frequency of asymptomatic cerebral emboli have been found. It is important to stress that these emboli do not cause immediate cerebral symptoms and that their clinical significance is unknown. These clinical situations include the following:

1. Invasive cardiovascular examinations such as cerebral angiography and cardiac catheterization.[5,7] It is hoped that the detection of asymptomatic emboli may help to determine how these procedures may be carried out with the lowest risk of embolic complications for the patient.
2. Cardiovascular surgery, such as cardiopulmonary bypass and carotid endarterectomy.[2,6,8,9,13-15] Cardiopulmonary bypass surgery is of special interest

because cerebral macroemboli and microemboli are a major cause of neurologic and neuropsychological dysfunction during this operation. Monitoring patients during surgery may alert the surgical team that emboli are entering the cerebral circulation so that immediate preventive or therapeutic steps can be taken.

3. Patients with carotid stenosis.[12,14] The detection of ipsilateral cerebral emboli in patients with carotid stenosis may help us move toward a more detailed understanding of the pathophysiologic mechanisms causing emboli formation in this patient group.
4. Patients with a potential cardiac embolic source, for example, following myocardial infarction, atrial fibrillation, and patients with prosthetic heart valves.[1,4,10,16] (Fig. 22-3; see also Plate 96) The detection of asymptomatic cerebral emboli in these patients may help in determining which of these patients have the greatest risk for embolic stroke, which will allow more individualized therapeutic and prophylactic decisions.

The duration of the examination depends on the clinical situation. Monitoring during surgery, especially cardiopulmonary bypass surgery, takes several hours. Nonsurgical patients should be monitored for at least 1 hour in that the frequency of emboli in these patients is extremely variable and may be as low as one per hour. It is now also apparent that the frequency of asymptomatic cerebral emboli differs greatly not only between different patient groups but also within the same patient group. Furthermore, it is clear that the Doppler intensity of the embolic signals may differ from one patient to the next, for example, much smaller relative intensity increases in patients with carotid stenosis compared to patients with prosthetic heart valves.

REFERENCES

1. Brækken SK, Russell D, Brucher R, Svennevig J: Cerebral emboli in prosthetic heart valve patients, *Stroke* 25:79, 1994.
2. Brækken SK, Russell D, Brucher R, Svennevig J: Cerebral embolus monitoring during open heart surgery, *Stroke* 25:251, 1994.
3. Brucher R, Russell D: The Doppler characteristics of solid and gaseous emboli, *Cerebrovasc Dis* 4:88, 1994.
4. Georgiadis D, Grosset D, Kelman A, et al: Prevalence and characteristics of intracranial microemboli signals in patients with different types of prosthetic cardiac valves, *Stroke* 25:587-592, 1994.
5. Grosset DG, Yi Yang, Georgiadis D, et al: *Ultrasound detection of emboli in the middle cerebral artery during cardiac catheterization.* Paper read at the fifth meeting of the Neurosonology Research Group, University of Toronto, September 1-3, 1993.
6. Jansen C, Vriens EM, Eikelboom BC, et al: Carotid endarterectomy with transcranial Doppler and electroencephalographic monitoring. A prospective in 130 operations, *Stroke* 24:665-669, 1993.
7. Markus H, Loh A, Israel D, et al: Microscopic air embolism during cerebral angiography and strategies for its avoidance, *Lancet* 341:784-787, 1993.
8. Newman S: The incidence and nature of neuropsychological morbidity following cardiac surgery, *Perfusion* 4:93-100, 1989.
9. Pugsley W, Klinger L, Paschalis C, et al: The impact of microemboli during cardiopulmonary bypass on neuropsychological functioning, *Stroke* 25:1393-1399, 1994.
10. Rams JJ, Davis DA, Lolley DM, et al: Detection of microemboli in patients with artificial heart valves using transcranial Doppler: preliminary observations, *J Heart Valve Dis* 2:37-41, 1993.
11. Seibler M, Sitzer M, Rose G, et al: Microembolus detection in patients with high-grade internal carotid artery stenosis, *Stroke* 25:745, 1994.
12. Siebler M, Sitzer M, Steinmetz H: Detection of intracranial emboli in patients with symptomatic extracranial carotid artery disease, *Stroke* 23:1652-1654, 1992.
13. Spencer MP, Lawrence GH, Thomas GI, Sauvage LR: The use of ultrasonics in the determination of arterial aeroembolism during open heart surgery, *Ann Thorac Surg* 8:489-497, 1969.
14. Spencer MP, Thomas GI, Nicholls SC, Sauvage LR: Detection of middle cerebral artery emboli during carotid endarterectomy using transcranial Doppler ultrasonography, *Stroke* 21:415-423, 1990.
15. Stump DA, Tegeler CH, Rogers AT, et al: Neuropsychological deficits are associated with the number of emboli detected during cardiac surgery, *Stroke* 24:509, 1993.
16. Tegeler CH, Leighton VJ, Barber CC, et al: Nonoperative clinical use of carotid artery Doppler emboli detection, *J Neuroimaging* 1:162, 1991.

23

Doppler Embolus Detection: Stroke Treatment and Prevention

Hugh Markus

CEREBRAL EMBOLISM AND STROKE

Stroke is the third leading cause of death, accounting for 10% to 12% of all deaths in industrialized countries.[4] It also represents a major cause of disability. Cerebral embolism is the underlying pathogenic mechanism in many cases of stroke. Emboli may arise from the heart, carotid plaques, aortic plaques, intracranial atherosclerotic stenoses, or systemic venous thrombosis in the presence of a vein-to-artery shunt. Earlier clinical studies estimated that about 15% of all ischemic strokes are cardioembolic,[8] but the advent of transesophageal echocardiography has allowed identification of more cardioembolic sources; in most stroke populations about one third of patients with ischemic stroke are shown to have a cardioembolic source if they are evaluated fully.[26] Important cardioembolic sources include atrial thrombus in individuals with atrial fibrillation, mural thrombus following myocardial infarction, and valvular heart disease, including bacterial endocarditis and prosthetic cardiac valves.[33] Internal carotid artery stenosis is associated with an increased risk of stroke in the arterial territory of the stenosed artery, and this is believed to be predominantly embolic.[15,48] More recently it has been

appreciated that aortic arch atheroma is an important source of cerebral embolism. This region can be well visualized by transesophageal echocardiography,[33] and an association with stroke has been reported.[69] Despite the proven benefit of pharmacologic and surgical treatments in the prevention of stroke, problems still exist in their application. These management problems may be reduced by the ability to detect asymptomatic emboli.

The detection of gaseous emboli by using ultrasound was reported in the 1960s,[1] and the technique has been successfully applied to study embolization during cardiopulmonary bypass and decompression sickness. However, it was only with the recent demonstration that solid, or formed, emboli such as platelet aggregates, thrombus, and atheroma can also be detected that the potential application of the technique to the much larger group of patients with cerebrovascular disorders was widely realized. In 1990 Spencer and associates reported that, while recording from the middle cerebral artery during carotid endarterectomy, Doppler signals similar to those resulting from air emboli occurred prior to any arterial opening, that is, before air could have been introduced into the circulation.[62] They deduced that these must

Table 23-1. Potential uses of embolic signal monitoring in the management of stroke and transient ischemic attack

Potential uses of embolic signal detection in management of stroke and transient ischemic attack
1. Localization of embolic source
2. Identification of at-risk patients
a. Carotid stenosis
b. Cardiac embolism
Prosthetic cardiac valves
Native valve disease
Atrial fibrillation
Postmyocardial infarction
Other cardiac embolic sources
3. Monitoring during procedures
a. Cardiopulmonary bypass
b. Carotid endarterectomy
c. Coronary angiography
d. Carotid angioplasty
4. Monitoring effectiveness of treatment
a. Anticoagulation
b. Antiplatelet therapy

represent solid emboli dislodged from the internal carotid artery plaque during surgical mobilization and manipulation of the carotid artery. Experimental studies, as described in Chapter 21, have confirmed that such embolic materials can be detected in animal and in vitro models.[31,38,41,54] The detection of emboli has a number of potential applications in the management of stroke (Table 23-1).

Improving the risk-benefit and cost-benefit ratios

Despite the effectiveness of warfarin in patients with atrial fibrillation, and of carotid endarterectomy in symptomatic carotid stenosis, a considerable number of patients need to be treated to prevent each stroke. In the case of primary prevention in patients with atrial fibrillation, one stroke is prevented for every 40 patient years of treatment with warfarin.[72] In patients with greater than 70% symptomatic carotid stenosis, between 5 and 10 patients must be operated on to prevent one stroke.[73] The situation for lesser degrees of symptomatic carotid stenosis and for asymptomatic carotid stenosis is even more difficult. The risk-benefit and cost-benefit ratios could be much improved if there were better methods for identifying patients who are at highest risk of subsequent stroke. Assuming asymptomatic emboli are predictive of an increased risk of subsequent clinical emboli, in a similar way to that in which transient ischemic attacks indicate increased stroke risk,[73] a method to detect circulating asymptomatic cerebral emboli might allow identification of those at highest risk

of stroke, enabling more specific targeting of treatment. This may be particularly useful in selecting individuals with asymptomatic carotid stenosis for surgery.

Diagnosis of the site of embolism

Management of embolic stroke is also limited by the difficulty in detecting and localizing an embolic site in individual patients. Current diagnosis of embolic stroke rests on an investigational approach of "guilt by association."

A lack of validated, reliable clinical diagnostic criteria for cardioembolic stroke hampers individual patient treatment, and challenges the accuracy of prevalence estimates. The likelihood of identifying a potential cardioembolic source for brain ischaemia clearly depends on how thoroughly patients are evaluated and what lesions are accepted as potentially cardioembolic.[9]

This may explain the widely differing prevalence of cardioembolic stroke in different studies. For example, in one large multicenter stroke data bank project,[17] a 19% prevalence of cardioembolic stroke was reported. However, within each of the four centers the prevalence varied from 13% to 34%. The situation is made even more complex by the coexistence of potential cardioembolic sources with cerebral atherosclerosis that may also be responsible for the stroke. A review of cerebral arteriograms performed in 50 consecutive patients with transient ischemic attacks (TIAs) who had a potential cardioembolic source found additional significant ipsilateral carotid atherosclerosis in 19 (38%).[3] By recording from multiple arterial sites, localization of the active embolic site should be possible.

Monitoring of potentially embolic procedures

In a number of surgical and neuroradiologic procedures, cerebral embolism is an important cause of morbidity. Carotid endarterectomy was associated with a risk of stroke of 5% to 7.5% in two recent trials,[15,48] and embolism may be an important contributing factor. Cardiopulmonary bypass is associated with a small risk of focal neurologic deficit and a much higher risk of neuropsychological deficit.[55] Embolism may contribute to the pathogenesis of both. Cerebral angiography is associated with a small but definite risk of stroke;[13,36] it has been suggested that emboli released during the procedure may account for at least some of these complications. Recently, carotid angioplasty has been suggested as an alternative to carotid endarterectomy but there has been concern over the possibility of distal embolization at the time of balloon deflation.

For each of these procedures, the ability to monitor circulating emboli would allow the investigation both of the role of embolization in the pathogenesis of operative complications and of methods to reduce embolization.

Monitoring of the effectiveness of treatment

Despite significantly reducing stroke risk, treatments such as aspirin and warfarin are not effective in all patients. Inadequate inhibition of thrombosis or platelet aggregation may occur in some individuals and result in the formation of potentially embolic material. Although complete inhibition of platelet aggregation was found in the majority of stroke patients on 325 mg aspirin daily, a minority were relatively resistant to the effects of aspirin, even at high dose.[27] Despite adequate anticoagulation with warfarin, some patients with prosthetic heart valves suffer clinical embolic events. In situations such as these, monitoring asymptomatic emboli might enable the identification of potential treatment failures before clinical embolism occurs.

TECHNICAL ASPECTS OF EMBOLIC SIGNAL DETECTION IN PATIENTS AT RISK OF STROKE
Equipment

Most studies have used standard transcranial Doppler machines with a 2 MHz transducer. Studies monitoring the carotid arteries have used 5 MHz probes. A variety of machines have been used. The characteristics of one machine, the EME TC2000, has been evaluated in detail in a flow model with glass microspheres as emboli.[61] Optimal separation of an embolic signal from the background signal was obtained with a low gain setting and a short sample volume. A low gain setting is important if embolic signals are to be differentiated from the background signal; this is a reflection of the limited dynamic range of most commercially available machines.

Arteries studied

The majority of studies have monitored the middle cerebral artery. This offers the advantage of allowing the probe to be held in place against the temporal bone by a headband, and prolonged monitoring is possible for periods of up to an hour, or even longer in cooperative patients. Fixation with a headband is important to reduce movement artifact. Monitoring of the anterior cerebral artery, the distal carotid artery, and the posterior cerebral artery can been performed through the temporal window, allowing fixation of the probe and prolonged monitoring in a similar manner to that for the middle cerebral artery. Fixation of the probe in one position for long periods is more difficult when monitoring the vertebral and basilar arteries through the suboccipital window, although it has been successfully performed. There has been some concern over prolonged monitoring through the transorbital route due to the potential effect of ultrasound on the eye. The common carotid artery has also been monitored; this has the potential advantage of monitoring a larger flow volume that will contain more cardiac emboli than an individual, more distal intracerebral vessel. However, the sensitivity of the technique may be reduced with the higher-frequency transducers usually used for extracranial ultrasound. Spencer and Granado applied multiple Doppler probes with frequencies ranging from 2 to 10 Hz over the internal and common carotid arteries of three patients with mechanical prosthetic valves and detectable embolic signals.[61] Probes using 2 and 2.7 MHz detected 12 times more embolic signals than those using 5 to 5.6 MHz; the 7 and 10 MHz probes failed to detect any embolic signals.

In order to localize an embolic source, recordings need to be taken from a number of sites. For example, recording from both middle cerebral arteries helps to differentiate carotid and cardiac embolic sources. A carotid source can be further localized by recording from the common carotid artery below the plaque and the internal carotid artery above the plaque. Recording from multiple sites is made much simpler with newer TCD machines allowing simultaneous recording from up to four arterial sites.

Recording time

Optimal protocols are not yet developed, and optimal time may vary for different conditions. In patients with mechanical prosthetic cardiac valves (discussed later in this chapter), embolic signals may be detected at high frequency, and monitoring times above 20 to 30 minutes do not greatly increase the proportion of patients in whom they are detected. In patients with carotid stenosis and atrial fibrillation, the frequency of embolic events is usually lower and may be less than three per hour. In these patients a recording time of 30 to 60 minutes is probably necessary. However, a preliminary study has suggested that, in patients with carotid stenosis, pickup may be increased more by repeating a 20-minute recording on a second day than by prolonging a single recording to 60 minutes.[46]

Analysis of signals

Embolic signals must be differentiated both from artifact and from background fluctuations in signal intensity, or "Doppler speckle." Embolic signals appear as short-duration, high-intensity signals, predominantly unidirectional in the direction of flow (Fig. 23-1; see also Plates 97 to 99). The intensity increase is frequency or velocity focused, although very intense signals may result in a spread of intensity over adjacent frequencies or even overloading of the receiver and aliasing, with an intensity increase at all frequencies or velocities. Embolic signals

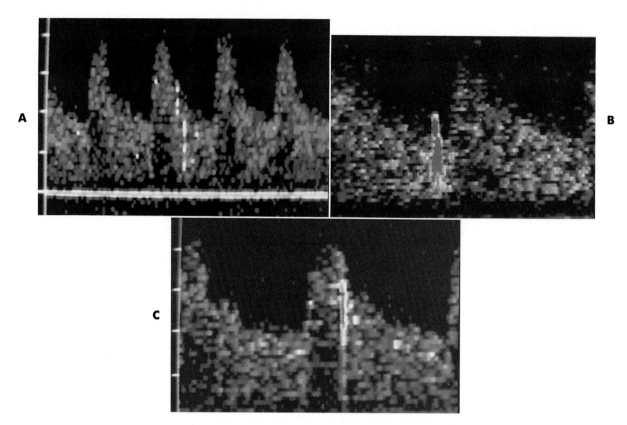

Fig. 23-1. Examples of embolic signals recorded during monitoring of the middle cerebral artery in patients with (**A**) a symptomatic carotid stenosis (two embolic signals are present), (**B**) a mechanical prosthetic valve, and (**C**) in the hour after a technically successful carotid angioplasty. The embolic signals appear as high-intensity signals. Intensity is color coded, with red indicating high intensity and blue, low intensity.

are accompanied by a characteristic audible "chirp." Duration can be expressed as the time for which the embolic signal has an relative intensity increase of more than 4 dB; using this intensity cutoff, mean signal duration was 12 ms for carotid stenosis, and duration rarely exceeded 30 to 40 ms, whereas for mechanical prosthetic cardiac valves, mean duration was 50 ms, and some embolic signals lasted 100 ms or occasionally even longer.[40] In contrast to embolic signals, artifact is bidirectional with the intensity increase predominantly at low velocity.[37] Usually embolic signals can be differentiated from artifact without great difficulty; however, embolic signals with a maximum intensity at low velocity or frequency can be difficult to differentiate from artifact, which on occasion can be predominantly unidirectional. Low-intensity embolic signals are sometimes difficult to distinguish from the background Doppler speckle. Random fluctuations in the intensity of the background Doppler signal of up to 4 dB occurred in one system, and an intensity cutoff at this level was used as a criterion for defining embolic signals.[44] Similar analyses need to be performed for other systems. It may be unreliable to transfer criteria developed on one system to another

system, particularly as methods for determining the relative intensity increase differ. A recent innovation is the use of a multigated Doppler that allows the same artery to be sampled at a number of depths. An embolus appears slightly later at a more distal point in the vessel, whereas artifact appears at the same time at all depths. This technique may markedly improve the differentiation of an embolic signal from artifact.

Despite the well-defined criteria for the identification of embolic signals, a recent examination of interobserver reproducibility produced disappointing results (Embolus Detection Research Group, presented at International Cerebral Haemodynamics meeting, Munster, Germany, 1994; unpublished). In contrast, a high degree of interobserver reproducibility has been reported in studies among trained observers.[44,58] Studies in the same disease states by different groups have produced markedly different proportions of patients in whom embolic signals are detected, as described later in this chapter. Differences between the characteristics of the patient groups may account for this variation, but there is always the concern that the interpretation of what constitutes an embolic signal varies between studies. For this reason, and to reduce unintentional bias, signals should be recorded onto audio or video tape and analyzed at a later date by an observer blinded to the diagnosis; in addition, each group should perform interobserver and intraobserver reproducibility studies. Replay of an audio signal allows evaluation of whether there is an accompanying characteristic sound; this is not possible if a copy of the analyzed signal is stored only as a processed image on the transcranial Doppler (TCD) machine. To date, these measures have been taken in a disappointingly small proportion of studies.

Automatic embolus detection

If the technique is to become widely used in routine clinical practice, an automatic system for detecting embolic signals and differentiating them from artifact will be necessary. This would ideally work in a similar fashion to 24-hour electrocardiographic monitoring, in which abnormal segments are identified for review. In an off-line system, using a computer algorithm, reliable differentiation of embolic signals from both the background signal and from artifact was possible for both experimental emboli in an animal model and embolic signals in patients.[37] This system detected the unidirectional frequency focused intensity increase seen with an embolus, added negative weighting for any bidirectional signal characteristic of an artifact, and computed an embolus probability score. An on-line version is currently being developed. An alternative approach is the use of a neural network that is trained to detect an embolic signal as defined by the trainer. Such a system has been developed and is highly specific for embolic signals, although its sensitivity for low-intensity signals needs to be improved.[58]

SPECIFIC DISEASE STATES
Potential embolic sources

Carotid stenosis. Carotid artery stenosis, both asymptomatic and symptomatic, is associated with an increased stroke risk.[10,15,48] This is believed to be embolic in origin in the majority of cases. Over the last 2 years, a number of studies have reported preliminary data on the incidence of embolic signals in both symptomatic and asymptomatic carotid stenosis, although many of the reports have been only in abstract form.

Although all studies have detected embolic signals in some patients with symptomatic carotid stenosis, the proportion of patients in whom embolic signals have been detected varies widely. A direct comparison between studies is difficult because of the heterogeneity of the different study populations; differences include the mean degree of carotid stenosis, the time interval from last clinical neurologic event, and the inclusion of patients with both cardiac and carotid embolic sources in some studies. Siebler and associates examined the

ipsilateral middle cerebral artery in 33 symptomatic high-grade (at least 70%) carotid stenoses and detected embolic signals in 27 (77%) at a mean rate of 14 per hour.[56] Antiplatelet therapy had been stopped in all patients for at least 5 days, although 25 were on heparin. Among 56 neurologically asymptomatic patients matched for degree of stenosis, embolic signals were significantly less common, occurring in only 9 (16%) at a mean rate of 0.35 per hour. Of the asymptomatic patients, 32 were on aspirin and 5 on warfarin. Babikian and colleagues retrospectively analyzed the results in patients in whom recording had been performed for 30 minutes from the ipsilateral middle cerebral artery.[2] Embolic signals were detected in 10 of 37 (27%) symptomatic extracranial carotid stenoses and 1 of 34 (2.9%) asymptomatic stenoses. Approximately equal numbers of patients were on antiplatelet agents or anticoagulants, and the interval between recording and symptoms was 12 days or less for approximately half of the symptomatic arteries. No correlation between the presence of embolic signals and time since last symptoms was published. Markus and associates found that during a single 20-minute ipsilateral middle cerebral artery recording, embolic signals were detected in none of 52 middle cerebral arteries of 26 normal controls, in 8 of 39 (21%) middle cerebral arteries ipsilateral to a symptomatic carotid stenosis, but in only 1 of 22 (4.5%) ipsilateral to an asymptomatic stenosis.[46] Considering only those subjects with symptomatic embolic signals detected, mean (median) number of embolic signals was 40.5 (3) per hour; (range 3 to 288). Recording from the middle cerebral artery for 30 minutes, Ries and co-workers detected embolic signals in 12 of 58 (21%) symptomatic carotid stenoses but in none of 29 asymptomatic stenoses.[52] Pharmacologic treatment, degree of stenosis, and time since stroke or TIA is not included in the abstract. Georgiadis and associates found embolic signals ipsilateral to 32 of 34 symptomatic unilateral carotid stenoses at a mean rate of 20 (range 8 to 24) during the 30-minute recording period.[21] Van Zuilen and colleagues noted embolic signals in 70% of 46 patients with carotid artery disease at a mean rate of 14 per hour; 43 of these patients had more than 70% stenosis, whereas 3 also had cardioembolic sources (2 atrial fibrillation, 1 prosthetic cardiac valve).[70] The recording time is not given in the abstract. Studies have reported both the association[2] and lack of association[46] between the degree of carotid stenosis and the detection of embolic. A number of studies have reported a relationship between time since last symptoms and presence of embolic signals[46,56,70]; signals were more common soon after a stroke or TIA. This is consistent with clinical data showing that the risk of a further stroke in the territory of a carotid stenosis is greatest soon after the initial stroke or TIA.[15]

The reason for the different proportions of patients with embolic signals found in these studies is unclear. A number of factors may be important, including different treatment regimens, time from last symptoms, time of recording and interpretation of what represents an embolic signal. A further factor is the temporal variability of embolic signals. In a preliminary study it has been shown that, whereas increasing recording time from 20 minutes to 60 minutes on a single occasion did not increase the proportion of patients with carotid stenosis who displayed embolic signals repeating the recording for 20 minutes on another day resulted in embolic signals being detected in additional patients. Therefore, detection rates are likely to be higher if recordings are repeated on a number of occasions. The optimal recording protocol needs to be investigated in further studies. An artifact is easily introduced into the recording by the use of a small probe or by scalp or jaw movements. Also, there has been some debate as to the nature of some of the high-intensity signals recorded.[28] Unintentional observer bias may occur, making blinded assessment of recordings important. In only one[46] of the studies reviewed here was the Doppler recording analyzed blinded to the diagnosis.

Limited information about embolus size can be derived from the intensity and duration of the embolic signals, but accurate sizing of emboli from their Doppler signals is not possible with currently available equipment if neither material or size is known.[41,53] The signals seen in the patients with carotid stenosis were less intense and of considerably shorter duration than those produced by platelet, thrombus, and atheroma emboli of 240 μ or greater diameter in a sheep model.[43] This suggests that the signals in patients are produced by emboli smaller than 240 μ.

The prognostic significance of embolic signals in patients with carotid disease remains to be determined. However, a number of lines of evidence suggest they may be important indicators of disease activity. All studies have shown an increased incidence in symptomatic as opposed to asymptomatic stenosis. Sitzer and colleagues reported a correlation between the presence of embolic signals preoperatively and intraluminal thrombus and plaque ulceration detected on histology of carotid endarterectomy specimens.[59] Following carotid endarterectomy, embolic signals are significantly less common.[58] In individual patients, embolic signals have disappeared after treatment with aspirin[45] and warfarin[42]; although the time course in these cases suggested a cause-and-effect relationship, the relationship was still circumstantial. Almost all embolic signals recorded have been asymptomatic; however, a recent case report describes a man with recurrent TIAs and a carotid bifurcation plaque in whom, during a reverberating compression maneuver of the common carotid artery, multiple embolic signals were detected in the middle cerebral artery. At the same time, the patient developed a hemiparesis and fundoscopy revealed retinal cholesterol emboli.[32] Further larger prospective studies with blinded data analysis are required to determine the frequency of embolic signals in patients with carotid artery stenosis, the factors influencing their frequency, and their prognostic significance.

Atrial fibrillation. Nonrheumatic atrial fibrillation affects 1.7% of persons aged 60 to 64 years and 11.6% of those older than 75.[34] The attributable risk of stroke from atrial fibrillation increases steadily and significantly with age from 1.5% in 50- to 59-year-olds to 23.5% in 80- to 89-year-olds.[74] The increased rate of stroke in patients with atrial fibrillation is mainly due to embolism, although in some individuals atrial fibrillation may act as a marker for other vascular risk factors that predispose to noncardioembolic stroke.

Few studies have monitored for embolic signals in patients with nonrheumatic atrial fibrillation. Tegeler and associates found embolic signals in 13 of 44 patients with recent stroke and atrial fibrillation when recording from the common carotid artery for 15 to 60 minutes.[66] The incidence of embolic signals may be lower in patients with atrial fibrillation but no recent neurologic event. The number of patients on anticoagulants or antiplatelet treatment is not given in the abstract. Tong and co-workers, recording from the middle cerebral artery for 30 minutes, found embolic signals in 2 of 13 patients with atrial fibrillation; 6 were on warfarin and 5 on aspirin treatment.[68] Eicke and colleagues reported embolic signals in 3 of 20 patients with nonrheumatic atrial fibrillation; the recording time and the presence or absence of any history of neurological event is not given in the abstract.[14]

The technique may be extremely useful in atrial fibrillation, both in selecting patients for anticoagulation and for monitoring the effectiveness of anticoagulation and antiplatelet therapy in individual patients. Further studies are required to determine the prevalence of embolic signals in patients with atrial fibrillation with and without neurologic events, the response to warfarin and aspirin, and, ultimately, the prognostic significance of the embolic signals.

Prosthetic cardiac valves. Thromboembolism is a major concern in patients with prosthetic cardiac valves. The risk of thromboembolism is greater with mitral valve replacement than with aortic valves.[7] The risk of embolization was particularly high with early prosthetic valves but has fallen with newer valve designs and the use of anticoagulation. Recent series report a risk of 1% to 4% with mechanical cardiac valves. In general, the incidence of thromboembolic complications is lower for tissue valves than for mechanical valves, and anticoagulation is not considered mandatory for this group of patients.

A number of studies have recorded embolic signals in patients with prosthetic cardiac valves, although many are only in abstract form. Comparison between the studies is complicated by the large number of different valve types studied and the different recording protocols used. All studies have demonstrated embolic signals in a large proportion of patients with mechanical heart valves and that they are more common in mechanical than bioprosthetic valves. Rams and associates detected embolic signals while recording from the middle cerebral artery of 14 of 26 subjects with mechanical cardiac valves.[51] The mean embolic rate (mean of left and right sides) shows that in those patients with embolic signals the mean number of embolic signals per hour was 29 (median 11). They stated that "the addition of intravenous heparin, low molecular weight dextran and saline or platelet inhibitors alone or in combination did not change the frequency and persistence of the 'blips,' " although no specific results or statistical analysis is provided. All patients with embolic signals had transthoracic echocardiography with no abnormal valvular or cavity findings. Georgiadis and co-workers, recording from the right middle cerebral artery for 30 minutes, found embolic signals in three different valve types with the following frequencies: Bjork Shiley monoleaflet tilting disk metallic valves, 76 of 85 subjects (89%), with a median frequency of 156 signals per hour; Medtronic-Hall mechanical valve, 28 of 56 (50%) with a median frequency of 2 per hour; Carpentier Edwards porcine bioprosthesis 20 of 38 (53%), with a median frequency of 2 per hour.[20] There was no relationship with international normalized ratio (INR) or time since valve insertion, and no relationship was found with a past history of neurologic events. Markus and colleagues, recording from both middle cerebral arteries for 20 minutes, detected embolic signals in 8 of 13 patients with Starr-Edwards or St. Jude mechanical valves but in only 1 of 11 (9%) with bioprosthetic valves (Carpentier-Edwards or Wessex).[44] In those mechanical valve patients with embolic signals, the mean (median) number of signals per hour was 52.8(24). Braekken and co-workers studied patients with Carbomedics metallic valves, recording for 30 minutes from the right middle cerebral artery; 5 days after valve insertion, embolic signals were detected in 22 of 29 (75%) patients, with a mean frequency of 10 (range 1 to 78) per 30 minutes.[5] In a separate group of patients studied 1 year following valve implantation, embolic signals were present in 26 of 29 (90%), with a mean frequency of 55 (range 1 to 353) per 30 minutes. Siwka and associates recorded for 15 minutes from the middle cerebral artery and noted embolic signals in 50 of 75 patients with St. Jude metallic

prostheses and 5 of 14 patients with Medtronic-Hall prostheses.[60] The frequency of embolic signals is not given in the abstract.

These results demonstrate that all groups have detected embolic signals in a proportion of patients with mechanical cardiac valves, but this varies from 50% to 90%. The proportion of patients with bioprosthetic valves who have embolic signals is much lower. The differences in frequencies between studies may be due to a number of reasons: Different valves types were studied in different positions, and different anticoagulation and antiplatelet regimens were used. Furthermore, as for carotid artery stenosis, the criteria for embolic signals may have differed. They are often not clearly stated, and in all but one study[46] the analysis of embolic signals was not blinded.

The origin of the embolic signals remains uncertain and may differ in patients with bioprosthetic and mechanical valves. In the former group, the frequency of signals is low, and there is little information on the effects of different anticoagulation and antiplatelet regimens. In patients with mechanical valves, circumstantial evidence suggests the embolic signals may result from neither platelet nor thrombus emboli. There is no relationship to degree of anticoagulation assessed on a single INR measurement.[20,51] In five patients with mechanical prosthetic cardiac valves and recent neurologic events in whom middle cerebral artery embolic signals were detected despite oral anticoagulation, the addition of intravenous and oral aspirin and intravenous heparin had no effect on the frequency of embolic signals.[64] No correlation has been found between the number of embolic signals and plasma concentrations of a number of coagulation markers (cross-linked D-dimer, antithrombin, and thrombin-antithrombin III complex).[22] Embolic signals in patients with metallic prosthetic valves have a higher intensity and longer duration than signals in patients with bioprosthetic cardiac valves and carotid stenosis.[25,44] This is consistent with them arising from emboli composed of a more echogenic material, and it has been suggested that they result from air bubbles. A possible mechanism is the formation of cavitation bubbles, which has been demonstrated in experimental models with mechanical valves.[4] Prospective follow-up studies are required to determine whether the presence of embolic signals is a marker for increased stroke risk that could be used clinically to decide on optimal anticoagulation and antiplatelet therapy or whether it may provide information on the relative merits of different valve designs.

Native valve disease and other cardiac embolic sources. Native heart valve disease is associated with an increased stroke risk, particularly in the case of mitral stenosis with associated atrial fibrillation. Natural history studies are now not possible because of the widespread use of anticoagulation in this condition, but in early studies prior to the widespread use of warfarin, systemic embolization was reported in 20% to 25% of patients with mitral stenosis,[30] with the primary determinants of embolization being age and the presence of atrial fibrillation. Weaker associations have been reported between stroke and mitral valve prolapse and other forms of valvular heart disease.[9] The prevalence of ischemic stroke in infective endocarditis ranges between 15% and 20%, with the majority of strokes occurring at, or shortly after, presentation;[9] embolism from valvular vegetations is believed to be the cause of most of these strokes. Left ventricular thrombus may form in the presence of impaired left ventricular function, either secondary to cardiomyopathy or acutely following myocardial infarction. This may embolize and result in stroke. The incidence of clinical emboli in patients with idiopathic cardiomyopathy has been estimated at about 4% per year.[9] About 2.5% of consecutive patients with acute myocardial infarction experience stroke within 2 to 4 weeks of the event, and this rate is much greater for anterior myocardial infarction, being about 6%, compared to 1% for inferior myocardial infarction.[9] This reflects the greater risk of left ventricular thrombus formation with anterior myocardial infarction.

Doppler embolus detection may prove useful in the management of patients with a variety of these cardioembolic sources, but there have been few studies in this area. Kitzam and colleagues prospectively studied 76 patients 3 to 10 days following their first myocardial infarction, of whom 70% had predominantly anterior myocardial infarction and 66% had Q waves; 21% of the patients had embolic signals detected on common carotid Doppler (C. Tegeler, personal communication).[65]

Monitoring during invasive procedures

The ability to detect asymptomatic emboli has obvious applications in identifying the importance of embolism as the cause of perioperative morbidity, studying the effectiveness of preventative measures, and assessing the effectiveness of surgical removal of an embolic source, such as in carotid endarterectomy. For each condition it has to be demonstrated that the asymptomatic signals detected are clinically important, either by correlating with neurologic or neuropsychological outcome or with changes on neuroimaging.

Cardiopulmonary bypass. Much of the pioneering work on Doppler embolus detection was performed in patients with cardiopulmonary bypass, and researchers in this area have led the way in correlating embolic signals with neuropsychological outcome. The effect of interventions, such as improved filters, has been correlated with a reduction in emboli count and improvement in neuropsychological outcome.[50] This topic is dealt with in detail in Chapter 24.

Carotid endarterectomy. Embolic signals have been recorded during carotid endarterectomy, particularly during dissection around the artery, on cross-clamp release, and during shunt insertion and removal.[60] A recent study found embolic signals in 37 of 40 subjects at some time during operation: in 14 during arterial dissection, in 19 at release of cross-clamps, and in 10 of 13 shunted patients during shunt insertion.[29] There was a significant relationship between the number of embolic signals detected during surgical dissection of the carotid artery and new subcortical lesions detected on magnetic resonance imaging. A correlation has also been reported between embolic signals during the dissection phase and postoperative neuropsychological decline.[18] The technique may allow early detection of postoperative thrombosis at the endarterectomy site.[19] This topic is covered in detail in Chapter 34.

Cerebral angiography. Cerebral angiography is associated with a small but definite risk of neurologic complications.[13] Estimates of the frequency of central nervous system complications vary from 1% to 14% in different studies, with transient deficits being more common than permanent deficits.[36] The risk of exacerbation of neurologic deficit following angiography in acute stroke is even higher.[16] Embolism is believed to be important in the pathogenesis of these complications; potential embolic particles include blood clot forming on the catheter and guide wires, material dislodged from atheromatous plaque by the angiographic catheter, particles introduced in contrast media and from the syringe, and inadvertent injection of air bubbles. Three studies have used transcranial Doppler ultrasound to monitor the middle cerebral artery for embolic signals in patients during cerebral angiography. In 1990 Staudacher and colleagues reported high-intensity signals while recording from the middle cerebral artery during injection of contrast media into the common carotid artery.[63] Simultaneously transient high-intensity signals were visualized in the internal carotid artery using B-mode ultrasound. Markus and associates studied seven patients during selective common carotid artery angiography.[39] During injection of the nonionic contrast medium iohexol into the carotid artery ipsilateral to the middle cerebral artery being insonated, numerous high-intensity signals, frequently resulting in overloading of the receiver, were seen (Fig. 23-2; see also Plate 100). These occurred with every one of the 38 contrast injections studied in the seven patients. During flushing of the catheter with saline, similar high-intensity signals were seen on some occasions; these occurred mainly when saline was injected rapidly rather than slowly. Occasional high-intensity signals, of duration less than 50 ms, were also detected. All embolic signals were asymptomatic. Dagirmanjian and co-workers detected embolic signals during all phases of bilateral carotid

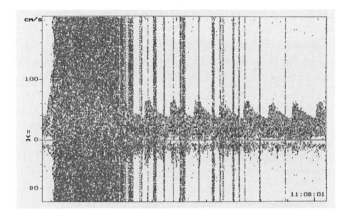

Fig. 23-2. Recording from the middle cerebral artery of a patient during cerebral angiography. Contrast has just been injected into the common carotid artery. There are multiple embolic signals, leading to overloading of the receiver and aliasing, with the intensity increase seen at all frequencies. Intensity is color coded, with red indicating high intensity and blue, low intensity.

arterial angiography; 25 middle cerebral arteries in 15 individuals were insonated.[11] Embolic signals occurred predominantly during catheter flushing and injection of contrast material but were also noted during manipulations of the catheter and guide wire. No neurologic complications were noted by nursing personnel during the study, although formal neurologic examination or psychometry was not performed.

Two experimental studies, one in a flow model[61] and the other in a sheep model,[39] have suggested that gaseous emboli are responsible for the majority of embolic signals during contrast injection. Air introduction can occur at the time of contrast being drawn up; microscopy revealed that freshly drawn-up contrast medium contained numerous small bubbles with a diameter less than 200 μ,[63] and injection of this contrast medium resulted in multiple embolic signals. Allowing the contrast to stand for 12 hours[63] or even 10 minutes[39] resulted in a marked reduction or abolition of embolic signals. This effect was more marked with more concentrated contrast media; with iohexol 350 there was a 66% reduction in embolic signal duration with contrast left to stand for 1 minute, and the reduction reached 96% for contrast left to stand for 10 minutes. For the less concentrated contrast medium Omnipaque 140 or with saline, there was no significant difference between contrast injected immediately and that left to stand for 5 minutes. It was suggested that air introduced at the time the contrast is drawn up may take longer to diffuse out from the more viscous concentrated contrast medium. Gaseous emboli may also be introduced at the time of injection of the contrast medium, and this is primarily found with fast speeds of injection. Contrast medium that had been left for 12 hours to ensure that it was gas-free resulted in high-intensity signals only if the speed of injection was greater than 2000 cm/s[63] and the speed of injection was

found to be important with contrast medium and saline in the sheep model.[39] This suggests that a rapid speed of injection resulted in cavitation bubbles.

The consequences of this air embolism are unknown. Despite the frequent air embolism noted during angiography, focal neurologic deficits did not occur at the same time. In patients undergoing cardiopulmonary bypass, a significant relationship has been found between embolic signals, thought to be predominantly due to air, and postoperative neuropsychological deficit.[50] Neuropsychological examination has not been performed after carotid angiography. In cases where the tissue is already vulnerable, such as an ischemic penumbra around a recent cerebral infarct, air embolism could result in more extensive focal cerebral injury, and this may explain the deterioration in neurologic status in some patients with acute stroke following cerebral angiography.

Although the predominant embolic material during cerebral angiography appears to be air, other materials, particularly dislodged atheromatous material or thrombus, are likely to be important, particularly in the pathogenesis of focal neurologic deficits. Current transcranial Doppler machines are unable to reliably differentiate solid from air emboli. Although it is likely that most of the individual embolic signals seen during angiography at times other than contrast injection also represent air bubbles accidentally introduced, they may on occasion represent particulate emboli. Furthermore, the multiple intense signals resulting from air emboli may obscure those of particulate emboli. New technologic advances may allow accurate characterization of emboli from the Doppler signal and resolve this difficulty,[45] allowing the true incidence and type of emboli in cerebral angiography to be determined.

Carotid angioplasty. Carotid angioplasty has been suggested as an alternative to carotid endarterectomy.

An understandable concern about distal embolization has led to a reluctance to use carotid angioplasty, in marked comparison to the situation with coronary angioplasty. No prospective studies have yet produced published data on the risks of clinical embolization with carotid angioplasty, but an overview of a number of retrospective studies including more than 100 cases suggested a stroke rate of less than 5%.[6]

The effect of carotid percutaneous transluminal angioplasty (PTA) on both immediate and short-term cerebral embolization, assessed by transcranial Doppler, has been evaluated in a prospective study in 10 patients undergoing technically successful carotid PTA.[42] Frequent embolic signals were detected during angiographic contrast injection. Multiple embolic signals were detected immediately following balloon deflation in 9 of 10 patients and usually persisted for two to five cardiac cycles. The signals tended to be most numerous following the first balloon deflation and less numerous with successive deflations. In contrast, neurologic symptoms (ipsilateral nondisabling stroke) occurred in only 1 of 10 patients, who was 1 of the 9 with embolic signals detected following balloon deflation.

Embolic signals were very common immediately following completion of the procedure and femoral catheter removal (80% of subjects) and 2 hours after angioplasty (83%) but became progressively less common after this, being present in 20% at 4 hours, 20% at 48 hours, and 17% at 7 days. A month after angioplasty, all subjects remained asymptomatic, and embolic signals were detected only in 1 (10%). The mean number of embolic signals per 20 minutes at each time point was immediately afterward, 6; 2 hours, 3.4; 4 hours, 0.4; 48 hours, 0.9; 7 days, 0.5; and 1 month, 0.2.

As described in the previous section, during carotid angiography multiple asymptomatic embolic signals can be detected by TCD, and experimental studies suggest that these represent air emboli. As it is not possible to definitively differentiate air bubbles from solid embolic material, it is uncertain whether individual embolic signals detected during passage of the balloon catheter through the stenosis represent dislodged solid emboli or residual air emboli from previous contrast injections, although it was felt that the multiple emboli released at the time of balloon inflation are likely to represent solid emboli for a number of reasons discussed in the paper.[41] The authors suggested that TCD monitoring will allow the study of the effectiveness of methods to reduce distal embolization at the time of balloon inflation, such as the triple coaxial catheter system with a distal balloon, and comparison of embolization occurring during PTA with that during equivalent procedures such as atherectomy or rotational thrombectomy.

Late ischemic events have also been reported after carotid angioplasty; in one study,[49] of 35 carotid dilations in 32 patients, there were no neurologic adverse events during the procedure, but in 3 patients contralateral sensorimotor deficits developed at 18, 24, and 36 hours postprocedure. After angioplasty with plaque rupture, a complex series of events takes place, including endothelial denudation, cracking and disruption of the atherosclerotic plaque, and stretching of the media and adventitia.[35] Embolization from platelet aggregates on this disrupted plaque may account for the risk of delayed stroke following carotid angioplasty. It was suggested that the use of TCD may allow the identification of patients in whom late embolization is occurring and enable the effectiveness of prophylactic pharmacologic treatments to be studied.[42]

LOCALIZATION OF EMBOLIC SOURCE IN STROKE

In patients with symptomatic carotid stenosis and no cardioembolic source, embolic signals are detected in the ipsilateral middle cerebral artery,[38] although signals have also been detected in the contralateral middle cerebral artery but only in the presence of angiographically demonstrated cross-flow.[58] Further localization should be possible by recording from the carotid system above and below the plaque. In contrast, in patients with prosthetic cardiac valves, signals are detected in all the major intracranial vessels,[23] whereas in atrial fibrillation signals are also detected in both middle cerebral arteries. This suggests that Doppler embolus detection will prove useful in localizing active embolic sources. In individual cases, embolus detection has assisted in the identification of internal carotid artery[43] and posterior cerebral artery[12] embolic sources. In 41 patients within 48 hours of stroke, embolic signals were found in all groups except in 8 patients with lacunar stroke; lacunar stroke usually does not involve embolism from large vessels.[24] Examples of the use of embolic signal detection in localizing a carotid and cardiac embolic source, respectively, are given below. Case 1 has been published previously.[43]

Case 1. A 44-year-old man who presented with an abrupt onset of weakness in the right arm was found to have a left lentiform nucleus infarct on CT scan. He recovered fully but experienced repeated transient symptoms in the right arm lasting a few minutes despite aspirin therapy, with at least 20 episodes occurring during a 6-month period. An angiogram showed only minimal irregularity of the wall contour at the right carotid bifurcation. Aspirin therapy (300 mg per day) alone was continued; however, he continued to experience transient ischemic attacks. With transcranial ultrasound, the Doppler signal was recorded from both middle cerebral arteries for a period of 20 minutes each. In the left middle cerebral artery, frequent embolic signals were seen. These embolic signals were noted at the very frequent rate of 4.8 per minute during the 20-minute recording period. No embolic signals were seen recording from the right middle cerebral artery. On reexamination of the carotid bifurcation using

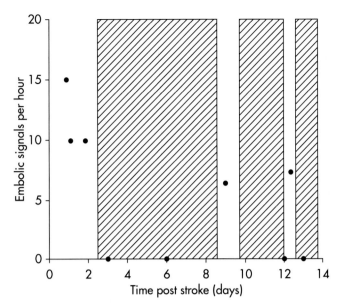

Fig. 23-3. Relationship between cerebral embolic signals detected in the left anterior cerebral artery and heparin anticoagulation in a patient with an anterior cerebral artery territory stroke. Periods of heparin administration are indicated by the hatched areas. (Modified from Siebler M, Nachtmann A, Sitzer M, et al: Anticoagulation monitoring and cerebral microemboli detection, *Lancet* 344:555, 1994 [letter].)

carotid Duplex ultrasound, a large smooth plaque was found in the bulb, but parallel with the carotid bulb wall, explaining the angiographic appearance. Warfarin was started, and transcranial Doppler recordings were repeated 1 month later; he had experienced only one TIA in the interim, at the time of which his international normalized ratio had been subtherapeutic at 1.3. In contrast to the previous recording, only one embolic signal was detected in the left middle cerebral artery during the whole 20 minutes; again, none was detected on the right side.

Case 2. A 63-year-old right-handed woman presented with two episodes of transient expressive dysphasia. Carotid duplex demonstrated a large plaque in the left proximal internal carotid artery but no velocity increase on Doppler. The right carotid artery was normal. She was taking 300 mg of aspirin daily. Transcranial Doppler recordings were made from each middle cerebral artery for 20 minutes each, according to the protocol in the first case history. Bilateral middle cerebral artery embolic signals were detected, three on the right side and two on the left, suggesting a cardiac source of emboli. Transesophageal echocardiography demonstrated a patent foramen ovale, and coagulation studies demonstrated protein S deficiency on two occasions. It was assumed she was having cardiac emboli, possibly paradoxical emboli from the venous circulation, and she was started on warfarin for her protein S deficiency.

Simultaneous recording from both cerebral hemispheres and from above and below a carotid stenosis improves the ability of the technique to localize embolic sources. No prospective studies have formally examined this application of asymptomatic embolus detection. These are now required to determine the additional information on embolic site that embolus detection gives

above conventional determination of embolic site using clinical history and examination, brain imaging, echocardiography, and carotid duplex.

Transcranial Doppler embolus detection now has an established use in the detection of a right-to-left cardiac or pulmonary shunt. The technique is similar to that of contrast echocardiography. Microscopic air bubbles are introduced into the venous circulation either in a blood-saline mix agitated with air or in a proprietary ultrasound contrast medium. In the presence of a shunt, high-intensity signals are detected in the middle cerebral artery and other cerebral vessels as the air microemboli pass through the vessel.[65]

PROGNOSTIC SIGNIFICANCE OF EMBOLIC SIGNALS IN PATIENTS AT RISK OF STROKE

The crucial question as to whether embolic signals have a prognostic significance similar to TIA in the prediction of subsequent stroke remains to be answered. The significance of embolic signals in the different conditions discussed previously may differ, and prospective studies are needed for each condition. Preliminary data suggest that, with the possible exception of embolic signals in patients with mechanical valves, embolic signals correlate with stroke risk in patients with carotid stenosis, as discussed previously. A response of embolic signals to anticoagulation has also been reported in a patient with an anterior cerebral artery territory stroke but no obvious stenosis[57]; cerebral embolic signals were noted only in the anterior cerebral artery and responded to heparin treatment but recurred each time the heparin was stopped (Fig. 23-3). Tegeler and colleagues monitored from the carotid artery using a 5 MHz continuous Doppler probe for 15 to 60 minutes in 155 patients admitted for ischemic stroke.[66] Phone follow-up in 66 patients at a mean follow-up time of 400 days was performed. End points of recurrent stroke, TIA, or death were more common in patients with embolic signals at baseline (10 of 41 versus 14 of 45). Prospective studies are required to confirm these findings.

PATHOPHYSIOLOGIC INFORMATION

In addition to its potential use in the management of stroke, Doppler embolus detection provides a unique tool for investigating the pathophysiology of stroke. The number of asymptomatic embolic signals occurring in individual patients is striking. The lack of a one-to-one association between embolus and stroke implies that other factors must be important in determining whether individual emboli cause symptoms. In addition to embolus size and composition, these factors may include collateral supply and the characteristics of the recipient vessel. Doppler embolus detection allows investigation of these factors. The factors involved in determining why a specific embolic source, such as a carotid plaque, becomes "active" or symptomatic is incompletely understood; embolus detection may provide a tool to examine these factors.

Whether there is a preferential distribution of cardiac emboli to any particular intracerebral arteries has been investigated by studying the intracranial distribution of embolic signals. Following the introduction of agitated saline introduced into a vein and passed through a patent foramen ovale in 12 patients, embolic signals were detected in all middle cerebral arteries and 75% of basilar arteries.[71] A similar study[23] has demonstrated the distribution of embolic signals in the carotid, middle cerebral, anterior cerebral, and vertebral arteries in patients with mechanical cardiac valves.

REFERENCES

1. Austen WG, Howry D: Ultrasound as a method to detect bubbles or particulate matter in the arterial line during cardiopulmonary bypass, *J Surg Res* 5:283-284, 1965.
2. Babikian VL, Hyde C, Pochay V, et al: Clinical correlates of high-intensity transient signals detected on transcranial Doppler sonography in patients with cerebrovascular disease, *Stroke* 25:1570-1573, 1994.
3. Bogousslavsky J, Hachinski VC, Boughner DR, et al: Cardiac and arterial lesions in carotid transient ischaemic attacks, *Arch Neurol* 43:223-228, 1986.
4. Bonita R: Epidemiology of stroke, *Lancet* 339:342-344, 1992.
5. Braekken SK, Russell D, Brucher R, et al: Cerebral emboli in prosthetic heart valve patients, *Stroke* 25:739, 1994 (abstract).
6. Brown MM: Balloon angioplasty for cerebrovascular disease, *Neurol Res* 14(suppl):159-163, 1992.
7. Campbell Cowan J: *Surgery for valvar heart disease*. In Hall RJC, Julian DG, editors: *Diseases of the cardiac valves*, Edinburgh, 1989, Churchill Livingstone.
8. Cerebral Embolism Task Force: Cardiogenic brain embolism, *Arch Neurol* 43:71-84, 1986.
9. Cerebral Embolism Task Force: Cardiogenic brain embolism: the second report of the Cerebral Embolism Task Force, *Arch Neurol* 46:727-743, 1989.
10. Chambers BR, Norris JW: Outcome in patients with asymptomatic neck bruits, *N Engl J Med* 315:860-865, 1986.
11. Dagirmanjian A, Davis DA, Rothfus WE, et al: Silent cerebral microemboli occurring during carotid angiography: frequency as determined with Doppler sonography, *AJR Am J Roentgenol* 161:1037-1040, 1993.
12. Diehl RR, Sliwka U, Rautenberg W, et al: Evidence for embolization from a posterior cerebral artery thrombus by transcranial Doppler monitoring, *Stroke* 24:606-608, 1993.
13. Dion JE, Gates PC, Fox AJ, et al: Clinical events following neuroangiography: a prospective study, *Stroke* 18:997-1004, 1994.
14. Eicke BM, Barth V, Kubowski B, et al: TCD monitoring in patients after valve replacement surgery and non-rheumatic atrial fibrillation, *Cerebrovasc Dis.* 4:22, 1994 (abstract).
15. European Carotid Surgery Trialists' Collaborative Group: MRC European Carotid Surgery Trial: interim results for symptomatic patients with severe (70-99%) or with mild (0-29%) carotid stenosis, *Lancet* 337:1235-1243, 1991.
16. Fieschi C, Argentino C, Lenzi GL, et al: Clinical and instrumental evaluation of patients with ischaemic stroke within the first six hours, *J Neurol Sci* 91:311-322, 1987.
17. Foulkes MA, Wolf PA, Price TR, et al: The Stroke Data Bank: design, methods, and baseline characteristics, *Stroke* 19:547-554, 1988.
18. Gaunt ME, Martin PJ, Smith JL, et al: Clinical relevance of intraoperative embolization detected by transcranial Doppler ultrasonography during carotid endarterectomy: a prospective study of 100 patients, *Br J Surg* 81:1435-1439, 1994.
19. Gaunt ME, Ratliff DA, Martin PJ, et al: On-table diagnosis of incipient carotid artery thrombosis during carotid endarterectomy by transcranial Doppler scanning, *J Vasc Surg* 20:104-107, 1994.
20. Georgiadis D, Grosset DG, Kelman A, et al: Prevalence and characteristics of intracranial microemboli signals in patients with different types of prosthetic cardiac valves, *Stroke* 25:587-592, 1994.
21. Georgiadis D, Grosset DG, Quin RO, et al: Detection of intracranial emboli in patients with carotid disease, *Eur J Vasc Surg* 8:309-314, 1994.
22. Georgiadis D, Mallinson A, Grosset DG, et al: Coagulation activity and emboli counts in patients with prosthetic cardiac valves, *Stroke* 25:1211-1214, 1994.
23. Grosset DG, Cowburn P, Georgiadis D, et al: Ultrasound detection of cerebral emboli in patients with prosthetic hart valves, *J Heart Valve Dis* 3:128-132, 1994.
24. Grosset DG, Georgiadis D, Abdullah I, et al: Doppler emboli signals vary according to stroke subtype, *Stroke* 25:382-384, 1994.
25. Grosset DG, Georgiadis D, Kelman AW, et al: Quantification of ultrasound emboli signals in patients with cardiac and carotid disease, *Stroke* 24:1922-1924, 1993.
26. Hart RG: Cardiogenic embolism to the brain, *Lancet* 339:589-594, 1992.
27. Helgason CM, Tortorice KL, Winkler SR, et al: Aspirin response and failure in cerebral infarction, *Stroke* 24:345-350, 1993.
28. Hennerici MG: High intensity transcranial signals (HITS): a questionable "jackpot" for the prediction of stroke risk, *J Heart Valve Dis* 3:124-125, 1994 (editorial).
29. Jansen C, Ramos LM, van Heesewijk JP, et al: Impact of microembolism and hemodynamic changes in the brain during carotid endarterectomy, *Stroke* 25:992-997, 1994.
30. Keen G, Leveaux V: Prognosis of cerebral embolism in rheumatic heart disease, *Br Med J* 2:91-92, 1958.

31. Kessler C, Kelly AB, Suggs WD, et al: Induction of transient neurological dysfunction in baboons by platelet microemboli, *Stroke* 23:697-702, 1992.

32. Khaffaf N, Karnik R, Winkler WB, et al: Embolic stroke by compression maneuver during transcranial Doppler sonography, *Stroke* 25:1056-1057, 1994.

33. Kronzen I, Tunick PA: Transoesophageal echocardiography as a tool in the evaluation of patients with embolic disorders, *Prog Cardiovasc Dis* 36:39-60, 1993.

34. Lake FR, Cullen KJ, de Klerk N: Atrial fibrillation and mortality in an elderly population, *Aust N Z J Med* 19:321-326, 1989.

35. Landau C, Lange RA, Hillis LD: Percutaneous transluminal coronary angioplasty, *N Engl J Med* 330:981-993, 1994.

36. Mani RL, Eisenberg RL, McDonald EJ, et al: Complications of catheter cerebral angiography: analysis of 5000 procedures. 1. Criteria and incidence, *AJR Am J Roentgenol* 131:861-865, 1978.

37. Markus H, Loh A, Brown MM: Computerized detection of cerebral emboli and discrimination from artifact using Doppler ultrasound, *Stroke* 24:1667-1672, 1993.

38. Markus H, Loh A, Brown MM: Detection of circulating cerebral emboli using Doppler ultrasound in a sheep model, *J Neurol Sci* 122:117-124, 1994.

39. Markus H, Loh A, Israel D, et al: Microscopic air embolism during cerebral angiography and strategies for its avoidance, *Lancet* 341:784-787, 1993.

40. Markus HS: Detection of circulating cerebral emboli using Doppler ultrasound; in vitro and in vivo validation and the application to the study of patients, DM thesis; 1994, University of Oxford.

41. Markus HS, Brown MM: Differentiation between different pathological cerebral embolic materials using transcranial Doppler in an in vitro model, *Stroke* 24:1-5, 1993.

42. Markus HS, Clifton A, Buckenham T, et al: Carotid angioplasty: detection of embolic signals during and following the procedure, *Stroke* 25:2403-2406.

43. Markus HS, Droste D, Brown MM: Ultrasonic detection of cerebral emboli in carotid stenosis, *Lancet* 341:1606, 1993 (letter; comment).

44. Markus HS, Droste DW, Brown MM: Detection of asymptomatic cerebral embolic signals with Doppler ultrasound, *Lancet* 343: 1011-1012, 1994.

45. Markus HS, Thomson ND, Brown MM: Asymptomatic cerebral embolic signals in symptomatic and asymptomatic carotid artery disease, *Brain* (in press).

46. Markus HS, Thompson N, Droste DW, et al: Cerebral embolic signals in carotid artery stenosis and their temporal variability, *Cerebrovasc Dis* 4:22, 1994 (abstract).

47. Moehring MA, Klepper JR: Pulse Doppler ultrasound detection, characterisation and size estimation of emboli in flowing blood, *Trans Biomedical Engineering* 41:35-44, 1994.

48. North American Symptomatic Carotid Endarterectomy Trial Collaborators: Beneficial effect of carotid endarterectomy in symptomatic patients with high-grade stenosis, *N Engl J Med* 325:445-453, 1991.

49. Porta M, Munari L, Belloni G, et al: Percutaneous angioplasty of atherosclerotic carotid arteries, *Cerebrovasc Dis* 1:265-272, 1991.

50. Pugsley W, Klinger L, Paschalis C, et al: The impact of microemboli during cardiopulmonary bypass on neuropsychological functioning, *Stroke* 25:1393-1399, 1994.

51. Rams JJ, Davis DA, Lolley DM, et al: Detection of microemboli in patients with artificial heart valves using transcranial Doppler: preliminary observations, *J Heart Valve Dis* 2:37-41, 1993.

52. Ries S, Schminke U, Daffertshofer M, et al: Emboli detection by TCD in patients with cerebral ischaemia, *Cerebrovasc Dis* 4:22, 1994.

53. Russell D, Brucher R, Madden K, et al: *The intensity of the Doppler signal caused by arterial emboli depends on embolus size.* In Oka M, von Reutern GM, Furuhata H, et al, editors: *Recent advances in neurosonology,* Amsterdam, 1992, Elsevier.

54. Russell D, Madden KP, Clark WM, et al: Detection of arterial emboli using Doppler ultrasound in rabbits, *Stroke* 22:253-258, 1991.

55. Shaw PJ, Bates D, Cartlidge NEF, et al: Early intellectual dysfunction following coronary bypass surgery, *Q J Med* 58:59-68, 1986.

56. Siebler M, Kleinschmidt A, Sitzer M, et al: Cerebral microembolism in symptomatic and asymptomatic high-grade internal carotid artery stenosis, *Neurology* 44:615-618, 1994.

57. Siebler M, Nachtmann A, Sitzer M, et al: Anticoagulation monitoring and cerebral microemboli detection, *Lancet* 344:555, 1994.

58. Siebler M, Sitzer M, Rose G, et al: Silent cerebral embolism caused by neurologically symptomatic high-grade carotid stenosis: event rates before and after carotid endarterectomy, *Brain* 116:1005-1015, 1993.

59. Sitzer M, Muller W, Siebler M, et al: Carotid plaque ulceration and lumen thrombus are the main sources of cerebral microemboli, *Cerebrovasc Dis* 4:20, 1994 (abstract).

60. Siwka U, Diehl R, Meyer B, et al: Significance of cerebral emboli in patients with heart valve prosthesis, *Cerebrovasc Dis* 4:239, 1994 (abstract).

61. Spencer M, Granado L: Ultrasonic frequency and Doppler sensitivity to arterial microemboli, *Stroke* 24:510, 1993 (abstract).

62. Spencer MP, Thomas GI, Nicholls SC, et al: Detection of middle cerebral artery emboli during carotid endarterectomy using transcranial Doppler ultrasonography, *Stroke* 21:415-423, 1990.

63. Staudacher T, Prey N, Sonntag W, et al: Zur grundlage der ultraschallphanomene wahrend der injektion von rontgenkontrastmitteln, *Radiologe* 30:124-129, 1990.

64. Sturzenegger M, Beer JH, Rihs F: The use of transcranial Doppler emboli detection and coagulation markers to monitor combined antithrombotic treatments in patients with prosthetic heart valves, *Cerebrovasc Dis* 5:15, 1994 (abstract).

65. Teague SM, Sharma MK: Detection of paradoxical cerebral echo contrast embolization by transcranial Doppler ultrasound, *Stroke* 22:740-745, 1991.

66. Tegeler CH, Burke GL, Dalley GM, et al: Carotid emboli predict poor outcome in stroke, *Stroke* 24:186, 1993 (abstract).

67. Tegeler CH: Personal communication,

68. Tong DC, Bolger A, Albers GW: Incidence of transcranial Doppler-detected cerebral microemboli in patients referred for echocardiography, *Stroke* 25:2138-2141, 1994.

69. Tunick PA, Perez JL, Kronzon I: The association between protruding atheromas in the thoracic aorta and systemic embolization, *Ann Intern Med* 115:423-427, 1991.

70. Van Zuilen EV, Mauser HW, van Gijn J, et al: The relationship between cerebral microemboli and symptomatic cerebral ischaemia: a study of transcranial Doppler monitoring, *Cerebrovasc Dis* 4:20, 1994 (abstract).

71. Venketasubramanian N, Sacco RL, Di Tullio M, et al: Vascular distribution of paradoxical emboli by transcranial Doppler, *Neurology* 43:1533-1535, 1993.

72. Warlow C: Non-rheumatic atrial fibrillation: warfarin or aspirin for all? Neurological comment, *Br Heart J* 68:647-648, 1992.

73. Warlow C: Secondary prevention of stroke, *Lancet* 339:724, 1992.

74. Wolf PA, Abbott R, Kannel WB: Atrial fibrillation as an independent risk factor for stroke: the Framingham study, *Stroke* 22:983-988, 1991.

24

Embolus Detection during Cardiopulmonary Bypass

David A. Stump
Stanton P. Newman

There have been major advancements in cardiac surgery over the past two decades, with a concomitant decrease in mortality and major morbidity. Partly because of the improved safety in cardiac procedures, there were 330,000 surgeries involving cardiopulmonary bypass (CPB) performed in the United States in 1992. In recent years it has been established that cardiac surgery poses significant risks to the brain in a proportion of patients.[15] The proportion of patients who have strokes declined for a period and then increased.[1] This pattern was attributed to the tendency in the United States to perform cardiac surgery on increasingly older patients.[3] A significant deterioration in neuropsychological functioning has also been reported in more than two thirds of patients prior to discharge and approximately one quarter to a third have been found to have deficits that persist.[5,7,11]

The mechanisms contributing to post-CPB neuropsychological deficits are uncertain. However, two major interrelated etiologic factors, hypoperfusion and microemboli, have been suggested. Microemboli in cardiac surgery may be either air or particulate in nature. The candidates for particulate matter include atheromatous matter, fat, and platelet aggregates. Recent neuropathologic studies have identified the occurrence of what has been termed *small capillary arteriolar dilatations* (SCADs) in the brains of humans who have succumbed in cardiac surgery as well as dogs undergoing cardiopulmonary bypass but not in those who have not been on extracorporeal circulation (Fig. 24-1).[4]

EMBOLUS DETECTION IN CARDIAC SURGERY

Early research using embolus detection during cardiac surgery established the occurrence of high-frequency signals.[8] These have been verified in the laboratory through the use of microspheres and other particulate matter and are considered to reflect the presence of emboli.[10] Many researchers are working on techniques to identify the material of the emboli, in particular to discriminate air from particulate matter, but to date, despite many claims to the contrary, no convincing data or accepted method has been identified.

In recent years both transcranial Doppler detection at the middle cerebral artery[9] and at the carotid[13] have

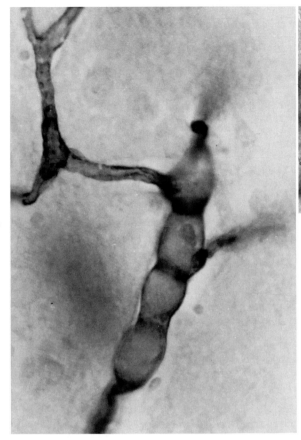

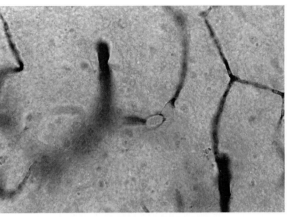

Fig. 24-1. A, *S*mall *C*apillary *A*rteriolar *D*ilitations (SCADs) in a 64-year-old woman after cardiopulmonary bypass. Alkaline phosphatase stain, light micrograph of a 100 μm thick section. Original magnification x 100. (From Moody DM et al: *ACTA Radiologica* suppl 369:139-142, 1986.) **B,** Aneurysmal dilatations in a brain capillary from a patient following cardiopulmonary bypass. The capillary arises from the arteriole that is out of focus to the left (100 μm thick celloidin section stain for alkaline phosphatase). (From Moody DM, Bue MA, Challa VR, et al: Brain microemboli during cardiac surgery or aortography, *Ann Neurol* 28: 477-486, 1990.)

been applied. Both of these techniques offer the ability to perform continuous measurement of emboli and the possibility to link the occurrence of emboli to activities in surgery. This, in turn, offers the possibility of reducing the numbers of emboli by altering technique and/or equipment during surgery. It is important, however, that the variety of equipment used makes it difficult to make comparisons across studies on the absolute number of emboli, as different equipment and techniques have produced markedly different counts of the occurrence of emboli.

WHEN DO EMBOLI OCCUR DURING CORONARY ARTERY BYPASS GRAFT SURGERY?

A number of studies have attempted to identify when emboli occur in cardiac surgery. In one study[12] of 196 patients undergoing routine coronary artery bypass graft (CABG) surgery a modified CME Dopscan 1070 continuous-wave ultrasound device was placed over the left common carotid artery throughout surgery. Thirteen different intraoperative tasks were noted and, if an embolic signal was detected in the 1-minute period following one of these tasks, the latter was considered to be associated with that event. The distribution of embolic signals is displayed in Figure 24-2.

Figure 24-2 shows that more than 60% of the emboli were detected during a period in which physical manipulation of the heart or aorta was in progress. More than 10% were detected in the 2 minutes following removal of the aortic cross-clamp. However, more than one third of the embolic signals were not associated with any specific period or surgical manipulation. This period occurred when the observer could not associate any act of the surgeon, perfusionist, or anesthesiologist as having a timely relationship with the signal.

These data suggest that there may be two separate major sources of emboli: (1) those secondary to surgical and manual manipulation of the heart and arteries and (2) emboli from a nonobvious source. It may be that the former are easier to reduce, as it may be possible to modify some of the manipulations of the heart and arteries. It remains important to be able to identify the composition of the emboli occurring at these different time periods, as the composition may offer information as to which may be preventable.

THE IMPACT OF EMBOLI ON NEUROPSYCHOLOGICAL OUTCOME

Neuropsychological techniques have been widely used to document the incidence of disturbance to the brain following cardiac surgery.[6] One important question is whether emboli detected during surgery have an impact on neuropsychological performance.

A study of 167 patients undergoing routine CABG surgery assessed patients prior to surgery and 5 to 7 days

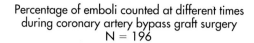

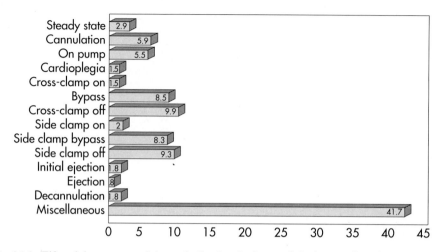

Fig. 24-2. Fifty-eight percent of the embolic signals detected during cardiopulmonary bypass were associated with specific surgical manipulations or time intervals. Forty-two percent of the embolic signals were not associated with one of the 13 categories listed in the figure. The miscellaneous events were often spontaneous and few in number. Embolic signals associated with surgical maneuvers were often detected in greater numbers.

postsurgery on a battery of 10 neuropsychological tests.[14] Emboli were counted during surgery in the left common carotid artery with a 5 MHz continuous-wave Carolina Medical Electronics Embolic Event monitor. Patients with neuropsychological deficits averaged more than twice the number of emboli compared to those without deficits. If the emboli count is dichotomized as an indicator of greater than 100 emboli detected, then it is significantly associated with deficit (Chi square = 4.8; p = 0.028). Of those patients with more than 100 emboli, 79% had a neuropsychological deficit, whereas only 63% of those with fewer than 100 emboli had a deficit.

Pugsley and colleagues[10] examined the relationship between microemboli and neuropsychological deficits at a longer time interval following surgery, when the deficits appear to be more stable. A transcranial Doppler (TC2-64, EME, Germany) recorded from the middle cerebral artery throughout surgery. Ninety-four patients who completed the neuropsychological assessment at 8 weeks had successful transcranial Doppler recordings. When the microemboli count was less than 200, only 5 of 58 patients (8.6%) exhibited a deficit at 8 weeks. When the count was higher than 1000, 3 of 7 (43%) patients were found to have a deficit in postoperative neuropsychological performance. These findings are displayed in Table 24-1.

Despite using different recording instruments and different sites and being unable to characterize emboli by size or composition, these two studies demonstrate

Table 24-1. Neuropsychological outcome 8 weeks after surgery and the number of microembolic events in surgery

Microemboli count during deficit cardiopulmonary bypass	Number of patients	Number with deficit	Percent
<200	58	5	9%
201-500	13	3	23%
501-1000	16	5	31%
>1000	7	3	43%

the clinical significance of emboli delivered to the brain during cardiac surgery.

SURGICAL TECHNIQUES TO REDUCE THE OCCURRENCE OF EMBOLI IN CARDIAC SURGERY
Filtration

Pugsley and associates showed that the introduction of an arterial line filter (40 microns) significantly reduced the numbers of microemboli assessed at the middle cerebral artery during routine CABG.[10] What was also important is that the introduction of the filter and the reduced microembolic count in the filtered patients resulted in a significantly lower incidence of neuropsychological deficits (8%) than in the nonfiltered patients (27%).

Venting

Venting to remove air is an important behavior of the surgeon that is likely to influence the generation of emboli. One study has investigated the different venting procedures in patients undergoing routine CABG.[2] Forty-two patients undergoing routine CABG were assessed for microemboli by means of a continuous-wave Doppler (modified CME Dopscan 1070) on the left common carotid artery. Two venting techniques were assessed: (1) A Sarns 20 Fr 9.5 cm curved left heart vent catheter was placed in the left superior pulmonary vein and positioned through the mitral valve into the left ventricle. It was attached to a 20-cm water pressure regulated suction. (2) A DLP 12-gauge, double-lumen cardioplegia cannula, with a flange, was placed in the proximal aorta and attached to low suction after cardioplegia administration. The mean number of emboli detected during surgery was 152 ± 231 for the aortic vent group and 86 ± 81 for the ventricular vent group. Given the wide range of emboli detected (4 to 1184), we looked at how many patients were above and below an arbitrary cutoff point of 100 emboli detected during the course of CABG. Of the 26 patients in the aortic vent group, 50% (13) had more than 100, and 50% had fewer. In the ventricular vent group, 81% (13) had fewer than 100 emboli, and only 3 (19%) had more than 100 emboli detected (Chi square, $p < 0.05$). The data from this study suggest that the embolic load delivered to the patient's brain during CABG may be reduced by altering the venting of the left heart during bypass, by avoiding aortic manipulation and suction, and by clearing air from the left ventricular cavity.

Both these studies illustrate that it is possible to reduce the incidence of microemboli during cardiac surgery. The impact of other variations in surgery on microembolic load are currently being assessed.

CONCLUSION

The detection of microemboli during cardiac surgery is now a well-established technique. It is important that the incidence of microemboli is related to neuropsychological outcome following surgery. This relationship should not be expected to be perfect as the impact of microemboli on cognitive performance is dependent upon many factors, including the size, composition, and brain location of the material. Future research to identify the composition of the emboli in the context of cardiac surgery may make it possible to see whether particulate matter is more damaging than gaseous material.

REFERENCES

1. Gardner TJ, Horneffer PJ, Manolio TA, et al: Stroke following coronary artery bypass grafting: a ten year study, *Ann Thorac Surg* 40:574-581, 1985.
2. Hammon JW, Stump DA, Hines M, Phipps JM: Prevention of embolic events during coronary artery bypass graft surgery, *Perfusion* (in press).
3. Mills S, Prough D: Neuropsychiatric complications following cardiac surgery, *Semin Thorac Cardiovasc Surg* 3:39-46, 1991.
4. Moody DM, Bell MA, Challa VR, et al: Brain microemboli during cardiac surgery or aortography, *Ann Neurol* 28:477-486, 1990.
5. Newman S: The incidence and nature of neuropsychological morbidity following cardiac surgery, *Perfusion* 4:93-100, 1989.
6. Newman S: Neuropsychological and psychological consequences of cardiac surgery. In Taylor K, Smith P, editors: *The brain and cardiac surgery,* Andrew Arnold, 1993.
7. Newman S, Klinger L, Venn G, et al: *The persistence of neuropsychological deficits twelve months after coronary artery bypass surgery.* In Wilner A, Rodewald G, editors: *Impact of cardiac surgery on the quality of life,* New York, 1990, Plenum.
8. Padayachee TS, Parsons S, Theobald R, et al: The detection of microemboli in the middle cerebral artery during cardiopulmonary bypass: a transcranial Doppler ultrasound investigation using membrane and bubble oxygenators, *Ann Thorac Surg* 44:298-302, 1987.
9. Pugsley W: The use of Doppler ultrasound in the assessment of microemboli during cardiac surgery, *Perfusion* 4:115-122, 1989.
10. Pugsley WB, Klinger L, Paschalis C, et al: Does arterial line filtration affect the bypass related cerebral impairment observed in patients undergoing coronary artery surgery? *Clin Sci* 75(suppl 19):30-31, 1988.
11. Stump DA, Newman S, Coker L, et al: Persistence of neuropsychological deficits following CABG, *Anesthesiology* 73:113, 1990, (abstract).
12. Stump DA, Rogers AT, Kon ND, et al: When emboli occur during coronary artery bypass graft surgery, *Anesthesiology* 79(suppl 3A):49, 1993.
13. Stump DA, Stein CS, Tegeler CH, et al: Validity and reliability of a device for detecting carotid emboli, *J Neuroimaging* 1:18-22, 1991.
14. Stump DA, Tegeler CH, Rogers AT, et al: Neuropsychological deficits are associated with the number of emboli detected during cardiac surgery, *Stroke* 24:509, 1993.
15. Taylor K, Smith P, editors: *The brain and cardiac surgery,* Andrew Arnold, 1993.

SECTION FIVE

Echocardiography

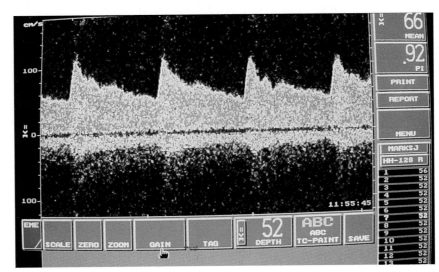

Plate 1 For legend, see Fig. 4-1 in text.

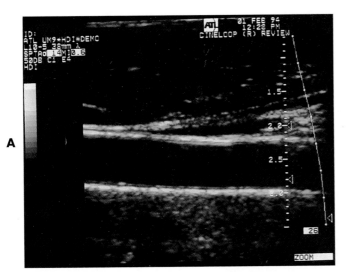

A

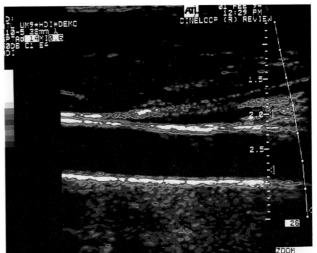

B

Plate 2 For legend, see Fig. 4-2 in text.

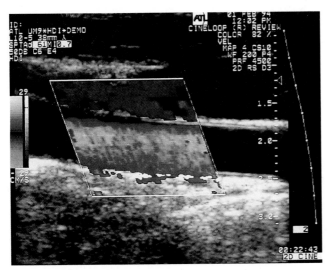

Plate 3 For legend, see Fig. 4-4 in text.

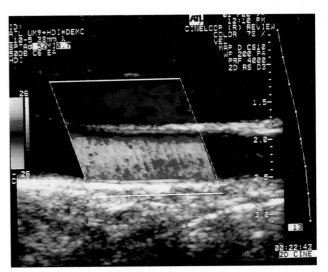

Plate 4 For legend, see Fig. 4-5, *A* in text.

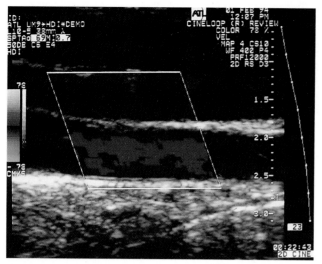

Plate 5 For legend, see Fig. 4-5, *B* in text.

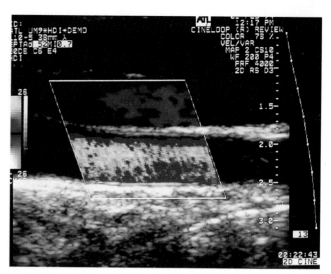

Plate 6 For legend, see Fig. 4-6 in text.

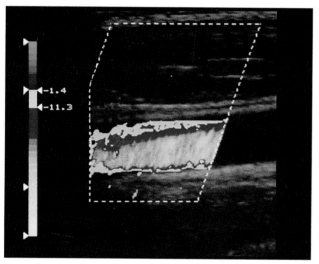

Plate 7 For legend, see Fig. 4-7, *A* in text.

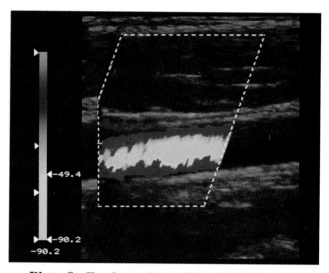

Plate 8 For legend, see Fig. 4-7, *B* in text.

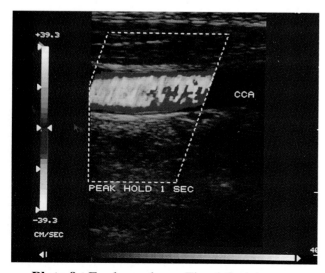

Plate 9 For legend, see Fig. 4-8, *A* in text.

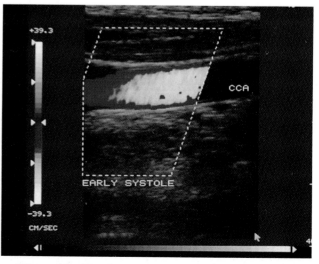

Plate 10 For legend, see Fig. 4-8, *B* in text.

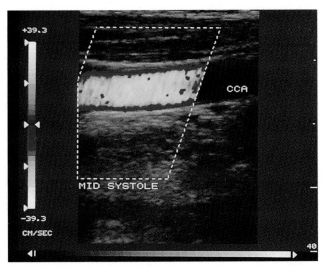

Plate 11 For legend, see Fig. 4-8, *C* in text.

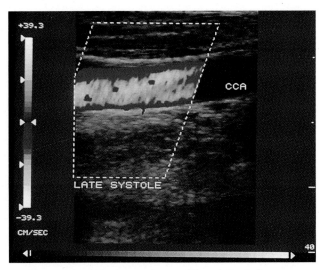

Plate 12 For legend, see Fig. 4-8, *D* in text.

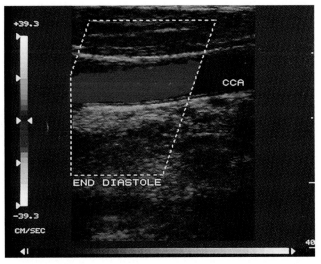

Plate 13 For legend, see Fig. 4-8, *E* in text.

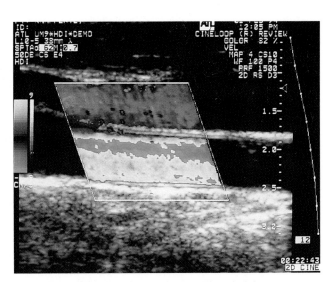

Plate 14 For legend, see Fig. 4-9 in text.

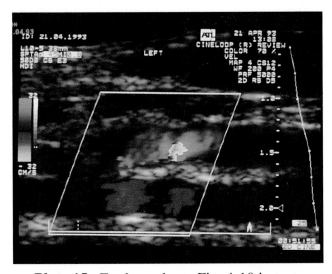

Plate 15 For legend, see Fig. 4-10 in text.

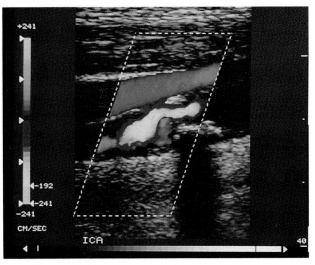

Plate 16 For legend, see Fig. 4-11, *A* in text.

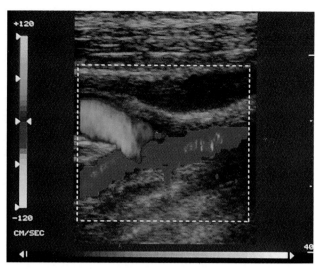

Plate 17   For legend, see Fig. 4-11, *B* in text.

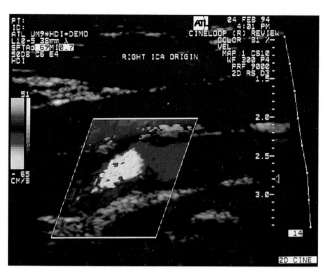

Plate 18   For legend, see Fig. 4-12, *A* in text.

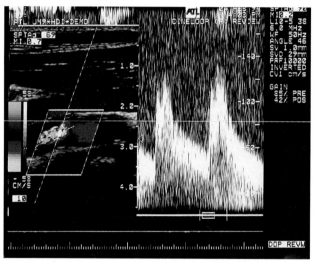

Plate 19   For legend, see Fig. 4-12, *B* in text.

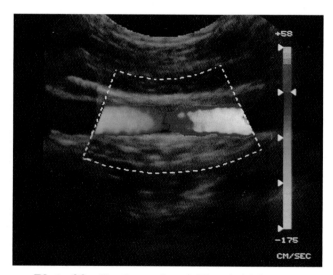

Plate 20   For legend, see Fig. 4-14 in text.

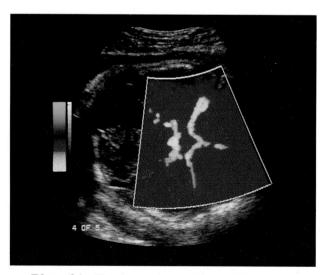

Plate 21   For legend, see Fig. 4-16 in text.

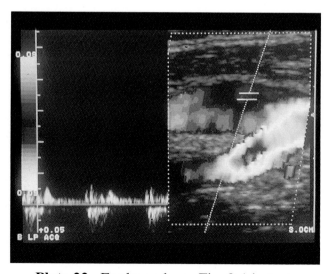

Plate 22   For legend, see Fig. 9-1 in text.

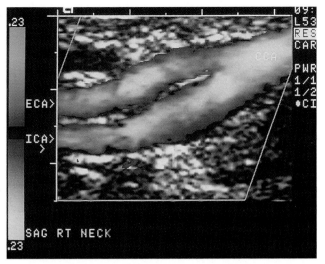

Plate 23 For legend, see Fig. 9-2 in text.

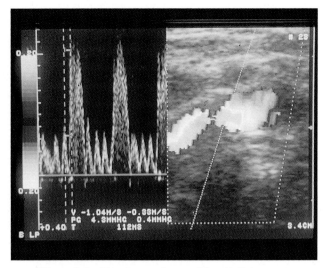

Plate 24 For legend, see Fig. 9-3 in text.

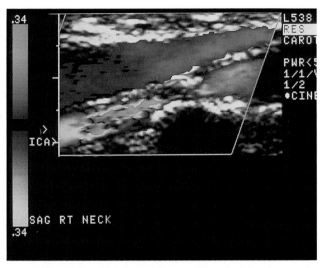

Plate 25 For legend, see Fig. 9-4 in text.

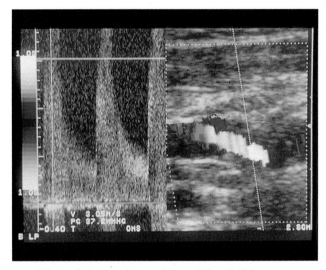

Plate 26 For legend, see Fig. 9-5 in text.

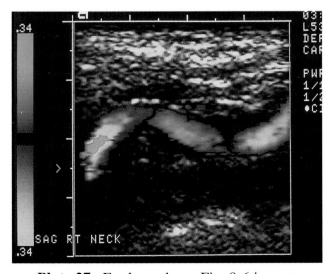

Plate 27 For legend, see Fig. 9-6 in text.

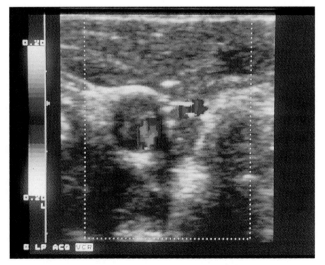

Plate 28 For legend, see Fig. 9-7 in text.

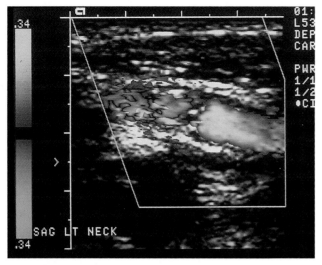

Plate 29 For legend, see Fig. 9-8 in text.

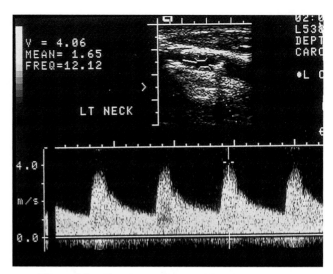

Plate 30 For legend, see Fig. 9-9 in text.

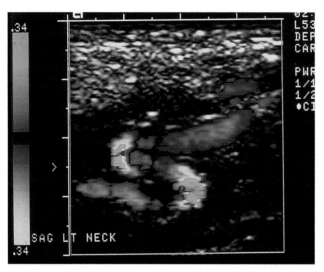

Plate 31 For legend, see Fig. 9-10 in text.

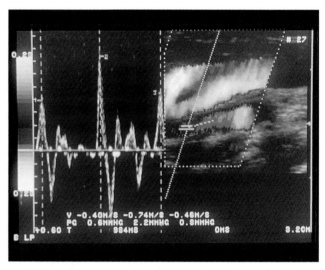

Plate 32 For legend, see Fig. 9-11 in text.

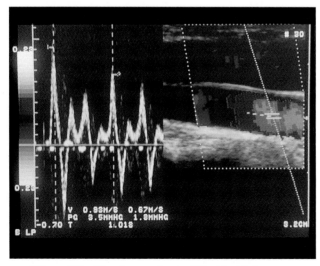

Plate 33 For legend, see Fig. 9-12 in text.

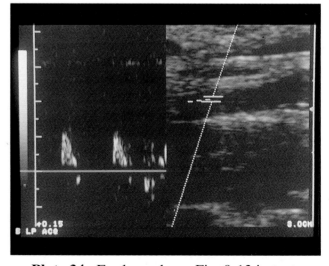

Plate 34 For legend, see Fig. 9-13 in text.

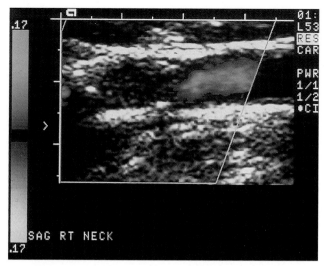

Plate 35 For legend, see Fig. 9-14 in text.

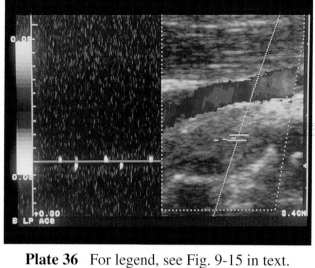

Plate 36 For legend, see Fig. 9-15 in text.

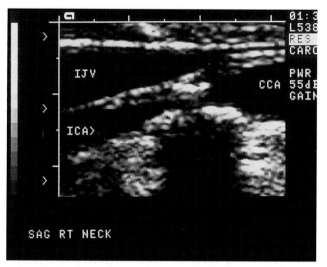

Plate 37 For legend, see Fig. 9-16 in text.

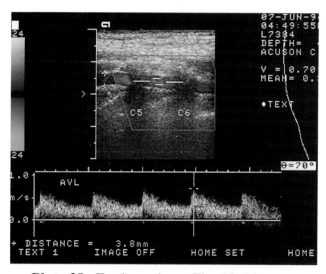

Plate 38 For legend, see Fig. 10-4 in text.

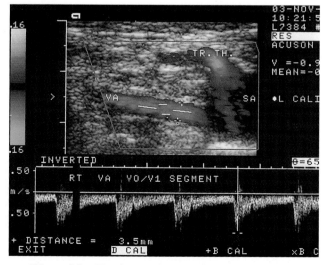

Plate 39 For legend, see Fig. 10-5 in text.

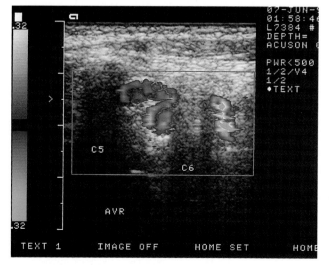

Plate 40 For legend, see Fig. 10-6 in text.

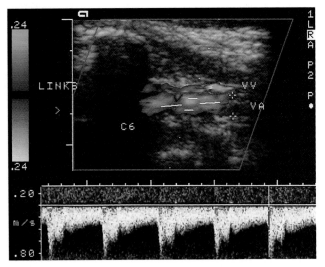

Plate 41 For legend, see Fig. 10-7 in text.

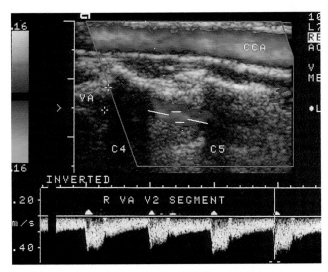

Plate 42 For legend, see Fig. 10-8 in text.

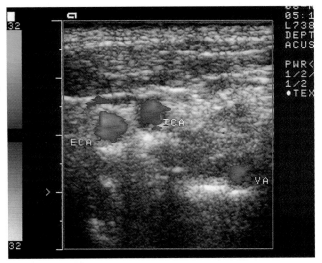

Plate 43 For legend, see Fig. 10-9 in text.

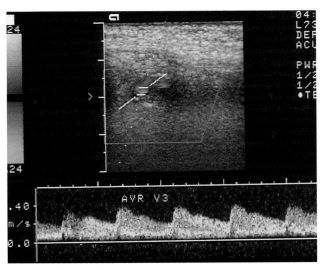

Plate 44 For legend, see Fig. 10-10 in text.

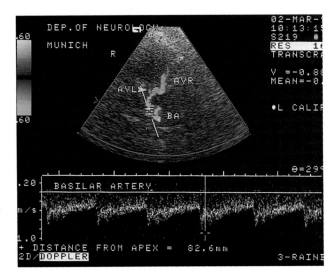

Plate 45 For legend, see Fig. 10-11 in text.

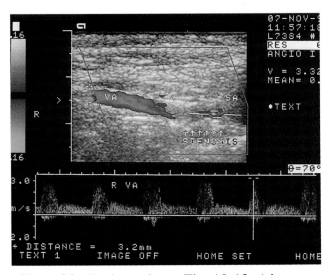

Plate 46 For legend, see Fig. 10-12, *A* in text.

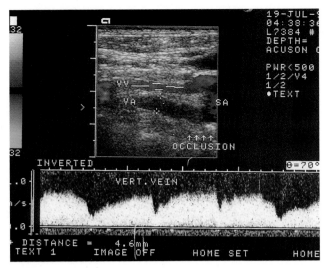

Plate 47 For legend, see Fig. 10-13, *A* in text.

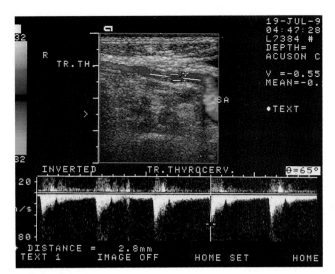

Plate 48 For legend, see Fig. 10-13, *B* in text.

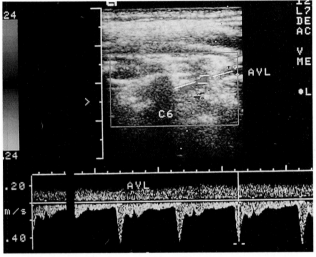

Plate 49 For legend, see Fig. 10-14, *A* in text.

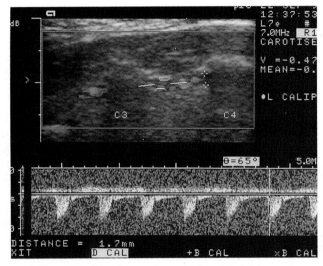

Plate 50 For legend, see Fig. 10-15 in text.

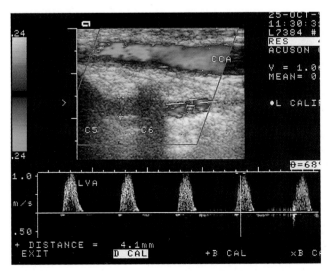

Plate 51 For legend, see Fig. 10-16, *A* in text.

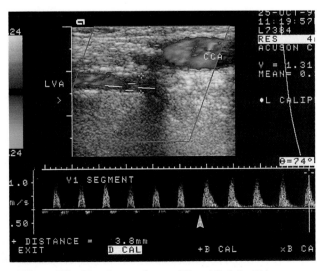

Plate 52 For legend, see Fig. 10-16, *C* in text.

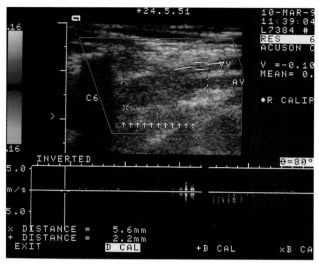

Plate 53 For legend, see Fig. 10-17, *A* in text.

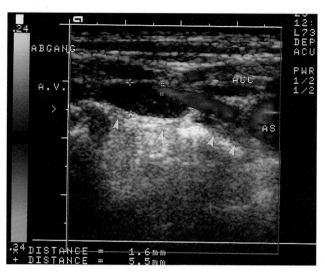

Plate 54 For legend, see Fig. 10-18, *A* in text.

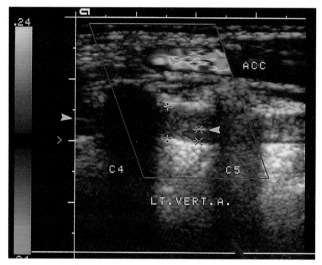

Plate 55 For legend, see Fig. 10-18, *B* in text.

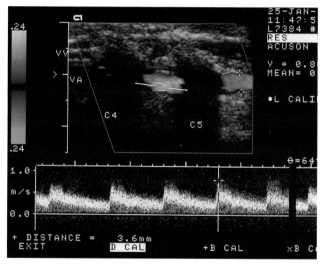

Plate 56 For legend, see Fig. 10-18, *D* in text.

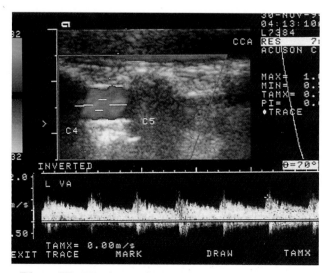

Plate 57 For legend, see Fig. 10-19, *A* in text.

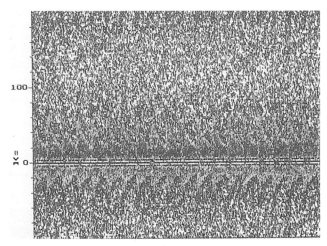

Plate 58 Middle cerebral artery flow velocity baseline values for a healthy subject undergoing cerebral vasoreactivity studies.

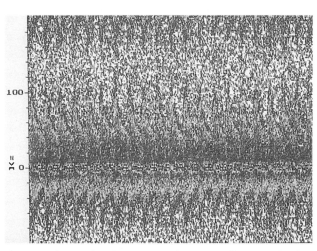

Plate 59 Middle cerebral artery flow velocity values after inhalation of 5% CO_2 for the healthy subject in Plate 58. Notice that flow velocity values have increased markedly.

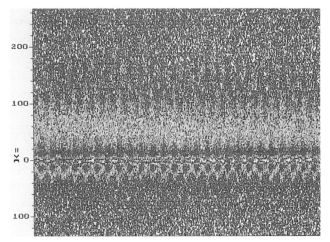

Plate 60 Middle cerebral artery flow velocity baseline values in a patient with bilateral severe carotid stenosis.

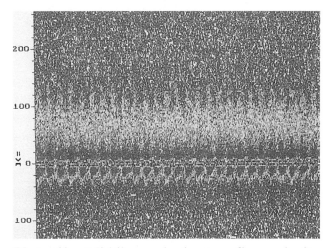

Plate 61 Middle cerebral artery flow velocity values for the patient in Plate 60 after inhalation of 5% CO_2. Notice that flow velocity values are increased only mildly.

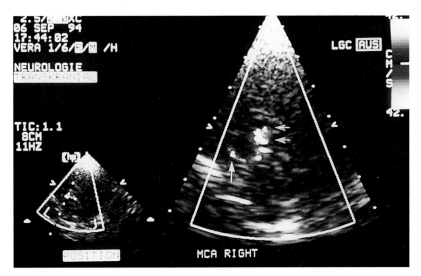

Plate 62 For legend, see Fig. 16-2 in text.

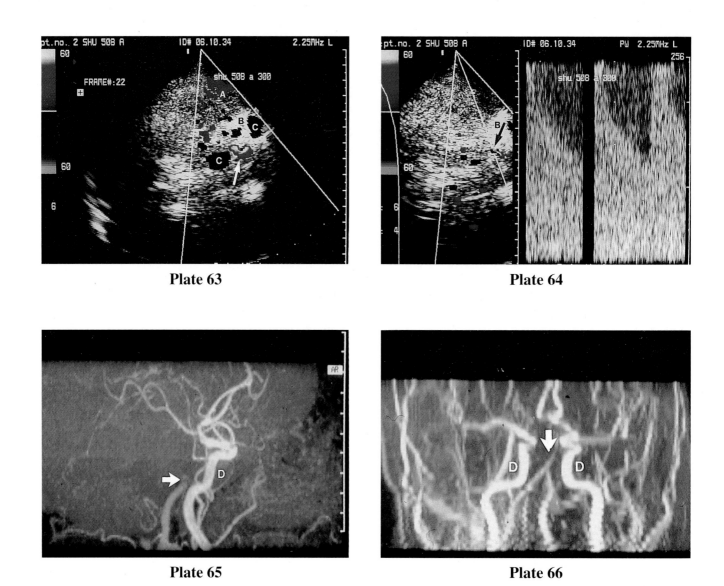

Plate 63   **Plate 64**

Plate 65   **Plate 66**

High-grade distal stenosis of the basilar artery detected by contrast-enhanced TCCS. **Plate 63,** Color Doppler image (semicoronal scan from a transtemporal approach) indicating turbulent high flow velocities in the distal basilar artery (arrow). **Plate 64,** Doppler sample from the stenotic portion of the basilar artery (arrow) demonstrating systolic Doppler flow velocities exceeding 256 cm/sec. Lateral, **Plate 65,** and coronal, **Plate 66,** views of the MRI angiogram of the same patient with loss of signal from the distal portion of the basilar artery indicating minimal net flow. *A* represents temporal lobe branches of the middle cerebral artery; *B* indicates the pyramidal bone; *C* denotes the bulb of the jugular vein; *D* marks the internal carotid artery.

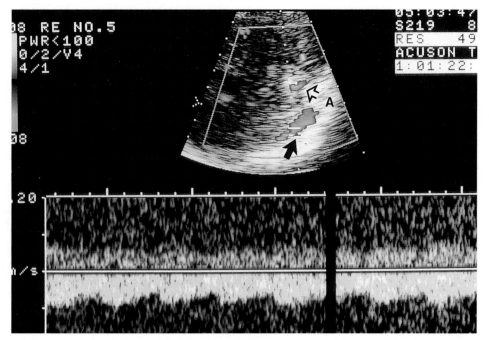

Plate 67

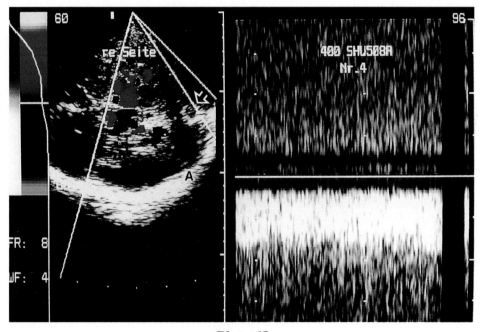

Plate 68

Imaging of the deep venous system by contrast-enhanced TCCS. **Plate 67,** Imaging of the contralateral transverse sinus (arrow) through a transtemporal approach; the open arrowhead denotes the confluence sinuum. **Plate 68,** Color Doppler image and Doppler spectrum of the confluens sinuum through the transtemporal approach (open arrowhead). *A* represents the occipital bone. Non–angle-corrected Doppler flow velocities are 10 and 28 cm/sec. Both studies were obtained after intravenous administration of the contrast agent Levovist (SHU 508 A).

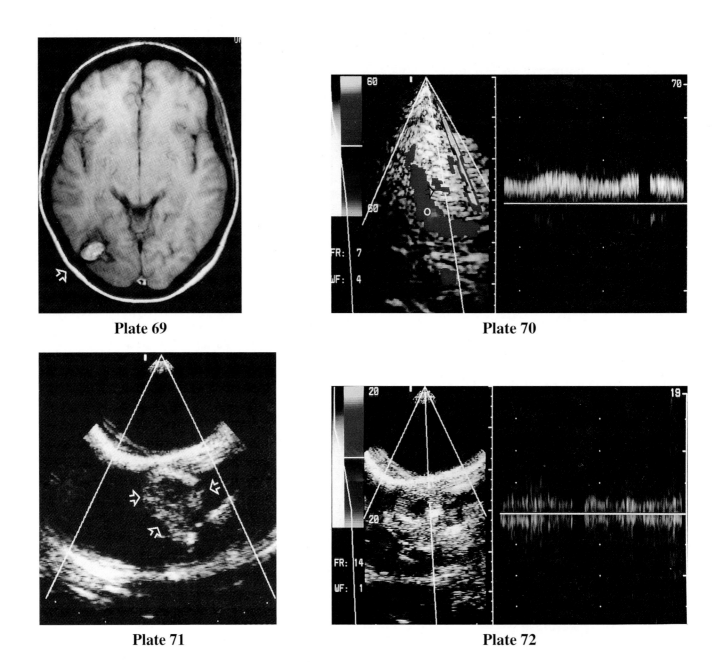

Plate 69

Plate 70

Plate 71

Plate 72

Imaging of intracerebral cavernomas by contrast-enhanced TCCS. **Plate 69,** Proton-density image of a right temporo-occipital cavernoma (arrowhead). **Plate 70,** Contrast-enhanced color Doppler image and Doppler spectrum of the same lesion. The ultrasound approach was through the temporo-occipital bone as indicated by the arrowheads in Plate 69. The Doppler flow velocity was approximately 12 cm/sec and had a venous flow pattern. **Plate 71,** Non–contrast-enhanced intraoperative B-mode and, **Plate 72,** color Doppler image and Doppler spectrum of this lesion (arrowheads in Plate 71). Without contrast-application even intraoperative insonation shows no color flow and marginal artery flow velocities of approximately 3 to 5 cm/sec. *O* denotes a normal cortical artery. The contrast-enhanced study was performed after intravenous administration of Levovist (SHU 508 A).

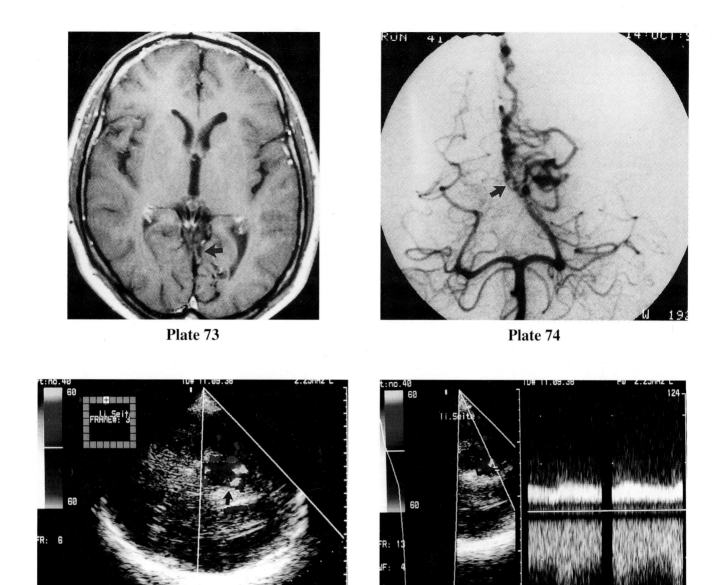

Plate 73

Plate 74

Plate 75

Plate 76

Imaging of intracerebral arteriovenous malformations (AVMs) by contrast-enhanced TCCS. **Plate 73,** Proton-density weighted MRI of a small left occipital paramedian AVM (arrow). **Plate 74,** Digital subtraction angiography of the same case displaying the small AVM (arrow) and a large draining vein. **Plate 75,** Contrast-enhanced color Doppler image of the same lesion (arrow), indicating turbulent flow. **Plate 76,** Doppler spectrum showing bidirectional arterial and venous flow within the AVM. The contrast-enhanced study was performed after intravenous administration of the ultrasound contrast agent Levovist (SHU 508 A).

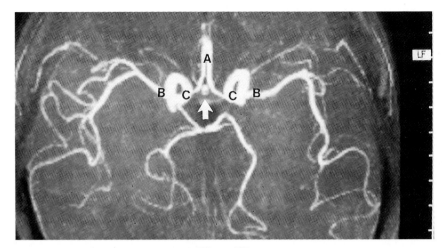

Plate 77

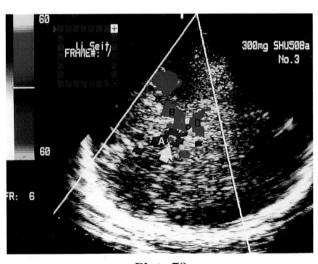

Plate 78

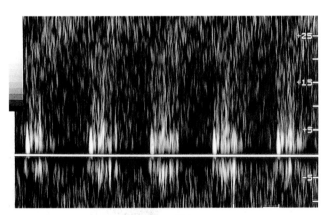

Plate 79

Imaging of intracerebral aneurysm by contrast-enhanced TCCS. **Plate 77,** MRI angiography of a 2.3 mm diameter anterior communicating artery aneurysm (arrow). **Plate 78,** Contrast-enhanced color Doppler image (axial scan) showing aneurysm (arrow). **Plate 79,** Example of a characteristic bidirectional systolic Doppler spectrum from the neck of an aneurysm showing the pulsating back-and-forth movement of the blood column. *A* denotes the anterior cerebral artery; *B* denotes the middle cerebral artery; *C* represents the internal carotid artery; *D* denotes the posterior cerebral artery; *o* marks the posterior communicating artery. The study was performed after intravenous administration of the contrast agent Levovist (SHU 508 A).

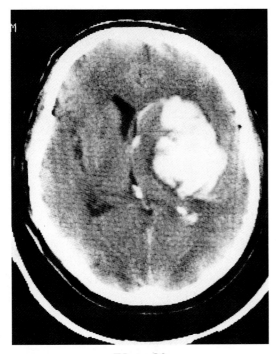

Plate 80

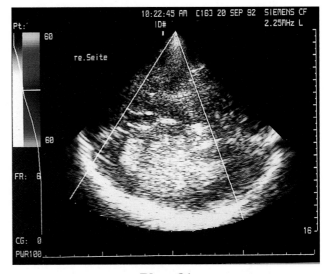

Plate 81

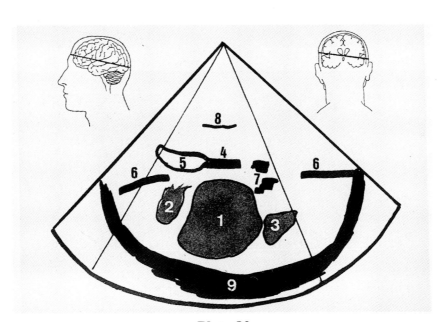

Plate 82

Transcranial color Doppler imaging of cerebral hemorrhages. **Plate 80,** CT image of an extensive hypertensive hematoma with ventricular extension and midline shift. **Plate 81,** TCCS image of the same hematoma. **Plate 82,** Schematic illustration of the TCCS findings: *1*, parenchymal hematoma; *2*, blood within the frontal horn; *3*, trigone of the lateral ventricle; *4*, third ventricle; *5*, contralateral frontal horn of the lateral ventricle; *6*, falx cerebri; *7*, pineal gland and supracerebellar cistern; *8*, sylvian fissure; *9*, contralateral skull.

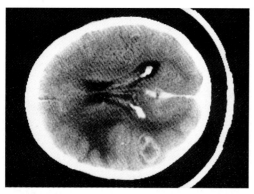

Plate 83

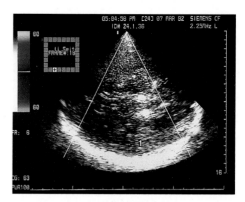

Plate 84

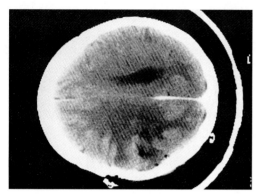

Plate 85

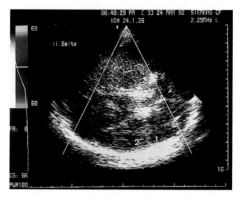

Plate 86

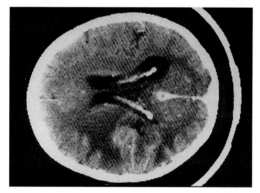

Plate 87

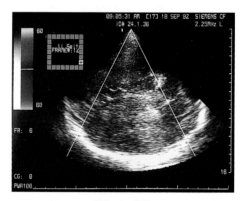

Plate 88

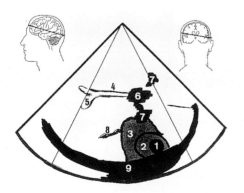

Plate 89

Transcranial color Doppler imaging of intracerebral neoplasms. Preoperative and postoperative CT and TCCS examinations of a patient with parietooccipital glioblastoma. **Plate 83,** Preoperative CT findings: ring-type contrast-enhancing parietooccipital lesion; low density of the white matter indicates peritumoral edema. **Plate 84,** Preoperative TCCS findings: left parietooccipital hyperechogenic lesion, *1*, with nonhomogeneous echotexture, surrounded by a thin hypoechogenic halo. **Plate 85,** Early postoperative CT (first postoperative day): contrast enhancement indicates residual tumor. **Plate 86,** Early postoperative TCCS: anechogenic resection cavity, *1*, surrounded by a hyperechogenic area; *2*, with a non-homogeneous echotexture. **Plate 87,** CT findings 6 months after surgery: extension of the irregular contrast enhancing area at the resection site indicates tumor regrowth. **Plate 88,** TCCS findings 6 months after surgery: large parietooccipital, hyperechogenic lesion closely corresponds to contrast enhancing area on CT and indicates tumor regrowth. **Plate 89,** Schematic illustration of TCCS images (Plates 86 and 88): *1*, resection cavity; *2*, hyperechogenic area after the first postoperative week indicating residual tumor; *3*, hyperechogenic area 6 months after surgery indicating tumor regrowth; *4*, third ventricle; *5*, frontal horn of a lateral ventricle; *6*, pineal gland and supracerebellar cistern; *7*, trigone; *8*, sylvian fissure; *9*, contralateral skull.

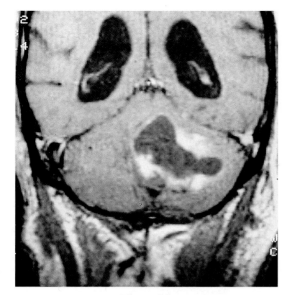

Plate 90

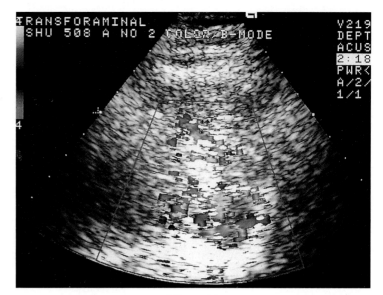

Plate 91

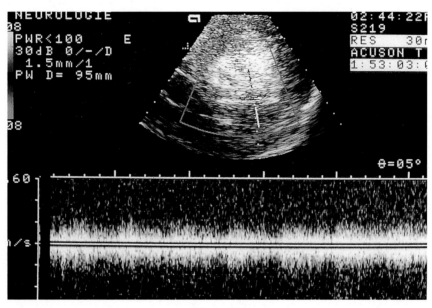

Plate 92

Imaging of intracranial neoplasms by contrast-enhanced TCCS. **Plate 90,** T1-weighted coronal MRI showing a cystic left cerebellar malignant ependymoma. **Plate 91,** Contrast-enhanced color Doppler image showing diffuse, irregular color pixels indicating blood flow in a multitude of directions and covering the hyperechogenic tumor. **Plate 92, upper frame:** the hyperechogenic tumor is seen in the color Doppler image through a transforaminal approach: color pixels covering the tumor are indicative of tumor vascularization; **lower frame:** Doppler spectrum from the tumor, showing atypical venous flow with a velocity of approximately 12 cm/sec.

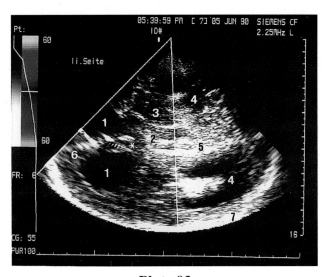

Plate 93

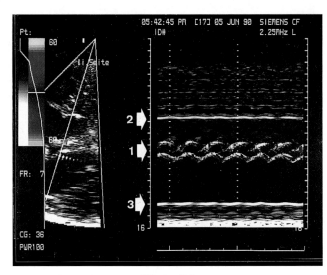

Plate 94

Transcranial color Doppler imaging of hydrocephalus. CT and TCCS findings in a patient with low pressure hydrocephalus. **Plate 93,** TCCS findings — axial scanning plane through the diencephalon: *1*, right and left frontal horns; *, septum pellucidum; *2*, third ventricle; *3*, thalamus; *4*, enlarged trigone and occipital horn of the lateral ventricle; *5*, quadrigeminal cistern; *6*, falx cerebri; *7*, skull. **Plate 94,** M-mode images illustrate a distinct deflection of the septum pellucidum during rotatory head shaking. *1*, septum pellucidum; *2*, ventricular wall of the ipsilateral frontal horn; *3*, ventricular wall of the contralateral frontal horn.

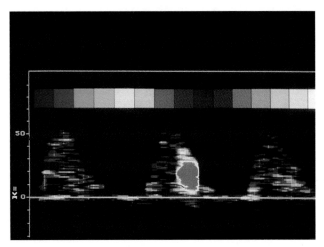

Plate 95   For legend, see Fig. 21-3 in text.

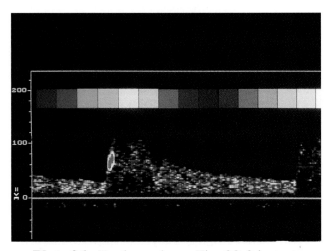

Plate 96   For legend, see Fig. 22-3 in text.

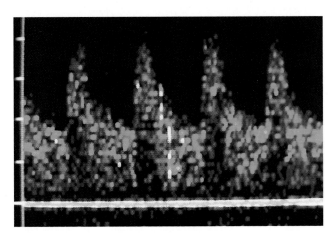

Plate 97 For legend, see Fig. 23-1, *A* in text.

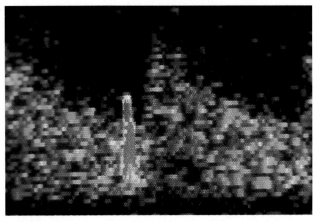

Plate 98 For legend, see Fig. 23-1, *B* in text.

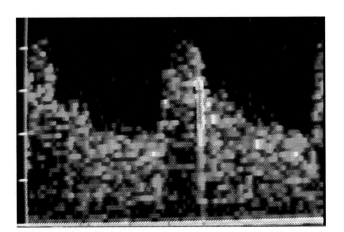

Plate 99 For legend, see Fig. 23-1, *C* in text.

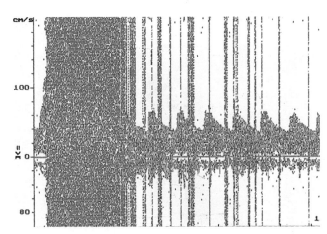

Plate 100 For legend, see Fig. 23-2 in text.

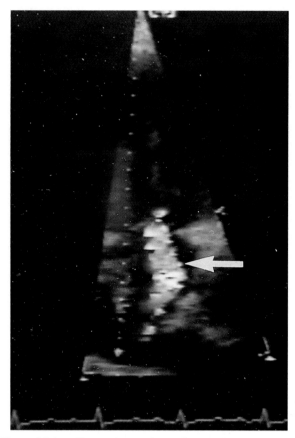

Plate 101 Transthoracic echocardiogram four-chamber view. Note the turbulent jet (arrow) in the left atrium consistent with moderate mitral regurgitation.

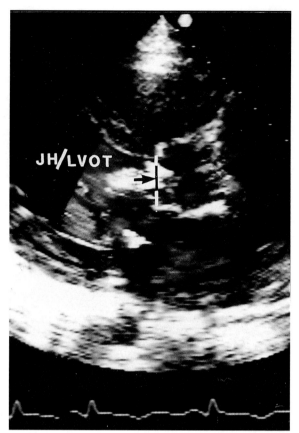

Plate 102 Transthoracic echocardiogram. Evaluation of aortic regurgitation severity. The severity of aortic regurgitation is estimated by color flow Doppler by measuring the ratio of the jet height (JH) divided by the left ventricular outflow tract diameter (LVOT).

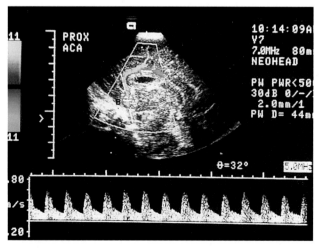

Plate 103 For legend, see Fig. 35-1 in text.

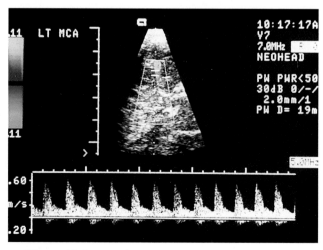

Plate 104 For legend, see Fig. 35-2 in text.

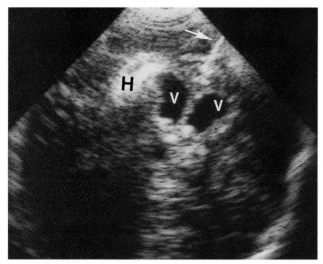

Plate 105   For legend, see Fig. 36-8, *A* in text.

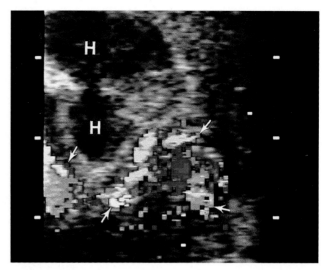

Plate 106   For legend, see Fig. 36-8, *B* in text.

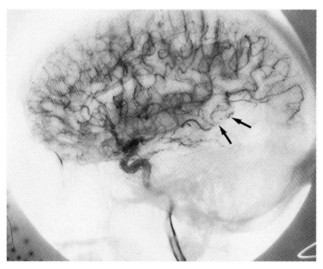

Plate 107   For legend, see Fig. 36-9, *A* in text.

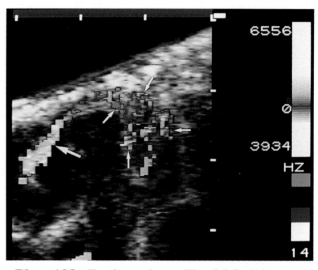

Plate 108   For legend, see Fig. 36-9, *B* in text.

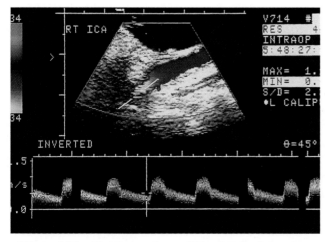

Plate 109   For legend, see Fig. 39-1, *A* in text.

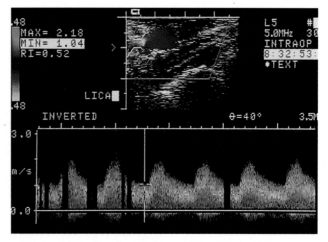

Plate 110   For legend, see Fig. 39-1, *B* in text.

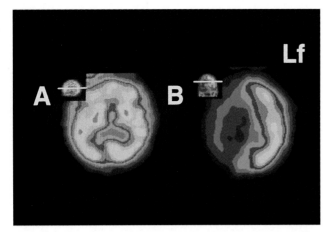

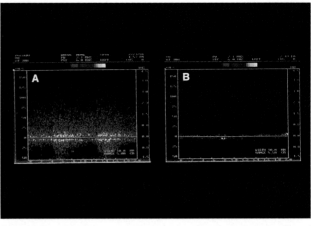

Plate 111 **A,** Single photon emission computed tomography (SPECT) scan of a patient with a right middle cerebral artery distribution infarct in association with a right cavernous carotid artery fistula. **B,** Following angioplastic balloon occlusion of the distal right internal carotid artery, there is more prominent hypoperfusion of the right cerebral hemisphere by SPECT scan.

Plate 112 **A,** The correlative transcranial Doppler ultrasound (TCD) study of the right middle cerebral artery in the patient in Plate 111 prior to occlusion. **B,** Loss of the transcranial Doppler signal of the right middle cerebral artery during the occlusive procedure.

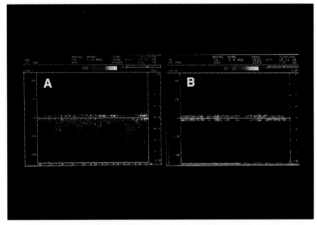

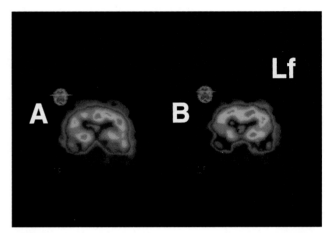

Plate 113 **A,** Transcranial Doppler study of the right ophthalmic artery, which demonstrates a normal flow pattern. **B,** Loss of the flow pattern of the right ophthalmic artery during test angioplastic balloon occlusion of the right internal carotid artery.

Plate 114 **A,** The correlative single photon emission computed tomography (SPECT) scan of the patient illustrated in Plate 113 prior to occlusion of the right internal carotid artery. **B,** The resultant right hemispheric hypoperfusion demonstrated by SPECT following test occlusion of the right internal carotid artery.

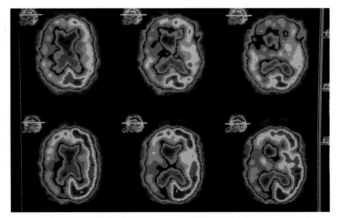

Plate 115 Single photon emission computed tomography (SPECT) scan of a patient with an acute right hemispheric ischemic stroke secondary to meningovascular syphilis. Despite a relatively small right subcortical infarct shown by computed tomographic (CT) brain scan, there is pronounced cerebral hypoperfusion, which is most prominent in the right middle cerebral artery territory. The degree of involvement shown by SPECT correlated with the diffuse nature of the vasculitic changes seen by cerebral arteriography.

25

Transthoracic and Transesophageal Echocardiography

Ramon Castello
Arthur J. Labovitz

Over the past two decades cardiac ultrasound imaging, or echocardiography, has become the technique of choice for noninvasive assessment of cardiac anatomy and function. M-mode, two-dimensional imaging, conventional Doppler, and color flow Doppler are some of the significant improvements in technical modalities that have become available over the years. Although each step improved the previous one, a comprehensive echocardiographic study in the 1990s should include all these modalities in an integrated fashion.

Traditionally, ultrasound evaluation of the heart was restricted to transthoracic studies. In the past few years a semiinvasive technique, transesophageal echocardiography, has become available and widely used in clinical practice. In addition, strictly invasive ultrasound imaging, intravascular echocardiography, has become increasingly popular, although its clinical utility is yet to be established.

In this review, we will discuss the indications and main clinical uses of transthoracic and transesophageal echocardiography.

TECHNICAL ASPECTS OF CARDIAC ULTRASOUND

The main echocardiographic imaging modalities are M-mode and two-dimensional echocardiography. M-mode was the first echocardiographic technique that became available in clinical practice. It has been compared to an ice pick traversing the different structures of the heart and displayed over time. The images are recorded on tape or on paper. By moving the transducer from the base to the apex of the heart, the ultrasound beam traverses different cardiac structures that can be analyzed.[8] Although largely replaced by two-dimensional echocardiography, M-mode recordings are still an essential part of every echocardiographic study. It is especially useful to obtain measurements and dimensions of the main cardiac structures. Also, because of the high frame rate sampling, it is the technique of choice to evaluate the timing of cardiac events. In clinical practice, the M-mode tracings are obtained guiding the ultrasound beam with two-dimensional imaging. The measurements most commonly obtained include the aortic root and the left atrial diameter, the left ventricular end-diastolic and end-systolic diameters, and the ventricular septum and posterior wall thicknesses. These measurements allow an estimation of left ventricular function and left ventricular mass.

Two-dimensional echocardiography is the primary imaging technique available. The ultrasound beam now moves in a sector and is displayed in tomographic two-dimensional "slices" of the heart. By placing the transducer in different positions (windows) and obtaining different orientations (planes), a three-dimensional reconstruction of the heart can be generated. In this way, most cardiac structures can be seen in real time, and not only the dimensions but also their functional anatomy can be evaluated.[24] The standard windows and planes are summarized in Table 25-1.

DOPPLER ECHOCARDIOGRAPHY

The use of Doppler in conjunction with two-dimensional imaging has revolutionized and certainly broadened the information that can be obtained noninvasively. The main advantage of the use of Doppler echocardiography is that hemodynamic information is available and can be added to the anatomic information obtained from the two-dimensional images.

Based on the Doppler principle, the direction and velocity of a moving target (red blood cells) along the ultrasound beam can be obtained. The information is extraordinarily important in the evaluation of valvular heart disease. Through the Doppler technique, pressure gradients derived from the peak and mean velocities through a stenotic valve can be easily calculated. In addition, the evaluation of valvular regurgitation is feasible and easily obtainable. Estimation of cardiac output and assessment of diastolic function can also be performed by using certain Doppler parameters.

Doppler echocardiography comprises three different modes: pulsed, continuous-wave Doppler, and color flow mapping.[24] Pulsed-wave Doppler permits the estimation of the velocity and direction of the blood at a certain point along the Doppler beam, which is determined by the location of the sample volume. The velocities that can be recorded with pulsed Doppler are limited by the pulse repetition frequency of the system. Thus, if the blood is moving very rapidly, as is the case through a stenotic valve, a phenomenon known as *aliasing* occurs, and neither the velocity nor the direction of the blood can be estimated. On the contrary, continuous-wave Doppler allows the estimation of the highest velocity along the Doppler beam. Continuous wave is thus necessary when very high velocities within the cardiovascular system are to be recorded and therefore is most suitable to estimate high pressure gradients between the cardiac or vascular structures (i.e., aortic stenosis).

Table 25-1. Main windows and planes for two-dimensional imaging

Window	Plane	Main cardiac structures
Parasternal	Long axis	Aortic root
		Aortic valve
		Left atrium
		Mitral valve
		Interventricular septum
		Posterior wall
	Short axis (2 levels)	Aortic valve
		Tricuspid valve
		Pulmonary valve
		Pulmonary artery
		Mitral valve
		Papillary muscles
		Left ventricle
Apex	4 chambers	Left and right ventricles
		Mitral, tricuspid, and aortic valves
		Right and left atria
	2 chambers	Mitral valve
		Left ventricle and atrium
	Long axis	Mitral valve
		Aortic valve
		Left ventricle and atrium
Subcostal	4 chambers	Aortic valve
		Tricuspid valve
		Pulmonary valve
		Pulmonary artery
		Mitral valve
		Papillary muscles
		Left and right ventricles
		Right and left atria
	Short axis (2 levels)	Left and right ventricles
		Mitral, tricuspid, and aortic valves
		Right and left atria
Suprasternal notch		Ascending and descending aorta and aortic arch
		Pulmonary artery

Color flow Doppler is a variety of pulsed-wave Doppler.[11] Color flow mapping is created by multiple Doppler gates that interrogate a certain area within the cardiac chambers. In color flow mapping, velocities are encoded in different shades of color, and the direction of the blood is displayed according to a color code. By convention, velocities away from the transducer are depicted in blue, and velocities toward the transducer are depicted in red. Turbulent flows are depicted as a mixture or mosaic of colors or as green (variance). Color flow mapping images can be superimposed on a two-dimensional image or M-mode recording. It is an excellent tool to assess the spatial distribution of flow and therefore is extremely useful for the evaluation of valvular regurgitation. Color flow mapping is also used in conjunction with the other Doppler modalities (pulsed- and continuous-wave) to align the ultrasound beam as parallel as possible to the flow of interest.

TRANSTHORACIC ECHOCARDIOGRAPHY
Technique and normal examination

Transthoracic echocardiographic examination is virtually painless and harmless to the patient. Performing an adequate examination requires a great deal of expertise by the operator, a systematic approach to the cardiac structures, and a careful search for the clinical question. Therefore, prior knowledge of the clinical characteristics of the patients is mandatory for an adequate echocardiographic examination.

Typically, the patient is positioned in the left-lateral decubitus, and the transducer is placed in four different positions or windows, including the left parasternal border, the apex, the subcostal, and the suprasternal notch. The planes or views that can be obtained are standardized into three planes including the long axis, the short axis, and the four-chamber plane. The combination of the four different windows and planes allows a thorough examination of the cardiac anatomy (Table 25-1).

The portability, accessibility, and low cost have made echocardiography a very valuable diagnostic tool, not only in the echocardiography laboratory but also in the emergency room, intensive care units, and the operating room setting. The indications for transthoracic echocardiographic studies are multiple and varied. When heart disease is suspected, echocardiographic studies are an essential part of the evaluation and assessment of the disease. This review summarizes the main indications in four large areas, including evaluation of ventricular function, ischemic heart disease, valvular heart disease, and cardiac masses and tumors.

Evaluation of ventricular mass and function

Left ventricular (LV) mass can be accurately calculated from M-mode-derived parameters.[21] In addition to the end-diastolic diameter (EDD), the septal (VST) and posterior wall diastolic thickness (PWT) are measured and arranged in the formula as follows:

$$\text{LV mass} = 0.83 \times [(\text{EDD} + \text{VST} + \text{PWT})^3 - \text{EDD}^3]$$

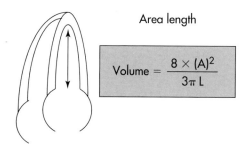

Fig. 25-1. Schematic representing the area-length method for calculating left ventricular volumes. The volume is directly proportional to the area (A) obtained from the four-chamber view, divided by the length (L) from the mitral annulus to the left ventricular apex.

The assessment of left and right ventricular function and performance is an essential part of the cardiac evaluation. Echocardiography provides a simple method to assess noninvasively the right and left ventricular function, and therefore multiple echocardiographic parameters have been developed over the years for this purpose.

When only M-mode echocardiography was available, the end-systolic diameter (ESD) and end-diastolic diameters were routinely obtained, and the shortening fraction was used as a rough estimate of left ventricular function and contractility. In patients with normal hearts, this parameter correlated closely with the ejection fraction obtained by angiographic or radionuclide methods. The shortening fraction is calculated as follows:

$$\text{Shortening fraction } (\%) = \frac{\text{EDD} - \text{ESD}}{\text{EDD}} \times 100$$

With the advent of two-dimensional echocardiography, a better assessment of the left ventricular walls and geometry could be obtained. By delineating the endocardium from two or three orthogonal planes, calculations of the left ventricular volumes can be obtained by applying certain geometric assumptions. One of the most popular methods is the area-length method. With two-dimensional echocardiography, this method is usually applied from the four-chamber view (Fig. 25-1). Another formula, the Simpsons rule, is especially attractive because it minimizes the effect of geometric shape for calculating volumes. The modified Simpsons formula includes the four-chamber view and two short axis views at the papillary muscle and the mitral valve level. By including all these planes, accurate calculations of left ventricular volumes, even in ventricles with distorted geometry, such as in valvular or ischemic heart disease, can be obtained.[1] When the systolic (ESV) and diastolic volumes (EDV) are known,

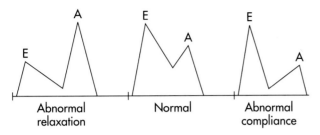

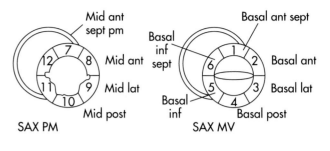

Fig. 25-2. A schematic of normal and abnormal patterns of mitral flow obtained by pulsed-wave Doppler. Note the difference between diastolic dysfunction due to abnormal relaxation or abnormal compliance (restrictive pattern).

the ejection fraction (EF) can be easily obtained by applying the formula:

$$EF\ (\%) = \frac{EDV - ESV}{EDV} \times 100$$

The ejection fraction is a very useful parameter in clinical practice and therefore is routinely obtained in every echocardiographic examination.

Evaluation of diastolic function

The diastolic phase of the cardiac cycle is a rather complex and multifactorial process that requires energy and is responsible for the adequate filling of the heart. Therefore, the evaluation of diastolic function has been difficult and characterized by the lack of simple and accurate indexes of such function. During the past decade there has been a substantial effort to evaluate diastolic function noninvasively. The analysis of the left ventricular inflow or mitral flow by Doppler echocardiography has been promising in such evaluation.

The normal left ventricular inflow pattern by pulsed-wave Doppler is characterized by an early (E) wave, corresponding to early left ventricular filling, and a late (A) wave, corresponding to atrial contraction. Diastolic abnormalities include abnormal relaxation or abnormal compliance of the left ventricle. Although with certain and well-known limitations, the analysis of the mitral inflow by Doppler echocardiography can be useful to estimate these abnormalities.[13]

The classic pattern for abnormal relaxation consists of a reduced E wave and an increased A wave resulting in a reduced E:A ratio (Fig. 25-2). This type of abnormality is most commonly seen in patients with left ventricular hypertrophy, hypertension, or coronary artery disease. The other classic abnormal pattern of left ventricular diastolic dysfunction—the restrictive or abnormal compliance pattern—is characterized by a high E wave and a low A wave, resulting in an abnormally increased E:A ratio. This restrictive pattern can be seen in patients with elevated left ventricular end-diastolic pressure, severe mitral regurgitation, or constrictive pericarditis. Unfor-

Fig. 25-3. Schematic representation for the regional wall motion analysis of the left ventricle. The segments are obtained from the short axis view at the papillary muscle level (SAX PM), the mitral valve level (SAX MV), and the apical level (SAX AP). *ant,* anterior; *mid,* midventricular; *inf,* inferior; *lat,* lateral; *post,* posterior.

tunately, the influence of filling pressure on transmitral flow patterns often makes interpretation difficult.

More recently, the analysis of the pulmonary vein flow in conjunction with the mitral inflow appears promising for a more detailed and comprehensive evaluation of left ventricular function by Doppler echocardiography.[5]

Ischemic heart disease: evaluation of global and segmental wall motion

Myocardial ischemia is known to induce abnormalities of the left ventricular wall mechanics and contractility. These wall motion abnormalities can be readily detected by two-dimensional echocardiography, and therefore the evaluation of the segmental wall motion has resulted in the widespread use of echocardiography in patients with coronary artery disease.

A resting echocardiogram can be useful to confirm the diagnosis in patients with suspected coronary artery disease by detecting severe regional wall motion abnormalities. More recently, two-dimensional echocardiography has been used in conjunction with exercise to detect ischemia-induced wall motion abnormalities during exercise. In patients unable to exercise, pharmacologic agents such as dipyridamole or dobutamine are used in conjunction with two-dimensional echocardiography for the stress-induced wall motion abnormalities.

For a thorough evaluation of left ventricular wall motion analysis, the ventricle is divided in segments related to the coronary artery supply (Fig. 25-3). To visualize every left ventricular segment, it is necessary to obtain different planes from different echocardiographic views. The contractility of each of these segments is evaluated, and a semiquantitative score is assigned to them. The most common assessment includes normal movement, hypokinesis, akinesis, and dyskinesis. In this fashion, the higher the left ventricular score, the poorer the left ventricular function. Advantages for using the score include the adequate comparison of preintervention and postintervention left ventricular contractility, or the follow-up of patients with certain regional wall motion abnormalities.[12]

A more accurate and precise way to evaluate regional wall motion is a computer-based quantitative approach. These methods, although accurate, are tedious and cumbersome. The most common ones evaluate the endocardial motion and express regional left ventricular function as shortening fraction or systolic wall thickening, which indicates the percent increase in thickness of the wall during systole. These calculations are traditionally done off-line and are quite time-consuming.

Recently, some of the commercially available ultrasound instruments have incorporated systems that automatically detect the endocardial borders and are able to compute and generate on-line ejection fractions, although they do not perform regional wall motion analysis.[19] The accuracy of these systems and therefore their widespread application in clinical practice are still under investigation.

Evaluation of valvular disease

In the past, the diagnosis and evaluation of patients with suspected valvular disease had been accomplished with cardiac catheterization and angiography. Unfortunately, patients with valvular disease require frequent examinations that ideally should be done noninvasively. Since the advent of cardiac ultrasound, special emphasis was placed on the ability of this technique to diagnose valvular heart disease. One of the earliest reported uses of M-mode echocardiography was the diagnosis of mitral stenosis. Two-dimensional echocardiography was also useful in the identification of the etiology and delineation of the anatomy of the cardiac valves. Because of the lack of hemodynamic information provided, only the impact of the pressure or volume overload on the cardiac chambers could be assessed by cardiac imaging.

The introduction of Doppler echocardiography resulted in a marked improvement in the evaluation of patients with valvular heart disease. By measuring the velocities across the valves by continuous-wave Doppler, the pressure gradients through a stenosed valve can be easily calculated, based on the Bernoulli equation. In addition, pulsed Doppler and color flow Doppler are extremely useful in the evaluation of patients with valvular regurgitation.

Mitral valve disease: mitral stenosis

The detection of mitral stenosis was the first clinical application of echocardiography. Rheumatic heart dis-

ease, the most common cause of mitral stenosis, produces thickening, decreased movement, and calcification of the mitral valve and the mitral valve apparatus. These abnormalities can be detected by M-mode echocardiography. Classical signs of mitral stenosis by M-mode echocardiography include high amplitude and multiple echoes on the mitral valve, suggesting thickening and calcification. The motion of the leaflets is typically restricted, and there is characteristic motion of the posterior leaflet during diastole, parallel to the anterior leaflet.

Two-dimensional echocardiography allows a better delineation of the mitral leaflets and especially of the mitral valve apparatus. The thickening and restricted motion are also noted, and the leaflets exhibit a characteristic doming during diastole. The presence of doming is very useful in distinguishing a truly stenotic valve from one that opens poorly due to low cardiac output. In addition, the mitral valve area can be planimetered from the short-axis view.

Two-dimensional echocardiography is also very useful to detect the consequences of these mitral valve abnormalities on the cardiac chambers. The left atrium is usually enlarged in patients with mitral stenosis, and the size can be measured from multiple planes. Two-dimensional echocardiography is also useful to detect left atrial thrombus, a common complication in patients with mitral stenosis and atrial fibrillation.

Doppler echocardiography provides the most accurate way to calculate the mitral valve area and pressure gradient through the mitral valve.[16] By placing the continuous-wave Doppler beam through the mitral valve, the highest velocities can be recorded. The classic pattern of mitral stenosis is characterized by high early velocities with a flattened decay throughout diastole, indicating a high gradient between the left atrium and the left ventricle during diastole. The mitral valve area can be calculated according to Hatle's formula as follows:

$$\text{Mitral valve area} = \frac{220}{\text{Pressure half-time}}$$

where the pressure half-time is the time it takes the earliest diastolic gradient to be halved. In addition to the mitral valve area, the peak instantaneous gradient and the mean gradient can be calculated by using the modified Bernoulli equation:

$$\text{Gradient (mm Hg)} = 4 \times \text{Velocity}^2$$

Mitral regurgitation

Ischemic heart disease, mitral valve prolapse, mitral annular calcification, and a dilated left ventricle are some of the most common causes for mitral regurgitation. Although two-dimensional echocardiography is certainly limited for the quantitation of mitral regurgitation, it is extremely useful for the identification of the etiology of the valvular insufficiency. In addition, both M-mode and two-dimensional echocardiography provide useful indices of the impact of the volume overload on the left ventricular size and function.

Mitral regurgitation is usually quantitated by color flow mapping. Mitral regurgitation is diagnosed in the presence of an abnormal turbulent color jet detected in the left atrium during systole (see Plate 101). Multiple methods have been used to quantitate mitral regurgitation by Doppler echocardiography. The most common is to obtain the highest regurgitant jet area to the left atrial area ratio from three orthogonal planes. A ratio of less than 20% is considered mild mitral regurgitation, a ratio between 20% and 40% is considered moderate, and above 40% is considered severe.

Because of the limitations and multiple factors affecting the color flow jet area, other new methods have recently been tested and employed in clinical practice. One of them is the calculation of the regurgitant fraction by Doppler echocardiography. It is easily obtained with pulsed-wave Doppler by calculating the stroke volume through the mitral valve and through the aortic valve.

A new method for quantitation of valvular regurgitation by color flow Doppler is being intensively studied. This method, based on the proximal isovelocity surface area (PISA), appears very promising because it is independent of some of the inherent limitations of color flow mapping. However, the clinical utility of this particular method is yet to be established.[3]

Aortic valve disease; aortic stenosis

Congenital bicuspid aortic valve, rheumatic heart disease, and degenerative calcific senile aortic valve are the most common etiologies for aortic stenosis. Two-dimensional echocardiography is useful to identify the etiology of aortic stenosis. Highly echogenic, thickened aortic cusps and restricted motion with decreased opening are some of the classic echocardiographic findings of this valvular abnormality. Before Doppler echocardiography was available, the estimation of the severity of the stenosis was roughly assessed by evaluating the degree of left ventricular hypertrophy. With the advent of Doppler echocardiography, the severity of aortic stenosis can be easily quantitated and expressed in terms of peak and mean transvalvular gradient and aortic valve area.

Peak and mean gradients are the most easily obtainable parameters to quantitate aortic stenosis. The noninvasive assessment of these transvalvular gradients is based on the modified Bernoulli equation:

$$\text{Gradient} = 4 \times (V_{MAX}^2 - V_{LVOT}^2)$$

where V_{MAX} = maximal velocity across the aortic valve and V_{LVOT} = velocity at the left ventricular outflow

tract. These gradients have been shown to correlate closely with the transvalvular gradients obtained at cardiac catheterization.

Patients with impaired left ventricular function may exhibit low transvalvular gradients despite the presence of severe stenosis. In these patients, calculation of the aortic valve area may actually better reflect the severity of the aortic valve stenosis. The calculation of this particular parameter is accomplished by applying the continuity equation and most accurately estimates the severity of aortic stenosis.[15]

Aortic regurgitation

Left ventricular dilatation, increased shortening fraction, fluttering of the anterior mitral leaflet, and shortening of the mitral valve opening are some of the classic M-mode signs of aortic regurgitation. Two-dimensional echocardiography is helpful in determining the etiology of aortic insufficiency and in evaluating the left ventricular response to the volume overload imposed by the aortic regurgitation.

Doppler echocardiography is extremely useful in the quantitation of aortic regurgitation. Pulsed- and continuous-wave Doppler and color flow mapping can be used in the estimation of aortic regurgitation severity. By mapping the left ventricle below the aortic valve, one may estimate the severity of aortic regurgitation by pulsed wave Doppler echocardiography. Continuous-wave Doppler is useful in separating mild from severe degrees of aortic regurgitation, by evaluating the steepness of the slope of the aortic regurgitation Doppler signal.

Color flow mapping is the most common method to estimate aortic regurgitation noninvasively.[20] By measuring the width of the regurgitant jet and its relation to the left ventricular outflow tract diameter, one may estimate and accurately identify mild, moderate, and severe aortic regurgitation (see Plate 102).

Infective endocarditis

Although a clinical diagnosis, echocardiography plays an increasing role in the diagnosis and management of this valvular disease. Echocardiography allows the visualization of vegetations that appear as echo-dense masses attached to the infected valve. The vegetations must be approximately 3 to 4 mm in diameter before they can be appreciated on a transthoracic echocardiogram.

In patients with suspected endocarditis, the clinical scenario has to be taken into account for the adequate use of the ultrasound examination. Active vegetations cannot be distinguished from chronic, healed vegetations echocardiographically. More important, in patients with myxomatous valve degeneration, thickened and highly mobile subvalvular structures may be difficult to distinguish from infected vegetations.

Echocardiography is not only useful in the diagnosis of this valvular disease but also in the early detection of complications.[22] One of the most challenging, the presence of intracardiac abscesses can be detected by echocardiography; they appear as echo-free spaces in the vicinity of the valve ring. In addition, some recent studies suggest that echocardiography may be useful in identifying patients who are more prone to sustain embolic events as a consequence of the disease. Size and mobility of the vegetations are useful indices for such risk stratification.

Cardiac tumors and thrombi

The identification of cardiac tumors and masses have been greatly enhanced by the use of echocardiography. The clinical importance of intracardiac thrombi lies primarily in their potential to embolize. Intracardiac thrombi rarely cause clinical manifestations independent of embolization, and therefore their identification places the patient in a higher-risk subgroup.

Thrombus formation usually requires stasis of the blood and a low flow state. In the cardiac chambers, thrombi are most commonly found in the left ventricle and atrium. Abnormal left ventricular function secondary to myocardial infarction or dilated cardiomyopathy favors the occurrence of left ventricular mural thrombus. In the left atrium, left atrial enlargement, mitral valve disease, and atrial fibrillation are the most common predisposing factors.

Left ventricular thrombi appear as discrete echo-dense masses along the endocardial surface in the left ventricle. Their acoustic density varies and is usually different from the adjacent myocardium. Thrombi occur most commonly at the cardiac apex (Fig. 25-4). Observing the thrombus in more than one echocardiographic view is usually required to make the diagnosis. Echocardiography is useful to estimate the age of the thrombus and probably its potential to embolize. Fresh thrombi exhibit and acoustic density that is very similar to that of the myocardium and usually have a tendency to change their shape. Chronic thrombi have well-defined borders and are sometimes calcified and therefore highly echogenic.

Echocardiography has been extensively used to assess the risk of embolization in patients with predisposing factors such as myocardial infarction. Studies have shown that protruding and highly mobile left ventricular thrombi are more likely to be associated with embolic phenomena. The presence of hyperkinesia in the adjacent myocardial walls is also considered a risk factor.[9]

Left atrial thrombi can be detected by transthoracic echocardiography, although the limitations of this technique have been long recognized. More important, the inability of transthoracic echocardiography to image the left atrial appendage adequately results in a consider-

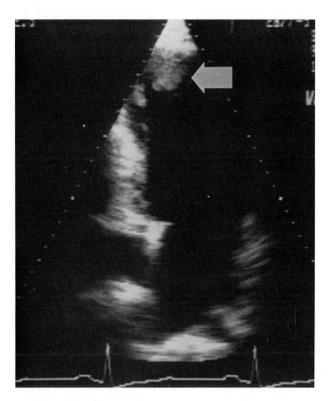

Fig. 25-4. Transthoracic echocardiogram four-chamber view. Note the highly echogenic mass *(arrow)* at the left ventricular apex consistent with thrombus.

able decrease in sensitivity, as left atrial thrombi frequently occur in this location. Numerous studies have shown that transesophageal echocardiography is consistently more sensitive than transthoracic echocardiography for diagnosing left atrial thrombus. Unlike left ventricular thrombi, which usually does not need further confirmation, patients with suspected left atrial thrombus by transthoracic echocardiography may undergo transesophageal echocardiography for confirmation.[17]

Although rare, most cardiac tumors can be detected by two-dimensional echocardiography. Myxomas are the most common primary benign tumors and are typically detected in the left atrium. Myxomas usually have a stalk attached to the interatrial septum (Fig. 25-5). They are highly mobile and may cause obstruction of the mitral valve. Myxomas can also occur in the left ventricle and right atrium and ventricle.

The histologic type of cardiac tumors cannot be determined by their echocardiographic appearance. However, some of the characteristics in relation to their location within the heart may be useful for the initial assessment of these tumors. Diagnostic confirmation often requires open-heart surgery.

TRANSESOPHAGEAL ECHOCARDIOGRAPHY

Introduced clinically in the United States in the late 1980s, transesophageal echocardiography has estab-

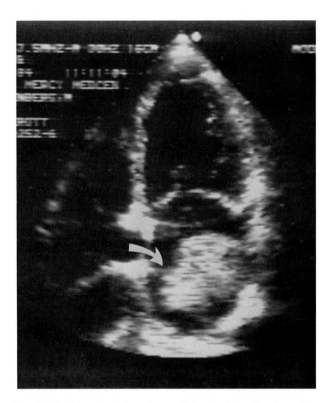

Fig. 25-5. Transthoracic echocardiogram, four-chamber view, showing a large left atrial myxoma. Note the characteristic thin attachment to the interatrial septum *(arrow).*

lished itself as a valuable diagnostic tool, particularly in the evaluation of patients in whom standard transthoracic echocardiography has significant limitations.

Technical aspects

Transesophageal echocardiography utilizes a transducer mounted at the tip of a modified flexible gastroscope. To obtain adequate imaging planes of the heart, the gastroscope is passed into the esophagus and stomach with controls to manipulate the probe tip in both the anteroposterior and lateral planes. Since its introduction, transesophageal echocardiography has rapidly evolved technologically. Single-plane transesophageal echocardiography was the first available, followed by biplane and currently by multiplane transesophageal probes. Common to all these three modalities is the transducer at the tip of the gastroscope and a handle mechanism to control the probe tip, which allows up to 90° of forward flexion or retroflexion. In most probes, another knob allows up to 65° of lateral rotation. The gastroscope is connected to a standard echocardiographic machine, and most current systems have M-mode and two-dimensional imaging capabilities, along with pulsed continuous wave and color flow Doppler.[14]

Performance of the study

Studies should be performed by a physician with adequate training in this particular technique. Patients are asked to fast for at least 4 to 6 hours prior to the procedure. In the operating room or intensive care unit setting, intubated patients can be imaged as well, even with a nasogastric tube in place.

Mild intravenous sedation is usually required and most commonly accomplished with midazolam, meperidine or a combination thereof. Anesthesia of the hypopharynx is obtained by spraying locally with lidocaine or benzocaine.

After inserting the biteblock and following lubrication, the probe is introduced into the esophagus. Images are obtained at the upper and lower esophageal level and from the stomach. By gentle manipulation of the probe, including rotation, flexion, and extension of the tip, the appropriate planes are obtained.

When the transesophageal study is performed, the main clinical question should be answered first. Thereafter, a thorough and detailed examination of the other structures of the heart should be attempted. Typically, a complete study lasts 15 to 30 minutes.

Clinical indications

There are a variety of clinical situations in which transesophageal echocardiography can provide important diagnostic information. In general, they involve regions of the heart or great vessels that may not be optimally visualized by other imaging techniques. The close proximity of the transducer, the relative lack of acoustic impedance, and the possibility of using high frequency transducers (5 MHz) are the main reasons why transesophageal echocardiography provides excellent imaging of the heart.

The clinical indications for transesophageal echocardiographic studies may vary from institution to institution. Figure 25-6 summarizes our experience in a consecutive series of 1000 cases.

Valvular heart disease

Mitral and aortic valve disease. The close proximity of the transesophageal transducer to the posterior aspect of the heart allows a very detailed and accurate visualization of the mitral valve. For mitral valve stenosis, the characteristics of the leaflets, such as thickening, calcification, and pliability, are evaluated similarly with transesophageal or transthoracic echocardiography. In the evaluation of the submitral apparatus, there is no substantial advantage of transesophageal over transthoracic echocardiography. Complications of mitral stenosis, such as left atrial or left atrial appendage thrombus, are much more frequently detected with transesophageal echocardiography.

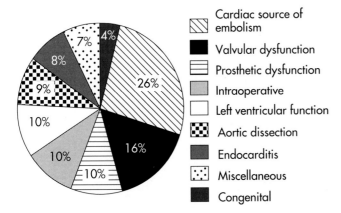

Fig. 25-6. Main indications for transesophageal echocardiographic studies at Saint Louis University Hospital.

In the evaluation of mitral regurgitation, transesophageal echocardiography is clearly superior to transthoracic echocardiographic studies.[4] Again, the proximity of the transducer to the left atrium and the fact that the mitral regurgitant jet is directed toward the transducer result in transesophageal studies being exquisitely sensitive to diagnose this abnormality. Actually, transesophageal echocardiography is more sensitive than cardiac catheterization to detect mitral regurgitation. As compared to transthoracic echocardiography, transesophageal studies provide a more accurate estimation of the severity of mitral regurgitation. In addition, in some cases, such as suspected papillary muscle rupture or flail mitral leaflet, transesophageal echocardiography can be more accurate to establish the etiology of mitral regurgitation. Quantitation of mitral regurgitation is usually based on the maximal regurgitant area. Evaluation of pulmonary venous flow, with special attention to the occurrence of systolic flow reversal, can be very useful in grading mitral regurgitation with this technique.[6]

The evaluation of the aortic valve can also be accomplished with transesophageal echocardiography. Although there is no clear-cut advantage of this technique over conventional transthoracic echocardiography for the assessment and quantitation of stenosis or regurgitation, morphologic assessment of the valve (e.g., two or three leaflets), as well as determination of structural abnormalities causing dysfunction, can be facilitated by transesophageal echocardiography.

Evaluation of prosthetic valves. Transthoracic echocardiography is limited in the evaluation of prosthetic mitral valves. The interaction of the ultrasound beam with the prosthetic material, especially in the case of mechanical prostheses, results in overshadowing of the left atrium, which precludes an adequate evaluation of mitral regurgitation.

Transesophageal echocardiography has been shown to be superior to transthoracic echocardiography in the evaluation of prosthetic mitral dysfunction. In a biologic valve prosthesis, the cusps can be very easily imaged, and abnormalities such as excessive thickening or torn cusps can be readily detected. With a mechanical prosthesis, the superiority of transesophageal echocardiography is even more evident. Because of lack of overshadowing and interference of the ultrasound beam with the material of the prosthesis, the evaluation of mitral regurgitation (perivalvular or valvular) can be easily accomplished.

An important complication of mechanical mitral prosthesis is thrombosis, which is also easily detected with transesophageal echocardiography because thrombi usually form on the atrial side of the prosthesis. Transesophageal echocardiography has been successfully used to manage patients with prosthetic thrombosis with thrombolytic therapy. Therefore, in patients in whom mitral prosthetic dysfunction is clinically suspected, a transesophageal echocardiogram is mandatory.[2]

Transesophageal echocardiography is also used to evaluate aortic valve prostheses, although the advantages over transthoracic studies are not as obvious as in the case of the mitral prosthesis.

Infective endocarditis. Both transesophageal and transthoracic echocardiography have been shown to be very useful in the evaluation of patients with suspected endocarditis. Both techniques can detect the presence of vegetations in both native and prosthetic valves. However, transesophageal echocardiography is more sensitive not only for the detection of the vegetations but also for the diagnosis of associated complications such as abscesses and fistulae. The better evaluation of the morphologic characteristics of the vegetations provides prognostic information with regard to emboligenicity of the vegetations (Fig. 25-7).

A very important advantage of transesophageal echocardiography is the detection of subaortic complications in patients with aortic valve endocarditis. Transesophageal studies have shown that these abnormalities are present in more than one third of these patients.[10]

Diseases of the thoracic aorta

Aortic dissection was one of the first clinical indications for transesophageal echocardiographic studies. The descending aorta, aortic arch, and most of the ascending aorta can be very accurately imaged with transesophageal echocardiography. Therefore, aortic dissection with its characteristic intimal flap is one of the clinical conditions in which transesophageal echocardiography can be most useful (Fig. 25-8). Transesophageal echocardiography has been shown to be more sensitive than computerized tomographic scan and aortography for this important diagnosis. A recent study showed that

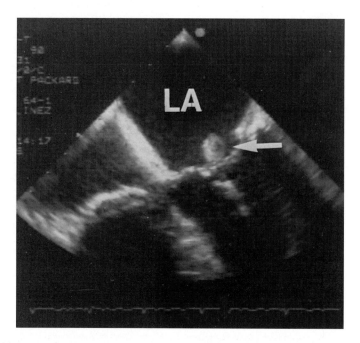

Fig. 25-7. Transesophageal echocardiogram modified four-chamber view. Note a highly echogenic mass at the left atrial side of the mitral valve consistent with infected vegetation.

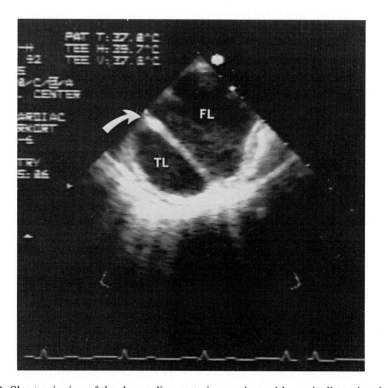

Fig. 25-8. Short-axis view of the descending aorta in a patient with aortic dissection. Note the intimal flap *(arrow)* dividing the true *(TL)* and the false lumen *(FL),* and the spontaneous echocardiographic contrast curling up within the false lumen, indicating a low flow state.

its sensitivity is comparable to that of magnetic resonance imaging and is approximately 98%. The portability and accessibility that allow performing studies in the emergency room have made transesophageal echocardiography the diagnostic tool of choice when aortic dissection is suspected. Importantly, recent studies have shown that certain transesophageal echocardiography characteristics of patients with aortic dissection, such as the presence of thrombus in the false lumen of the aorta, may have an important prognostic implications for the management of these patients.[7]

Evaluation of cardiac source of embolism

Transesophageal echocardiography has revolutionized the assessment of patients with a suspected cardiac source of embolism. Transesophageal echocardiography is more sensitive in detecting well-known and definite cardiac sources of embolism such as left atrial appendage thrombus. In addition, a number of transesophageal echocardiographic-related findings appear to reflect an increased embolic risk, such as spontaneous contrast, atrial septal aneurysm, patent foramen ovale, and the presence of aortic debris. The importance and prognostic significance of these findings are discussed in detail in Chapter 26.

Intraoperative indications

Transesophageal echocardiography was initially used to monitor left ventricular function in the operating room setting. Anesthesiologists have found transesophageal echocardiography to be very useful in the evaluation of anesthetic drugs that depress left ventricular contractility, to detect ongoing myocardial ischemia, or to detect the presence of intracardiac air as a potential source of embolism.

Transesophageal echocardiography has been found to be more sensitive than electrocardiography in detecting myocardial ischemia. It has also been useful in evaluating the effect of coronary revascularization on improvement of regional left ventricular contractility. Finally, it is an excellent means, in managing patients with hypotension, to determine whether the primary problem is poor left ventricular contractility or hypovolemia.

Another very important indication for transesophageal studies in the operating room setting is the evaluation of mitral valve repair. This surgical technique has been increasingly used because the preservation of left ventricular geometry and function obtained with it results in an increased survival of these patients. The adequate performance of mitral valve repair requires prompt verification of the results, and therefore intraoperative transesophageal echocardiographic studies in these patients are mandatory. Transesophageal echocardiography, when performed routinely in the operating

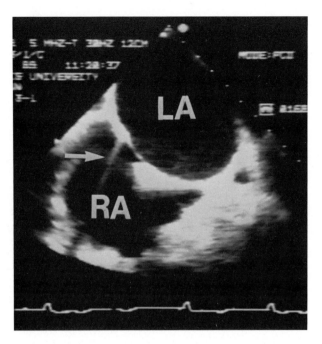

Fig. 25-9. Transesophageal echocardiographic study guiding the catheter *(arrow)* for a transseptal puncture at the cardiac catheterization laboratory.

room, leads to modification of planned valve surgery in approximately one third of the patients.[23] The impact of the technique is even greater in mitral valve surgery, where it may lead to major surgical decisions in up to 40% of the patients.

Interventional transesophageal echocardiography

Transesophageal echocardiography can be very useful as an adjunct technique to other diagnostic or therapeutic cardiology procedures.

Patients undergoing mitral balloon valvuloplasty should have a transesophageal echocardiogram prior to the procedure to exclude the presence of left atrial thrombus. In addition, transesophageal echocardiography can be useful during the procedure itself to guide the transseptal puncture and evaluate the immediate results (Fig. 25-9). It can also be useful to detect uncommon but important procedure-related complications, such as mitral valve rupture.

Transesophageal echocardiography has been successfully used to allow a safe closure of a patent foramen ovale. Temporary closure of a patent foramen ovale in patients with acute and sudden elevation of right-sided pressures and subsequent systemic oxygen desaturation may be necessary. Transesophageal echocardiography is useful in guiding the percutaneous closure of a patent foramen ovale by using a transseptal balloon catheter.[18]

Finally, transesophageal echocardiography can be used in conjunction with radio frequency catheter ablation of accessory pathways for the treatment of dysrhythmias. This technique involves a certain risk of damaging the mitral valve apparatus, especially in the case of left-sided bypass tracts. Transesophageal echocardiography has been used by some investigators to guide the catheters into the coronary sinus and to prevent damage of the mitral valve apparatus by inadvertently producing fulguration of the mitral leaflet surface, with the consequent perforation of the valve.

Transesophageal echocardiography in the intensive care unit

Transesophageal echocardiography has been shown to be a useful diagnostic tool in the critically ill patient. These patients, often on mechanical ventilation, are technically difficult to examine by transthoracic echocardiography. Diagnostic yields in patients with unexplained hypotension and suspected mechanical complications of myocardial infarction are quite high and justify selected use of transesophageal echocardiography in this setting.

ACKNOWLEDGMENTS

The authors are very grateful to Lissanne Hayman for her superb secretarial work.

REFERENCES

1. Borow K: An integrated approach to the noninvasive assessment of left ventricular systolic and diastolic performance. In Sutton MS, Oldershaw P, editors: *Textbook of adult and pediatric echocardiography and Doppler,* Boston, 1989, Blackwell Scientific.
2. Castello R: Echocardiographic evaluation of prosthetic mitral valve dysfunction, *Cardio* 35-44, October 1993.
3. Castello R, Labovitz AJ: Evaluation of mitral regurgitation by echocardiography, *Echocardiography* 121:1347-1352, 1991.
4. Castello R, et al: Comparison of transthoracic and transesophageal echocardiography for the assessment of left sided valvular regurgitation, *Am J Cardiol* 68:1677-1680, 1991.
5. Castello R, et al: Evaluation of pulmonary venous flow by transesophageal echocardiography in subjects with normal hearts: comparison to transthoracic echocardiography, *J Am Coll Cardiol* 18:65-71, 1991.
6. Castello R, et al: Quantitation of mitral regurgitation by transesophageal echocardiography with Doppler color flow mapping: correlation with cardiac catheterization, *J Am Coll Cardiol* 19:1516-1521, 1992.
7. Erbel R, et al: Echocardiography in the diagnosis of aortic dissection, *Lancet* 1:457-461, 1989.
8. Feigenbaum H: *Echocardiography,* ed 5, Philadelphia, 1994, Lea & Febiger.
9. Judgutt BI, et al: Prospective two-dimensional echocardiographic evaluation of left ventricular thrombus and embolus after acute myocardial infarction, *J Am Coll Cardiol* 13:554-564, 1989.
10. Karalis DG, et al: Transesophageal echocardiographic recognition of subaortic complications in aortic valve endocarditis: clinical and surgical implications, *Circulation* 86:353-362, 1992.
11. Kisslo J, Adams DB, Belkin RN: *Doppler color flow imaging,* New York, 1988, Churchill Livingstone.
12. Labovitz AJ: *Stress echocardiography.* In Froelicher VF, Myers J, Follansbee WP, Labovita AJ, editors: *Exercise and the heart,* ed 3, St Louis, 1993, Mosby–Year Book.
13. Labovitz AJ, Pearson AC: Evaluation of left ventricular diastolic function: clinical relevance and recent Doppler echocardiographic insights, *Am Heart J* 114:836-851, 1987.
14. Labovitz AJ, Pearson AC: *Transesophageal echocardiography: basic principles and clinical applications,* Philadelphia, 1993, Lea & Febiger.
15. Labovitz AJ, Williams GA: *Aortic valve pathology.* In *Doppler echocardiography,* ed 3, Philadelphia, 1992, Lea & Febiger.
16. Labovitz AJ, Williams GA: *Mitral valve pathology.* In *Doppler echocardiography,* ed 3, Philadelphia, 1992, Lea & Febiger.
17. Mügge A, Kühn H, Daniel WG: The role of transesophageal echocardiography in the detection of left atrial thrombi, *Echocardiography* 10:405-417, 1993.
18. Ofili EO, et al: Usefulness of transesophageal echocardiography during invasive intracardiac procedures, *J Am Coll Cardiol* 17:315A, 1991.
19. Perez JE, et al: On-line assessment of ventricular function by automatic boundary detection and ultrasonic backscatter imaging, *J Am Coll Cardiol* 19:313-320, 1992.
20. Perry GJ, et al: Evaluation of aortic insufficiency by Doppler color flow mapping, *J Am Coll Cardiol* 9:952-959, 1987.
21. Sahn DJ, et al: The Committee on M-mode Standardization of the American Society of Echocardiography: recommendations regarding quantitation in M-mode echocardiography: result of a survey of echocardiographic measurements, *Circulation* 58:1072-1083, 1978.
22. Sanfilippo AJ, et al: Echocardiographic assessment of patients with infectious endocarditis: prediction of risk for complications, *J Am Coll Cardiol* 18:1119-1191, 1991.
23. Sheikh KH, et al: The utility of transesophageal echocardiography and Doppler color flow imaging in patients undergoing cardiac valve surgery, *J Am Coll Cardiol* 15:363-372, 1990.
24. Weyman AE: *Principles and practice of echocardiography,* ed 2, Philadelphia, 1994, Lea & Febiger.

26

Echocardiography in the Evaluation of Patients with Ischemic Stroke

Camilo R. Gomez
Ramon Castello
Arthur J. Labovitz

The role of clinicians in caring for victims of ischemic stroke is twofold: to provide treatment for the acute event and to identify its cause and mechanism. The latter allows for the more logical implementation of measures for secondary prevention. In general, three categories of tests are available for evaluating the various potential causes of ischemic stroke: tests designed to assess the cerebral vasculature (e.g., ultrasound and angiography), tests that permit the diagnosis of hematologic abnormalities (e.g., protein C, protein S), and, finally, tests that allow the identification of cardiac sources of cerebral embolism. Among these, echocardiography has been the most extensively used in the evaluation of patients with ischemic strokes or transient ischemic attacks (TIA). The following is a review of the role that echocardiography plays in the assessment of patients with cerebrovascular disorders. It is our intention to emphasize the changes that have taken place over the course of the years in the rationale for its application. In addition, we will address issues of patient selection, impact upon management, and cost-effectiveness.

TRANSTHORACIC ECHOCARDIOGRAPHY: A BEGINNING

The use of M-mode and two-dimensional echocardiography as screening procedures in unselected stroke patient populations was reported as early as 1981.[19] In this first study, two definite cardiac sources of cerebral embolism (i.e., left ventricular thrombi) were found among a subgroup of 48 patients (the total population included 95 patients) with previous evidence of heart dysfunction. Following this report, other groups began to publish their experiences using transthoracic echocardiography (TTE) in the assessment of selected[24,31] or unselected[5] populations of stroke patients (Table 26-1). The results of these early publications were somewhat disappointing and led to the traditional teaching that echocardiography is relatively insensitive for the detection of cardiac sources of cerebral embolism and that its use should be confined to patients with clinical evidence of cardiac dysfunction.[28] Over time, a more selective utilization of TTE in the assessment of stroke patients resulted in its use only when cardiac disorders were

Table 26-1. Early reports of the use of transthoracic echocardiography in the evaluation of cardiogenic sources of embolism (CSE)

Reference	Number of patients	Patient selection	Heart disease	CSE
Greenland et al (1981)[19]	48	None	Yes	2
	47	None	No	0
Lovett et al (1981)[31]	138	Yes*	Some	41
Hofmann et al (1990)[24]	138	Yes†	Some	27
Bergeron and Shah (1981)[5]	184	None	Some	5

*Cardioembolism suspected or no other cause found.
†Young patients (mean age = 42 years).

Table 26-2. Summary of the existing reports comparing to transthoracic echocardiography (TTE) and transesophageal echocardiography (TEE) in the evaluation of cardiogenic sources of embolism (CSE)

Source	Number of patients	Heart disease TEE+ / TTE+ (%)	No heart disease TEE+ / TTE+ (%)	CSE TEE/TTE
Zenker et al (1988)[43]	40			25/20
Pop et al (1990)[38]	72	32/5	9/2	1/0
Pearson et al (1991)[35]	79	73/22	38/19	31/13
Cujec et al (1991)[12]	63	79/38	22/0	7/1
Lee et al (1991)[30]	50	66/0	33/0	4/0
Black et al (1991)[6]	63	78/0	17/8	9/2

present, when patients were younger than "expected" for a stroke victim, or when no other finding explaining the cause and mechanism of the stroke was detected (the so-called cryptogenic strokes). As discussed later in this chapter, however, this restricted approach to the echocardiographic evaluation of stroke patients was bound to change as a result of technologic advances. Some of the changes that have taken place, in fact, have forced clinicians to reassess the concept of "cryptogenic" stroke.

TRANSESOPHAGEAL ECHOCARDIOGRAPHY: UNCOVERING CAUSES OF STROKE

In 1977, Hisanaga and colleagues reported for the first time a new method for acquiring ultrasonic cardiac images by having the probe located at the tip of an esophagoscope, giving birth to transesophageal echocardiography (TEE).[23] At first, the technique was not widely accepted for diagnostic purposes, mainly because of technical limitations. Later, the introduction of minuscule electronic phased-array transducers led to the growth and development of an ultrasound field that is most suitable for the evaluation of victims of ischemic stroke.

The first report comparing the sensitivity of TEE with that of TTE in patients with stroke was that of Zenker and associates.[43] They studied 40 patients under the age of 45 years who suffered cerebral ischemic events. The major focus of this study was mitral valve prolapse, which was found slightly more frequently by TEE. Two years later, Pop and co-workers published their study of 72 consecutive patients with TIA or minor stroke.[38] In general, the yield of TEE, although small (approximately 13%), was greater than that of TTE. Of interest is the fact that TEE revealed abnormalities in four patients who had no clinical evidence of cardiac dysfunction, whereas TTE missed all four lesions. Pearson and colleagues were the first to compare TEE and TTE in an

unselected population of stroke patients using routine contrast TEE.[36] Potential cardiac sources of embolism were found almost four times more frequently by TEE. In fact, the yield of TEE in patients devoid of clinical cardiac abnormalities was about twice that of TTE.[36] Since the publication of that study, three other groups of investigators have compared TEE and TTE in the assessment of stroke patients.[6,12,30] Their findings have been similar, demonstrating that TEE is indeed more sensitive than TTE in detecting cardiac sources of embolism and that it uncovers patients at risk for cardiogenic stroke, even if no clinical evidence of cardiac dysfunction exists (Table 26-2).

In this context, it is a matter of controversy whether all cardiac abnormalities detected by TEE are risk factors for stroke or not.[17] Obviously, the etiologic diagnosis of stroke subtype is always presumptive, and TEE findings form part of a continuum whose extremes differ only in how compelling they are as proof of cardiogenic stroke (Fig. 26-1). For example, the finding of a dilated left atrium and a left atrial thrombus represents very strong evidence of the possibility of cardiogenic brain embolism. By contrast, the finding of isolated left atrial spontaneous contrast or an atrial septal aneurysm is a weaker indicator for such a diagnosis. In any case, it seems that patients with abnormal TEE, regardless of the finding, are at greater risk to develop further cerebral ischemic events than those with normal TEE.[9]

ECHOCARDIOGRAPHIC FINDINGS IN PATIENTS WITH ISCHEMIC STROKE

Ischemic stroke results from occlusion of a cerebral artery by a blood clot that either forms in situ or that

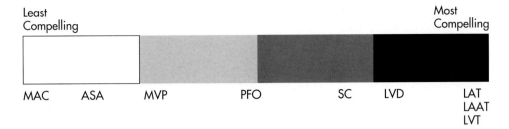

Fig. 26-1. Continuum of the significance of transesophageal echocardiography (TEE) findings as potential cardiogenic sources of brain embolism. (*MAC,* Mitral annulus calcification; *ASA,* atrial septal aneurysm; *MVP,* mitral valve prolapse; *PFO,* patient foramen ovale; *SC,* spontaneous contrast; *LVD,* left ventricular dysfunction; *LAT,* left atrial thrombus; *LAAT,* left atrial appendage thrombus; *LVT,* left ventricular thrombus.)

originates somewhere else in the body. Echocardiography plays a role not only in the detection of thrombi that have formed within the heart but also in uncovering abnormalities that can predispose to thrombus formation or that allow emboli originating in the venous system to reach the cerebral circulation. The principal echocardiographic findings associated with ischemic stroke follow.

Intracardiac thrombi

The most significant echocardiographic finding in patients with cerebral ischemic events is that of a thrombus in one of the left-sided chambers. Left atrial thrombi (LAT) are very frequent in patients with mitral stenosis, especially in those with left atrial enlargement and atrial fibrillation.[4,20,34,42] They typically appear as round or ovoid echodense masses with a clear delineation from the surrounding blood and a broad base of attachment to the atrial wall (Fig. 26-2, *A*). Their surface may be smooth or irregular, and they may be flat or immobile. Thrombi can also form in the left atrial appendage (LAA), where their incidence seems to have been previously underestimated. Recently, TEE has allowed easier identification of LAA thrombi. Factors that seem to contribute to the formation of LAA clots include increased LAA size[15] and decreased LAA motion[37] and flow.[39] Intracardiac thrombi can also form within the left ventricle (LV), usually as a result of wall motion abnormalities associated with dyskinetic segments or LV aneurysmal dilatation. Two major types of LV thrombi have been described: mural (i.e., intracavitary margin is parallel to endocardium) and protruding (i.e., intracavitary margin is convex). The latter are more commonly associated with embolic events.[22,25,26,41]

Potential sources of intracardiac thrombus formation

In the majority of instances in which stroke patients undergo echocardiographic evaluation, a thrombus is not identified. Somehow, this fact has been interpreted as evidence for the patient not having had a cardiogenic brain embolism. However, it must be pointed out that it is frequently possible to document cardiac derangements *capable* of leading to thrombus formation (e.g., atrial myxomas) without actually imaging the clot itself. Furthermore, the inability to image intracardiac thrombi may be related to the size of the clots, sufficiently large to induce cerebral ischemic events but too small for the resolution of echocardiographic instruments. In addition, abnormalities of the cardiac valves (e.g., mitral stenosis) and chambers (e.g., left atrial enlargement), of myocardial wall motion (e.g., apical hypokinesis), or of intracardiac hemodynamics (e.g., spontaneous contrast) are more likely markers of conditions that predispose to thrombus formation (Fig. 26-2, *A*).[3,10,11]

In addition to all of the preceding lesions, others also deserve special attention because their implication as potential sources of cardiogenic embolism is controversial. Among them, atrial septal aneurysm, mitral annular calcification, and mitral valve prolapse are probably the most widely recognized. Of these, atrial septal aneurysm, a bulging of the interatrial septum involving the region of the fossa ovalis (Fig. 26-2, *B*), is being increasingly recognized in patients with ischemic stroke.[35] The incidence of this finding is approximately four times greater in patients undergoing TEE for evaluation of ischemic cerebral events.[35] It is important to keep an open mind regarding the role that these lesions may play in the pathogenesis of stroke.

Aortic atherosclerosis

Perhaps one of the most exciting developments associated with the performance of TEE in stroke patients is the ability to identify potential atherogenic sources of cerebral embolism in the thoracic aorta.[2,40] In the past, clinicians who cared for stroke victims concentrated on the assessment of the carotid arteries and, to a lesser extent, the vertebrobasilar system. At present, however, TEE allows a truly comprehensive ultrasound assessment of the only portion of the cerebral circulation system that could not be properly studied in the past. The ascending aorta and the aortic arch can be the source of embolic material. The plaques observed in the

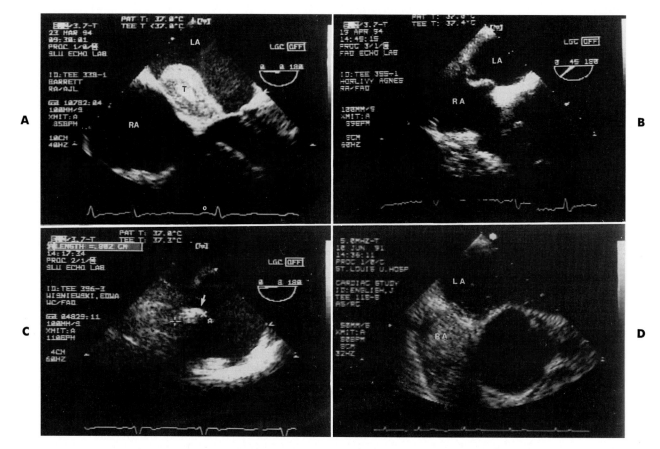

Fig. 26-2. A, Modified four-chamber transesophageal echocardiographic (TEE) view showing a large thrombus *(T)* and spontaneous contrast in the left atrium *(LA)*; *(RA,* Right atrium). **B,** Short-axis TEE view of an atrial septal aneurysm. *(LA,* Left atrium; *RA,* right atrium). **C,** Short-axis TEE view of the thoracic aorta. Note a large protruding mobile atherosclerotic plaque *(arrow).* **D,** Short-axis TEE view showing a patent foramen ovale. Note microbubbles crossing from the right atrium *(RA)* into the left atrium *(LA).*

patients reported in the literature have been described as protruding, ulcerated, and prone to the formation of cholesterol emboli (Fig. 26-2, *C*). The best therapeutic approach to patients with this type of vascular pathology remains unknown. However, the continued use of TEE to study the thoracic aorta in patients with stroke is likely to provide significant information about its role in the pathogenesis of stroke.

Paradoxical cerebral embolism

Blood clots that form within the venous system have not been traditionally considered likely to reach the cerebral circulation. In fact, under most circumstances, emboli originating in the deep veins of the lower limbs are trapped within the pulmonary circulation, where they may lead to respiratory symptoms. The recent introduction of TEE and contrast echocardiography, however, has led to the realization that patent foramina ovale (PFO) are more frequent than previously suspected, and that right-to-left shunting may also be a relatively prevalent factor predisposing to paradoxic

brain embolism (Fig. 26-2, *D*).[36] The main reservation in assessing the significance of PFO in patients with stroke concerns their high prevalence at routine autopsy (approximately 25% to 35%).[21] The advent of TEE, however, has also allowed the recognition that, in patients with ischemic stroke (particularly the young), PFO are approximately four times more frequent than in controls.[29] An additional problem in the diagnosis of paradoxic brain embolism, even when a PFO is identified, resides in the documentation of the venous source of embolism. Venous ultrasound may not be sensitive enough to detect smaller thrombi. For this reason, some authors have suggested the use of venography. Also, regardless of the diagnostic technique, the chances of finding a thrombus diminish when testing is delayed.

CARDIOGENIC ISCHEMIC STROKE: CURRENT STATUS

Traditionally, ischemic strokes have been considered to be most commonly the result of atherosclerosis of the cerebral blood vessels, sometimes leading to in situ thrombosis and sometimes to artery-to-artery embolism.[8,14,33] This idea was based upon the findings of large stroke data banks that included thousands of patients with ischemic strokes. These studies have suggested that only a minority (approximately 10% to 15%) of patients with ischemic stroke are victims of cardiogenic brain embolism.[8,14,33] It must be pointed out, however, that these studies were conducted at a time when the diagnosis of stroke relied heavily upon clinical criteria (i.e., neurologic phenomenology) and when TEE was not readily available. The absence of TEE among the evaluating tools used in these studies makes their criteria for the diagnosis of cardiogenic embolism inadequate by today's standards. Recently, several authors have shown that, considering the fact that TEE is more sensitive for detecting cardiac sources of embolism, this category of ischemic stroke is likely to have been previously underestimated.[18] In fact, it is even possible that strokes that in the past were considered "cryptogenic" or lacunar may have been caused by emboli of cardiac origin.[7,18,32] The evolution of our understanding of the etiopathogenesis of ischemic stroke, as well as the impact of TEE in the evaluation of these patients, gives rise to a controversial issue: Which stroke patients should undergo TEE evaluation? The answer to this question is not a simple one, and opinions are bitterly divided. On the one hand, some feel that only patients with clinical evidence of cardiac abnormalities, those who are relatively young, or those with "cryptogenic" strokes should be subjected to TEE. On the other hand, however, some feel that TEE should be now considered the gold standard and that, in the absence of compelling reasons, every stroke patient should be considered for TEE assessment.[16,18] Although our group favors the latter approach, it is important to acknowledge both positions and their rationale.

Undoubtedly, patients with clinical evidence of cardiac disorders (i.e., history or physical examination) are more likely to show abnormalities by TEE.[6,12,30,36,38] However, does this mean that individuals without evidence of cardiac dysfunction will not have abnormal TEE studies? The answer is obviously no! In fact, the literature just reviewed points exactly to the contrary.[6,12,30,36,38] It is precisely in patients without clinically evident cardiac dysfunction that TEE has the greatest yield and uncovers cardiac pathology that otherwise may go undiagnosed. It is also suggested that the evaluation of younger stroke victims using TEE is likely to be more productive. Again, this argument cannot be reversed to indicate that older stroke patients only rarely have relevant TEE findings. Finally, there is the issue of patients with "cryptogenic" stroke: who they are, how they can be identified, and how TEE fits into their evaluation scheme.

Table 26-3. Changes in the character of cryptogenicity of ischemic strokes according to the stage of evaluation

Clinical stage	Cryptogenicity	Reason
Upon admission	Absolute	Not enough information
During evaluation	Relative	Evaluation incomplete
Upon discharge	Specific	Only those without findings

"CRYPTOGENIC" STROKE: A RELATIVE TERM

The term *cryptogenic* can be broken down into two components: *crypto-* from the Latin *crypta* and the Greek *kruptos,* meaning "hidden", and *-genic* from the Latin *genea,* meaning "origin." It is a term applied to clinical conditions of unknown or obscure meaning. It is very important to point out that the latter two are not equivalent and that an ischemic stroke caused, for example, by excessive factor VIII activity[27] certainly has an obscure cause, but one that is known. Then again, patients who undergo extensive yet unyielding evaluation, using all available diagnostic tools, truly have strokes of unknown etiology. The existing literature does not present an uniform view of what constitutes a "cryptogenic" stroke, and definitions as simple as one that includes all patients "without significant carotid atherosclerosis" can be found among the published material. Not only does this create a considerable problem when assessing the role of TEE in the evaluation of stroke patients but also it overlooks a situation we have come to call *double jeopardy.* The latter refers to patients who are excluded from echocardiographic evaluation simply because they have noncardiac lesions such as carotid atherosclerosis and because it is assumed that a cardiac source of embolism cannot coexist with the already identified pathology. This is not the case at all, and we have recently shown that TEE demonstrates intracardiac thrombi in 8% and potential cardiac sources of emboli in 33% of patients with moderate carotid atherosclerosis.[13]

Even when one uses a specific definition of *cryptogenic* stroke (i.e., only patients who do not have an obvious cause for stroke following thorough investigation), it is clear that the term has a temporal relativity because the degree of "cryptogenicity" of a stroke progressively changes between the moment it occurs and the time when it has been completely evaluated (Table 26-3). From this point of view, strokes assessed in emergency departments must be considered to be *absolutely* cryptogenic because no etiopathogenic evaluation has been undertaken. Even in cases in which the patient has preexisting risk factors, one cannot make inferences about the cause-effect relationship until the diagnostic evaluation is completed. Stroke should be considered *relatively* cryptogenic throughout the course of the evaluation, before all tests are completed. Finally, upon the patient's discharge, those strokes whose etiology is not found despite extensive investigation should be considered *specifically* cryptogenic. A special subgroup of patients is formed by individuals whose evaluation has uncovered more than one potential cause, making it difficult for the clinician to decide which one of these entities was the acting causative mechanism.[1] This also constitutes double jeopardy and, beyond what has been discussed, is a subject beyond the scope of this presentation.

ROLE AND APPLICATION OF TRANSESOPHAGEAL ECHOCARDIOGRAPHY IN CLINICAL PRACTICE

Several important conclusions can be derived from the preceding concepts: (1) that TEE is more sensitive than TTE in detecting cardiac sources of embolism in patients with stroke, (2) that the presence or absence of clinical evidence of cardiac disorders does not allow one to predict whether TEE will be normal or abnormal, (3) that some TEE findings have a stronger clinical impact than others, and (4) that "cryptogenic" stroke is a relative term that should be used with caution. Based upon these considerations, we now consider the practical utilization of TEE in the assessment of patients with stroke, taking into account the impact of test results upon management and cost-effectiveness.

Impact upon management

In order to be clear about the repercussions of using TEE in clinical practice, one must first consider management changes that directly result from the TEE results. In general, it is not uncommon for clinicians to ask if the results of a test will influence management. Unfortunately, when it comes to TEE, this question has become, Is the TEE result going to determine whether a patient is treated with warfarin? Obviously, this oversimplification represents a naive view of what the management of a stroke patient encompasses. Such a view fails to recognize that stroke management is a comprehensive task, only part of which deals with the selection of medications. The results of the etiopathogenic evaluation usually lead to decisions about immediate therapy, the necessity for additional evaluation and follow-up strategy, and may even have implications regarding the management of future cerebrovascular events. In addition, the understanding of the prognosis depends significantly upon the etiopathogenic mechanism uncovered. From this perspective, clinicians face a variety of issues regarding the future of their patients when they consider the diagnostic data acquired and not simply a choice of drugs. Therefore, the less comprehensive and complete the diagnostic database is, the more guessing the clinician has to do. This underscores the necessity for comprehensive evaluation of stroke patients and supports the role of TEE in the diagnostic process.

Finally, the assessment of any test's impact on patient management is relatively easy if the test has a fairly limited and fixed number of possible results. Tests whose results fall within an all-or-none (i.e., positive or negative) dichotomy are a good illustration of this concept. For example, it is relatively easy for the clinician to predict the impact that cryptococcal antigen assay results in the cerebrospinal fluid will have upon management. However, TEE has the potential of providing a wide variety of findings that, when combined in different patterns, may lead to very different decisions regarding care. This characteristic of the test must be considered when trying to decide a priori whether its results will change the patient's management.

Cost-effectiveness

Cost-effectiveness is a concept that was foreign to most physicians until the 1970s, when it began to creep from the desks of health care administrators into the medical wards, and it has since become part of the day-to-day jargon. Theoretically, cost-effectiveness helps to assess the worth of a diagnostic test (or other form of clinical intervention) by comparing its cost with its impact on the care of the population (not on the individual patient). In today's health care climate, cost-effectiveness translates into "For the health care system, is it worth spending a certain amount of money to pay for a test (or procedure) associated with a specifically documented outcome?"

There are no good data regarding the cost-effectiveness of TEE. However, we could consider hypothetical situations and use them as a means to generate discussion. The average cost of a TEE is approximately a thousand dollars. If we were to estimate that, by using TEE, clinicians could find information that would help prevent disabling strokes in 2 of every 100 patients, we may conclude that, with a yield of 2%, TEE is not cost-effective. Nevertheless, let us consider that the approximate cost of the TEEs for 100 patients is $100,000 and that the cost of caring for 2 patients who would have suffered disabling strokes approximates $50,000-70,000 per year. Simple calculations suggest that savings incurred by the prevention of two disabling strokes in 100 patients, based upon the TEE findings, are more than enough to cover the expense of performing the TEE studies in the other 98. Furthermore, if TEE allows the prevention of significant disability in more than 2% of the stroke population (which many of us think it does), the test is, in fact, leading to greater savings.

CONCLUSIONS

In summary, the etiopathogenic assessment of stroke victims is a comprehensive task that requires the application of multiple diagnostic techniques, among which echocardiography has gained greater importance in recent years.[16,17] Indeed, cardiogenic cerebral embolism may be more frequent than it has been traditionally suspected,[18] and TEE is the most sensitive test available today to uncover cardiac abnormalities in patients with stroke.[6,12,30,36,38] From this perspective, the care of stroke patients must include TEE as one of the evaluation tools, particularly when there are no more powerful or compelling reasons not to use the test.[16]

REFERENCES

1. Adams HP, Bendixen BH, Kapella LJ, et al: Classification of subtype of acute ischemic stroke: definitions for use in a multicenter clinical trial, *Stroke* 24:35-41, 1993.
2. Amarenco P, Duyckaerts C, Yzourio C, et al: The prevalence of ulcerated plaques in the aortic arch in patients with stroke, *N Engl J Med* 326:221-225, 1992.
3. Beppu S, Nimura Y, Sakakibara H, et al: Smoke-like echo in the left atrial cavity in mitral valve disease: its features and significance, *J Am Coll Cardiol* 6:744, 1985.
4. Beppu S, Park Y, Sakakibara H, et al: Clinical features of intracardiac thrombosis based on echocardiographic observation, *Jpn Circ J* 48:75-82, 1984.
5. Bergeron GA, Shah PM. Echocardiography unwarranted in patients with cerebral ischemic events, *N Engl J Med* 304:489, 1981 (correspondence).
6. Black IW, Hopkins AP, Lee LCL, et al: Role of transesophageal echocardiography in evaluation of cardiogenic embolism, *Br Heart J* 66:302-307, 1991.
7. Bogousslavsky J: The plurality of subcortical infarction, *Stroke* 23:629-631, 1992.
8. Bogousslavsky J, Van Melle G, Regli F: The Lausanne Stroke Registry: analysis of 1,000 consecutive patients with first stroke, *Stroke* 19:1083-1092, 1988.
9. Camp A, Pearson AC, Sullivan NA, et al: Evaluation of patients with transesophageal echocardiography following cerebral ischemic events: follow up experience, *J Am Coll Cardiol* 17:315A, 1991.
10. Castello R, Pearson AC, Labovitz AJ: Prevalence and clinical implications of atrial spontaneous contrast in patients undergoing transesophageal echocardiography, *Am J Cardiol* 65:1149, 1990.
11. Chia BL, Choo MH, Yan PC, et al: Intra-atrial smoke-like echoes and thrombi formation, *Chest* 95:912, 1989.
12. Cujec B, Polasek, P, Voll C, et al: Transesophageal echocardiography in the detection of potential cardiac source of embolism in stroke patients, *Stroke* 22:727-733, 1991.
13. Dressler F, Meric M, Castello R, et al: Frequency of cardiac sources of emboli in patients with cerebral ischemia and moderate carotid artery stenosis, *J Am Soc Echocardiogr* (in press).
14. Foulkes MA, Wolf PA, Price TR, et al: The Stroke Data Bank: design, methods and baseline characteristics, *Stroke* 19:547-554, 1988.
15. Garcia-Fernandez MA, Torrecilla EG, Roman DS, et al: Left atrial appendage Doppler flow patterns: implications on thrombus formation, *Am Heart J* 124:955-961, 1992.
16. Gomez CR: Diagnostic evaluation of patients with cerebral ischemic events. In Adams HP, editor: *Handbook of cerebrovascular diseases,* New York, 1993, Marcel Dekker.
17. Gomez CR, Labovitz AJ: Transesophageal echocardiography in the etiologic diagnosis of stroke, *J Stroke Cerebrovasc Dis* 1:81-87, 1991.
18. Gomez CR, Tulyapronchote R, Malkoff MD, et al: Changing trends in the etiologic diagnosis of stroke, *J Stroke Cerebrovasc Dis* 4(3): 169-173, 1994.
19. Greenland P, et al: Echocardiography in diagnostic assessment of stroke, *Ann Intern Med* 95:51-53, 1981.
20. Gross RI, Cunningham JN, Shively SL, et al: Long term results of open radical mitral commissurotomy: ten year follow up study of 202 patients, *Am J Cardiol* 47:821-827, 1987.
21. Hagen PT, Scholz DG, Edwards WD: Incidence and size of patent foramen ovale during the first 10 decades of life: an autopsy study of 965 normal hearts, *Mayo Clin Proc* 59:17-20, 1984.
22. Haugland JM: Embolic potential of left ventricular thrombi detected by two-dimensional echocardiography, *Circulation* 70:588-598, 1984.
23. Hisanaga K, Hisanaga A, Nagata K, Yoshida S: A new transesophageal real-time two dimensional echocardiographic system using a flexible tube and its clinical application, *Proc Jpn Soc Ultrason Med* 32:43-44, 1977.
24. Hofmann T, Kasper W, Meinertz T, et al: Echocardiographic evaluation of patients with clinically suspected arterial emboli, *Lancet* 336:1421-1424, 1990.
25. Johannessen KA, et al: Risk factors for embolization in patients with left ventricular thrombi and acute myocardial infarction, *Br Heart J* 60:104-110, 1988.
26. Keren A, et al: Natural history of left ventricular thrombi: their appearance and resolution in the post-hospitalization period of acute myocardial infarction, *J Am Coll Cardiol* 15:790-800, 1990.
27. Kosik KS, Furie B: Thrombotic stroke associated with elevated plasma Factor VII, *Ann Neurol* 8:435-437, 1980.
28. Larson EB, Stratton JR, Pearlman AS: Selective use of two-dimensional echocardiography in stroke syndromes, *Ann Intern Med* 95:112-114, 1981 (editorial).
29. Lechat PH, Mas JL, Lascault G, et al: Prevalence of patent foramen ovale in patients with stroke, *N Engl J Med* 318:1148-1152, 1988.
30. Lee RJ, Bartzokis T, Tiong-Keat Y, et al: Enhanced detection of intracardiac sources of cerebral emboli by transesophageal echocardiography, *Stroke* 22:734-739, 1991.
31. Lovett JL, Sandok BA, Givliani ER, et al: Two-dimensional echocardiography in patients with focal cerebral ischemia, *Ann Intern Med* 95:1-4, 1981.
32. Millikan C, Futrell N: The fallacy of the lacunar hypothesis, *Stroke* 21:1251-1257, 1990.
33. Mohr JP, Caplan LR, Melski JW, et al: The Harvard Cooperative Stroke Registry: a prospective registry, *Neurology* 28:754-762, 1978.
34. Nichols HT, Blanco G, Morse DP, et al: Open mitral commissurotomy: experience with 200 consecutive cases, *JAMA* 182:268-270, 1962.
35. Pearson AC, Labovitz AJ, Tatineni S, et al: Superiority of transesophageal echocardiography in detecting cardiac source of embolism in patients with cerebral ischemia of uncertain etiology, *J Am Coll Cardiol* 17:66-72, 1991.
36. Pearson AC, Nagelhout D, Castello R, et al: Atrial septal aneurysm and stroke: a transesophageal echocardiographic study, *J Am Coll Cardiol* 18:1223-1229, 1991.
37. Pollick C, Taylor D: Assessment of left atrial appendage function by transesophageal echocardiography: implications for the development of thrombus, *Circulation* 84:223-231, 1991.
38. Pop G, Sutherland GR, Koudstaal PJ, et al: Transesophageal echocardiography in the detection of intracardiac embolic

sources in patients with transient ischemic attacks, *Stroke* 21:560-565, 1990.

39. Pozzoli M, Febo O, Torbicki A, et al: Left atrial appendage dysfunction: a cause of thrombosis? Evidence by transesophageal echocardiography — Doppler studies, *J Am Soc Echocardiogr* 4:435-441, 1991.

40. Tunick PA, Kronzon I: Protruding atherosclerotic plaque in the aortic arch of patients with systemic embolization: a new finding seen by transesophageal echocardiography, *Am Heart J* 120:658-660, 1990.

41. Vissler CA, et al: Embolic potential of left ventricular thrombus after myocardial infarction: a two-dimensional echocardiographic study of 119 patients, *J Am Coll Cardiol* 5:1276-1280, 1985.

42. Wallach JB, Lukash L, Angrist AA: An interpretation of the incidence of mitral thrombi in the left auricle and appendage with particular reference to mitral commissurotomy, *Am Heart J* 45:252-254, 1953.

43. Zenker G, Erbel R, Kramer G, et al: Transesophageal two dimensional echocardiography in young patients with cerebral ischemic events, *Stroke* 19:345-348, 1988.

27

Intravascular Ultrasound in Neurosonology

Marc D. Malkoff
Camilo R. Gomez
Morton J. Kern

Intravascular ultrasound (IVUS) encompasses several diagnostic techniques developed during the last decade. The interest in IVUS stems from the proliferation of percutaneous interventional procedures such as balloon angioplasty, as well as from the need to study atherosclerotic plaques more extensively than simply using conventional imaging techniques. As early as 1956, reports of the use of single-element echo catheters to measure cardiac chamber sizes in animals began to appear in the literature.[6] Several years later, a more sophisticated four-element catheter was used to attempt to generate similar but more detailed images.[7] By the early 1980s, several groups had begun to develop dedicated IVUS imaging systems, and the first studies addressing the use of IVUS in the study of atherosclerotic plaques were presented at the meeting of the American College of Cardiology in 1988.[14,21] The first clinical images of the application of IVUS to the evaluation of the peripheral vessels were made available by Yock and associates,[20] and its use in assessing the coronary circulation was described by two other groups.[11,15] All of these early developments have been followed by a significant wave of clinical research of the applications of IVUS in clinical medicine.

The possibility of applying these techniques to the study of cerebrovascular disorders is part of evolution of the field of interventional neurology. Although widely practiced by neuroradiologists (i.e., interventional neuroradiology) and by neurosurgeons (i.e., endovascular neurosurgery), the utilization of catheter technology for the diagnosis and treatment of neurologic patients is also within the scope of neurology as one of its subspecialty fields (Fig. 27-1).[9] This chapter is a summary of the most important principles that govern IVUS, both as an imaging and as a hemodynamic (i.e., Doppler) diagnostic tool, as well as some general ideas about its potential role in the practice of vascular and interventional neurology.

INTRAVASCULAR ULTRASOUND IMAGING
Basic principles

The cross-sectional imaging of blood vessels using IVUS systems is performed by sweeping the ultrasound beam numerous times through a series of adjacent and sequential radial positions within a cross-sectional plane.

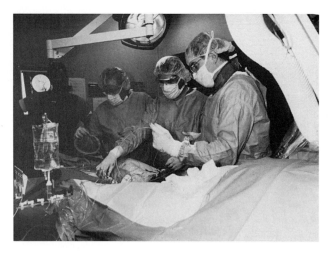

Fig. 27-1. Neurointerventional team composed of individuals from multiple specialties, including two of the authors (CRG, center; MJK, right).

For each of the positions of the transducer, the echoes generated are stored in a scan converter memory, on a line that represents the direction of the ultrasound beam at the moment the echoes were created. This process assures that all the echoes form a real-time, cross-sectional, and tomographic image of the vessel. The technical basis for the IVUS imaging system is either a mechanically rotated acoustic element (the transducer or a mirror) or a set of several electronically switched acoustic elements (Fig. 27-2).

The rotating transducer and rotating mirror IVUS catheters are characterized by very flexible shafts that contain the electric wires for the transducer. In the former, the transducer element is positioned in such a way that there is no transmission pulse effect (ring-dome artifact) in the display, allowing imaging very close to the vessel wall (i.e., there is no "dead zone").[19] The dome of the catheter must be acoustically transparent. Catheters with rotating mirrors also include a flexible shaft and a transparent dome (Fig. 27-2). However, the fact that the transducer is immobile avoids the need to have electric wires rotate. In addition, the mirror may have one of various shapes and focuses.

The electronically switched (i.e., phased-array) catheter uses many small acoustic elements (usually 32 or 64) positioned cylindrically around the catheter tip (Fig. 27-2). The construction of these catheters allows their introduction into the vessel studied using a central guide wire. Another feature of this type of device is that subgroups of adjacent elements are provided with time delays that essentially make them act like a single larger echo-transducer. This principle allows aperture variations and focusing. Alternatively, imaging reconstruction can be performed a posteriori, but this is a more time-consuming method.

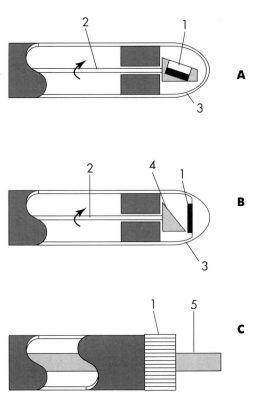

Fig. 27-2. Schematic drawing of the tips of the existing catheter designs for IVUS. Their engineering bases are **(A)**, mechanical rotational transducer, **(B)**, mechanical rotational mirror, and **(C)** phased array. (1. Ultrasonic element; 2. rotating shaft; 3. transparent dome; 4. focusing mirror; 5. guide wire.)

Technical limitations

As with any other type of ultrasonic system, IVUS has some technical limitations. The first one is the acoustic dead zone (Fig. 27-3). Essentially, if the time between pulses is too short, the transducer elements are saturated when some of the echoes (i.e., those closer to the transducer) return and are not able to receive them or display them. Catheters with rotating mirrors have the shortest dead zone. Another potential problem is the need to balance the shaft's flexibility (required for navigation through arterial curvatures and tortuosities) with its rigidity (required for torsional effects). In addition, IVUS is not an exception to other ultrasound techniques, requiring a compromise between increased frequency to provide better axial resolution and the consequent decreased penetration. The latter translates into increased difficulty in imaging larger vessels (e.g., the aorta). For IVUS, the practical axial resolution approximates 0.1 mm, and the lateral resolution varies between 0.3 and 0.5 mm.

Clinical experience

The use of IVUS imaging systems in clinical medicine has added a new dimension to the study of specific

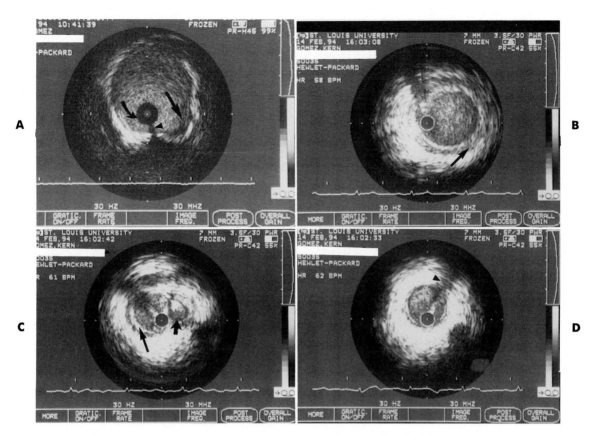

Fig. 27-3. Intravascular ultrasound (IVUS) of some of the large arteries that supply the brain. It is possible to identify the acoustic dead zone *(curved arrow)* and the guide wire artifact *(arrowhead)*. **A,** Imaging of the aortic arch provides visualization of the origin of the innominate *(arrow),* left common carotid, and left subclavian arteries. **B,** Imaging of the common carotid artery in a patient with dissection discloses an unusually thickened media *(arrow).* **C,** In the same patient, IVUS imaging of the common carotid artery bifurcation clearly displays both the internal *(long arrow)* and external carotid *(short arrow)* arteries. **D,** The internal carotid artery is engaged next, using the IVUS catheter.

arterial systems, in particular, the coronary circulation. In fact, its use has been characterized as an in vivo histologic study of the coronaries. The main advantage of using IVUS imaging is that it provides information that cannot be obtained angiographically. Indeed, in the past, comparisons between vascular ultrasonography and angiography have given rise to significant controversy and unclear data. The principal reason is that both techniques are so different in the type of information they generate. Angiography, which we could also consider "lumenography," provides images of a column of dye within the lumen of the vessel, outlining irregularities of the endothelial surface. The morphology of the vascular wall, by contrast, has to be inferred. Contrary to this, ultrasound provides adequate information about this variable.

There are several potential advantages for the utilization of IVUS in the assessment of atherosclerotic lesions. The cross-sectional perspective allows visualization of the full 360° circumference of the vessel wall, not

just two surfaces. Therefore, measurement of lumen area does not depend upon the radiographic projection but can be determined by planimetry of the tomographic image. The tomographic orientation also permits better visualization of bifurcation sites, notoriously difficult to image by radiography because of vessel overlap. As with any other form of ultrasound, the penetration of tissue allows imaging of normal and abnormal anatomy, including measurements of the thickness and echogenicity of vessel wall layers. Also, the tomographic perspective permits assessment of lumen shape, a characteristic of significant importance in the evaluation of eccentric atherosclerotic lesions.

INTRAVASCULAR DOPPLER
Technical aspects

The technology currently available for the application of intravascular Doppler has mostly resulted from developments in the field of interventional cardiology. The utilization of catheters and guide wires specially fitted with Doppler transducers on their tips provides clinicians with accurate and continuous determinations of blood flow velocity. In the coronary circulation, which we will use as a descriptive model, two types of catheters are currently available for the performance of intravascular Doppler: nonselective and subselective.

The subselective catheters are placed over 0.014-inch angioplasty guide wires, allowing the measurement of blood flow velocity within individual branches of the coronary arteries. In general, they consist of a single 20-MHz piezoelectric crystal, which is mounted on the tip or the side of an Fr 3 catheter.[18,19] The side-mounted crystal generates an ultrasound beam at 30° to 45° from the long axis of the catheter. In general, the end-mounted catheters may be superior for serial measurements with repeated insertions, whereas the catheter with the side-mounted crystal may detect peak velocity more readily. The Doppler catheter is usually introduced coaxially through a standard Fr 8 angioplasty guide catheter.

Nonselective Judkins-style Doppler-tipped angiographic catheters are made of polyvinyl chloride, have an Fr 8 diameter, and are fitted with a 20-MHz ultrasound crystal in their distal tip.[12] Measurements of flow velocity are comparable to those achieved with the subselective Doppler catheters. This catheter has been found to be particularly useful in the assessment of patients without focal atherosclerotic lesions, as well as in those with cardiac transplantation.

The most recently introduced device is an angioplasty-type ultrasonic guide wire. This very attractive instrument allows measurements not only in the most distal branches of the coronary arteries but also during the performance of angioplasty procedures. The currently available Doppler guide wire is 0.018 inch, and it has a 12-MHz ultrasonic transducer on its tip. It can be placed through a balloon angioplasty catheter, and it generates a uniform beam of pulsed Doppler ultrasound with a 20° spread. This device provides on-line spectral display of flow velocity, which is a more precise and easily identifiable method to detect flow velocity.

Clinical experience

The bulk of the existing experience on the use of intravascular Doppler derives from work performed in the coronary circulation. In general, the intravascular Doppler technique has been used as an adjunct to coronary angiography in selected groups of patients: those with chest pain syndromes and normal coronary arteries, those with coronary stenosis of intermediate (40% to 60%) severity, and those with suspected transplant rejection. In addition, the techniques are being used to monitor the progress of angioplasty and other coronary interventions.

The clinical syndrome of chest pain in the context of normal coronary arteriogram is a relatively common medical problem. Approximately 10% to 20% of these patients are found to have evidence of coronary ischemia by noninvasive testing. It is postulated that disturbances of the microcirculation are responsible for this process. These patients are candidates for invasive evaluation using intravascular Doppler and pharmacologic challenges with ergonovine (to provoke spasm in susceptible individuals) and/or vasodilators (to assess the flow reserve capacity).[1-5,17]

Arteriographic quantitation of coronary artery narrowing does not always allow adequate assessment of patients with lesions of intermediate severity. In contrast, the assessment of patients with such lesions with intravascular Doppler and flow reserve measurement has provided additional information about this topic.[10,16] It has been shown that lesions associated with a coronary flow reserve of less than 3.5 times the resting flow are of clinical significance.[10,16] The reasons for the variability in vascular reserve are presumed to be hypertrophy, infarction, and microcirculatory abnormalities.

In the context of coronary angioplasty, intravascular Doppler is an ideal tool for monitoring the procedure, as well as for assessing its physiologic effects. It has been noted that, in the absence of restenosis, coronary reserve ratios normalize in most patients at approximately 8 months after angioplasty.[13]

APPLICATIONS IN NEUROSONOLOGY

Based upon the concepts noted earlier in this chapter, it is reasonable to ask if there is a role for IVUS imaging and Doppler in neurosonology. The answer to this question must be considered in the context of the current availability of well-developed ultrasonic imaging techniques capable of providing anatomic and physiologic information about the cerebral arteries, extracranially and intracranially. From this perspective, the application of IVUS imaging of the cerebral blood vessels will require the technique to have a unique role (Fig. 27-3). This role directly relates to the clinical and pathologic characteristics of the atherosclerotic involvement of the cerebral arteries.

In general, the two characteristics of atherosclerotic plaques that make them prone to cause cerebral ischemia are their histologic composition and the degree of luminal area reduction that they cause.[8] The use of IVUS helps in the assessment of the endothelial integrity of regions of the cerebral vasculature that are not yet accessible to conventional ultrasound imaging. In addition, endothelial integrity and plaque composition represent important variables in the application of revascularization techniques, particularly those that are nonsurgical (e.g., balloon angioplasty). As it does in the

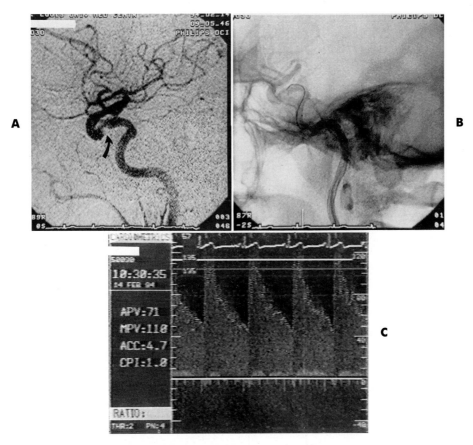

Fig. 27-4. Intravascular Doppler assessment of an intracavernous internal carotid artery stenosis. **A,** Angiography clearly displays the atherosclerotic lesions *(arrow),* narrowing the lumen diameter by approximately 50%. **B,** Fluoroscopic placement of the Doppler guide wire across the lesion. The carotid artery can be faintly visualized because of residual contrast material. **C,** Doppler waveform obtained as the Doppler guide wire is placed across the narrowed lumen (Mean Peak Velocity [Vm] = 110 cm/s).

peripheral and coronary circulations, it is conceivable that IVUS will also help direct the decision of what type of interventional procedure to use in specific patients, for example, balloon versus laser angioplasty versus rotational atherectomy. Finally, IVUS provides the means for immediate intraoperative assessment of the effects of these procedures, as well as the opportunity to discover aspects about nonatherosclerotic vascular disorders such as spontaneous dissection (Fig. 27-3).

The utilization of intravascular Doppler in the assessment of neurologic patients is also appealing. Obviously not a technique to be used for screening purposes, intravascular Doppler provides additional information about flow characteristics at specific points in the cerebral vasculature and under specific circumstances (Fig. 27-4). In spite of the availability of a variety of neurovascular Doppler techniques, there are potential advantages to the selective utilization of intravascular Doppler. For example, there are portions of the cerebral arterial system (e.g., the petrous segment of the

internal carotid artery) that cannot be reached with conventional Doppler instruments, including transcranial Doppler (TCD). Also, in approximately 15% of the population, the ultrasound beam cannot effectively cross the skull and allow assessment of the circle of Willis by using TCD. Furthermore, the use of an external ultrasound transducer during monitoring of endovascular procedures is somewhat cumbersome and often impractical. Also, the localization of the intravascular Doppler sample volume is extremely precise because the device can be positioned fluoroscopically (Fig. 27-4). Finally, concurrent measurement of vascular diameter using other imaging techniques (i.e., angiography or IVUS) may allow the determination of hemodynamic variables (e.g., cerebrovascular impedance) not yet explored (CA Giller, personal communication).

Intravascular Doppler also provides a practical method for the assessment of the cerebral flow reserve of the vascular bed supplied by the catheterized artery. Based on the flow and pressure relationship in the

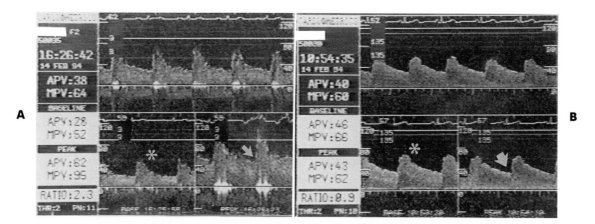

Fig. 27-5. Comparison between normal and abnormal cerebrovascular reserve as measured using intravascular Doppler and intraarterial nitroglycerin injections. **A,** Response in a normal vascular territory; note the increased blood flow velocities following injection *(arrow)*. **B,** Abnormally blunted response obtained from a system without any reserve *(arrow)*. (Asterisk, baseline tracings before injection of nitroglycerin.)

cerebral circulation, downward changes in pressure result in proportional reductions in resistance in order to maintain constant flow. Such changes in resistance are part of the autoregulation mechanism and can compensate only up to a certain point, beyond which flow progressively decreases. Under normal circumstances, the intraarterial administration of short-acting vasodilators such as papaverine, adenosine, or nitroglycerin results in distal arterial dilation, decreased distal resistance, and increased Doppler blood flow velocities (Fig. 27-5). The same maneuver repeated by injecting a similar vasodilator into an artery that supplies a hemodynamically compromised territory results in few or no Doppler velocity changes, due to the lack of cerebral flow reserve of this territory (Fig. 27-5). Combined with translesional pressure gradient measurements, intravascular Doppler adds a new dimension to the assessment of cerebrovascular insufficiency due to atherosclerotic lesions.

CONCLUSIONS

Intravascular ultrasound is a relatively new field of medicine that offers significant potential advantages for the assessment of patients with cerebrovascular disorders. The application of the techniques of IVUS imaging and Doppler requires a team of individuals with sufficient knowledge about the pathologic processes being investigated as well as the technology behind the devices being applied. Furthermore, these specialists have to have expertise in the performance of endovascular catheter procedures, including supraselective catheterization of the cerebral blood vessels. Although the traditional concept has been that neuroradiologists perform such procedures, the field is sufficiently unexplored to warrant the participation of qualified individuals from other specialties including neurosurgery, neurology, and cardiology.

REFERENCES

1. Arbogast R, Bourassa MG: Myocardial function during atrial pacing in patients with angina pectoris and normal arteriograms, *Am J Cardiol* 32:257-263, 1973.
2. Cannon RO, Epstein S: Chest pain and "normal" coronary arteries: role of small coronary arteries, *Am J Cardiol* 55:50B-60B, 1985.
3. Cannon RO, Schenke WH, Leon M, et al: Limited coronary flow reserve after dipyridamole in patients with ergonovine-induced coronary vasoconstriction, *Circulation* 75:163-174, 1987.
4. Cannon RO, Watson RM, Rosing DR, Epstein SE: Angina caused by reduced vasodilator reserve of the small coronary arteries, *J Am Coll Cardiol* 1:1359-1373, 1983.
5. Cannon RO, Bonow RO, Bacharach SL: Left ventricular dysfunction in patients with angina pectoris, normal epicardial coronary arteries, and abnormal vasodilator reserve, *Circulation* 71:218-226, 1985.
6. Cieszynski T: Intracardiac method for investigation of structure of the heart with the aid of ultrasonics, *Arch Immunol Ter Dow* 8:551-553, 1960.
7. Eggleton RC, Townsend C, Kossoff G, et al: *Computerized ultrasonic visualization of dynamic ventricular configurations.* Presentation at the eighth annual meeting of the ICMBE, Chicago, July 1969.
8. Gomez CR: Carotid plaque morphology and the risk of stroke, *Stroke* 21:148-151, 1990.
9. Gomez CR, Kern MJ: Cerebral catheterization: back to the future! *J Stroke Cerebrovasc Dis* (in press).
10. Gould KL, Kelley KO, Bolson EL: Experimental validation of quantitative coronary arteriography for determining pressure-flow characteristics of coronary stenosis, *Circulation* 66:930-937, 1982.
11. Graham SP, Brands D, Sheehan H, et al: Assessment of arterial wall morphology using intravascular ultrasound in vitro and in patients, *Circulation* 80(suppl 2):56, 1989 (abstract).
12. Kern MJ, Courtois M, Ludbrook P: A simplified method to measure coronary blood flow velocity in patients: validation and application of a Judkins-style Doppler-tipped angiographic catheter, *Am Heart J* 120:1202-1212, 1990.

13. Kern MJ, Deligonul U, Vandormael M, et al: Impaired coronary vasodilator reserve in the immediate postcoronary angioplasty period: analysis of coronary artery flow velocity indexes and regional cardiac venous efflux, *J Am Coll Cardiol* 13:860-872, 1989.

14. Mallery J, Griffith J, Gessert J, et al: Intravascular ultrasound imaging catheter assessment of normal and atherosclerotic arterial wall thickness, *J Am Coll Cardiol* 11:22A, 1988.

15. Marco J, Fajadet J, Robert G, et al. Intracoronary ultrasound imaging: initial clinical trials, *Circulation* 80(suppl 2):374, 1989 (abstract).

16. Marcus ML, Harrison DG, White CW, et al: Assessing the physiologic significance of coronary obstructions in patients: importance of diffuse undetected atherosclerosis, *Prog Cardiovasc Dis* 31:39-56, 1988.

17. Marcus ML, White CW: Coronary flow reserve in patients with normal coronary angiograms, *J Am Coll Cardiol* 6:1254-1256, 1985.

18. Sibley DH, Millar HD, Hartley CJ, et al: Subselective measurement of coronary blood flow velocity using a steerable Doppler catheter, *J Am Coll Cardiol* 8:1332-1340, 1986.

19. Wilson RF, Laughlin DE, Ackell PH, et al: Transluminal, subselective measurement of coronary artery blood flow velocity and vasodilator reserve in man, *Circulation* 72:82-92, 1985.

20. Yock P, Linker D, Saether O, et al: Intravascular two-dimensional catheter ultrasound: initial clinical studies, *Circulation* 78(suppl 2):21, 1988 (abstract).

21. Yock PG, Linker DT, Thapliyal HV, et al: Real-time two-dimensional catheter ultrasound: a new technique for high resolution intravascular imaging, *J Am Coll Cardiol* 11:130A, 1988 (abstract).

SECTION SIX

Pediatric Neurosonology

28

Neonatal Neurosonography: Techniques and Normal Anatomy

Asma Fischer
Paul Maertens

The major advantages of neurosonography over other neuroimaging techniques include the apparent safety of ultrasound, the relative low cost, and the fact that the instrumentation is portable. This noninvasive bedside procedure is well tolerated by even the sickest and smallest premature infants, provided that care is taken to leave the infant warm and undisturbed during the entire examination. State-of-the-art neurosonography demands from the sonographer good hand-eye coordination and a thorough understanding of equipment capabilities, acoustic windows, normal anatomy, and neuropathology. Neurosonographic diagnosis has proven to correlate well with examinations obtained by computed sonography and autopsy studies.[6,7] This chapter provides guidelines critical in obtaining consistently high-quality neurosonographic images.

TECHNIQUE

The equipment should ideally be chosen on its merits for safety, high resolution, and sensitivity to visualizing structures at depth.[8] The machine should be small and mobile so it can be operated without difficulty in the crowded space of the neonatal units. Real-time imaging is achieved rapidly with either mechanical or phased-array transducers. The transducers should be short and small, so they could be applied to the head via the porthole of the incubator. The surface of the transducer head should preferably be short and convex to allow better contact with the infant's head. Sector transducers have a definite advantage over linear-array transducers and are best suited for neuroimaging in this setting. Through a small acoustic window, their field of view is maximum at higher depth. A 5-MHz transducer is generally adequate for the evaluation of most neonatal brains. Higher-frequency transducers, such as 7.5- or 10-MHz transducers, are necessary to evaluate superficial structures, such as the cortical surface and the extracerebral spaces. A 7.5-MHz transducer is preferred to a 5-MHz transducer in small, premature infants. Occasionally, a 3-MHz transducer is needed to ensure adequate penetration, especially in infants with big heads or closing fontanelles.[4] Sonographic imaging of the brain can be performed through various acoustic windows where the calvaria has not been ossified (Fig. 28-1) or where a craniotomy was performed. The anterior fontanelle (bregma), metopic suture, and sag-

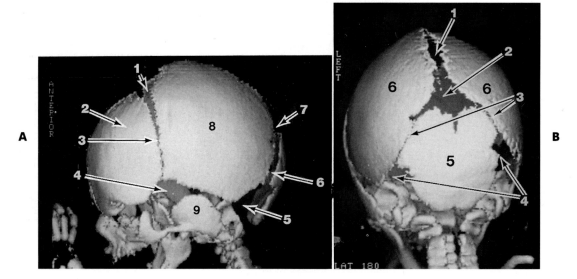

Fig. 28-1. Three-dimensional computerized tomography imaging of the normal neonatal skull. **A,** Lateral view: *1,* anterior fontanelle (bregma); *2,* frontal bone; *3,* coronal plane; *4,* anterolateral fontanelle (pterion); *5,* posterolateral fontanelle (asterion); *6,* lambdoid suture; *7,* posterior fontanelle (lambda); *8,* parietal bone; *9,* temporal squama. **B,** Posterior view: *1,* sagittal suture; *2,* posterior fontanelle (lambda); *3,* lambdoid suture; *4,* posterolateral fontanelle (asterion); *5,* occipital squama; *6,* parietal bone.

ittal suture are the most useful windows for grading intracranial hemorrhages and assessing the integrity of the corpus callosum. The anterior fontanelle is usually available for neurosonographic imaging through the first year of life; other acoustic windows generally close within the first few months after term. The anterolateral or temporal fontanelles (pterion) and coronal sutures are useful in assessing the vascular structure of the circle of Willis and in identifying extracerebral fluid collections not visualized through the anterior fontanelle. Scanning through the posterior fontanelle (lambda) is helpful in visualizing posterior cerebral structures and the posterior fossa. Posterolateral or mastoid fontanelles can be used an adjuncts in evaluating the posterior fossa.

At the beginning of the examination, the date, name of patient, and other identifying information are entered on the monitor. The selected transducer(s) is (are) carefully cleaned with a nonallergenic disinfectant, and aqueous gel is placed on the acoustic window to allow acoustic coupling between the transducer and the skin. After the transducer is positioned, the scanner output and receiver sensitivity must be adjusted for optimal imaging. The depth gain compensation should be adjusted so that similar structures have similar brightness, regardless of depth.

NORMAL SONOGRAPHIC ANATOMY

Ultrasound can be used to demonstrate fine anatomic details of the brain. This is best achieved by using two or more acoustic window. By positioning the transducer immediately close to the structure of interest, higher-

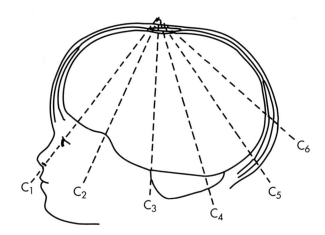

Fig. 28-2. Six coronal planes obtained through the anterior fontanelle.

frequency transducers can be used to produce higher-resolution images. Furthermore, by changing the angle at which the sound beam strikes interfaces between soft tissue structures of different acoustic densities, different structures of interest are highlighted because of changes in the brightness of their reflective surfaces.

Anterior fontanelle sonography

During any one study the entire brain is visualized in real time. Standardized views are documented in planes that have the best chance of demonstrating a pathologic process.[9] These planes are photographed with a hard-copy camera.

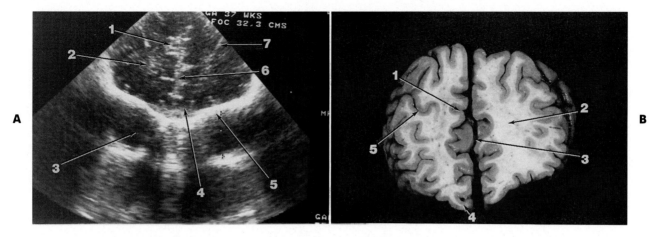

Fig. 28-3. First coronal plane (C1a). **A,** Sonogram: *1,* cingulate sulcus; *2,* rostral corona radiata; *3,* eye; *4,* straight gyrus; *5,* roof of the orbit; *6,* interhemispheric fissure; *7,* inferior frontal sulcus. **B,** Brain section: *1,* cingulate sulcus; *2,* rostral centrum semiovale; *3,* interhemispheric fissure; *4,* straight gyrus; *5,* inferior frontal sulcus.

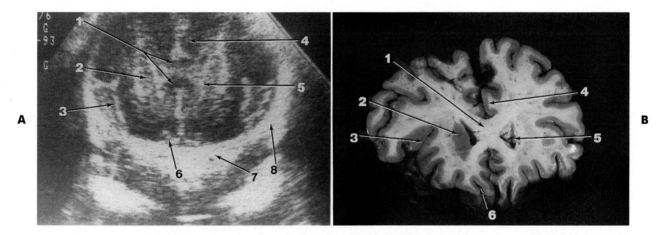

Fig. 28-4. Second coronal plane (C1b). **A,** Sonogram, and **B,** brain section: *1,* genu of corpus callosum; *2,* caudate nucleus; *3,* lateral sulcus; *4,* cingulate gyrus; *5,* lateral ventricle; *6,* straight sulcus; *7,* greater wing of the sphenoid; *8,* frontal bone.

Coronal and modified coronal studies. The transducer head should be centered on the anterior fontanelle at its widest diameter at the level of the coronal suture. During the entire procedure, care should be taken to obtain symmetric images. This is accomplished by using the skull and sutures as landmarks. Six coronal planes are obtained through the anterior fontanelle (Fig. 28-2). For each coronal plane, the structures of the cranial base generate a typical configuration.

In the first coronal plane (C1a, plane passing through the frontal lobe), the transducer is angled anteriorly toward the bright concave echoes of the orbital roofs. This produces a section through the frontal lobes, separated in the middle by the echogenicity of the falx and interhemisphere fissure. The rostral centrum semiovale appears hyperechoic (Fig. 28-3). The lateral ven-

tricles are normally not seen on this section unless they are enlarged.

In the second coronal plane (C1b, plane passing through the frontal lobe), the transducer is angled slightly posteriorly toward the posterior edge of the anterior fossa at the junction between the greater wings of the sphenoid and the frontal bone. This section crosses the genu of the corpus callosum, cingulate gyri, gyri recti, and lateral sulci. The rostral portion of the anterior horn of the lateral ventricles appears as a nonechogenic slit on either side of the midline echo of the interhemispheric fissure. The caudate nuclei constitute the inferior and lateral walls of the lateral ventricles (Fig. 28-4).

In the third coronal plane (C2, plane passing through the temporal parietal lobe), the transducer is almost

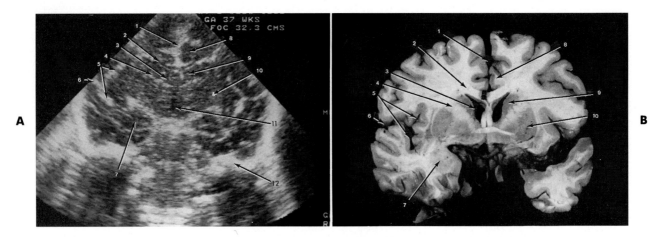

Fig. 28-5. Third coronal plane (C2): **A,** Sonogram, and **B,** brain section: *1,* interhemispheric fissure; *2,* corpus callosum; *3,* lateral ventricle; *4,* internal capsule; *5,* insula; *6,* lateral sulcus; *7,* amygdala; *8,* cingulate gyrus; *9,* caudate nucleus; *10,* lentiform nucleus; *11,* third ventricle; *12,* temporal squama.

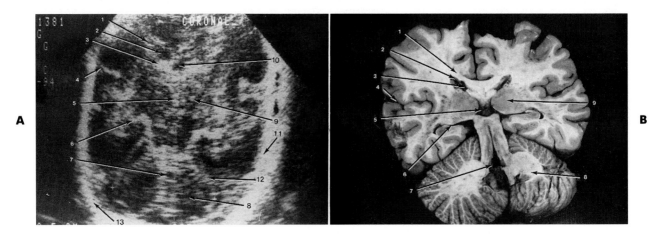

Fig. 28-6. Fourth coronal plane (C3): **A,** Sonogram, and **B,** brain section: *1,* corpus callosum (body); *2,* lateral ventricle; *3,* choroid plexus of lateral ventricle; *4,* lateral sulcus; *5,* third ventricle; *6,* hippocampal sulcus; *7,* fourth ventricle; *8,* cerebellar hemisphere; *9,* pulvinar; *10,* cisterna magna; *11,* parietal bone; *12,* tentorium; *13,* occipital squama.

vertical and angled toward the pituitary fossa just behind the lesser wings of the sphenoid. This section is at the level of the foramen of Monro. In this plane, the outline of the corpus callosum, a thin nonechogenic structure, is best delineated by two thin, parallel echogenic lines. The hyperechoic interhemispheric fissure demarcates the midline and is perpendicular to the callosal sulci, which delineate the superior edge of the corpus callosum and the inferior edge of the hypoechoic cingulate gyri. The cingulate sulci, which first appear at 18 weeks of gestation, delineate the upper border of the cingulate gyri. Below the corpus callosum, the lateral ventricles are slitlike and anechoic. They are separated in the midline by the parallel leaves of the septi pellucidi. Occasionally, small, echogenic, dotlike structures corresponding to the columnae fornices are seen at the inferior portion of the septi pellucidi. The third ventricle, below the fornices, is frequently seen as an echogenic midline slit. Laterally, the caudate nuclei form the lateral wall of the lateral ventricles. Immediately lateral and inferior to the caudate nuclei are the putamen and globus pallidus. More laterally, the echogenic sylvian fissure insula separates frontal lobe from temporal lobe (Fig. 28-5).

In the fourth coronal plane (C3, midcoronal plane passing through the temporo-occipital lobe and cerebellum), the transducer is angled posteriorly toward the occipital squama, just behind the foramen magnum. In this plane, the hypoechoic cerebellar hemispheres are seen at their widest diameter, below the highly echogenic tentorium. The bodies of the lateral ventricles now lie

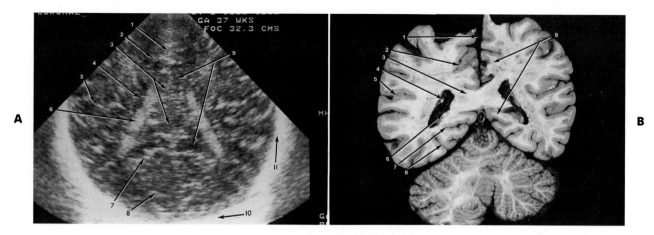

Fig. 28-7. Fifth coronal plane (C4): **A,** Sonogram, and **B,** brain section: *1,* interhemispheric fissure; *2,* cingulate sulcus; *3,* splenium of the corpus callosum; *4,* atrium of the lateral ventricle; *5,* lateral sulcus; *6,* choroid plexus; *7,* calcarine fissure; *8,* occipitotemporal sulcus; *9,* cingulate gyrus; *10,* occipital squama; *11,* parietal bone.

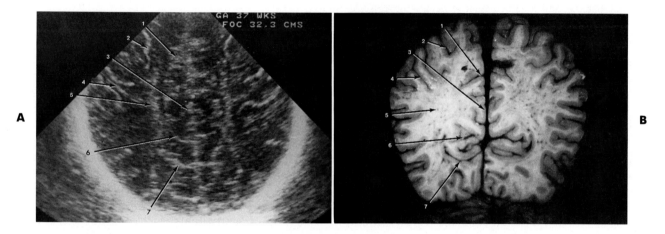

Fig. 28-8. Sixth coronal plane (C5): **A,** Sonogram, and **B,** brain section: *1,* cingulate sulcus; *2,* superior frontal sulcus; *3,* interhemispheric fissure; *4,* centralis sulcus; *5,* corona radiata; *6,* parietooccipital sulcus; *7,* calcarine fissure.

more laterally. The hyperechoic choroid plexi make the floor of the body of the lateral ventricles, the inner aspect of the temporal horns, and the roof of the third ventricle. The lateral recesses of the lateral ventricles are bordered by the echogenic bodies of the caudate nuclei. The corpus callosum makes the roof of the lateral ventricles. The echogenic thalami lie laterally to the third ventricle. Inferior to the thalami are the hypoechoic cerebral peduncles. The insula, interhemispheric fissure, and parahippocampal gyri are also seen in this plane (Fig. 28-6). On a slightly more posterior view, the highly echogenic quadrigeminal cistern is visualized superior to the echogenic cerebellar tentorium.

In the fifth coronal plane (C4, mid-posterior coronal plane passing through the occipital lobe and cerebellum), the transducer is angled further posteriorly at the

level of the midline insertion of the tentorium on the occipital squama. This section is at the level of the nonechogenic atria of the lateral ventricles. The atria contain the hyperechoic divergent glomi of the choroid plexi. Lateral to both atria are normal areas of evenly increased periventricular echogenicity. The degree of echogenicity of the normal periventricular halos is less than that of the choroid plexus. Above the level of the lateral ventricles, the midline hyperechoic interhemispheric fissure is crossed horizontally by the echogenic cingulate sulci. At the level of the lateral ventricles, the interhemispheric fissure is crossed superiorly by the echogenic callosal sulci above and below the hypoechoic splenium of the corpus callosum and inferiorly by the echogenic calcarine fissures. Above and below the splenium of the corpus callosum, the cingulate gyri are

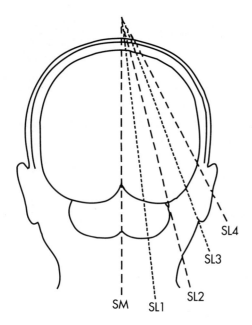

Fig. 28-9. Sagittal and modified sagittal planes through the anterior fontanelle.

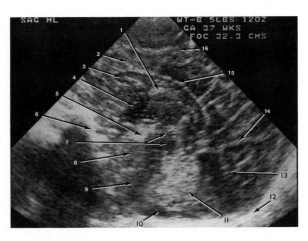

Fig. 28-10. Midline sagittal plane (SM): *1,* tela choroidea; *2,* cingulate gyrus; *3,* corpus callosum (genu); *4,* third ventricle; *5,* interpeduncular gyrus; *6,* clivus; *7,* aqueduct of Sylvius; *8,* basis pontis; *9,* medulla; *10,* cerebellar vermis; *11,* cisterna magna; *12,* occipital squama; *13,* calcarine fissure; *14,* parietooccipital sulcus; *15,* callosal sulcus; *16,* cingulate sulcus.

delineated by the echogenic cingulate sulci and calcarine fissures, respectively. Below the calcarine fissures, the occipital lobes are separated from the temporal lobes by the occipitotemporal sulci. Laterally the parietal lobes are separated from temporal lobes by sylvian fissures (Fig. 28-7).

In the sixth coronal plane (C5, plane passing through the occipital lobe), the transducer is angled superiorly in an almost transverse plane of section. At this level, there are no ventricles. The medium echogenicity of the centrum semiovale is seen on either side of the midline hyperechoic interhemispheric fissure. The interhemispheric fissure is crossed horizontally by the echogenic cinglate sulci superiorly and parietooccipital sulci inferiorly (Fig. 28-8).

Sagittal and modified sagittal studies. The sagittal images are obtained by rotating the transducer on the anterior fontanelle 90° from the coronal plane.

The clivus, the foramen magnum, and the occipital squama form the far field landmarks of the sagittal midline plane (SM). This section should demonstrate the interhemispheric fissure, the corpus callosum, cavum septi pellucidi and cavum vergae if present, choroid plexus of the third ventricle, third ventricle, aqueduct of Sylvius, brainstem, and cerebellar vermis. At the level of the interhemispheric fissure, the echogenic sulcal details are usually prominent with best visualization of the cingulate sulcus, callosal sulcus, and parietooccipital sulcus. Two thin, parallel, crescentic echogenic lines delineate the contour of the genu, body, and splenium of the hypoechoic corpus callosum. The cavum septi

pellucidi appears as an anechoic structure immediately below the genu of the corpus callosum. The anechoic cavum vergae is visualized more posteriorly and inferior to the body of the corpus callosum. It communicates anteriorly with the cavum septi pellucidi. Just below the cavum, the tela choroidea is a curvilinear hyperechoic structure forming the roof of the third ventricle. The anechoic foramen of Monro is anterior to the tela choroidea and inferior to the fornix. The supraoptic and pituitary recesses of the third ventricle are shown as triangular nonechogenic structures extending inferiorly and anteriorly toward the suprasellar region. The floor of the third ventricle appears as an echogenic line in continuity with the less echogenic aqueduct of Sylvius. The hyperechoic posterior commissure is inferior to pineal and suprapineal recesses of the third ventricle. In normal conditions, the third ventricle is slightly echogenic at the level of the thalami (posteriorly and superiorly), and the massa intermedia is not visualized. Inferior to the third ventricle, the hypoechoic midbrain is delineated by the medium echogenicity of the fossa interpeduncularis anteriorly and of the quadrigeminal cistern posteriorly. The aqueduct of Sylvius appears as a medium echogenic line separating the tectum from the tegmentum. The dorsal portion of the hypoechoic pontine tegmentum is in continuity with the mesencephalic tegmentum. It is recognized by the presence of the hyperechoic basis pontis anteriorly and of the hyperechoic cerebellar vermis posteriorly. The hyperechoic basis pontis has a half-circle convex surface that points to the clivus and is located above the medullary cistern and below the interpeduncular cistern. The hyperechoic cerebellar vermis resembles a Pacman with

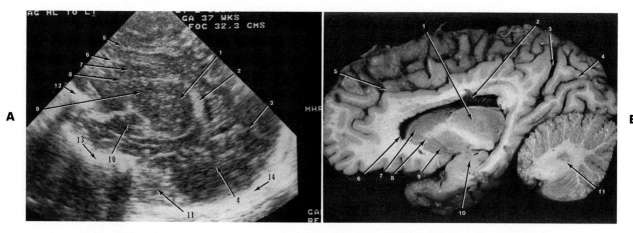

Fig. 28-11. Second modified sagittal plane (SL2): **A,** Sonogram, and **B,** brain section: *1,* thalamus; *2,* choroid plexus of the atrium; *3,* parietooccipital sulcus; *4,* calcarine fissure; *5,* cingulate sulcus; *6,* frontal horn of the lateral ventricle; *7,* caudate nucleus; *8,* internal capsule; *9,* ventricular nucleus; *10,* amygdala; *11,* cerebellar hemisphere; *12,* sphenoidal bone; *13,* temporal squama; *14,* occipital squama.

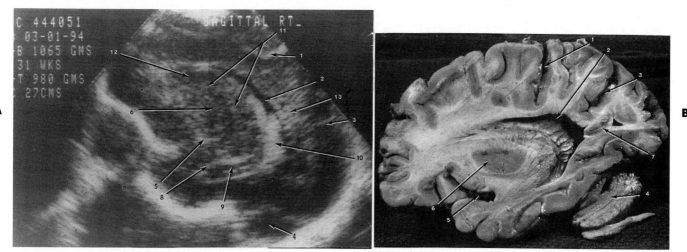

Fig. 28-12. Third modified sagittal plane (SL3): **A,** Sonogram, and **B,** brain section: *1,* cingulate sulcus; *2,* lateral ventricle; *3,* parietooccipital sulcus; *4,* cerebellar hemisphere; *5,* lateral sulcus; *6,* lenticular nucleus; *7,* calcar avis; *8,* hippocampal sulcus; *9,* fimbria hippocampi; *10,* glomus of the choroid plexus; *11,* internal capsule; *12,* caudate nucleus; *13,* corona radiata.

an echogenic small mouth corresponding to the fourth ventricle. The cerebellar vermis is separated from occipital bone by an anechoic space corresponding to the cisterna magna. The hypoechoic medulla is in continuity with the dorsal pontine tegmentum (Fig. 28-9). After study of the midline, the transducer is angled to the side (left or right) in four parasagittal planes.

The first parasagittal plane (SL1; indicates parasagittal left and SR, parasagittal right) should be close to the midline, demonstrating in the far field the base of the anterior, middle, and posterior cranial cavities located behind each other in a highly echogenic cascade. This view shows the narrow, nonechogenic, reversed-C shape

of the frontal horn, body, atrium, and temporal horn of the lateral ventricle. The floor of the frontal horn is made by the head of the caudate nucleus and does not contain any hyperechoic material. Posterior to the foramen of Monro, the hyperechoic choroid plexus separates the body, atrium, and temporal horn of the lateral ventricle, the choroid plexus is very thin (2 to 3 mm in height). It appears to end at the thalamocaudate groove. In premature infants, the germinal matrix is located immediately anterosuperiorly to the thalamocaudate groove. The roof of the frontal horn and body of the lateral ventricle is made by the cingulate gyrus (and corpus callosum). The floor of the temporal horn is made by the

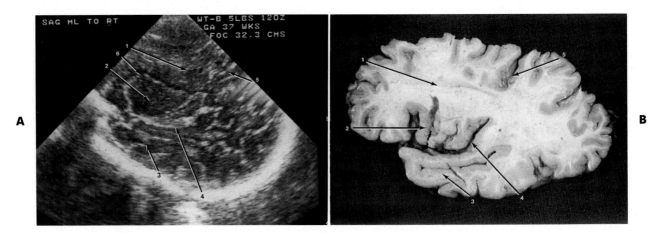

Fig. 28-13. Fourth modified sagittal plane (SL4): **A,** Sonogram, and **B,** brain section: *1,* centrum sulcus; *2,* corona radiata; *3,* temporal pole; *4,* lateral sulcus; *5,* central sulcus; *6,* circular insular sulcus.

minimally echogenic cornu Ammonis. A slightly more median section shows the hypoechoic fimbria surrounded by parallel echogenic lines instead of showing the temporal horn of the lateral ventricle. The low echogenicity of the amygdala is located just anterior to the temporal horn. Anterior to the thalamus and inferior to the caudate nucleus is the medium echogenicity of the internal capsule, which frames the low echogenicity of the globus pallidus. In the posterior fossa, the low echogenicity of the cerebellar hemisphere is covered by the hyperechoic tentorium (Fig. 28-10).

The second parasagittal plane (SL2) is made slightly lateral to the first image. In the far field, the hyperechoic occipital squama appears relatively shorter. This section demonstrates the triangular nonechogenic occipital horn of the lateral ventricle. The calcar avis may produce an echogenic impression on the anterior aspect of the occipital horn. The white matter superior to the occipital horns is normally hyperechogenic, producing a periventricular halo. More anteriorly, the trigone of the lateral ventricle is partially filled with the smooth contour of the choroid glomus. The body of the caudate nucleus bulges inside the lateral ventricle. No choroid plexus is seen in the outer edge of the lateral ventricle's temporal horn. The outer edge of the cerebellar hemisphere is still seen (Fig. 28-11).

The third parasagittal plane (SL3) is made slightly lateral to the second. In the far field the occipital squama is in continuity with the temporal bone. This section demonstrates the periventricular vascularity of white matter, which appears uniformly hyperechogenic (Fig. 28-12). Further lateral angulation of the transducer produces a section through SL4, the inner aspect of the insula (Fig. 28-13).

Imaging of the subarachnoid space, superior sagittal sinus, falx, and cerebral surface through the anterior fontanelle is best performed with a high-frequency transducer. Color Doppler imaging effectively visualizes internal carotid arteries, middle cerebral artery, anterior cerebral artery, basilar artery, and internal cerebral vein.[10,19] When duplex is not available, pulsation of the cerebral arteries is easily recognizable. Special attention should be paid to the symmetry of pulsations.[18]

Posterior fontanelle sonography

Most patients younger than 2 months of age have a patent posterior fontanelle.[13] The posterior fontanelle approach is particularly useful in distinguishing peritrigonal hyperechoic blush from periventricular leukomalacia, in imaging small hemorrhages in the occipital horns, and in visualizing exquisite details of the brainstem and other posterior fossa structures.

Posterior fontanelle midline sagittal plane. The clivus, the foramen magnum, and the occipital squama make the far field landmarks. The medial aspect of the parietal and occipital lobes is interposed between the transducer and the posterior fossa. The parietooccipital sulcus is easily identified as an echogenic line going toward the transducer. This section should demonstrate the integrity of the midline ventricular system from the third ventricle to the cisterna magna. The low echogenicity of the midbrain is separated in the tectum and tegmentum by two parallel echogenic lumina of the aqueduct of Sylvius. Normally the anteroposterior diameter of the aqueduct of Sylvius is 0.2 mm (± 0.05 mm). At the pontine level, the floor of the fourth ventricle displays an echogenic dorsal convexity corresponding to the level of the facial colliculus. The echogenic pattern of the posterior tegmentum is similar to the one seen through the anterior fontanelle. At the medullary level, the fourth ventricle is reduced to a virtual space due to the echogenicity of the tela choroidea, which is normally immediately adjacent to the floor of the fourth ventricle. The medulla is hypoechoic. The roof of the non-

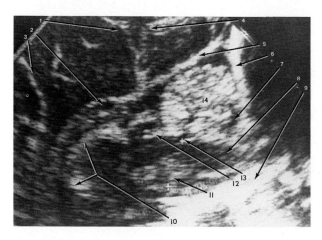

Fig. 28-14. Posterior fontanelle midline sagittal plane (PF-SM) sonogram: *1,* parietooccipital sulcus; *2,* splenium of corpus callosum; *3,* cingulate sulcus; *4,* calcarine fissure; *5,* tentorium; *6,* occipital squama; *7,* cisterna magna; *8,* medulla oblongata; *9,* clivus; *10,* tela choroidea; *11,* pons; *12,* aqueduct of Sylvius; *13,* fourth ventricle; *14,* cerebellar vermis.

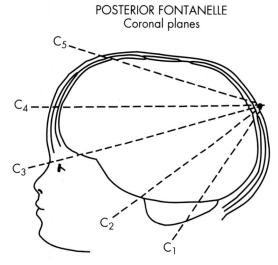

Fig. 28-15. Five coronal planes obtained through the posterior fontanelle.

echogenic pontine fourth ventricle extends toward an apex within the hypoechoic cerebellar vermis known as the *fastigium.* Through the posterior fontanelle, the nonechogenic quadrigeminal cistern and cisterna magna outline the contours of the cerebellar vermis. Anterior to the brainstem, the pulsatile motion of the basilar artery is seen in real time (Fig. 28-14).

Posterior fontanelle coronal and modified coronal planes. The transducer head is centered on the posterior fontanelle at its wider diameter at the level of the lambdoid suture. Using the skull as a landmark to monitor symmetric images, four "coronal" planes are obtained (Fig. 28-15).

In the first coronal plane (PF-C1), the transducer is angled posteriorly toward the foramen magnum, surrounded by the highly echogenic occipital squama. This section demonstrates the tent-shaped hyperechoic tentorium, which separates the supratentorial compartment from infratentorial compartment. The nonechogenic sinuses are found along the attached edges of the tentorium, the straight sinus at the upper edge, and the transverse sinuses at the lateral edges. At the infratentorial level, the triangular shape of the moderately echogenic cerebellar hemispheres is separated in the middle by the more echogenic cerebellar vermis. Below the vermis, the low echogenicity of the medulla is sectioned obliquely while it enters the foramen magnum. At the supratentorial level, the hyperechoic falx cerebri and interhemispheric fissure intervene between the low echogenicity of the occipital lobes. The interhemispheric fissure is crossed horizontally by the calcarine fissure (Fig. 28-16).

In the second coronal plane (PF-C2), the transducer is angled anteriorly toward the clivus. The section

demonstrates the insertion of the tentorium on the petrous temporal bone. The infratentorial space is narrow and contains the moderately echogenic paleo-cerebellum (anterior), the nonechogenic fourth ventricle, the hypoechoic dorsal pontine tegmentum, and the hyperechoic basis pontis. In the supratentorial space, temporal lobes occupy the middle cranial fossa; the occipital lobes are easily recognizable in the parasagittal region by the calcarine fissures (Fig. 28-17). The occipital horns are nonechogenic.

The third "coronal" plane (PF-C3) is almost transverse, showing the hyperechoic tentorial notch and its insertion on the anterior clinoid processes. The tentorial notch is crossed by the hypoechoic midbrain. On the anterior surface of the midbrain, the large hypoechoic cerebral peduncles are separated by the hyperechoic interpeduncular cistern. Close to the quadrigeminal plate, the small nonechogenic lumen of the aqueduct of Sylvius is surrounded by an echogenic circular rim. Posterior to the quadrigeminal plate is the narrow nonechogenic quadrigeminal or superior cistern. Anterior to the midbrain lies a space containing the non-echogenic cavernous sinuses, the echogenic internal carotid arteries, and the echogenic basilar artery. Lateral to the tentorial notch are the hypoechoic temporal lobes. Posterior to the tentorial notch, the hypoechoic occipital lobes are connected on the midline by the hypoechoic splenium of the corpus callosum. Lateral to the quadrigeminal cisterns are the pulvinars (Fig. 28-18).

The fourth "coronal" plane (PF-C4) goes through the atria of the lateral ventricles, which are almost completely filled with hyperechoic choroid plexus. Anterior to the choroid plexus are the thalami, which are separated from the basal ganglia by the slightly hyperechoic internal capsules. Laterally, the lateral sulci

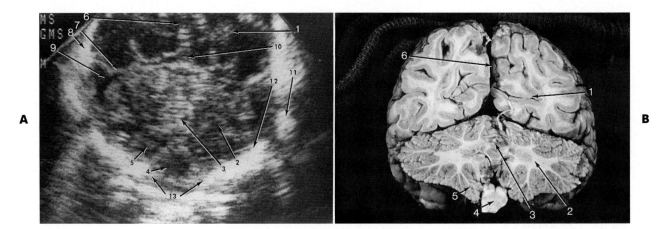

Fig. 28-16. First posterior fontanelle coronal plane (PF-C1): **A,** Sonogram, and **B,** brain section: *1,* calcarine fissure; *2,* cerebellar hemisphere; *3,* cerebellar vermis; *4,* spinal medulla; *5,* cerebellar tonsils; *6,* interhemispheric fissure and falx cerebri; *7,* tentorium; *8,* parietal bone; *9,* transverse sinus; *10,* straight sinus; *11,* temporal squama; *12,* occipital squama; *13,* foramen magnum.

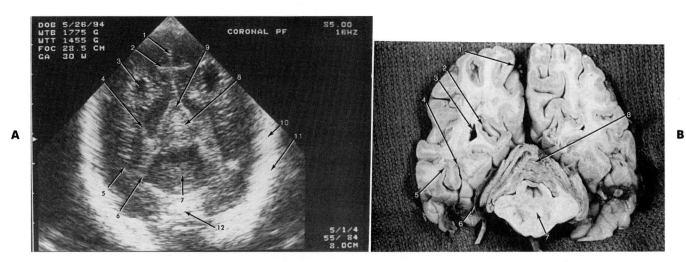

Fig. 28-17. Second fontanelle coronal plane (PF-C2): **A,** Sonogram, and **B,** brain section: *1,* interhemispheric fissure; *2,* calcarine fissure; *3,* occipital horn of the lateral ventricle; *4,* occipitotemporal sulcus; *5,* temporal lobes; *6,* tentorium (anterior insertion); *7,* pons; *8,* cerebellar vermis; *9,* straight sinus; *10,* parietal bone; *11,* temporal squama; *12,* clivus.

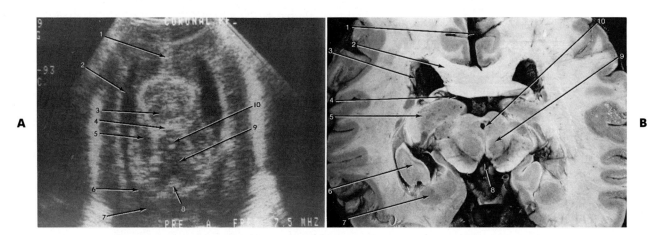

Fig. 28-18. Third posterior fontanelle coronal plane (PF-C3): **A,** Sonogram, and **B,** brain section: *1,* interhemispheric fissure; *2,* occipital horn of the lateral ventricle; *3,* splenium of the corpus callosum; *4,* quadrigeminal cistern; *5,* pulvinar; *6,* hippocampal formation; *7,* amygdaloid complex; *8,* interpeduncular cistern; *9,* midbrain; *10,* aqueduct of Sylvius.

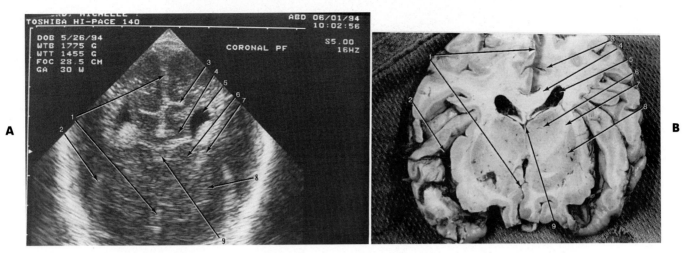

Fig. 28-19. Fourth posterior fontanelle coronal plane (PF-C4): **A,** Sonogram, and **B,** brain section: *1,* interhemispheric fissure; *2,* lateral sulcus; *3,* parieto-occipital sulcus; *4,* splenium of the corpus callosum; *5,* atrium of the lateral ventricle; *6,* choroid plexus; *7,* internal capsule; *8,* lentiform nucleus; *9,* third ventricle.

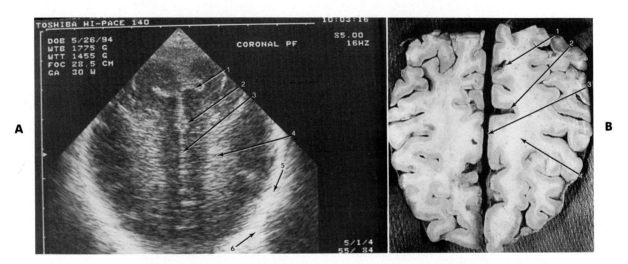

Fig. 28-20. Fifth posterior fontanelle coronal plane (PF-C5): **A,** Sonogram, and **B,** brain section: *1,* parieto-occipital fissure; *2,* cingulate sulcus; *3,* interhemispheric fissure; *4,* corona radiata; *5,* parietal bone; *6,* frontal bone.

separate the temporal lobes from the frontal lobes (Fig. 28-19).

In the fifth "coronal" plane (PF-C5), the transducer is angled superiorly above the lateral ventricles toward the highly echogenic frontal and parietal bones. This section demonstrated the normal echogenicity of the peritrigonal white matter and the hyperechoic inter-hemispheric fissure.[2] In the near field, the parieto-occipital sulci are perpendicular to the interhemispheric fissure (Fig. 28-20).

Lateral fontanelle sonography

Axial sonograms are done in special instances to obtain cuts in a plane that correlate directly with computed tomographic planes. For the axial sonogram, the transducer is placed in front of the ear and superior to the zygomatic process, over the anterolateral (pter-ion) fontanelle. With this approach, images of the circle of Willis anterior to the hypoechoic midbrain are easily obtained (Fig. 28-21). Slight oblique and posterior angulation of the transducer produces an image of the

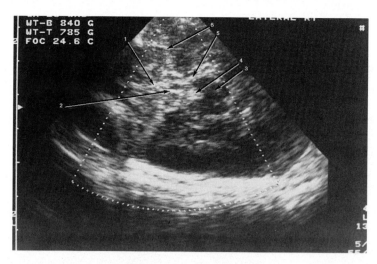

Fig. 28-21. Axial sonogram through the anterolateral fontanelle: *1,* anterior cerebral artery; *2,* infundibulum; *3,* midbrain; *4,* basilar artery; *5,* posterior cerebral artery; *6,* middle cerebral artery.

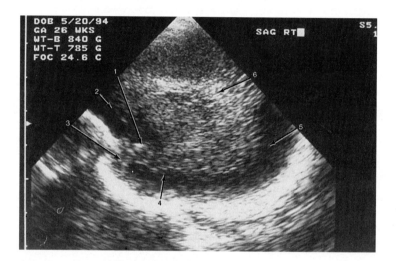

Fig. 28-22. Sonogram of a 26-week normal premature infant, lateral sagittal right (SR4): *1,* anterior lateral sulcus; *2,* frontal pole; *3,* subarachnoid space; *4,* temporal lobe; *5,* occipital pole; *6,* corona radiata.

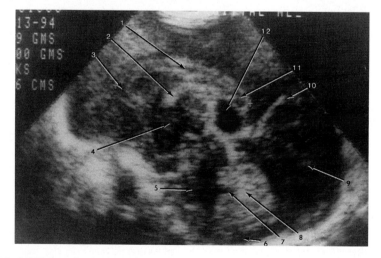

Fig. 28-23. Midline sagittal sonogram (SM) of a 27-week normal premature infant: *1,* body of corpus callosum; *2,* tela choroidea; *3,* genu of corpus callosum; *4,* third ventricle; *5,* pons; *6,* cisterna magna; *7,* fourth ventricle; *8,* cerebellar vermis; *9,* calcarine fissure; *10,* parietooccipital sulcus; *11,* splenium of corpus callosum; *12,* cavum vergae.

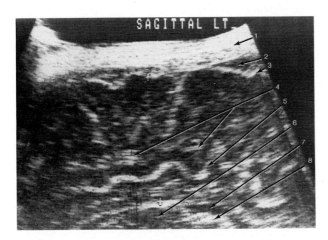

Fig. 28-24. Near field parasagittal (SL1) sonogram in a 30-week gestation premature infant (using a 7.5-MHz transducer): *1,* skin; *2,* subarachnoid space; *3,* cortical surface; *4,* white matter; *5,* cingulate sulcus; *6,* caudate; *7,* lateral ventricle; *8,* choroid plexus. Note brain thickness: between the two calipers (+).

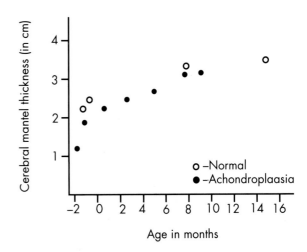

Fig. 28-25. Relationship between age from term in months and brain thickness in centimeters at the level of the foramen of Monro in 174 normal and 4 achondroplastic infants.

frontal horns, third ventricle, temporal horns, and cerebellar hemispheres.

NORMAL VARIANTS: CHANGES WITH MATURITY
Subarachnoid space

When a high-frequency transducer is applied to the anterior fontanelle, the subarachnoid space is well visualized. Using this technique in healthy normocephalic premature infants and term newborns, the normal anechoic subarachnoid space is crossed by small vessels. The shortest distance between the lateral wall of the triangular anechoic superior sagittal sinus and the outer surface of the adjacent cerebral cortex measures 2 mm or less. In older, healthy, normocephalic infants, the subarachnoid space does not exceed 3 mm in diameter.[11] In infants 3 to 5 months old, a subarachnoid space ranging from 3 to 5 mm may be observed without associated brain pathology. In other areas, the subarachnoid space is more variable in its dimension and configuration, depending on gestational age. In premature infants 25 weeks or less, widening of the subarachnoid space is seen at the level of the insula, calcarine fissure, and cisterna magna. At 3 months of gestation, the insula appears as a depressed area at the inferolateral portion of each hemisphere. Adjacent cortical regions progressively overlap the insula to form the parietal operculum, temporal operculum, and, finally, frontal operculum. At 20 to 26 weeks, there is a large subarachnoid space in front of temporal lobes without associated pathology (Fig. 28-22). The opercula delineate the hypoechoic sylvian fossa in which runs the pulsatile hyperechoic middle cerebral artery. Abundant subarachnoid fluid separates the brain from the parietal skull. Between 26 to 30 weeks, the insula is gradually

covered by the parietal and temporal opercula. At birth, the insula is nearly completely covered. The sylvian fissure appears as an echogenic line that runs horizontally from the laterally located parietal squama toward the center and forks in a Y-shaped configuration at the level of the insula. The insula is completely submerged by the end of the first year of life.

In 20- to 25-week premature infants, the medial surface of the occipital lobes is separated by a wide interhemispheric fissure. The indentation of the calcarine fissure is quite shallow but already produces an impression on the occipital horn of the lateral ventricle. After 25 weeks of gestation, there is a progressive narrowing of the interhemispheric fissure, while the calcarine fissure deepens and becomes prominent. The cisterna magna is a hypoechoic space separating cerebellum from occipital squama. It is larger in premature infants than in term newborns.

Cerebral cortex

In 20- to 25-week premature infants, the cerebral cortex is smooth, thick, and low in echogenicity. The calcarine fissure, parieto-occipital sulcus, and Sylvian fissure are developing. The gyrus rectus, hippocampal gyrus, and anterior part of the cingulate gyrus are forming. In 25- to 30-week premature infants, the whole cingulate sulcus, rolandic (central) sulcus, and superior and inferior temporal sulci are readily observed. After 30 weeks, all of the insular sulci, most of the secondary sulci from the cingulate sulcus, and all the tertiary sulci develop. As the cortical organization advances, a nearly normal adult sulcal pattern is reached by the last trimester. At term, the sulci are formed but are not as deep as they become in the next several weeks. The low-echogenicity cortical ribbon is relatively thinner than in premature infants.

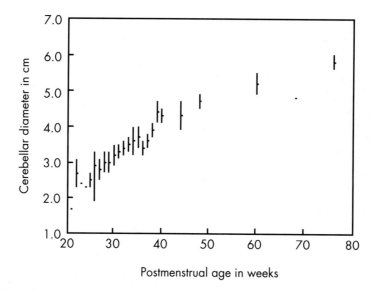

Fig. 28-26. Relationship between postmenstrual age in weeks and cerebellar diameter in centimeters in 174 normal infants.

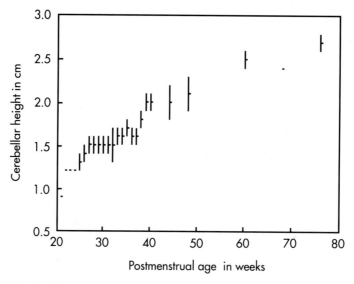

Fig. 28-27. Relationship between postmenstrual age in weeks and vermis height (distance between central lobule and uvula) in centimeters in 174 normal infants.

Ventricles and choroid plexi

The ventricles of premature infants appear relatively larger than those of term infants.[5] This is partially due to the fact that the ventricular size decreases relative to the size of the brain with increasing fetal age. In fact, the internal diameter of the atrium does not vary after 20 weeks of gestation. From 20 weeks to term, a measurement of 1 cm or less is indicative of normality.[17] Similarly, the internal diameter of the frontal horn of the lateral ventricle does not vary in relation to gestational age.

During the first few days of life, the frontal horns are small and slitlike. By the end of the first week of life, a rapid increase in size occurs probably in association with the increase in cerebrospinal fluid volume.[15] The width of the lateral ventricles at the level of the foramen of Monro, defined as the shortest distance between the caudate nucleus and the corpus callosum, normally does not exceed 3 mm. The occipital horns of the lateral ventricles of premature infants are larger than the occipital horns of full-term infants.

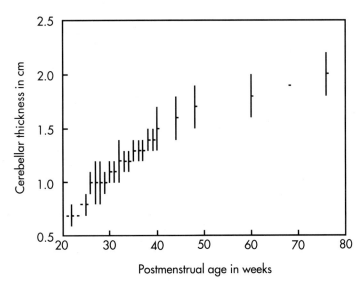

Fig. 28-28. Relationship between postmenstrual age in weeks and vermis thickness (distance between fastigium and posterior edge) in centimeters in 174 normal infants.

In normal infants, lateral ventricles diverge from the frontal region to the temporal region. In infants with a large cavum septi pellucidi, the distance between the most lateral walls of the frontal horns of the lateral ventricles may not be increased.

Third and fourth ventricles are small. The third ventricle is frequently reduced to a virtual space and normally never exceeds 2 mm of diameter in coronal planes. Rostrocaudal measurements of the third ventricle (from the supraoptic recess to the suprapineal recess) are most sensitive to rapid changes in ventricular size.[9] The fourth ventricle is best seen through the posterior fontanelle. Its anteroposterior size at the level of the fastigium is less than 5 mm in full-term neonates.

The size of the choroid plexus in relation to the lateral ventricles decreases as gestation advances. Small cysts are occasionally visualized in the choroid plexus during the second trimester. Normally, these cysts involute by 26 weeks of gestation.[1] Such cysts are usually of no clinical significance. They are frequently seen, however, in trisomy 18 and 21. The choroid plexus of the lateral ventricle can sometimes be asymmetric. The fourth ventricle and plexus appear like a Pacman's tongue when sonographically visible.

Cavum septi pellucidi, cavum vergae, cavum veli interpositi

The cavum septi pellucidi and cavum vergae are normally found in the fetus. The cavum vergae begins to close in a caudorostral fashion during the sixth month of gestation. The cavum septi pellucidi begins to close just before term; it may exist in 62% of premature infants and

42% of all newborns.[3] Closure is complete in most infants by 2 months of postterm life.[16]

The cavum velum interpositum is visualized only when the cavum vergae is prominent. It is an anechoic space situated posterior and inferior to the cavum vergae, posterior to the echogenic quadrigeminal cistern, and anterior to the splenium of the corpus callosum. This space is separated from the cavum vergae by a septation (Fig. 28-23 on p. 300).

Corpus callosum

The corpus callosum begins to form in the midportion of the genu at 8 weeks of gestation. It then extends in an anterior-posterior direction with the exception of the rostrum, which is formed after the splenium. At 20 weeks of gestation, the corpus callosum thickness is uniform (2 mm) except for the splenium, which is thinner. During pregnancy, the genu and splenium increase in thickness while the body remains unchanged. At birth, the bulbous enlargement of the splenium is thicker than that of the genu. A slight depression is frequently seen at the junction of body and splenium by 9 months of age.

Cerebral growth

Cerebral growth is best assessed through the anterior fontanelle by measuring the distance between cortical surface and roof of the lateral ventricle at the level of the foramen of Monro (Fig. 28-24). A rapid growth of the cerebral hemispheres is demonstrated during the second trimester and at the beginning of the third trimester. Cerebral thickness in a full-term infant normally ranges from 2.2 to 2.4 cm (Fig. 28-25).

Cerebellar growth

The cerebellar vermis forms from the fusion of the developing cerebellar hemispheres. The fusion begins when the cerebellar hemispheres meet superiorly in the middle at 9 weeks of gestation. The vermis extends inferiorly as the hemispheres grow. The cerebellar vermis is normally formed by the end of the week 15 of gestation. The cerebellar hemisphere's width correlates well with gestational age and is not much affected by growth retardation.[14] Further, if the measurement is expressed in millimeters, the value is very similar to the gestational age (Fig. 28-26). A more accelerated growth in cerebellar width occurs after 34 weeks. The antero-posterior distance and superoinferior distance of the central vermian area are best assessed through the posterior fontanelle. Such measurements have shown that vermis growth is linear until term and decelerates thereafter[12] (Figs. 28-27 and 28-28).

REFERENCES

1. Chudleigh P, Pearce JM, Campbell S: The prenatal diagnosis of transient cysts of the fetal choroid plexus, *Prenat Diagn* 4:135-137, 1984.
2. DiPietro MA, Brody BA, Teele RL: Peritrigonal echogenic "blush" on cranial sonography: pathology correlates, *AJR Am J Roentgenol* 146:1067-1072, 1986.
3. Farrugia S, Babcock D: Cavum septi pellucidum: its appearance and incidence with cranial ultrasonography in infancy, *Radiology* 139:147-150, 1981.
4. Fischer AQ , Livingston AL: Transcranial Doppler and real-time sonography in neonatal hydrocephaly, *J Child Neurol* 4:64-69, 1989.
5. Fischer AQ, et al, editors: Basic principles of ultrasound. In Fischer AQ, et al, editors: *Pediatric neurosonography: clinical, tomographic, and neuropathologic correlates,* New York, 1985, Churchill Livingston.
6. Fischer AQ, et al: Normal anatomy: 24-27 weeks gestation, sonographic-anatomic correlates. In Fischer AQ, et al, editors: *Pediatric neurosonography: clinical, tomographic, and neuropathologic correlates,* New York, 1985, Churchill Livingston.
7. Fischer AQ, et al: *Pediatric neurosonography: clinical, tomographic, and neuropathologic correlates,* New York, 1985, Churchill Livingston.
8. Fischer AQ, et al: Selection and safety of equipment. In Fischer AQ, et al, editors: *Pediatric neurosonography: clinical, tomographic, and neuropathologic correlates,* New York, 1985, Churchill Livingston.
9. Fischer AQ, et al: Sonographic planes and anatomical landmarks. In Fischer AQ, et al, editors: *Pediatric neurosonography: clinical, tomographic, and neuropathologic correlates,* New York, 1985, Churchill Livingston.
10. Gomez CR, Fischer AQ, Gomez SM: Color flow imaging in neurosonology: technical background and clinical application, *J Islamic Med Assoc* 20:141-145, 1988.
11. Govaert P, Pauwels W, et al: Ultrasound measurement of the subarachnoid space in infants, *Eur J Pediatr* 148:412-413, 1989.
12. Huang CC, Lu CC: The differences in growth of cerebellar vermis between appropriate-for-age and small-for-gestational-age newborns, *Early Hum Dev* 33:9-19, 1993.
13. Maertens P: Imaging through the posterior fontanelle, *J Child Neurol* 4:562-567, 1989.
14. Reece EA, Goldstein I, Pilu G, et al: Fetal cerebellar growth unaffected by intrauterine growth retardation: a new parameter for prenatal diagnosis, *Am J Obstet Gynecol* 157:632-638, 1987.
15. Saliba E, Bertrand P, Gold F, et al: Area of lateral ventricles measured on cranial ultrasonography in preterm infants: reference range, *Arch Dis Child* 65:1033-1037, 1990.
16. Shaw C, Alvord E: Cava septi pellucidi and vergaw: their normal and pathologic states, *Brain* 92:213-224, 1969.
17. Siedler DE, Filly RA: Relative growth of the higher fetal brain structures, *J Ultrasound Med* 6:573-576, 1987.
18. Williams JL: Intracranial vascular pulsations in pediatric neurosonology, *J Ultrasound Med* 2:485-488, 1983.
19. Wong WS, Tsuruda JS, Liberman RL, et al: Color Doppler imaging of the intracranial vessels in neonates, *AJNR Am J Neuroradiol* 10:425-430, 1989.

Acquired Brain Pathology

Paul Maertens
Asma Fischer

This chapter discusses the sonographic pattern of various pathologic processes affecting the brain at or after birth. The distinction between acquired brain pathology and congenital brain pathology is quite arbitrary. Some acute pathologic processes (intracranial hemorrhages, intracranial infections, focal or diffuse cerebral ischemia) may be congenital when the insult occurs in utero,[29] although more commonly these lesions are acquired postnatally.[9] Similarly, some chronic pathologic processes (hypoplasia of the corpus callosum, porencephaly, encephalomalacia, hydrocephalus, atrophy, and intracranial calcifications) can be due to the immaturity of their brains, which respond differently than term newborns to these pathologic processes. Chronic pathologic processes such as periventricular leukomalacia and colpocephaly may occur almost exclusively in preterm newborns before or after birth. Most pathologic processes affecting the premature brain are discussed in the chapter dealing with congenital brain pathology. In this chapter, we limit our discussion to intracranial hemorrhages, hypoxic ischemic brain lesions, brain death, intracranial infections, hydrocephalus, and brain atrophy.

INTRACRANIAL HEMORRHAGES

Intracranial hemorrhages can occur in both premature and term infants. In premature infants, intracranial hemorrhages are associated most frequently with hypoxic-ischemic injury. In term infants, intracranial hemorrhage can result from a bleeding disorder, trauma, arteriovenous malformation, or hemorrhagic infarction.

Intracranial hemorrhages are discussed here under nine major clinically important categories: (1) germinal matrix and choroid plexus hemorrhages, (2) intraventricular hemorrhages, (3) periventricular hemorrhages, (4) thalamic and basal ganglia hemorrhages, (5) intracerebral cortical and subcortical hemorrhages, (6) intracerebellar and brainstem hemorrhages, (7) subdural and epidural hemorrhages, (8) subarachnoid hemorrhages, and (9) cavum septi pellucidi and vergae hemorrhages.

Germinal matrix and choroid plexus hemorrhages

Germinal matrix hemorrhages. The area of the germinal matrix is most extensive in size early in gestation and progressively decreases in size with maturity, with only remnants of germinal matrix present at term. Hemorrhage into the subependymal germinal matrix is primarily a problem of the premature infant but may occur in 4% of term newborns.[28] Subependymal germinal matrix hemorrhages may be associated with intraventricular hemorrhage. The most popular classification of intracranial hemorrhage was developed by Papile and associates.[46] According to their criteria, a grade I hemorrhage is confined to the subependymal germinal matrix. Sonographically, a subependymal germinal matrix hemorrhage appears as a hyperechoic bulge in the caudothalamic groove just anterior to the termination of the choroid plexus; it is best seen on parasagittal sections (Fig. 29-1). Caution should be taken not to confuse a subependymal germinal matrix hemorrhage with normal specular reflections from the ventricular floor or with normal choroid plexus. Most subependymal hemorrhages leave a thin, hyperechoic

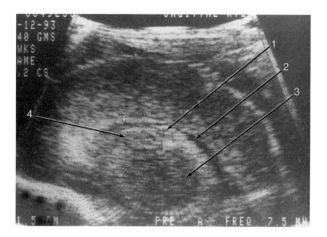

Fig. 29-1. Parasagittal sonogram (SR1) in a 23-week-gestational infant with grade I intracranial hemorrhage: *1,* acute right subependymal germinal matrix hemorrhage; *2,* body of lateral ventricle; *3,* thalamus; *4,* head of caudate nucleus.

bulge behind, whereas others undergo central liquefaction, resulting in formation of a subependymal "cyst" (Fig. 29-2). Subependymal "cysts" are also seen in congenital infections and metabolic disorders (e.g., Zellweger syndrome and Alexander's disease).[17,30,40]

Choroid plexus hemorrhages. Choroid plexus hemorrhages frequently accompany germinal matrix hemorrhages in premature infants.[47] In term infants, choroid plexus hemorrhages frequently indicate trauma or bleeding diathesis. In the premature infant, choroid plexus hemorrhages are frequently associated with intraventricular hemorrhages and physiologic stress. Sonographically, choroid plexus hemorrhages present as an enlargement of the tela choroidea at the roof of the third ventricle or as an irregular enlargement of the glomus at the level of the trigone. Transient enlargement of the choroid plexus may occur because of venous congestion without hemorrhage. Subacute hemorrhages may undergo central liquefaction and appear as "cysts" in the choroid plexus (Fig. 29-3). Other hemorrhages continue to give an irregular contour to the choroid plexus.

Intraventricular hemorrhage

In premature infants, intraventricular hemorrhages frequently result from the rupture of germinal matrix hemorrhages into the lateral ventricles. A grade II intracranial hemorrhage is a small, intraventricular hemorrhage. Blood clots do not distend the ventricular systems. They usually settle in the occipital horns, although on occasion they remain in the frontal horns. If small amounts of hyperechoic material are seen in the lateral ventricles anterior to the foramen of Monro, diagnosis of grade II intracranial hemorrhage can be made (Fig. 29-4). If the ultrasound is performed several

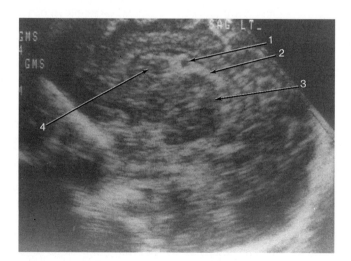

Fig. 29-2. Parasagittal sonogram (SL1) in a 32-week-gestational infant with grade I intracranial hemorrhage: *1,* chronic left subependymal germinal matrix hemorrhage (cystic); *2,* choroid plexus (glomus); *3,* thalamus; *4,* head of caudate nucleus.

days after the event, the ventricle is usually slightly enlarged, and the ependymal surface is irregularly echogenic. The posterior fontanelle approach is useful for differentiating choroid plexus hemorrhage from occipital horn blood clots (Fig. 29-5).[1]

Grade III intracranial hemorrhage is a massive intraventricular hemorrhage. The ventricle is distended by a large, hyperechoic, castlike blood clot (Fig. 29-6). An intraventricular hemorrhage is frequently asymmetric. The third and fourth ventricles, the aqueduct of Sylvius, and the posterior fossa cisterns (Fig. 29-7) are frequently filled with blood. With time, the hematoma decreases in echogenicity and is surrounded by a well-defined hyperechoic rim. The ependymal surface remains hyperechoic. Hydrocephalus is more likely to develop with obstruction of the aqueduct of Sylvius on the foramen of Monro. In neonates from 32 weeks to term, intraventricular hemorrhages seem to originate primarily from the choroid plexus.

Periventricular hemorrhage

Periventricular hemorrhages occurring in prematures with severe intraventricular hemorrhage are usually unilateral and are on the same side as the ventricular hemorrhage. Such patients are usually described as having grade IV intracranial hemorrhages.[46] Hemorrhagic periventricular leukomalacia may mimic grade IV intraventricular hemorrhage but occurs independently of it.[31]

Acutely, periventricular hemorrhages are suspected on ultrasound when there is increased echogenicity in the deep white matter adjacent to the external angle of the lateral ventricle. Acute periventricular hemorrhages are easy to differentiate from normal periventricular echogenic halos. The hyperechoic lesions are large, coarse, and heterogeneous (Fig. 29-8).[31] In

chronic periventricular hemorrhages, cysts develop in the periventricular region. The cysts are large and thick-walled and may contain echogenic clot fragments (Fig. 29-9). In some cases, the ependymal surface degenerates, producing the appearance of a ventricular outpouching. Sequelae of periventricular hemorrhages include focal cerebral atrophy or porencephaly, varying degrees of ventriculomegaly,[41] and thinning of the posterior body and splenium of the corpus callosum (Fig. 29-10).

Basal ganglia and thalamic hemorrhage

Basal ganglia and thalamic hemorrhages may occur in premature infants in association with intraventricular or

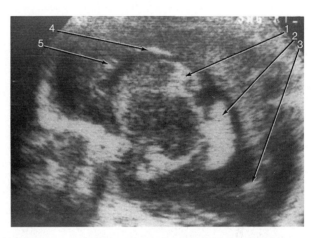

Fig. 29-4. Parasagittal sonogram (SL1) in a 28-week-gestational infant with grade II intracranial hemorrhage: *1,* germinal matrix hemorrhage; *2,* choroid plexus (glomus) hemorrhage; *3,* blood in occipital horn; *4,* specular reflection from the ventricular roof; *5,* small amount of blood in frontal horn.

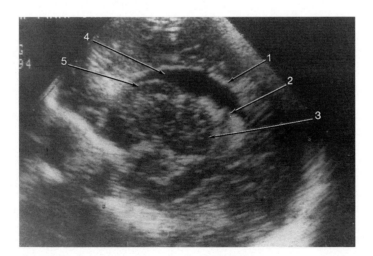

Fig. 29-3. Parasagittal sonogram (SL1) in a 30-week-gestational infant with grade II intracranial hemorrhage: *1,* residual blood along ependymal surface; *2,* choroid plexus "cyst" at the level of the glomus; *3,* thalamus; *4,* body of lateral ventricle; *5,* caudate nucleus.

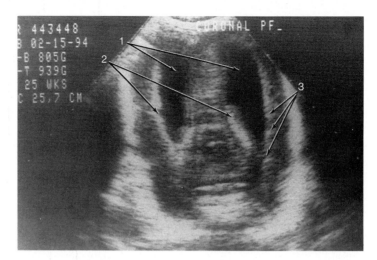

Fig. 29-5. Coronal posterior fontanelle (PF-C3) sonogram in a 25-week-gestational infant with old grade II intracranial hemorrhage: *1,* occipital horns; *2,* choroid plexus; *3,* irregular echogenicity of the ependymal surface.

A 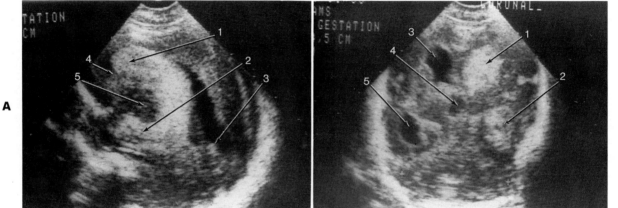 B

Fig. 29-6. A, Parasagittal sonogram (SL1) in a 24-week-gestational infant with grade III intracranial hemorrhage: *1,* blood clot occupying anterior horn of the lateral ventricle; *2,* blood clot occupying temporal horn; *3,* blood in occipital horn; *4,* head of caudate nucleus; *5,* thalamus. **B,** Coronal sonogram (C3) in the same infant: *1,* blood clot occupying body of left lateral ventricle; *2,* blood clot occupying left temporal horn; *3,* enlarged body of right lateral ventricle; *4,* enlarged third ventricle; *5,* enlarged temporal horn of right lateral ventricle.

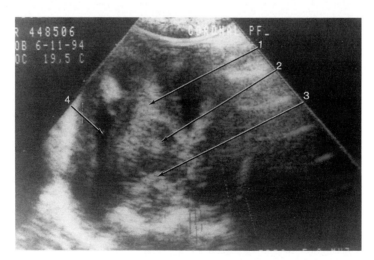

Fig. 29-7. Coronal posterior fontanelle sonogram (PF-C3) in a 28-week-gestational infant with grade III intracranial hemorrhage: *1,* subarachnoid blood in quadrigeminal cistern; *2,* blood clot in aqueduct of Sylvius; *3,* blood in interpeduncular cistern; *4,* enlarged temporal horn.

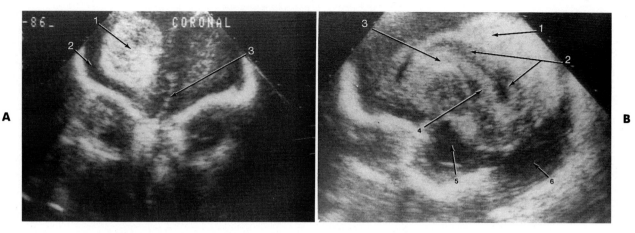

Fig. 29-8. A, Coronal sonogram (C1a) in a 26-week-gestational infant with grade IV intracranial hemorrhage: *1,* periventricular hemorrhage anterior to frontal horn of the right lateral ventricle; *2,* spared left cerebral cortex; *3,* shift of interhemispheric fissure to the left. **B,** Parasagittal sonogram (SL2) in another 25-week-gestational infant with grade IV intracranial hemorrhage: *1,* parietal periventricular hemorrhage; *2,* intraventricular hemorrhage; *3,* germinal matrix subependymal hemorrhage; *4,* choroid plexus; *5,* severely distended temporal horn; *6,* severely distended occipital horn.

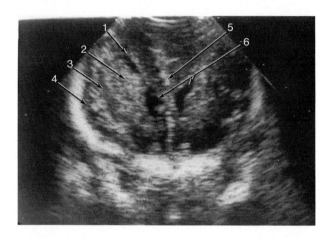

Fig. 29-9. Coronal sonogram (C1b) in a 29-week-gestational infant with 2-week-old grade IV intracranial hemorrhage: *1,* echogenic rim of forming porencephalic cyst; *2,* decreased echogenicity and retraction of previous periventricular hemorrhage; *3,* spared cerebral cortex; *4,* widened subarachnoid spare with residual blood clots; *5,* shift of interhemispheric fissure to left; *6,* frontal horns of lateral ventricles.

germinal matrix hemorrhages. Large germinal matrix hemorrhages are frequently associated with hemorrhages of the head of the caudate nucleus on the same side (Fig. 29-11). Extension of the hemorrhage to the putamen and thalamus is seen on the side of maximum intraventricular hemorrhage in nearly all cases (Fig. 29-12).[41] Unilateral basal ganglia and thalamic hemorrhages in prematures have been associated with venous flow obstruction secondary to the presence of

a large quantity of blood in the lateral ventricle. These hemorrhages in prematures are currently classified as grade IV.[46]

Basal ganglia and thalamus hemorrhages occur in term infants and early infancy with or without mass effect. Hemorrhage with mass effect is frequently associated with intraventricular hemorrhage. Unilateral thalamic hemorrhage producing a midline shift and associated with intraventricular extension has been reported in intracerebral deep venous thrombosis.[24] Unilateral putaminal hemorrhage producing a midline shift and also associated with intraventricular hemorrhage has been observed in congenital fibrinogen deficiency.[57] Bilateral hemorrhage without mass effect may indicate hemorrhagic infarction due to asphyxia or hypoglycemia. Such hemorrhages frequently spare the caudate nucleus and are not associated with intraventricular extension.[5,36,59] Basal ganglia and thalamus hemorrhages may also occur in diffuse ischemic injury.

Sonographically, basal ganglia and thalamus hemorrhages appear as areas of increased echogenicity. They may involve the internal capsule. When the latter is spared, it appears less echogenic than the thalamus and lenticular nucleus (Fig. 29-13). In patients with bleeding disorders, primary hemorrhagic lesions have an irregular echogenic pattern and can resolve with little damage. Secondary hemorrhagic lesions due to infarction are more homogeneous and are characterized by decreased vascular pulsation in the acute phase. In premature infants, large lesions tend to undergo liquefaction 1 to 2 weeks after the hemorrhage and appear hypoechoic, with a well-defined echogenic rim. The necrotic tissue

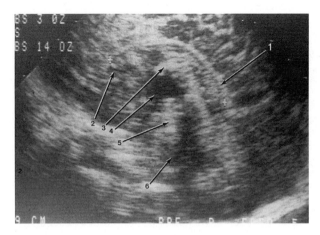

Fig. 29-10. Midline sagittal sonogram in a 29-week-gestational infant with 2-month-old parietal periventricular hemorrhage: *1,* thinning of splenium of the corpus callosum; *2,* genu of the corpus callosum; *3,* tela choroidea; *4,* third ventricle; *5,* interpeduncular cistern; *6,* pons.

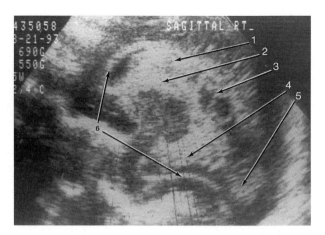

Fig. 29-11. Parasagittal sonogram (SR1) in a 26-week-gestational infant with a 2-week-old grade III intracranial hemorrhage and caudate nucleus hemorrhage: *1,* large blood clot in frontal horn of lateral ventricle; *2,* head of the caudate nucleus hemorrhage; *3,* liquefication of blood clot in trigone; *4,* blood clot in temporal horn; *5,* blood clot in occipital horn; *6,* increased echogenicity of ependymal surface.

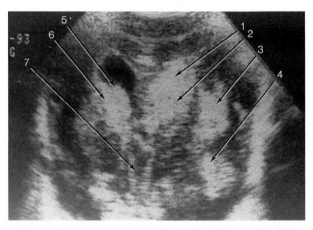

Fig. 29-12. Coronal sonogram (C2) in a 28-week-gestational infant with grade IV intracranial hemorrhage: *1,* large blood clot in left frontal horn; *2,* left caudate nucleus hemorrhage; *3,* hemorrhage in left putamen and left claustrum; *4,* blood clot in left temporal horn; *5,* blood clot in right frontal horn; *6,* right caudate nucleus hemorrhage; *7,* dilated third ventricle.

progressively resolves, and an area of encephalomalacia may develop. In term infants, the third and lateral ventricles become enlarged because of atrophy of the surrounding tissues. Thalamus and basal ganglia become small and remain echogenic.[60] Status marmoratus may develop.

Cerebral cortical and subcortical hemorrhage

Cerebral cortical and subcortical hemorrhage is uncommon in premature infants. In term newborns and young infants, three types of these hemorrhages can be distinguished: (1) hemorrhagic infarction in an arterial territory, (2) subcortical hemorrhagic venous infarction, and (3) cerebral contusion.

Hemorrhagic infarction in an arterial territory. This type of hemorrhage may be focal or multifocal.

Focal. Focal ischemic injury can occur in any of the major arterial territories but is most common in the distribution of the middle cerebral artery. Acute focal hemorrhagic infarctions appear inhomogeneously hyperechoic with loss of sulcal differentiation in the region of the infarction. As the infarction ages, the echogenic area resolves into an area of multicystic encephalomalacia or a porencephalic cyst. The ventricle on the side of the infarction may passively enlarge to occupy the space, and a widening of the subarachnoid space may develop. In the first year of life, subtle findings such as enlargement of the subarachnoid space may disappear with the growing brain.[12]

Multifocal. Acute multifocal hemorrhagic infarcts are visualized sonographically as dime-shaped hyperechoic lesions studded over many arterial territories. They may be hemorrhagic or ischemic. These lesions are usually secondary to a shower of emboli, originating from congenital heart lesions or occurring at the time

of heart catheterization procedures.[11] On occasion, multifocal hemorrhagic lesions have no embolic source and may be associated with hypoxia or alloimmune thrombocytopenia.[49]

Venous infarctions. Venous infarctions are frequently associated with thrombosis of the major venous sinuses and may be due to dehydration, trauma, or meningitis. They are generally subcortical and multifocal, have irregular margins, and are hemorrhagic in 20% of the cases. Thrombosis of venous sinuses is difficult to demonstrate by ultrasound unless the posterior fontanelle approach is used (Fig. 29-14) or the thrombus

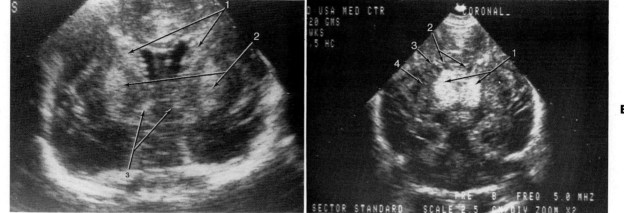

Fig. 29-13. A, Coronal sonogram (C2) in a term infant with status marmoratus (ischemia and hemorrhage of deep cerebral gray matter): *1,* symmetric caudate nucleus damage; *2,* symmetric putamen damage; *3,* symmetric thalamus damage. **B,** Coronal sonogram (C3) in a severely asphyxiated term infant: *1,* "bright thalami" due to hemorrhagic necrosis; *2,* slit lateral ventricles; *3,* normal echogenicity of caudate nucleus; *4,* normal echogenicity of putamen.

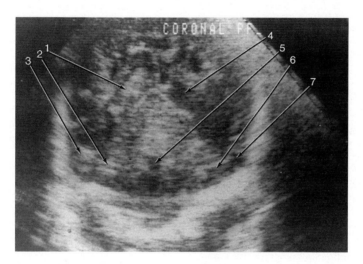

Fig. 29-14. Coronal posterior fontanelle sonogram (PF-C1) in a 32-week-gestational infant: *1,* hemorrhagic venous infarction in the medial occipitotemporal gyrus; *2,* transverse sinus thrombosis; *3,* subarachnoid hemorrhage; *4,* normal medial occipital gyrus; *5,* fourth ventricle; *6,* normal transverse sinus; *7,* normal subarachnoid space.

extends to the level of the anterior fontanelle. Doppler sonography is necessary to document venous thrombosis.

Cerebral contusions. Cerebral contusions are bruises of the brain caused by direct "coup" or contrecoup injury on the rough edges of the skull in the anterior temporal and inferofrontal regions. The cortical surface is always more involved than the underlying white matter. Subarachnoid and subdural hemorrhages are frequently associated with cerebral contusions. Cerebral contusions can also be associated with shear injuries; they occur most commonly at the junction of the gray and white matter and in the corpus callosum. Sonographically, they are heterogeneous hyperechoic lesions seen in the peripheral cerebral parenchyma. They may be visible by

sonography before their appearance on computed tomographic scan.[18] The anterior lateral fontanelle is particularly valuable in demonstrating these lesions.[44]

Brainstem and cerebellar hemorrhages

In infants up to 30 weeks of gestation, intracerebellar hemorrhages arise in the cerebellar germinal plate, a highly vascularized tissue. In premature infants they may be unilateral or bilateral. Although frequently associated with mild intracranial hemorrhages, they should not be classified as grade IV intracranial hemorrhages. In the acute phase, cerebellar hemorrhage appears as a well-defined area of increased echogenicity involving the lateral surface of the cerebellar hemisphere (Fig. 29-15).

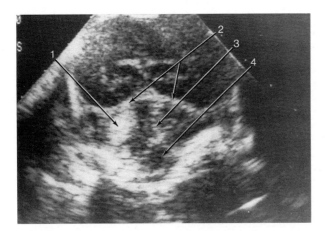

Fig. 29-15. Coronal posterior fontanelle sonogram (PF-C1) in a 22-week-gestational infant: *1,* increased echogenicity of lateral surface of cerebellar hemisphere; *2,* tentorium; *3,* cerebellar vermis; *4,* medulla.

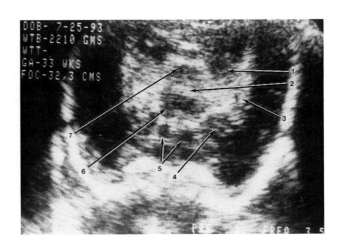

Fig. 29-17. Coronal posterior fontanelle sonogram (PF-C3) in a 33-week-gestational asphyxiated infant: *1,* pulvinar; *2,* hemorrhage in midbrain tegmentum; *3,* choroid plexus of lateral ventricle; *4,* amygdala; *5,* mamillary bodies; *6,* crus cerebri; *7,* superior colliculi.

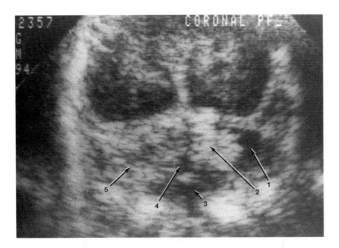

Fig. 29-16. Coronal posterior fontanelle sonogram (PF-C2) in a 24-week-gestational infant with a 2-month-old left cerebellar hemorrhage: *1,* enlarged subarachnoid space; *2,* increased echogenicity and decreased size of left cerebellar hemisphere; *3,* pons; *4,* large fourth ventricle; *5,* normal right cerebellar hemisphere.

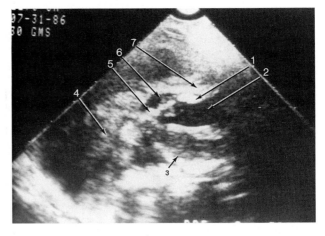

Fig. 29-18. Sagittal posterior fontanelle sonogram (PF-SM) in a 25-week-gestational infant with old cerebellar vermis contusion: *1,* residual cerebellar vermis; *2,* large fourth ventricle; *3,* pons; *4,* residual blood in the third ventricle; *5,* blood in aqueduct of Sylvius; *6,* quadrigeminal plate; *7,* tentorium.

Two weeks later, it becomes relatively hypoechoic. The long-term sequelae include cerebellar hemispheric atrophy (Fig. 29-16).[38] Brainstem hemorrhage in premature infants may be limited to basis pontis[3] or inferior colliculi (Fig. 29-17). Such lesions are frequently associated with hypoxic-ischemic lesions elsewhere. Cerebellar vermis hemorrhagic necrosis rarely occurs in premature infants (Fig. 29-18).

In term newborns, the cerebellar vermis is the initial site of the lesion. The mechanism is assumed to be compression of the occiput, which causes a contusion or laceration of the underlying cerebellum.[57] Subdural hemorrhage in the posterior fossa is frequently seen with these lesions. Damage of the vertebral arteries during

difficult delivery can result in hemorrhagic infarction of the brainstem, cerebellum, and occipital cortex.[62] In term infants experiencing hypoxic-ischemic lesions, neuronal insult may be restricted to the brainstem and thalami.[61]

Subdural and epidural hemorrhage

Epidural hemorrhages are extremely rare in infants because the middle meningeal artery is not encased in bone and is free to move. Subdural hemorrhage is more frequent in full-term infants than in premature infants. In the neonate, it is most commonly a traumatic lesion. Subdural hemorrhage may be massive in bleeding tendencies and may be supratentorial or infratentorial.[32]

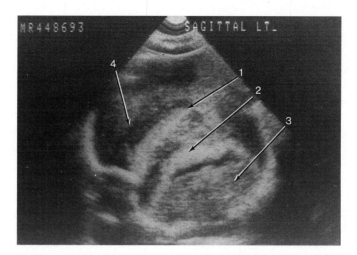

Fig. 29-19. Parasagittal sonogram (SL4) in a 28-week-gestational infant with traumatic delivery: *1,* subarachnoid blood in lateral fissure; *2,* contusion of inferior surface of left temporal lobe; *3,* subdural hematoma; *4,* frontal lobe.

Supratentorial subdural hemorrhage is likely to be secondary to falx laceration or to tearing of bridging veins. The laceration usually occurs near the falcial tentorium. The source of bleeding is most commonly the inferior sagittal sinus. With falx laceration, the subdural hematoma collects over the inferior aspect of the interhemispheric fissure and above the tentorium (Fig. 29-19). Tearing of bridging veins results in hematoma formation over the cerebral convexity, which is usually unilateral in the neonate and bilateral in older infants. When unilateral, large convexity subdural hematomas are easily seen on sonography. The surface of the brain is depressed inferiorly and medially, the lateral ventricle is compressed, and there is displacement of the midline structure to the contralateral side (Fig. 29-20). High-frequency transducers are useful in identifying medial extension of convexity subdurals. The lateral and posterior fontanelle approach is used to identify small convexity hematomas not visible through the anterior fontanelle. Infratentorial subdurals are secondary to tearing of the tentorium or to traumatic separation of the squamous portion of the occipital bone and the enchondral portion of the occipital bone (occipital osteodiastasis). They are frequently associated with cerebellar contusion. Large hematomas may compress the cerebellum and brainstem.[25] Scanning in the axial plane through the lateral posterior fontanelle is sometimes helpful in assessing the presence and extent of these lesions.[43]

When a subdural hematoma is acute, the subdural space appears echogenic.[22] As the hematoma evolves, it becomes hypoechoic relative to the brain and eventually anechoic (subdural hygroma). The highly echogenic and pulsatile dura covers the flattened gyri, which are displaced away from the cranial vault, falx, or tentorium. The dura also bridges sulci, which may be widened (Fig.

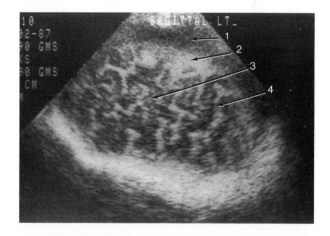

Fig. 29-20. Parasagittal sonogram (lateral to SL4) in a term infant with 1-week-old convexity subdural hematoma: *1,* relatively hypoechoic subdural hematoma; *2,* highly echogenic dura; *3,* frontal cortex; *4,* central sulcus.

29-21). Subdural hematomas cannot be differentiated from empyemas without clinical information.

Subarachnoid hemorrhage

Subarachnoid hemorrhage often accompanies intraventricular hemorrhage, cerebral or cerebellar contusion or anoxia-ischemia, or subdural hemorrhage and has also been associated with vascular disorders. In the acute phase, the hemorrhage manifests as increased echogenicity of the subarachnoid space.[43] At the infratentorial level, a subarachnoid hemorrhage should be suspected when the cerebellar contour is poorly visualized and pericerebellar cisterns (cisterna magna, quadrigeminal cistern) are filled with echogenic material. There, hemorrhages are best demonstrated through the anterior fontanelle (Fig. 29-18).[35] At the supratentorial level, subarachnoid hemorrhage is suspected when the inter-hemispheric fissure, sylvian fissure, and choroid fissure are widened, and hyperechoic blood is seen to extend into the enlarged cerebral sulci. A high-frequency transducer is necessary to visualize subarachnoid blood at the level of the interhemispheric fissure (Table 29-1). Subarachnoid hemorrhage cannot be differentiated sonographically from acute bacterial meningitis without clinical information.

Cavum septi pellucidi and vergae hemorrhage

Cavum septi pellucidi and vergae hemorrhage occurs almost exclusively in premature infants. During the acute phase, ultrasonography shows highly echogenic material displacing the corpus callosum upward, the tela choroidea downward, and the lateral ventricles laterally (Fig. 29-22). In the chronic phase, such lesions liquefy and may become cystic or disappear.

HYPOXIC-ISCHEMIC LESIONS

Hypoxic-ischemic lesions presenting as intracranial hemorrhage (periventricular hemorrhage, thalamic hemorrhage, cerebellar hemorrhage, or hemorrhagic strokes) have been discussed in the section on intracranial hemorrhages. The type and location of ischemic lesion depend on etiology and maturation of the vascular supply of the infant brain.

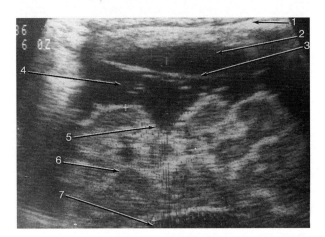

Fig. 29-21. Parasagittal sonogram (SR1) in a term infant with subdural hygroma: *1*, skin; *2*, subdural hygroma; *3*, dura mater; *4*, wide subarachnoid space with arachnoid trabeculae; *5*, widened sulcus; *6*, cingulate sulcus; *7*, body of lateral ventricle.

Six types of hypoxic-ischemic lesions can be distin-guished: (1) periventricular leukomalacia, (2) subcortical parasagittal white matter necrosis with ulegyria, (3) nonhemorrhagic infarction, (4) gyral infarction, (5) diffuse ischemic injury, and (6) brain death.

Periventricular leukomalacia

Periventricular leukomalacia consists of ischemic infarction of axons traversing the deep white matter at the external margins of lateral ventricles.[51] In premature infants, the periventricular region represents the arterial borderzone between the penetrating ventriculopedal (anterior, middle, and posterior cerebral arteries) and deep ventriculofugal (choroidal) arteries. Hypotension or hypoperfusion can result in bilateral, occasionally asymmetric, periventricular lesions. The most common locations of periventricular leukomalacia include the white matter adjacent to the trigone, the optic radiations, and the white matter adjacent to the foramen of Monro.[51]

The sonographic appearance of periventricular leu-komalacia evolves during the months that follow the ictus.[10,20] In the acute stage, small, discrete, linear, and irregular hyperechogenicities located superolaterally to the lateral ventricle are seen (Table 29-2). The diagnosis may be difficult when lesions are symmetric during this stage[7] (Fig. 29-23). Five to 73 days after the acute stage, the lesions become cavitary. This stage is characterized by small, discrete, single or multiple cysts that never communicate with the lateral ventricles (Fig. 29-24). The cysts usually disappear between 2 and 5 months after the acute stage. In the postcystic stage, there is mild ventriculomegaly and severe impairment in myelination on magnetic resonance imaging.

Subcortical parasagittal white matter necrosis

In term neonates, subcortical parasagittal white matter necrosis with ulegyria refers to ischemic lesions involving the borderzones between the three major cerebral arteries. These lesions are ascribed to sharply reduced cerebral blood flow and can be associated with periventricular leukomalacia. They are bilateral and can be asymmetric in the superomedial aspects of the cerebral convexity. They are most commonly seen in the frontal and parietooccipital regions and may be hemor-rhagic. In severe cases, necrosis may extend to large

Table 29-1. Differentiation of subdural and subarachnoid space lesions

Ultrasound	Subdural hemorrhage	Subdural hygroma	Subarachnoid hemorrhage
Echogenicity	+++	Anechoic	+++
Brain surface	Flattened	Flattened	Large sulci and normal gyri
Pulsatility	Close to cortical surface	Close to cortical surface	Between skull and cortical surface

portions of the cerebral convexity, especially in the parietooccipital regions. Sonographically, the parasagittal areas may be difficult to evaluate. To visualize posterior lesions through the anterior fontanelle, the transducer should be angled posteriorly. A high-frequency transducer may be necessary to visualize frontal regions. During the acute phase, diffuse ischemic lesions are characterized by highly echogenic areas within the cerebral cortex, poor definition of gyral-sulcal interfaces, and absent vascular pulsation (Fig. 29-25). Ultrasound testing cannot determine the extent of the damage during this period. Repeat testing 14 days later may show a return to near normal or, in those patients with a guarded prognosis, widening of the interhemispheric fissure, decreased brain thickness, and ventricular enlargement suggesting atrophy. Subcortical cysts may appear.[58] The cortical surface becomes irregular, with enlarged brain sulci surrounding somewhat shrunken, mushroom-shaped gyri in the borderzone region (ulegyria).

Gyral infarction

Gyral infarction can be seen in patients with meningitis or acute and severe asphyxia.[2,11] Increased echogenicity is seen in the region of the cortical gray matter, causing an alteration of the gray-white interface and an

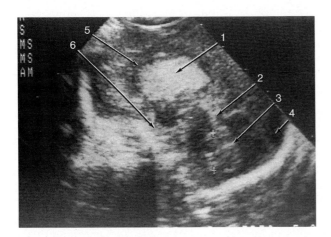

Fig. 29-22. Midline sagittal sonogram (SM) in a 26-week-gestational infant with grade III intracranial hemorrhage: *1,* cavum septi pellucidi and vergae hemorrhage; *2,* quadrigeminal cistern; *3,* cerebellar vermis; *4,* occipital lobe; *5,* superiorly displaced corpus callosum; *6,* blood clot in infundibulum of third ventricle.

inversion of the normal sonographic relationship (Fig. 29-26). These lesions are best seen within 1 week from the onset of meningitis and are frequently associated with widening of the subarachnoid space. Cortical laminar necrosis can be documented by ultrasound (Fig. 29-27). The long-term sequelae of such lesions include brain atrophy.[13]

Nonhemorrhagic strokes

Nonhemorrhagic strokes are the result of acute focal cerebral ischemia associated with thrombotic, embolic, or vasospastic arterial stenosis or occlusion. Their presence is suggested when there is a unilateral reduction of the pulsation in a cerebral artery or a shift of the falx is detected. There may be no mass effect initially. A few days after the onset of symptoms, a homogeneously increased echogenicity of the subcortical white matter with loss of gyral-sulcal interfaces may be seen (Fig. 29-28). In the acute stages, the area of infarction may be outlined by a hyperechoic rim, which may represent the edema–compressed brain interface or the area of luxury perfusion.[11] In the chronic stage, a nonhemorrhagic stroke may appear as a small area of localized brain atrophy or porencephaly.

Diffuse cerebral insults

Diffuse cerebral insults are more common in term infants than in premature infants. Timing of the sonographic examination in relation to hypoxic or hypoglycemic injury is important in determining their sonographic appearance. Within 1 or 2 days from the onset of symptoms, cellular disruption results in generalized increased parenchymal echogenicity, and most anatomic landmarks are obscured because of loss of most gray/matter–white matter interfaces (Fig. 29-29). Gyri along the interhemispheric fissure are flattened. Although ventricles are usually effaced if herniation occurs, they become entrapped and progressively enlarge. Pulsation of cerebral vessels is markedly reduced. A few days later, repeat sonography may show a more irregular echogenic pattern, with areas of increased echogenicity adjacent to areas of hypoechogenicity imparting a "Swiss cheese" configuration to the brain parenchyma. The ventricles, subarachnoid space, and cortical sulci progressively become enlarged. Long-term sequelae include cerebral atrophy and/or multicystic encephalomalacia.[56] Diffuse cerebral insults may lead to brain death.

Table 29-2. Sonographic differentiation of periventricular hemorrhage and periventricular leukomalacia

Ultrasound	Periventricular hemorrhage	Periventricular leukomalacia
Configuration	Continuous with intraventricular hemorrhage	Patchy and discontinuous
Laterality	Unilateral	Usually bilateral

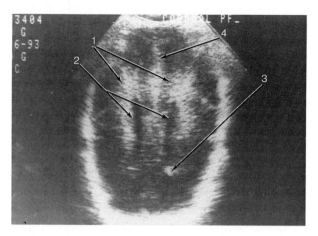

Fig. 29-23. Posterior fontanelle coronal sonogram (PF-C5) in a 31-week-gestational infant with early signs of periventricular leukomalacia: *1,* bilateral irregular and linear hyperechogenic lesions in the corona radiata; *2,* body of the lateral ventricles; *3,* small germina matrix hemorrhage; *4,* interhemispheric fissure.

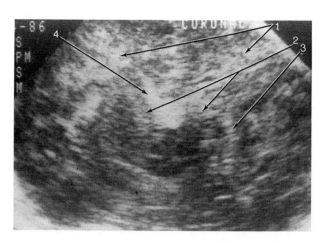

Fig. 29-25. Coronal sonogram (C2) in a term infant with subcortical parasagittal white matter necrosis: *1,* increased echogenicity of parasagittal subcortical white matter; *2,* increased echogenicity of caudate nucleus; *3,* increased echogenicity of putamen; *4,* intraventricular hemorrhage.

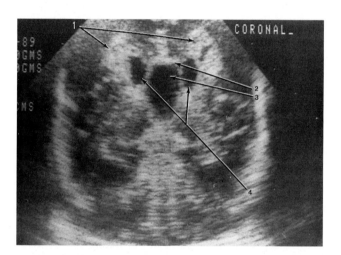

Fig. 29-24. Coronal sonogram (C3) in a 29-week-gestational infant with periventricular leukomalacia: *1,* symmetric cavitary periventricular hyperechogenicities; *2,* thin corpus callosum; *3,* enlarged cavum pellucidi; *4,* enlarged atrophic body of the lateral ventricles.

Brain death

Brain death is a permanent, irreversible, extensive brain insult that precludes recovery of any brain function. Along with other conventional methods, ultrasound is helpful in making the diagnosis of brain death. The sonographic features of the condition are variable, depending on its etiology and the timing of the ultrasound. Real-time ultrasound is helpful in discerning the etiologies of coma in infants and differentiating hypoxic-ischemic insults from other etiologies. Acutely, brain death is suggested sonographically by extensive changes

in brain echogenicity accompanied by loss of landmarks, loss of pulsation,[12] and effacement of posterior fossa cisterns with brainstem compression and cerebellar tonsil herniation (Fig. 29-30). Transcranial Doppler is helpful in assessing the degree and extent of vascular compromise.[15,42] None of these findings is pathognomic of brain death,[16] and at least one child who had no cerebral pulsations survived.[23] Temperature, among other factors, influences the outcome. Clinical correlation is always required before making the sonographic diagnosis of brain death.

INTRACRANIAL INFECTIONS

The sonographic distinction between intracranial infection and intracranial hemorrhage may be difficult in the absence of adequate clinical information.

Purulent meningitis

In its early stages, purulent meningitis frequently results in increased echogenicity and widening of the sulci and fissures and in a mild increase of ventricular size (Fig. 29-31). The gyri usually have normal echogenicity.[27] Meningitis may also be associated with subdural empyema or hygroma, cerebral edema, ventriculitis, hydrocephalus, brain abscess, and ischemic changes.

Ventriculitis

The sonographic picture of acute, purulent ventriculitis is characterized by particulate echoes floating freely within the enlarged ventricles.[53] The ependymal surface is irregular and hyperechoic, and choroid plexus are lined with echogenic debris (Fig. 29-32). A bidirectional pulsatile motion may be detected in the aqueduct of

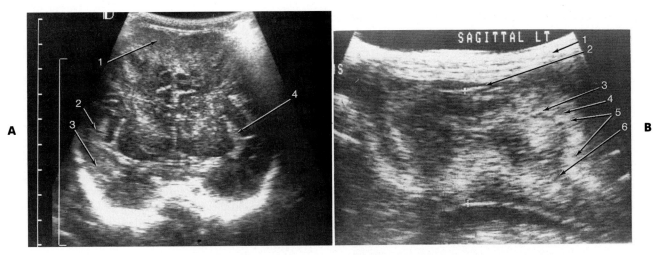

Fig. 29-26. A, Coronal sonogram (C2) in a 2-month-old term infant with pneumococcal meningitis and multiple gyral infarction: *1,* increased echogenicity of right superior and middle frontal gyri; *2,* pus in right lateral sulcus; *3,* increased echogenicity of right superior and middle temporal gyri; *4,* pus covering left insular cortex. **B,** Parasagittal sonogram (SL1) using a 7.5-MHz transducer demonstrating gyral infarction due to asphyxia in a term infant: *1,* skin; *2,* subarachnoid space; *3,* sulci; *4,* normal superficial cortical layers; *5,* highly echogenic deep cortical layers; *6,* relative sparing of subcortical white matter.

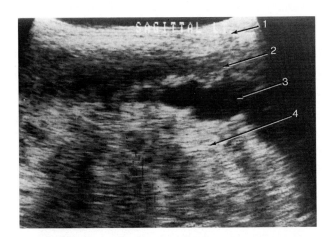

Fig. 29-27. Parasagittal sonogram (SL1) using a 7.5-MHz transducer demonstrating cortical laminar necrosis: *1,* skin; *2,* cortex; *3,* anechoic space separating superficial cortical layers from deeper cortical layers; *4,* irregular echogenicity of subcortical white matter.

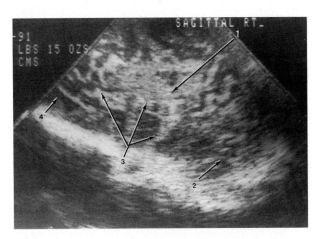

Fig. 29-28. Parasagittal sonogram (SR3) in a term infant with recent right middle cerebral artery stroke: *1,* homogeneous increased echogenicity of the cortex at the level of the insular ribbon; *2,* occipital cortex; *3,* circular sulcus of the insula; *4,* frontal cortex.

Sylvius.[39] During the chronic phase, intraventricular fibrous septa may lead to sequestered compartments within the ventricles (Fig. 29-33).[48]

Brain abscess

Brain abscesses are uncommon in neonates. They may be single or multiple and are usually located in the cerebral hemispheres. The frontal lobes are affected frequently. The developing abscess appears as a homogeneous echogenic mass compressing adjacent structures. After 7 to 14 days, the center of the echogenic mass becomes hypoechoic and contains low-amplitude

small echoes that represent collections of inflammatory cells.[33,37] The wall of the abscess is irregular in echogenicity, and its thickness varies, decreasing in response to antibiotic therapy. During the chronic stage, porencephaly may appear in the space previously occupied by the abscess. Aspiration of abscesses can be undertaken under sonographic guidance to establish an etiologic diagnosis and reduce mass effect.

TORCH infections

In the neonate, the most common causative organisms of meningoencephalitis are *Toxoplasma gondii,* rubella virus, cytomegalovirus, and herpes simplex virus, often collectively called TORCH. The spectrum of sonographic features of TORCH infections includes dystrophic calcification, cystic degeneration, ventricular enlargement, and echogenic vasculature in the basal ganglia.[19,21,54] Dystrophic calcifications appear as brightly echogenic foci with or without shadowing. Their presence implies that the responsible insult must have occurred at least 2 to 4 weeks earlier.[8] Their distribution varies with the causative organism and the severity of the encephalitis.[26] In central nervous system toxoplasmosis, calcifications are small and diffuse throughout the brain parenchyma (Fig. 29-34). In rubella meningoencephali-

tis, calcification may involve the periventricular white matter and the cerebral cortex. In herpes simplex type II infection, calcifications tend to be large, involving diffusely the brain parenchyma. The pial surface of the temporal lobe may be calcified (Fig. 29-35). In cytomegalovirus meningoencephalitis, calcifications are scattered in the periventricular regions. Cystic degeneration associated with TORCH infections may be subependymal, similar to lesions resulting from germinal matrix or periventricular parenchymal hemorrhage. Ventricular enlargement may be secondary to atrophy or hydrocephalus. Mineralized or hypercellular arterial walls look like a branched candlestick because of increased echogenicity of the basal ganglia and thalamic vessels.[55]

HYDROCEPHALUS

Hydrocephalus is a condition characterized by excessive cerebrospinal fluid (CSF) accumulation in the head. It may be associated with increased intracranial pressure. When associated with increased intracranial pressure, it is referred to as "dynamic" hydrocephalus, which may either be active or arrested. "Active" hydrocephalus refers to an imbalance between CSF formation and absorption. "Arrested" hydrocephalus occurs when CSF production and resorption are balanced. "Passive" hydrocephalus is without increased pressure; it usually results from craniocerebral disproportion.

"Dynamic" hydrocephalus

With the exception of hydrocephalus secondary to choroid plexus papillomas, overproduction of CSF is not a recognized cause of dynamic hydrocephalus, which almost always results from inadequate resorp-

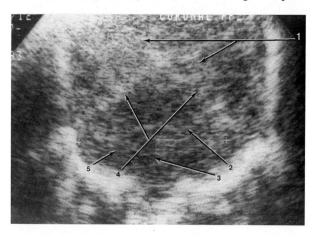

Fig. 29-29. Posterior fontanelle coronal sonogram (PF-C1) in a term asphyxiated infant: *1,* loss of most gray matter–white matter interfaces at the supratentorial level; *2,* left cerebellar hemisphere; *3,* cerebellar vermis (relatively less echogenic than cerebral parenchymal); *4,* tentorium; *5,* right cerebellar hemisphere.

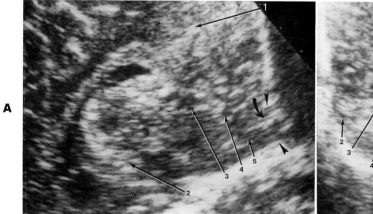
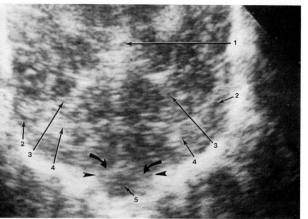

Fig. 29-30. A, Posterior fontanelle midline sagittal sonogram (PF-SM) cerebellar vermis herniation *(curved arrow)* through foramen magnum *(arrowheads): 1,* tentorium; *2,* echogenic (compressed) third ventricle; *3,* narrow (compressed) aqueduct of Sylvius; *4,* hyperechoic (necrotic) cerebellar hemisphere; *5,* medulla. **B,** Posterior fontanelle coronal sonogram (PF-C3) showing cerebellar tonsils herniation *(curved arrow)* through foramen magnum *(arrow heads): 1,* Straight sinus; *2,* sigmoid sinus; *3,* tentorium; *4,* hyperechoic cerebellar hemisphere; *5,* medulla.

tion. Dynamic hydrocephalus is classified as either "communicating" or "obstructive." In communicating hydrocephalus, CSF absorption or circulation within the subarachnoid space is impaired. In obstructive hydrocephalus, CSF flow within the ventricular system is decreased or absent.

Communication hydrocephalus. Communicating hydrocephalus is the most common form of acquired hydrocephalus. Typical causes of communicating hydrocephalus include subarachnoid hemorrhage, meningitis, and increased intracranial venous pressure from sinus thrombosis, arteriovenous malformation, narrowing of jugular foramen (achondroplasia), bilateral jugular cath-

eterization, or increased intrathoracic pressure (bronchopulmonary dysplasia).

Sagittal plane ultrasound images of communicating hydrocephalus show enlargement of the third and fourth ventricles and increased distance between the genu of the corpus callosum and the choroid plexus of the third ventricle. Coronal sections at the level of the foramen of Monro reveal frontal horns that are concentrically enlarged, round, and bulging above the level of the corpus callosum (Fig. 29-36). The temporal horn dilation is commensurate to that of the bodies of the lateral ventricles. Subarachnoid space and cortical sulci are frequently enlarged. Brain thickness may be increased, normal, or decreased. In achondroplasia, for instance, it is frequently increased (megaloencephaly); it is decreased when communicating hydrocephalus is associated with atrophy.

Obstructive hydrocephalus. Obstructive hydrocephalus may hinder cerebral blood flow, cause cerebral and cerebellar herniation, and compromise brainstem function. It requires prompt treatment by CSF diversion. Ultrasound is particularly useful in assessing (1) the obstruction's site, (2) the obstruction's cause, (3) the ventricular size, (4) the distortion of the brain and ventricular system, (5) the impact of intracranial pressure on cerebral perfusion, and (6) the effectiveness of therapeutic maneuvers.

Obstructive hydrocephalus usually produces ventriculomegaly rostral to the site of CSF obstruction. Vulnerable sites for blockage include the foramen of Monro, aqueduct of Sylvius, third ventricle, and the fourth ventricle's outflow foramina. As a rule, the temporal horns of the lateral ventricles are always distended in obstructive hydrocephalus. When both the aqueduct of

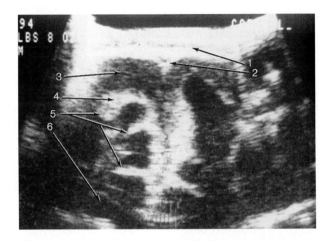

Fig. 29-31. Coronal sonogram (C2) using a 7.5-MHz transducer in a 2-month-old term infant with *Haemophilus influenzae* meningitis: *1,* skin; *2,* sagittal sinus; *3,* pus in subarachnoid space; *4,* hyperechoic pial surface; *5,* enlarged cortical sulcus; *6,* large lateral ventricle.

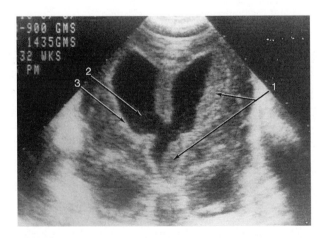

Fig. 29-32. Coronal sonogram (C2) in a 32-week-gestational infant with *Citrobacter* ventriculitis: *1,* collection of pus along the inferior wall of the ventricles (infant laying on the left side); *2,* particulate echoes floating freely within the dilated body of the lateral ventricle; *3,* hyperechoic irregular ependymal surface.

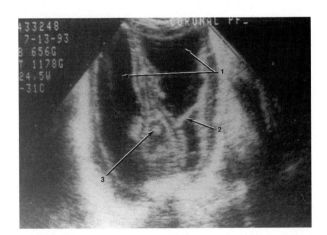

Fig. 29-33. Posterior fontanelle coronal sonogram (PF-C3) in a 25-week-gestational infant with Gram-negative ventriculitis: *1,* large occipital horns; *2,* fibrous septum connecting the choroid plexus to the ependymal surface of the left temporal horn; *3,* pus in the aqueduct of Sylvius.

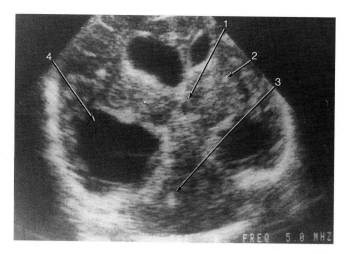

Fig. 29-34. Coronal sonogram (C3) in a term infant with central nervous system toxoplasmosis: *1,* small third ventricle with hyperechoic ependymal surface; *2,* left putaminal calcification; *3,* right cerebellar hemisphere calcification; *4,* markedly dilated right temporal horn.

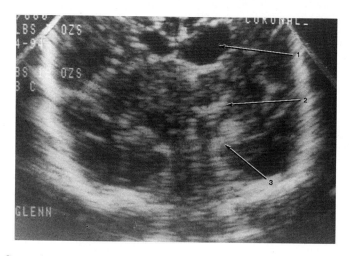

Fig. 29-35. Coronal sonogram (C2) in a term infant with congenital herpes encephalitis: *1,* enlarged body of the left lateral ventricle (atrophy); *2,* left thalamic calcification; *3,* calcified pial surface of the left temporal lobe.

Sylvius and the fourth ventricle outflow foramina are occluded, the isolated fourth ventricle progressively becomes distended because of continued CSF production by the choroid plexus of the fourth ventricle. Obstructive hydrocephalus can be caused by congenital defects, neoplasias, infections, hemorrhages, and uncal herniation.

Severe obstructive hydrocephalus causes distortions of the brain and ventricular system. At the supratentorial level, severe hydrocephalus can stretch the corpus callosum, displace the tela choroidea downward, fenestrate the septum pellucidum,[6] stretch the massa intermedia, decrease parenchymal thickness, and delay cingulate sulcus development.[52] The lateral ventricle is the most common site of ventricular herniation. The latter occurs through the choroidal fissure into the supracerebellar and quadrigeminal cisterns, producing

an atrial diverticulum.[34] This diverticulum can compress the mesencephalic tectum and can be mistaken for arachnoid cysts. Demonstration of continuity of the diverticulum with the trigonal ventricular wall establishes the diagnosis. Other sites of herniation of the ventricular wall include the suprapineal and anterior recesses of the third ventricle. The suprapineal diverticulum expands into the posterior incisural space, displacing the pineal gland inferiorly, compressing the quadrigeminal plate, and elevating the vein of Galen. It is frequently seen in the Arnold-Chiari type II malformations. The anterior recesses of the third ventricle (chiasmal and infundibular recesses) enlarge and extend inferiorly into the suprasellar cistern. Anterior recess diverticula can cause visual impairment and hypothalamic pituitary dysfunction.

At the infratentorial level, the brainstem, cerebellum,

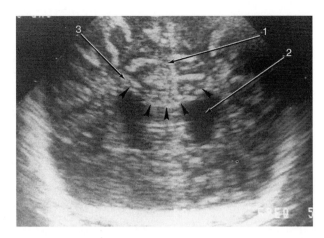

Fig. 29-36. Coronal sonogram (C1) in a term infant with communicating hydrocephalus: *1,* widening of interhemispheric fissure and cortical sulci; *2,* dilated frontal horns of the lateral ventricles; *3,* superior displacement of the lateral edge of the corpus callosum *(arrowheads).*

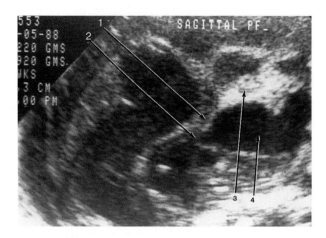

Fig. 29-38. Midline sagittal sonogram through the posterior fontanelle (PF-SM) in a 30-week-gestational infant without outlet foramina occlusion: *1,* posterior displacement of the quadrigeminal plate; *2,* distended aqueduct of Sylvius; *3,* cerebellar vermis; *4,* markedly distended fourth ventricle.

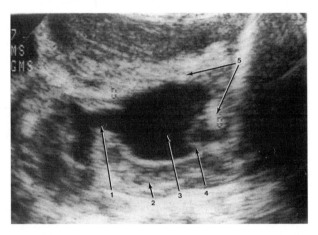

Fig. 29-37. Midline sagittal sonogram through the posterior fontanelle (PF-SM) in a 28-week-gestational infant with outlet foramina occlusion: *1,* dilated aqueduct of Sylvius; *2,* compressed pons; *3,* dilated third ventricle; *4,* membrane obstructing foramina; *5,* thin cerebellar vermis.

and ventricular system are best examined through the posterior midline and lateral fontanelles. The midbrain is adequately seen in a transverse plane through the anterior lateral fontanelle. Midbrain compression frequently results in aqueductal stenosis. Compression of the ventral midbrain causes an increase in the interpeduncular distance. Compression of the dorsal midbrain distorts the tectum. In uncal or hippocampal herniation, the midbrain is narrow. The aqueduct of Sylvius is best assessed through the midline posterior fontanelle. A dilated aqueduct indicates normal flow between the third and fourth ventricle unless the aqueduct's distal portion is stenotic or occluded. A stenotic aqueduct is usually associated with a small fourth ventricle unless the fourth ventricular outflow foramina are occluded. A

large, rounded anechoic fourth ventricle compressing the pons anteriorly and the cerebellar vermis posteriorly can be seen in fourth ventricular outlet foramina occlusion and in communicating hydrocephalus (Fig. 29-37). A large fourth ventricle communicating with a large cisterna magna excludes fourth ventricular outlet foramina occlusion (Fig. 29-38).

Severe obstructive hydrocephalus is best treated by ventricular fluid diversion. A ventriculostomy tube is inserted through a small hole in the calvaria. Ultrasonography is useful in determining the tube's position and monitoring for complications during and after the tube placement. Furthermore, recent studies have shown that Doppler is particularly helpful in determining the efficacy of CSF diversion in the presence of hydrocephalus.[14,45,50]

"Passive" hydrocephalus or craniocerebral disproportion

The sonographic pattern of passive hydrocephalus or craniocerebral disproportion must be differentiated from that of communicating hydrocephalus. In these conditions, the subarachnoid space and cortical sulci are enlarged, and there is an anterior widening of the interhemispheric fissure.[13]

Passive hydrocephalus can occur in two distinct clinical settings. In a patient with a small brain enclosed in a normal-sized cranium, the condition is referred to as *brain atrophy* when it is acquired. If the condition is static and congenital, it is referred to as *brain hypoplasia* (see Chapter 30). Clinically, these children tend to develop slowly, and their head circumferences tend to be in the low-normal range. Sonographically, the lateral ventricles are prominent in the frontal region with only minimal enlargement of the temporal horns. The roofs of the

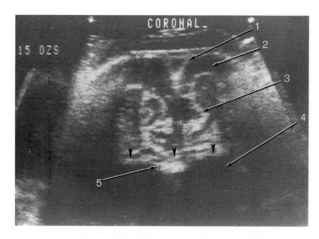

Fig. 29-39. Coronal sonogram (C2) using a 7.5-MHz transducer in a 3-month-old term infant with cerebral atrophy: *1,* large sagittal sinus; *2,* wide subarachnoid space; *3,* wide cortical sulci; *4,* flat corpus callosum *(arrowheads); 5,* large body of the lateral ventricle.

lateral ventricles remain at the level of corpus callosum unless white matter loss has occurred. Parenchymal thickness at the level of the foramen of Monro is markedly decreased (Fig. 29-39).

When a normal-sized brain is contained in a large cranium, the condition is referred to as *external hydrocephalus.* Clinically, these children tend to have a high-normal head circumference at birth that increases rapidly during the first few months of life. There is frequently a family history of large heads in adults. Although developmental milestones may be delayed in early life, the long-term neurologic outcome is normal. Sonographically, external hydrocephalus is characterized by relatively normal ventricles and normal parenchymal thickness.[4]

SUMMARY

Cranial sonography, using the natural sonic windows, is an invaluable tool for clinicians for diagnosing a wide array of acquired neurologic diseases in infancy. It is especially helpful in diagnosing and monitoring the evolution of secondary complications, thus allowing clinicians to tailor their management on the actual state of brain insults.

REFERENCES

1. Anderson N, Fulton J: Technical note: sonography through the posterior fontanelle in diagnosing neonatal intraventricular hemorrhage, *AJNR Am J Neuroradiol* 12:368-370, 1991.
2. Babcock DS, Han BK: Sonographic recognition of gyral infarction in meningitis, *AJR Am J Roentgenol* 6:119-122, 1985.
3. Barmada MA, Moosy J, Painter M: Pontosubicular necrosis and hypoxemia, *Pediatrics* 66:840-847, 1980.
4. Bode H, Strassburg HM: Craniocerebral disproportion: a contribution to the significance of extracerebral fluid collections in infancy, *Clin Pediatr (Phila)* 199:399-402, 1987.
5. Cabanas F, Pellicer A, Perex-Higueras A, et al: Ultrasonographic findings in thalamus and basal ganglia in term asphyxiated infants, *Pediatr Neurol* 7:211-215, 1991.
6. Cohen HL, Holler JO, Pollock A: Ultrasound of the septum pellucidum: recognition of evolving fenestration in the hydrocephalic infant, *J Ultrasound Med* 9:377-383, 1990.
7. Dipietro MA, Brody BA, Teele RL: Periventricular echogenic "blush" on cranial sonography: pathologic correlates, *AJNR Am J Neuroradiol* 7:305-310, 1986.
8. Eicke M, Briner J, Willi V, et al: Symmetrical thalamic lesion in infants, *Arch Dis Child* 67:15-19, 1992.
9. Fischer AQ: Pediatric application of clinical ultrasound, *Neurol Clin* 8:759-774, 1990.
10. Fischer AQ, Anderson GC, Shuman RN: The ultrasound appearance of early periventricular leukomalacia with neuropathologic correlation, *J Islamic Med Assoc* 17:34-37, 1985.
11. Fischer AQ, Anderson JC, Shuman RM: The evolution of ischemic cerebral infarction in infancy: a sonographic evaluation, *J Child Neurol* 3:105-109, 1988.
12. Fischer AQ, Anderson JC, et al:*Brain death.* In Fischer AQ, et al, editors: *Pediatric neurosonography: clinical, tomographic, and neurosonographic correlates,* New York, 1985, Churchill Livingston.
13. Fischer AQ, Aziz E: Diagnosis of cerebral atrophy in infants by nearfield cranial sonography method, *Am J Dis Child* 140:774-777, 1986
14. Fischer AQ, Livingston JN II: Transcranial Doppler and real-time sonography in neonatal hydrocephalus, *J Child Neurol* 4:64-69, 1989.
15. Fischer AQ, Truemper EJ: *Trancranial Doppler findings in infants with suspected brain death, Ann Neurol* 28:432, 1990 (abstract).
16. Fischer AQ, Truemper EJ: *Transcranial Doppler applications in the neonate and child.* In Wechsler L, Babikian V, editors: *Transcranial Doppler ultrasonography,* St Louis, 1993, Mosby–Year Book.
17. Fischer AQ, et al: *Intracranial hemorrhages.* In Fischer AQ, et al, editors: *Pediatric neurosonography: clinical, tomographic, and neuropathologic correlates,* New York, 1985, Churchill Livingston.
18. Fischer AQ, et al: *Trauma.* In Fischer AQ, et al, editors: *Pediatric neurosonography: clinical, tomographic, and neuropathologic correlates,* New York, 1985, Churchill Livingston.
19. Fischer AQ, et al: *Subependymal cysts of the germinal matrix.* In Fischer AQ, et al, editors: *Pediatric neurosonography: clinical, tomographic, and neuropathologic correlates,* New York, 1985, Churchill Livingston.
20. Flodmark O, Roland EH, Hill A, et al: Periventricular leukomalacia: radiologic diagnosis, *Radiology* 162:119-124, 1987.
21. Frank JL: Sonography of intracranial infection in infants and children, *Neuroradiology* 28:440-451, 1986.
22. Franze I, Forrest TS: Sonographic diagnosis of a subdural hematoma as the initial manifestation of hemophilia in a newborn, *J Ultrasound Med* 7:149-152, 1988.
23. Furgiule TL, Frank LM, Riegle C, et al: Prediction of cerebral death by cranial sector scan, *Crit Care Med* 12:1, 1984.
24. Govaert P, Achten E, Vanhaesebrouck P, et al: Deep cerebral venous thrombosis in thalamoventricular hemorrhage of term newborn, *Pediatr Radiol* 27:123-127, 1992.
25. Grant EG, Schellinger D, Richardson JD: Real-time ultrasonography of the posterior fossa, *J Ultrasound Med* 2:73-87, 1983.
26. Grant EG, White EM, Schellinger D, Slovis TL: Ultrasound calcification in the infants and neonate: evaluation by sonography and CT, *Radiology* 157:63-68, 1985.
27. Han BK, Babcock DS, McAdams L: Bacterial meningitis in infants: sonographic findings, *Radiology* 154:645-650, 1985.
28. Hayden CK, Shattuck KE, Richardson CJ, et al: Subependymal germinal matrix hemorrhage in full-term neonates, *Pediatrics* 75:714-718, 1985.
29. Herman JH, Jumbelic MI, Ancona RJ, Kickler TS: In utero

cerebral hemorrhage in alloimmune thrombocytopenia, *Am J Pediatr Hematol Oncol* 8:312-317, 1986.

30. Hess DC, Fischer AQ, Yaghmai F, et al: Comparative neuroimaging of CNS abnormality in Alexander's disease, *J Child Neurol* 5:248-252, 1990.

31. Hill A, Nelson GL, Clark B, Volpe JJ: Hemorrhagic PVL: diagnosis by real-time ultrasound and correlates with autopsy findings, *Pediatrics* 69:282-284, 1982.

32. Huang C-C, Shen E-Y: Tentorial subdural hemorrhage in term newborns: ultrasonographic diagnosis and clinical correlates, *Pediatr Neurol* 7:171-177, 1991.

33. Johnson SC, Kazzi NJ: *Candida* brain abscess: a sonographic mimicker of intracranial hemorrhage, *J Ultrasound Med* 4:237-239, 1993.

34. Karnaze MG, Shackelford GD, Abramson CL: Atrial ventricular diverticulum: sonographic diagnosis, *AJNR Am J Neuroradiol* 8:721-723, 1987.

35. Kazam E, Rudelli R, Monte W, et al: Sonographic diagnosis of cisternal subarachnoid hemorrhage in the premature infant, *AJNR Am J Neuroradiol* 15:1009-1020, 1994.

36. Kreusser KL, Schmidt RE, Shackelford GD, Volpe JJ: Values of ultrasound for identification of acute hemorrhage necrosis of thalamus and basal ganglia in an asphyxiated term infant, *Ann Neurol* 16:361-363, 1984.

37. Lam AH, Berry A, de Silva M, Williams G: Intracranial *Serratia* infection in pre-term newborn infants, *AJNR Am J Neuroradiol* 5:447-451, 1984.

38. Maertens P: Intracerebellar hemorrhages in premature infants, *J Neuroimaging* 1:54, 1991.

39. Maertens P, Johnson WH, Melhem RE, Duncan V: Real-time echoenchoencephalography and Doppler study of cerebrospinal fluid dynamics (abstract 9C). In Aaslid R, editor: Proceedings of second international conference on transcranial Doppler sonography, Salzburg, 1986, The Christian Doppler Institute.

40. Maertens P, Zellweger M, Simon N: Echoencephalography in inborn errors of metabolism, *J Ultrasound Med* 9(suppl 55) 1990. (abstract 1501)

41. McMenamin JB, Shackelford GD, Volpe JJ: Outcome of neonatal intraventricular hemorrhage with periventricular echodense lesions, *Ann Neurol* 15:285-290, 1984.

42. McMenamin JB, Volpe JJ: Doppler ultrasonography in the determination of neonatal brain death, *Ann Neurol* 14:302-307, 1983.

43. Mercker JM, Blumhagen JD, Brewer DK: Echographic demonstration of extracerebral fluid collections with the lateral technique, *J Ultrasound Med* 2:265-269, 1983.

44. Mercker JM, Blumhager JD, Brewer DK: Sonography of a hemorrhagic cerebral contusion, *AJNR Am J Neuroradiol* 6:115-116, 1985.

45. Norelle A, Fischer AQ, Flannery AM: Transcranial Doppler: a non-invasive method to monitor hydrocephalus, *J Child Neurol* 4(suppl):87-90, 1989.

46. Papile LA, Burstein J, Burstein R, et al: Incidence and evolution of subependymal hemorrhage: a study of infants with birth weights less than 1500 grams, *J Pediatr* 92:529-534, 1978.

47. Reeder JD, Kaude JV, Setzer ES: Choroid plexus hemorrhage in premature neonates: recognition by sonography, *AJNR Am J Neuroradiol* 3:619-622, 1982.

48. Reeder JD, Sanders RC: Ventriculitis in the neonate: recognition by sonography, *AJNR Am J Neuroradiol* 4:37-41, 1983.

49. Riley TF, Morrison S: Radiological case of the month, *Ach Pediatr Adolesc Med* 148:951-952, 1994.

50. Seibert JJ, McCowan TC, Chadduck WM, et al: Duplex pulsed Doppler ultrasound versus intracranial pressure in neonate: clinical and experimental studies, *Radiology* 171:155-159, 1989.

51. Shuman RM, Leech RW: *Special topics.* In Leech RW, editor: *Neuropathology: a summary for students,* Philadelphia, 1982, Harper & Row.

52. Slagle TA, Oliphant M, Gross SJ: Cingulate sulcus development in preterm infants, *Pediatr Res* 26:598-602, 1989.

53. Stannard MW, Pearrow J: Ultrasound diagnosis of purulent ventriculitis, *J Ultrasound Med* 3:143-144, 1984.

54. Teele RL, Hernanz-Schulman M, Sotrel A: Echogenic vasculature in the basal ganglia of neonates: a sonographic sign of vasculopathy, *Radiology* 169:423-427, 1988.

55. Toma P, Magnano GM, Mazzano P, et al: Cerebral ultrasound images in prenatal cytomegalovirus infection, *Neuroradiology* 31:278-279, 1989.

56. Volpe JJ: *Hypoxic-ischemic encephalopathy.* In Volpe JJ, editor: *Neurology of the newborn,* Philadelphia, 1987, WB Saunders.

57. Volpe JJ: *Intracranial hemorrhage.* In Volpe JJ, editor: *Neurology of the newborn,* Philadelphia, 1987, WB Saunders.

58. de Vries LS, Dubowitz LM, Pennock JM, Bydder GM: Extensive cystic leukomalacia: correlation of cranial ultrasound, magnetic resonance imaging and clinical findings in sequential studies, *Clin Radiol* 40:158-166, 1989.

59. de Vries LS, Smet M, Goemans N, et al: Unilateral thalamic hemorrhage in the pre-term and full-term newborn, *Neuropediatrics* 23:153-156, 1992.

60. Wang HS, Huang SC: Infantile panthalamic infarct with a striking sonographic finding: the "bright thalamus," *Neuroradiology* 35:92-96, 1993.

61. Wilson ER, Mirra SS, Schwartz JF: Congenital diencephalic and brainstem damage: neuropathologic study of three cases, *Acta Neuropathol (Berl)* 57:70-74, 1982.

62. Yates PO: Birth trauma to the vertebral arteries, *Arch Dis Child* 34:436-441, 1959.

Congenital Brain Pathology

Paul Maertens

Most central nervous system (CNS) anomalies can now be visualized prenatally and during the early months of life by using ultrasound. Ultrasound screening appears indicated for infants with multiple congenital anomalies, macrocephaly, microcephaly, and neurotube defects. However, congenital brain anomalies are not always associated with other structural anomalies. The neurologic exam or clinical history can provide additional clues. Some congenital lesions (e.g., tumors) may remain asymptomatic for extended periods of time.

Congenital CNS anomalies can be classified in two major groups: (1) congenital brain malformations and (2) congenital pathology without malformation (discussed in Chapter 29). Congenital brain malformations are extremely common in humans and represent the most common congenital anomalies.[11] They are best classified based on the stages of brain development[30] and can be divided into eight categories (box).

DISORDERS OF NEUROTUBE CLOSURE
Anencephaly

Anencephaly (Greek *an*, "without"; *enkephalon*, "brain") results from failure of the rostral neuropore to close during the fourth week of development. As a result, the forebrain is exposed or extrudes from the skull, a condition known as *exencephaly*. The embryonic exencephalic brain undergoes degeneration. Two types of

anencephaly are recognized. In holoanencephaly, there is complete absence of brain. This malformation is associated with craniorachischisis 80% of the time. The cervical spine is often retroflexed. In meroanencephaly, rudiments of the basal ganglia, brainstem, and cranial vault are replaced by an amorphous vascular-neural mass (area cerebrovasculosa). Anencephaly can be diagnosed in utero during routine obstetric ultrasound testing. On coronal views, there is absence of calvaria and brain above the level of the orbits.[20] The cerebrovasculosa may be seen in utero as a solid, cystic, or mixed echo mass, which may appear brainlike.[17]

Iniencephaly

Iniencephaly (Greek: *inion*, "nape of the neck"; *enkephalon*, "brain") results from failure of maturation of the ventral and dorsal paravertebral precartilaginous sclerotomes in the cervical and upper thoracic region. As a result, there is a severe retroflexion of the head and shortening and webbing of the neck, the nape of the neck is enclosed within an enlarged head with a low-set posterior hairline, the ears are always low-set and small, the jaw is small, and the chest is hypoplastic with short sternum and rib agenesis. In addition, there is rachischisis of variable extent and a deficiency of the occiput, with enlargement of the foramen magnum. Two types of iniencephaly are recognized. In iniencephaly clausus, the

Congenital brain pathology

Disorders of neurotube closure

Anencephaly
Iniencephaly
Cephaloceles
Chiari II malformation
Congenital cranial dermal sinus
Dysgenesis of the corpus callosum
Hypoplasia of the corpus callosum
Lipoma of the corpus callosum

Disorders of diverticulation

Holoprosencephalies
Hypoplasia of the corpus callosum
Septooptic dysplasia

Disorders of proliferation

Microcephaly vera
Cerebellar hypoplasia/aplasia

Disorders of cerebral cortex morphogenesis

Schizencephaly
Lissencephaly
Hemimegaloencephaly
Polymicrogyria

Destructive brain lesion

Hydranencephaly
Multicystic encephalomalacia
Porencephaly
Intracranial calcification

Congenital cystic lesions

Brain neoplasias

Disorders of histogenesis

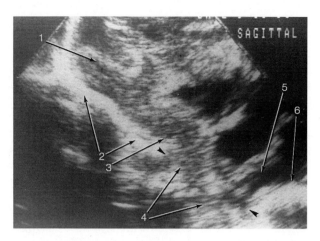

Fig. 30-1. Midline sagittal sonogram (SM) in a term infant with iniencephaly clausus: *1,* holospheric telencephalon; *2,* platybasia; *3,* hypoplastic brainstem; *4,* spinal cord exposed to cranial cavity content through a large foramen magnum (*between arrowheads*); *5,* large posterior fossa cyst; *6,* occipital squama.

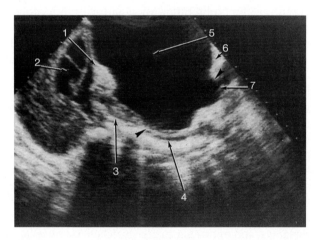

Fig. 30-2. Posterior fontanelle midline sagittal sonogram (PF-SM) in a term infant with iniencephaly apertus: *1,* hypoplastic cerebellar vermis; *2,* fenestration of septum pellucidum and superior displacement of the corpus callosum due to severe hydrocephalus; *3,* hypoplastic brainstem; *4,* spinal cord exposed to cranial cavity content through a large foramen magnum (*between arrowheads*); *5,* large posterior fossa cyst; *6,* occipital squama; *7,* cervical meningocele.

foramen magnum lies at the thoracic or lumbar level. The entire brain is enclosed in the cranium (Fig. 30-1). In iniencephaly apertus, there is an occipital cranium bifidum and an occipital meningocele (Fig. 30-2). In both forms of iniencephaly, the posterior fossa is filled with cerebrospinal fluid (CSF). Neuropathologic data regarding iniencephaly are limited. Aleksic and associates reported numerous brain anomalies such as holoprosencephaly and Dandy-Walker syndrome.[2]

Cephaloceles

Cephaloceles are defects in the cranium (cranium bifidum) and the dura mater with extracranial herniation of intracranial structures. The term *cranial meningocele* refers to herniation of the meninges only. The term *encephalocele* refers to herniation of both brain tissue and meninges. The etiology of cephaloceles varies with their location. Cephaloceles through the membranous calvaria may be secondary to defective induction of the bone or to pressure erosion of the bone by an intracranial mass or cyst.[10] Cephaloceles through the endochondral skull base result usually from faulty closure of the neural tube[10,46] or from faulty coalescence of endochondral ossification centers.[40]

Encephaloceles are classified according to the anatomic site of the cranial defect.[41] Occipital cephaloceles lie between the lambda and the foramen magnum. Parietal cephaloceles lie between the bregma and the lambda. Sincipital (frontoethmoidal) cephaloceles are sited at some point between the bregma and the anterior margin of the ethmoid bone. Basal cephaloceles herniate through the ethmoid or sphenoid bones into the nasopharynx, orbital cavity, and pterygopalatine fossa. Basal cephaloceles are usually occult. Both sincipital and basal cephaloceles can be associated with hypertelorism.

Occipital cephaloceles are the most common variety in the Western Hemisphere. Sincipital cephaloceles are particularly frequent in Southeast Asia. Parietal and basal cephaloceles are rare. Cephaloceles may occur as isolated lesions or as a part of a number of genetic and nongenetic syndromes.[9]

Ultrasonography is essential to demonstrate the content of the cephalocele, to search for the exceedingly common additional intracranial malformations, and to visualize the bony defect in the calvaria of the skull base. The cortex of the cerebral tissue within the encephalocele sac may be normal or show dysplastic changes. Neural tissue may be totally disorganized or show only polymicrogyria. Zones of ischemic change, hemorrhage, porencephaly, proliferation of abnormally thin-walled vascular channels, and dystrophic calcifications indicate recent or remote infarction. The neurologic prognosis, as a rule, is directly related to the presence of cerebral tissue in the cephalocele, to the presence of any hydrocephalus, and to additional cerebral malformations. True encephaloceles with massive external protrusion of brain tissue are frequently associated with microcephaly. Holoprosencephaly, agenesis of the corpus callosum, lissencephaly, polymicrogyria, and hydrocephalus are the most common associated primary cerebral dysplasias.* Lipomas of the corpus callosum have also been reported with frontal encephaloceles.[10] In sphenoid encephaloceles, the third ventricle, hypothalamus, and optic chiasm are stretched as they extend into the sac, resulting almost always in hypothalamic-pituitary dysfunction.[10,46] Posterior fossa abnormalities are more frequent in occipital encephaloceles. The brainstem may have a partial cleft in the midline and herniate into the sac. In other cases it is flattened and enlarged. Aqueductal stenosis or forking is common. The cerebellar vermis is frequently involved as well; it may be hypoplastic or even aplastic. Chiari III malformations are characterized by caudal displacement of the fourth ventricle and herniation of the cerebellar vermis through the enlarged foramen magnum into the occipital defect (Fig. 30-3).

Chiari II malformation

Chiari II malformation (Arnold-Chiari deformity) is the most common congenital brain malformation associated with spinal dysraphisms, such as meningoceles

*References 9, 10, 16, 40, 41, 46.

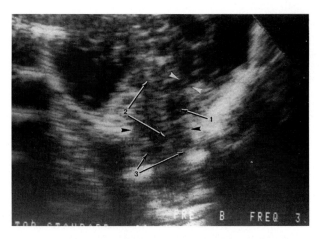

Fig. 30-3. Posterior fontanelle coronal sonogram (PF-C1) in a 36-week-gestational infant with occipital encephalocele and Chiari III malformation: *1*, dysplastic occipital lobe protruding through left tentorial defect (*between white arrowheads*) and filling most of the encephalocele; *2*, elongated cerebellar vermis; *3*, narrow cerebellar hemispheres extending below a wide foramen magnum (*between black arrowheads*).

and myelomeningoceles. Sonographically, a Chiari II malformation is best visualized through the posterior fontanelle approach. The sagittal hallmarks include elongation of the cerebellar vermis, caudal displacement, narrowing and elongation of the fourth ventricle and brainstem, vermian herniation through the enlarged foramen magnum, absence of cisterna magna, low insertion of the tentorium, and midbrain tectal beaking (Fig. 30-4). The coronal hallmarks include small size of the posterior fossa, towering of the tentorium, narrowing of the cerebellar hemisphere diameter, wrapping of the cerebellum around the medulla, herniation of the cerebellar tonsils, and widening of the foramen magnum (Fig. 30-5). The lumen of the aqueduct of Sylvius is not visualized in 70% of the patients.

Supratentorial cerebral abnormalities are seen in more than 90% of the patients and are best visualized through the anterior fontanelle. In the sagittal plane, the most common abnormalities are dysgenesis of the corpus callosum, absence of septum pellucidum, enlargement of the massa intermedia, and an abnormal gyral pattern in the medial aspect of the occipital lobes (Fig. 30-6). In the coronal plane, the most common cerebral abnormalities are dysgenesis of the corpus callosum, partial or complete absence of the septum pellucidum, abnormal configuration of the lateral ventricles, fenestration of the falx cerebri with interdigitation of gyri across the interhemispheric fissure, and large massa intermedia and caudate heads. Dysgenesis of the corpus callosum usually consists of hypoplasia or absence of the splenium and absence of the rostrum (Fig. 30-7). The distance between the most lateral walls of the lateral ventricles in

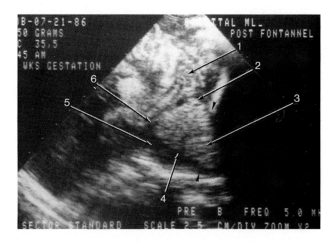

Fig. 30-4. Posterior fontanelle midline sagittal sonogram (PF-SM) in a term infant with Chiari II malformation: *1,* multiple small gyri on medial surface of occipital lobes; *2,* low insertion of tentorium; *3,* elongated cerebellar vermis protruding through large foramen magnum (*between arrowheads*); *4,* caudal position of fourth ventricle; *5,* narrow brainstem; *6,* beaking of tectal midbrain.

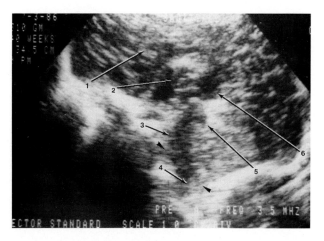

Fig. 30-6. Midline sagittal sonogram (SM) in a term infant with Chiari II malformation: *1,* flat and short corpus callosum (no rostrum); *2,* large massa intermedia; *3,* narrow brainstem; *4,* cerebellar vermis extending below large foramen magnum (*between arrowheads*); *5,* beaking of the midbrain; *6,* large suprapineal recess.

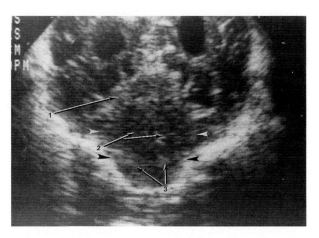

Fig. 30-5. Posterior fontanelle coronal sonogram (PF-C1) in a term infant with Chiari II malformation: *1,* towering of the tentorium; *2,* narrow cerebellar hemispheres (*between white arrowheads*); *3,* cerebellar tonsils below wide foramen magnum (*between black arrowheads*).

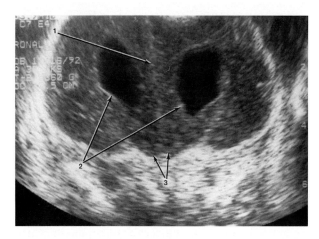

Fig. 30-7. Coronal sonogram (C1b) in a 35-week-gestational infant with Chiari II malformation: *1,* interhemispheric fissure that is not interrupted by rostral corpus callosum; *2,* widely separated frontal horns of the lateral ventricles with "squared-off" superolateral angle and sharply pointed inferomedial angle; *3,* gyri recti.

the frontal region frequently approaches that between the lateral walls of the temporal horns. The frontal horns typically have a squared roof and a medially pointed floor, giving a "batwing configuration" (Fig. 30-8). The occipital horns are often disproportionately enlarged. Hydrocephalus may be present at birth.

Ventricular enlargement can be seen in infants with microcephaly. Brain thickness is frequently decreased. An abnormal cranial configuration is best demonstrated in a transverse view above the ventricular level, using the posterior fontanelle approach. Anteriorly to the coronal suture, the frontal bones are displaced medially (scal-

loping) and have a concave contour with frontal bossing, producing the "lemon" sign (Fig. 30-9).

The majority of fetuses with spinal dysraphism exhibit in utero a decreased biparietal diameter, an enlargement of the atria of the lateral ventricles, a lemon sign, and an "banana" sign. In utero, the lemon sign is best demonstrated during the second trimester on axial scans obtained at the level of the biparietal diameter.[32,33] Demonstration of this sign should prompt a more detailed examination of the fetal spine[14] when a spinal defect is not immediately identified. The banana sign is best shown on suboccipital bregmatic views of the fetal

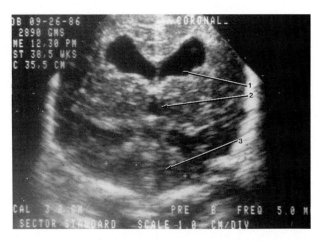

Fig. 30-8. Coronal sonogram (C3) in a 38-week-gestational infant with Chiari II malformation: *1,* "batwing configuration" of the widely spaced bodies of the lateral ventricles; *2,* slightly dilated (despite severe hydrocephalus) suprapineal recess of the third ventricle; *3,* narrow cerebellar hemispheres.

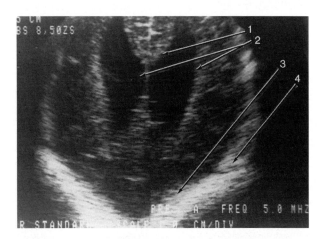

Fig. 30-9. Posterior fontanelle coronal sonogram (PF-C5) in a term infant with Chiari II malformation: *1,* splenium of corpus callosum; *2,* enlarged lateral ventricles that are parallel and pointed anteriorly; *3,* medial displacement and concave contour of frontal bone, producing the "lemon" sign; *4,* coronal suture.

head. The cerebellum obliterates the cisterna magna and appears as a crescent, with the concavity pointing anteriorly around the brainstem, producing the characteristic findings of the banana.[32]

Congenital cranial dermal sinus

A congenital cranial dermal sinus results from the failure of the neural ectoderm to separate from the overlying cutaneous ectoderm by the time neurulation is completed at 28 days.

Congenital cranial dermal sinuses are epithelium-lined dural tubes that extend from the shin surface to deeper tissues within the cranial cavity. Most cranial dermal sinuses form in the midline anywhere from the

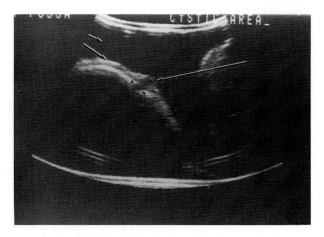

Fig. 30-10. Midline sagittal sonogram of an occipital dermal sinus using a 7.5-MHz transducer: *1,* stand-off pad; *2,* skin; *3,* dermal sinus crossing occipital bone (*between arrowheads*).

nasion to the foramen magnum and are frequently located near the external protuberance of the occipital bone. The epithelial tract in the occipital area always extends obliquely through the inion, ending intracranially below the tentorium cerebelli. Dermoids may be anywhere in the midline between the fourth ventricle and the extradural space. Symptoms usually arise from the chemical meningitis secondary to leakage of the contents of the cysts into the CSF or from infection and abscess formation. Hydrocephalus may result from arachnoiditis. Ultrasonography can demonstrate the epithelial tract crossing the occipital bone (Fig. 30-10). When a dermoid cyst is located in the cerebellar vermis, its demonstration is somewhat difficult because of the high echogenicity of the surrounding normal tissue. A dermoid cyst is, however, globular and more densely echogenic due to its fat content (Fig. 30-11).

Dysgenesis of the corpus callosum

The corpus callosum is composed of four portions: rostrum, genu, body, and splenium. At 5 weeks of gestation, the dorsal portion of the lamina terminalis becomes densely cellular and is called the lamina reuniens of His. At 6 weeks of gestation, fibers passing through the ventral part of the lamina reuniens form the anterior commissure. A week later, fibers that unite the hippocampal formations extend through the dorsal part of the lamina. During the eighth week, the lamina folds along its dorsal part, forming a medial groove (sulcus medianus telencephali medii) between the anterior and the hippocampal commissures.

During the ninth week, while the lamina reuniens continues to fold dorsally, the sulcus is filled by migrating cells of the lamina reuniens. By the tenth week, the ventral sulcus is obliterated and forms the massa commissuralis. The latter grows in a dorsal direction over the ensuing 5 to 7 weeks. It sends out chemotactic

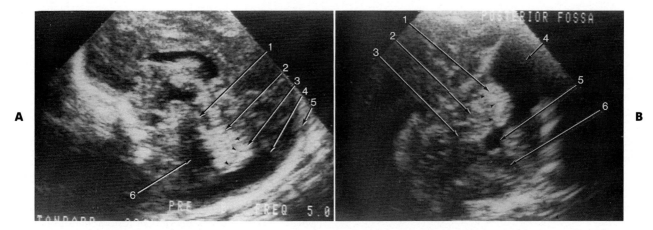

Fig. 30-11. A, Midline sagittal sonogram (SM) through anterior fontanelle in a term infant with congenital dermal sinus: *1,* aqueduct of Sylvius; *2,* hypoplastic cerebellar vermis; *3,* dermoid cyst (*outlined by arrowheads*); *4,* large cisterna magna; *5,* dermal sinus crossing defect in occipital bone; *6,* large fourth ventricle. **B,** Midline sagittal sonogram (PF-SM) through posterior fontanelle in the same infant: *1,* dermoid cyst (*outlined by arrowheads*); *2,* hypoplastic cerebellar vermis; *3,* aqueduct of Sylvius; *4,* large cisterna magna; *5,* fourth ventricle; *6,* brainstem.

factors to the developing cerebral hemispheres that induce developing axons to cross the midline and form the corpus callosum. The genu is formed by 11 to 13 weeks. The body and splenium are formed between 13 and 18 weeks. The rostrum is formed last, slightly after the splenium, between 18 and 20 weeks.[36]

Dysgenesis of the corpus callosum can be complete or partial. In the partially formed corpus callosum, the genu is always present, the body is found less frequently, and the splenium and rostrum are frequently absent. In complete agenesis (absence) of the corpus callosum, axons that would normally cross it turn instead at the interhemispheric fissure and run parallel to that fissure, forming the longitudinal callosal bundles of Probst. The hippocampal commissure is almost always absent. Both callosal bundles are connected to medial rudimentary fornices. Although a septum pellucidum may form, rarely cingulate gyri remain everted and the cingulate sulci remain unformed. The lateral ventricles have a distinctive pattern on coronal sections: Their frontal horns and bodies are widely separated. Their medial borders are convex, and their superolateral margins are pointed, giving a "double horn" appearance to the frontal horns and bodies. The occipital horns are relatively larger than the frontal horns (colpocephaly). There is frequently an incomplete formation of the horn of Ammon (Fig. 30-12). The foramina of Monro are frequently enlarged. The roof of the third ventricle is formed by the tela choroidea. In the absence of hydrocephalus, the tela choroidea approximates the level of the cingulate gyrus's lower border (Fig. 30-13). With hydrocephalus, the distance between tela choroidea and cingulate gyri increases. An interhemispheric

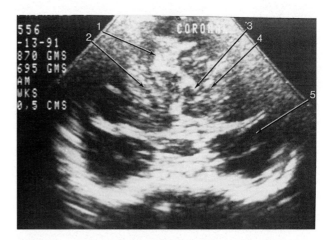

Fig. 30-12. Coronal sonogram (C2) in a 34-week-gestational infant with trisomy 18 and agenesis of the corpus callosum: *1,* sinuous interhemispheric fissure due to interdigitation of sulci (defective falx cerebri); *2,* right lateral ventricle; *3,* bundle of Probst; *4,* left lateral ventricle; *5,* dysplastic temporal lobe.

cyst displaces the cingulate gyri laterally while the choroid plexus continues to run anteriorly and superiorly to the massa intermedia (Fig. 30-14). In some patients with hydrocephalus, the tela choroidea may be deficient or displaced upward. In a sagittal plane, no corpus callosum is seen and, in the absence of an interhemispheric cyst, medial cerebral sulci radiate perpendicularly to the narrow inferior margin of the hemispheres (Fig. 30-15). Corpus callosum dysgenesis can be diagnosed in utero.[21]

Dysgenesis of the corpus callosum may be an isolated malformation, or it may occur in association with other abnormalities. Intracranial abnormalities may include hypoplasia or absence of the falx cerebri,[35] cephaloceles (nasofrontal, transphenoidal, or parietal), defects of neuronal migration (subependymal heterotopias, polymicrogyria, pachygyria), aqueductal stenosis, choroid plexus cysts (Aicardi's syndrome),[37] and cerebellar dysplasias (Dandy-Walker syndrome). The etiology of corpus callosum agenesis is diverse.[1]

Lipomas of the corpus callosum

These congenital tumors form as a result of faulty disjunction of the neuroectoderm from cutaneous ectoderm during the process of neurulation. Callosal lipomas are almost always associated with anomalies of the

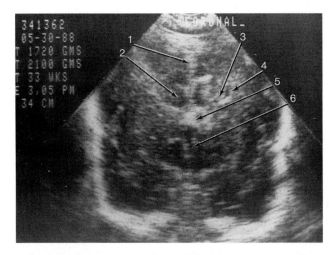

Fig. 30-13. Coronal sonogram (C2) in a 33-week-gestational infant with agenesis of the corpus callosum: *1,* interhemispheric fissure; *2,* cingulate gyrus; *3,* bundle of Probst; *4,* lateral ventricle; *5,* tela choroidea; *6,* third ventricle.

corpus callosum. They may be pericallosal or involve any portion of the corpus callosum. No callosal fibers are seen dorsal to the lipoma unless they involve the rostrum of the corpus callosum (Fig. 30-16). Lipomas are highly echogenic lesions.[24]

DISORDERS OF DIVERTICULATION
Holoprosencephalies

The holoprosencephalies are a group of disorders characterized by deficient cleavage of the prosencephalon at the rostral end of the primitive neural tube into distinct cerebral hemispheres. The majority of patients with holoprosencephalies have some facial dysmorphism. De Myer has divided holoprosencephalies into three subcategories: alobar, semilobar, and lobar.[31] These conditions are associated with absent olfactory tracts and bulbs (arrhinencephalia).

Alobar holoprosencephaly. Sonographically, alobar holoprosencephaly is diagnosed when a single midline horseshoe or crescent-shaped ventricle surrounds the fused thalami and basal ganglia anteriorly and the fused choroid plexus posteriorly, and when the hemispheres are completely fused on the surface anteriorly (holosphere).[5] A shallow midline groove can be seen posteriorly. The gyri recti are absent. Gray matter pachygyria or polymicrogyria are usually present. The falx cerebri and sagittal sinus are absent. The dorsal ventricular surface consists of a thin membrane and generally a dorsal sac, which may be small if further growth of the holospheric brain occurs. Cerebellar tentorium and straight sinus are absent (Fig. 30-17). A large single ventricle communicates directly with the aqueduct. Diagnosis can be made in utero.[13,34]

Semilobar holoprosencephaly. Sonographically, semi-

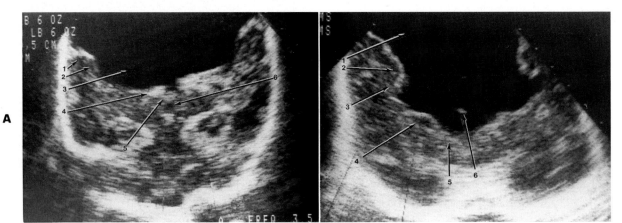

Fig. 30-14. A, Coronal sonogram (C3) in a term infant with congenital hydrocephalus and agenesis of the corpus callosum: *1,* cingulate gyrus; *2,* bundle of Probst; *3,* interhemispheric cyst; *4,* choroid plexus of the lateral ventricle; *5,* tela choroidea; *6,* third ventricle. **B,** Coronal sonogram (C2) in another term infant with congenital hydrocephalus and agenesis of the corpus callosum: *1,* interhemispheric cyst; *2,* cingulate gyrus; *3,* bundle of Probst; *4,* caudate nucleus; *5,* choroid plexus of the lateral ventricle; *6,* tela choroidea.

lobar holoprosencephaly resembles alobar holoprosencephaly. The single ventricle persists although the occipital and temporal horns may be separated. The distinction between semilobar and alobar forms is based on the demonstration of some sagittal separation of the holosphere.

In semilobar holoprosencephaly, there is a rudimentary third ventricle, and the posterior interhemispheric fissure, straight sinus, falx cerebri, and superior sagittal sinus are variably developed. The dorsal roof of the single ventricle is indented downward at the midline. Posteriorly, the velum interpositum connects both hemispheres. The interhemispheric fissure may extend in the frontal region but does not involve the entire brain thickness (Fig. 30-18).

Lobar holoprosencephaly. In lobar holoprosencephaly, there is nearly complete separation of the hemispheres, with development of a falx and an interhemispheric fissure, but a small portion of cortex remains fused anterior to the narrow single ventricular body. The brain has no corpus callosum, no septum pellucidum, and no fornices. Thalami and caudate nuclei are partially fused. Hydrocephalus is the most common anatomic aberration associated with holoprosencephaly. If the head size is small, hydrocephalus is more likely due to cerebral hypoplasia (Fig. 30-19). When the head is enlarged, hydrocephalus due to aqueductal stenosis is suspected. Prenatal diagnosis of lobar holoprosencephaly can be made.[22]

Septooptic dysplasia

Septooptic dysplasia is characterized by agenesis of the septum pellucidum and hypoplasia of the optic nerves. The anterior recess of the third ventricle is enlarged. In a coronal plane, the roof of the single ventricle is flat, and frontal horns have a squared shape. The fornices, falx, interhemispheric fissure, and corpus callosum are present. Hypopituitarism is frequently associated with this syndrome. Absence of septum pellucidum is also seen in holoprosencephaly, callosal dysgenesis, schizencephaly, porencephaly, and severe chronic hydrocephalus (Fig. 30-20).

DISORDERS OF PROLIFERATION

In the cerebrum, proliferation leads to the separation of the deeper germinal matrix from a more superficial cerebellar layer in the 5- to 6-week-old fetus. In the cerebellum, proliferation starts along the cortical surface. Neuroblasts and glioblasts are initially indis-

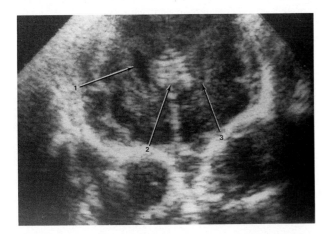

Fig. 30-15. Midline sagittal sonogram (SM) in a 36-week-gestational infant with agenesis of the corpus callosum: *1,* radial relationship of medial cerebral gyri and sulci (*arrowheads*); *2,* large massa intermedia; *3,* third ventricle.

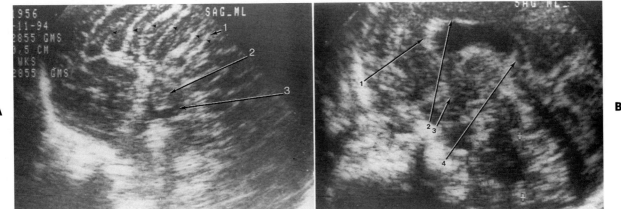

Fig. 30-16. A, Midline sagittal sonogram (SM) in a 28-week-gestational infant with a lipoma of the rostral corpus callosum: *1,* lipoma of the rostral corpus callosum; *2,* body of corpus callosum; *3,* third ventricle; *4,* splenium of corpus callosum. **B,** Coronal sonogram (C1a) in the same infant: *1,* frontal horn of the right lateral ventricle; *2,* lipoma of the rostral corpus callosum; *3,* frontal horn of the left lateral ventricle.

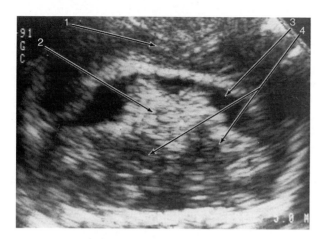

Fig. 30-17. Coronal sonogram (C3) in a term infant with alobar holoprosencephaly: *1,* midline telencephalon; *2,* choroid plexus; *3,* telencephalic cavity; *4,* cerebellar hemispheres.

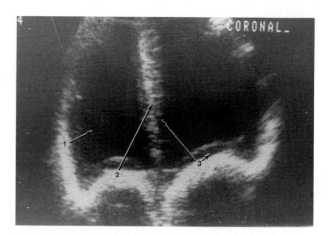

Fig. 30-19. Coronal sonogram (C1a) in a term microcephalic infant with lissencephaly type II and no olfactory tract: *1,* large frontal horns of the lateral ventricles, which are pointed at their inferiomedial angle; *2,* interhemispheric fissure; *3,* neopallia hypoplasia (thin cerebral mantle).

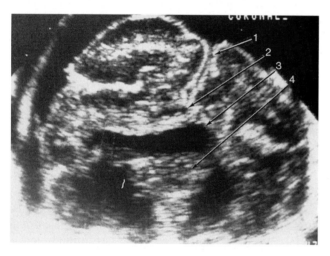

Fig. 30-18. Coronal sonogram (C2) in a term infant with semilobar holoprosencephaly and iniencephaly clausus: *1,* interhemispheric fissure partially separating the telencephalon; *2,* midline indentation of the dorsal roof of the single ventricle; *3,* telencephalic cavity; *4,* undivided thalami.

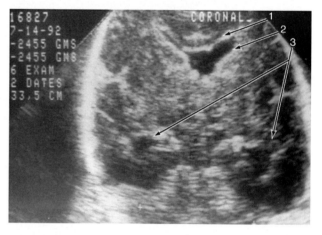

Fig. 30-20. Coronal sonogram (C3) in a 32-week-gestational infant with septooptic dysplasia: *1,* body of corpus callosum; *2,* asymmetric single ventricle (absence of septum pellucidum); *3,* large and asymmetric temporal horns of the lateral ventricles.

tinguishable. Proliferation continues till about the twentieth week of gestation. Defects in proliferation lead to delayed cortical morphogenesis. They occur in the absence of defects in neurulation and prosencephalic cleavage.

Brain hypoplasia

Brain hypoplasia is seen in microcephaly vera and in conditions associated with chromosomal defects. Sonographically the brain is small and immature (Fig. 30-21).

Hypoplasia of the corpus callosum

Hypoplasia of the corpus callosum occurs when axons fail to colonize the glial membrane forming the commissural bed. A complete hypoplasia of the corpus callosum

is associated with agyria (Fig. 30-22). Hypoplasia of the corpus callosum can occur in association with a number of unrelated inborn errors of metabolism (Zellweger syndrome, Canavan's disease, Alexander's disease, nonketotic hyperglycinemia, congenital mitochondrial encephalopathies) (Fig. 30-23).

Cerebellar aplasia/hypoplasia

Absence or underdevelopment of all or part of the cerebellum can be divided into three categories.

Total agenesis/hypoplasia. Total agenesis is rare and usually associated with other CNS pathology (e.g., Meckel-Gruber syndrome).[15] Cerebellar hypoplasia is more common. It may result from chromosomal aberration,[39] prenatal infection (cytomegalovirus) exposure

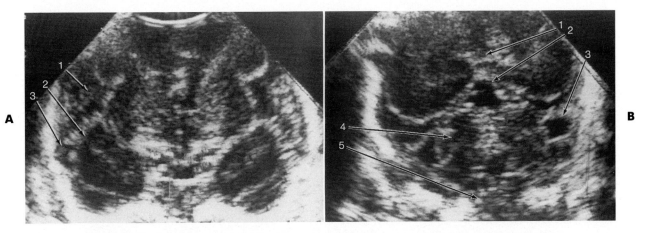

Fig. 30-21. A, Coronal sonogram (C2) in a 28-week-gestational infant with triploidy: *1,* large subarachnoid space; *2,* absence of operculation of the insula; *3,* thick cortex. **B,** Posterior fontanelle coronal sonogram (PF-C1) in the same infant: *1,* wide interhemispheric fissure at the level of the calcarine sulci; *2,* straight sinus; *3,* hypoplastic cerebellum; *4,* large transverse sinus; *5,* medulla.

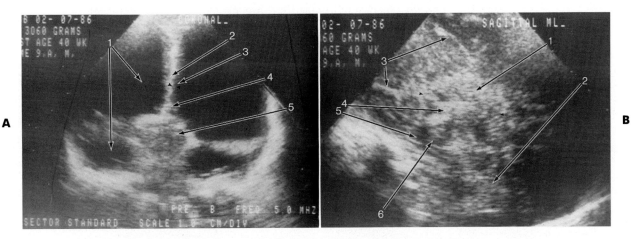

Fig. 30-22. A, Coronal sonogram (C2) in a term normocephalic infant with Barth syndrome: *1,* large lateral ventricles; *2,* interhemispheric fissure; *3,* neopallial hypoplasia (*between arrowheads*); *4,* hypoplastic (membranous) corpus callosum; and *5,* undivided thalami. **B,** Midline sagittal sonogram (SM) in the same infant: *1,* hypoplastic (membranous) corpus callosum (*between arrowheads*); *2,* hypoplastic cerebellar vermis; *3,* gyri radiating toward third ventricle; *4,* tela choroidea; *5,* third ventricle; *6,* massa intermedia.

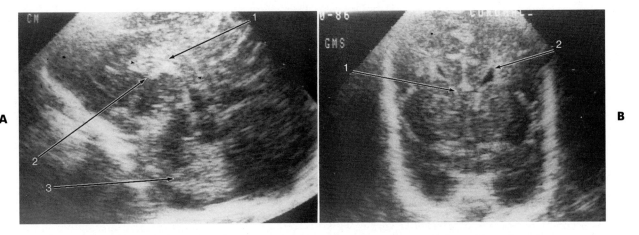

Fig. 30-23. A, Midline sagittal sonogram (SM) in a 39-week-gestational infant with nonketotic hyperglycinemia: *1,* short and thin corpus callosum (*between arrowheads*); *2,* tela choroidea (*short distance from corpus callosum*); *3,* hypoplastic cerebellar vermis. **B,** Coronal sonogram (C2) in the same infant: *1,* thin hypoplastic corpus callosum *2,* squared frontal horns.

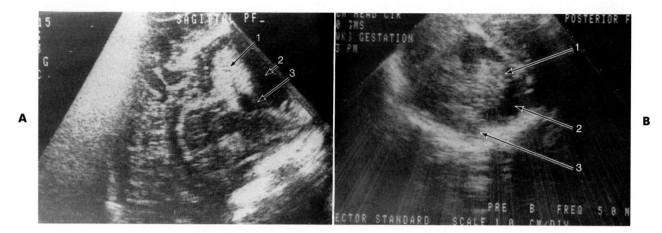

Fig. 30-24. A, Posterior fontanelle sagittal midline sonogram (PF-SM) in a 23-week-gestational infant with trisomy 18: *1,* hypoplastic cerebellar vermis; *2,* large cisterna magna in a normal-sized posterior fossa; *3,* large fourth ventricle. **B,** Posterior fontanelle coronal sonogram (PF-C1) in another infant with trisomy 18: *1,* hypoplastic cerebellar hemispheres with prominent folia; *2,* large cisterna magna in a normal-sized posterior fossa; *3,* medulla.

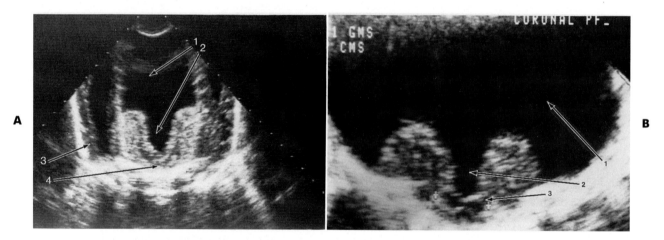

Fig. 30-25. A, Posterior fontanelle coronal sonogram (PF-C2) in a term infant with iniencephaly apertus and Dandy-Walker malformation: *1,* large posterior fossa cyst extending superiorly between the temporal lobes; *2,* large fourth ventricle communicating with posterior fossa cyst; *3,* temporal lobes; *4,* flattened brainstem. **B,** Posterior fontanelle coronal sonogram (PF-C1) in a term infant with classic Dandy-Walker malformation: *1,* large posterior fossa cyst; *2,* large fourth ventricle communicating with posterior fossa cyst; *3,* flattened brainstem.

to toxin (alcohol), metabolic disturbance (nonketotic hyperglycinemia, infantile Refsum's disease), or genetic disorder (Marinesco-Sjögren syndrome). Cerebellar hypoplasia can also be associated with other CNS pathology (e.g., lissencephaly with neopallial hypoplasia).[6]

Sonography shows a prominent cisterna magna, a large fourth ventricle, and a small cerebellum with prominent folia (Fig. 30-24). The posterior fossa is normal or small.

Vermis agenesis/hypoplasia. In Joubert's syndrome, there is a complete absence of cerebellar vermis with apposition of the cerebellar hemispheres on the midline.[25] This may simulate the appearance of an intact vermis. However, the fourth ventricle communicates superiorly and inferiorly with the arachnoid space.

In the Dandy-Walker syndrome, there is a large, fluid-filled posterior fossa cyst that is actually a ballooned fourth ventricle. A hypoplastic cerebellar vermis is attached superiorly to the midbrain tectum. The posterior fossa is enlarged because of an upward elevation of the tentorium. The straight sinus and transverse sinuses are also elevated. The cerebellar hemispheres, which may be normal in size or hypoplastic, are pushed superiorly and laterally by the midline cyst. The brainstem is frequently flattened against the clivus by the cyst. Hydrocephalus is a common feature

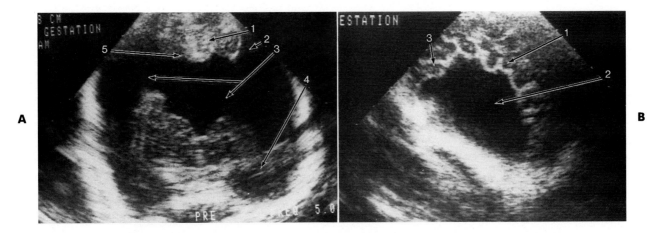

Fig. 30-26. A, Coronal sonogram (c2) in a term infant with schizencephaly: *1,* hypoplastic frontal lobe; *2,* wide subarachnoid space; *3,* bilateral transcerebral clefts; *4,* hypoplastic temporal lobe; *5,* corpus callosum. **B,** Parasagittal sonogram (SL4) in the same infant: *1,* gyri surrounding transcerebral cleft; *2,* transcerebral cleft; *3,* frontal lobe.

(Fig. 30-25). The Dandy-Walker malformation is, occasionally, associated with agenesis of the corpus callosum, cephalocele, iniencephaly, aqueductal stenosis, cerebral migratory defects, and lipomas.

Hemisphere aplasia-hypoplasia. Hemispheric aplasia-hypoplasia, when unilateral, is frequently associated with vermian hypoplasia.

DISORDERS OF CEREBRAL CORTEX MORPHOGENESIS

Morphogenesis of the cerebral cortex can be divided into two overlapping stages: migration and organization. Cell migration begins shortly after neuroblast histogenesis begins. Neurons pass through the future white matter in successive waves. The later waves pass through earlier and deeper waves to become more superficial cortical neurons. Neuronal migration continues till about 25 weeks of gestation. Gyral development commences at 14 weeks of gestation and is completed at about 2 years of age.

Disorders of cerebral cortex morphogenesis are usually characterized by abnormal development of the cortical mantle, which becomes too thick, too flat, and too folded. The abnormality may be focal, multifocal, or generalized; bilateral or unilateral; and symmetric or asymmetric. Disorders of cerebral cortex morphogenesis may be a feature of various hereditary or acquired conditions.

Schizencephaly

Schizencephaly is a congenital malformation believed to develop in the second month of gestation. A focal insult to the primitive brain wall prevents a portion of the wall from differentiating. A segment of the germinal matrix fails to form. The result is a cleft through the full thickness of the brain, and the pial surface is continuous with the ependyma. The gray matter lining the cleft is abnormal, usually displaying polymicrogyria or pachygyria. The cleft is most commonly located near the precentral and postcentral gyri. It may be unilateral or bilateral. Its lip may be fused or open. Clefts with fused lips are difficult to diagnose by sonography. Open lip clefts appear as large, fluid-filled spaces extending from the subarachnoid space to the ventricle. A cleft's edges are echogenic and have underlying hypoechoic gray matter. The septum pellucidum is absent in 80% to 90% of patients. The ventricles are frequently enlarged. Agenesis of the corpus callosum is common (Fig. 30-26). The basal ganglia, brainstem, and cerebellum are usually spared.

Lissencephaly

Lissencephaly results from incomplete migration of immature neurons to the cerebral cortex during the third and fourth gestational months. Consequently, the cerebral cortex is smooth without gyral formation (agyria) or with broad gyri (pachygyria). Lissencephaly can be divided into at least two types. In lissencephaly type I, the cerebellum is normal or slightly reduced in size, and most patients have no other birth defects or present typical facial changes (Miller-Dieker syndrome).[12] These classic forms of lissencephaly are due to a deletion of chromosome 17. Type II lissencephaly does not occur as an isolated malformation. It is frequently associated with a hypoplastic cerebellum and grossly dilated ventricles. Among type II lissencephaly, autosomal recessive inheritance has been observed in the Barth syndrome, the Neu-laxova syndrome (ichthyosis, hypoplasia genitalis), and the cerebrooculomuscular group of syndromes. Nongenetic causes of lissencephaly include intrauterine infections and exposure to alcohol, isoretinoin, and valproate.

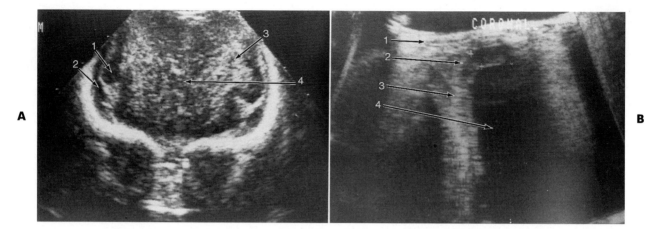

Fig. 30-27. A, Coronal sonogram (C1b) in a term infant with lissencephaly type I: *1,* cortex without sulci; *2,* dilated subarachnoid space; *3,* increased echogenicity of white matter; *4,* corpus callosum. **B,** Coronal sonogram (c2) using a 7.5-MHz transducer in a term microcephalic infant with lissencephaly type II: *1,* skin; *2,* argyric and hypoplastic neopallium; *3,* interhemispheric fissure; *4,* markedly enlarged lateral ventricles.

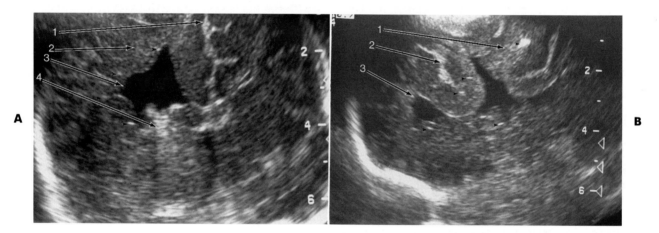

Fig. 30-28. A, Coronal sonogram (C2) in a term infant with hemimegaloencephaly: *1,* shift of interhemispheric fissure from right to left; on the right, there is a relative absence of sulci; *2,* irregular contour of the enlarged right lateral ventricle; *3,* increased echogenicity of the white matter with small calcification (*arrowheads*); *4,* irregular and calcified choroid plexus of right lateral ventricle. **B,** Parasagittal sonogram (SR2) in the same infant: *1,* increased echogenicity of the white matter (*small calcifications indicated by arrowheads*); *2,* deep sulcus without secondary sulci (pachygyria); *3,* irregular contour of the right lateral ventricle.

Sonographic findings differ in type I and type II lissencephaly. In type I lissencephaly, the sylvian fissures and subarachnoid space are widened, and the cortical surface of the brain is smooth and has a thick hypoechoic cortex[4] (Fig. 30-27, *A*). In the classic form, the occipital region ventricles are prominent. The corpus callosum may be normal. A cavum septi pellucidi is very common. Small midline calcifications in the region of the septum occur in about half of patients with the Miller-Dieker syndrome. The brainstem and cerebellum are usually normal. In type II lissencephaly, the third and fourth ventricles are grossly dilated and the cerebellum is dysplastic. Olfactory elements may be absent. The septum pellucidum is absent. The corpus callosum is absent or hypoplastic (Fig. 30-27, *B*). In nongenetic cases, CNS changes are more variable.

Hemimegalencephaly

Hemimegalencephaly results from a hamartomatous overgrowth of all or part of a cerebral hemisphere, with migration defects in the affected hemisphere. Pathologically, the cortex displays pachygyria and polymicrogyria (excessive number of gyri), and the white matter is characterized by heterotopias and gliosis. On sonography, there is a shift of midline structures due to the enlargement of the affected cerebral hemisphere. The lateral ventricle is enlarged on the affected side. The affected cortex is thickened with broad and shallow gyri.

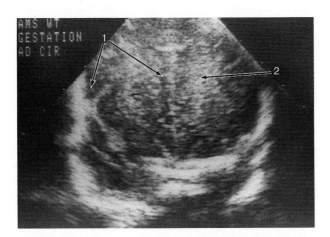

Fig. 30-29. Coronal sonogram (C1b) in a 36-week-gestational infant with Zellweger syndrome: *1,* irregular cortical surface due to decreased gyral width and depth (polymicrogyria); *2,* increased echogenicity of white matter.

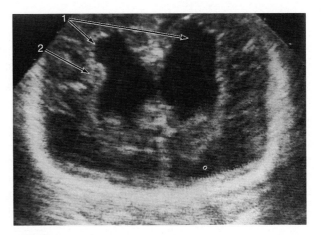

Fig. 30-30. Coronal sonogram (c1b) in a term infant with heterotopias: *1,* irregular contour of enlarged lateral ventricles; *2,* periventricular heterotopic gray matter.

Small calcifications can be seen in the white matter[26] (Fig. 30-28).

Polymicrogyria

Polymicrogyria is an abnormality of migration during the fifth and sixth month of fetal life. Neurons reaching the cortex distribute abnormally, forming multiple small gyri. The sulcal depth is variable, and the cortical surface is frequently abnormally thick. The most common location of polymicrogyria is around the sylvian fissure, suggesting that hypoxia may be a cause in many patients. Polymicrogyria may be found in congenital infections (e.g., cytomegalovirus) and single-gene syndromes (e.g., Zellweger's cerebrohepatorenal syndrome). Sonographically, the cortical surface is smooth, thick, and hypoechoic. Only a few gyri are seen. In the Zellweger syndrome, neurosonographic findings are relatively specific, with larger than normal parasylvian gyri, hypoplasia of the corpus callosum, and bilateral subependymal cysts at the level of the germinal matrix (Fig. 30-29).

Heterotopias

Gray matter heterotopias are collections of nerve cells in the white matter. They are more commonly seen in the subependymal region. Heterotopias are nonspecific and related to compromise of the integrity of the molecular-mesenchymal boundaries. Sonographically, heterotopias are nodular areas of hypoechoic gray matter in the subependymal region (Fig. 30-30). Subtle neuronal atopias cannot be diagnosed with ultrasound.

DESTRUCTIVE BRAIN ANOMALIES

The embryologic status of the brain at the time of an insult leads to well-defined morphologic changes that can be differentiated from one another on neurosonog-

raphy. Etiologic factors can be vascular, inflammatory, or traumatic.

Hydranencephaly

Hydranencephaly is a condition where most of the cerebral hemispheres are replaced by a thin-walled, membranous sac containing CSF. The sac's outer layer is composed of leptomeninges and glial tissue, with few neurons. A crescent of cerebral tissue is often seen at the inferior aspects of the frontal lobes and the inferomedial aspect of the temporal and occipital lobes. The thalami are atrophic, and the basal ganglia are not consistently present. The posterior fossa is usually normal except for an atrophic brainstem.

Sonographic features corresponding to hydranencephaly are (1) an incomplete falx cerebri, (2) a large anechoic collection of CSF replacing the cerebrum, (3) midline around hypeochoic structures at the cranial base representing the thalami and portions of the basal ganglia, (4) an anechoic third ventricle, and (5) a normal cerebellum, tentorium, and straight sinus. The differential diagnosis includes external hydrocephalus with schizencephaly, agenesis of the corpus callosum, holoprosencephaly, and severe hydrocephalus (Fig. 30-31). The diagnosis of hydranencephaly can be made prenatally.[28]

Multicystic encephalomalacia

Multicystic encephalomalacia is the result of an insult subsequent to neuronal migration and sustained during late gestation, during delivery, or after birth. The cerebral parenchyma is replaced by cysts of varying size. Lesions are located in the peripheral white matter or in the cortex. Many of the cysts are separated from each other by only thin, gliotic membranes or trabeculations. Both hemispheres are involved equally. The inferior temporal lobes are usually spared. Concomitant asymmetric ventricular dilatation and midline shift are frequently present. The thalami are small and hyperechoic. Calcifications may be present and suggest a viral etiology. Sparing of the cerebellum is usual[43] (Fig. 30-32). The cortex may show ulegyria.

Porencephaly

Porencephaly has been subdivided into agenetic and encephaloclastic categories. Agenetic porencephaly has been discussed under Schizencephaly. Encephaloclastic porencephaly results from insults occurring following neuronal migration but before the brain has acquired the

capacity for glial reaction (during the first half of gestation).

Typically, porencephaly appears as a unilocular, smooth-walled, anechoic cavity surrounded by white matter. The term *external porencephaly* applies if the ventricular wall is intact and the cavity communicates with the subarachnoid space. The term *internal porencephaly* is used when the cortex is intact and the cavity communicates with the ventricles. Porencephalic cysts are cystic defects of the white matter without communication with the ventricles or the subarachnoid space. In encephaloclastic porencephaly, the surrounding cortex has a normal gyral pattern.

Intracranial calcifications

Intracranial calcifications are rare and, when associated with microcephaly, ventriculomegaly, or destructive brain lesions, are frequently the consequence of fetal infection. They occur in areas of cell necrosis and are more commonly found along the ependymal surface and the cerebral parenchyma (basal ganglia or cortex). Calcifications appear as bright echogenic foci with or without shadowing (Fig. 30-33). The differential diagnosis includes fetal infections, teratomas, Sturge-Weber syndrome, tuberous sclerosis, brain tumors, lissencephaly, and hemimegalencephaly.[18]

CONGENITAL CYSTIC LESIONS

Congenital cystic lesions are fluid-filled cavities within or adjacent to the brain. Care must be taken not to confuse intracranial cystic masses with normal cystic areas, such as the cisterna magna and cavum septi pellucidi and vergae.

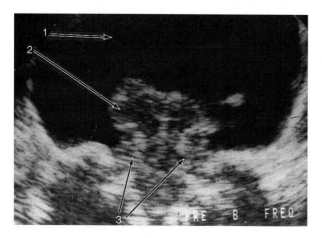

Fig. 30-31. Coronal sonogram (c2) in a 33-week-gestational infant with hydranencephaly: *1,* large anechoic space filling most of the cranium; *2,* preservation of thalami, third ventricle, and portion of basal ganglia; *3,* remnants of uncus.

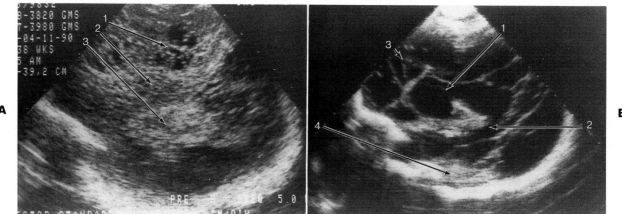

Fig. 30-32. A, Parasagittal sonogram (SR4) in a 38-week-gestational infant with early signs of multicystic encephalomalacia: *1,* irregular small cortical and subcortical cyst in frontoparietal region; *2,* insula; *3,* increased echogenicity of temporal lobe. **B,** Parasagittal sonogram (SR2) in a term infant with advanced encephaloclastic encephalomalacia: *1,* enlarged right lateral ventricle; *2,* choroid plexus of the lateral ventricle; *3,* membranes and trabeculations replacing most cerebral tissue; *4,* cerebellum.

Arachnoid cysts

Arachnoid cysts are fluid-filled cavities contained entirely within a splitting of the arachnoid. The most common sites are the cisterns around the sella turcica, the quadrigeminal plate, the cerebellum (retrocerebellar or cerebellopontine angle), the temporal fossa, and the sylvian fissure. However, they can also occur within the interhemispheric fissure and over the convexity of the brain. Adjacent brain tissue tends to be compressed and invaginated but not destroyed (Fig. 30-34).

Choroid plexus "cysts"

Choroid plexus "cysts" can be associated with trisomy 18. Sonographically, a large, anechoic, round mass is seen within the choroid plexus at the level of the trigone. Other features of trisomy 18 include hypoplasia of the vermis and corpus callosum.

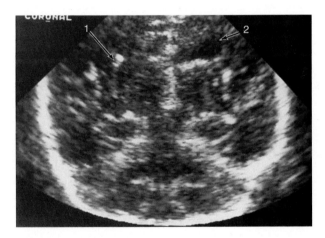

Fig. 30-33. Coronal sonogram (C3) in a term infant with congenital herpes simplex infection: *1*, calcification with shadowing in right putamen; *2*, enlarged lateral ventricle.

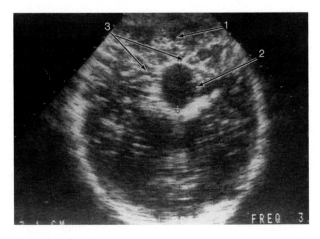

Fig. 30-34. Coronal sonogram through foramen magnum in a 6-year-old child with arachnoid cyst: *1*, cerebellum; *2*, arachnoid cyst of the quadrigeminal cistern; *3*, occipital lobes.

Germinal matrix subependymal cyst

Large germinal matrix subependymal cysts are found in patients with Zellweger syndrome (Fig. 30-35). Other features suggestive of the syndrome include corpus callosum hypoplasia and cerebral migratory defects. Subependymal cysts frequently are caused by prenatal germinal matrix hemorrhages or viral infections.

BRAIN NEOPLASIA

Most tumors presenting before 1 year of age are congenital.[8] They usually present with signs and symptoms of hydrocephalus and increased intracranial pressure. Seizures are rarely seen. Sonographically, most neoplasms are large and easily identified. They are highly echogenic relative to the surrounding brain.[42] The only exception is the cystic ependymoma of the lateral ventricle.[19] Tumor site, size, and composition are accurately diagnosed by ultrasound. Sonography may also allow prenatal diagnoses.[45] Supratentorial neoplasms are more common than infratentorial tumors during the first year of life.

Supratentorial tumors

The most common supratentorial tumors are astrocytomas teratomas that are primitive neuroectodermal and choroid plexus tumors. Astrocytomas usually arise from the hypothalamus and are grade II to III. These masses are infiltrative and echogenic relative to surrounding cerebral tissues; they demonstrate increased vascular flow on Doppler studies. Areas of necrosis are uncommon. Primitive neuroectodermal tumors and teratomas are usually quite large and produce marked distortion of the normal anatomy, with displacement of midline structures. Their border is sharply demarcated by edema. Areas of cystic necrosis appear as anechoic

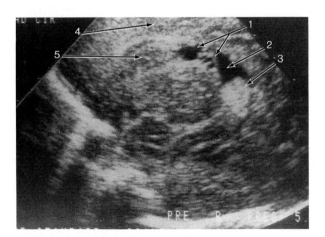

Fig. 30-35. Parasagittal sonogram in a 36-week-gestational infant with Zellweger syndrome: *1*, germinal matrix subependymal cysts; *2*, enlarged lateral ventricle; *3*, choroid plexus; *4*, increased echogenicity of periventricular white matter; *5*, head of caudate nucleus.

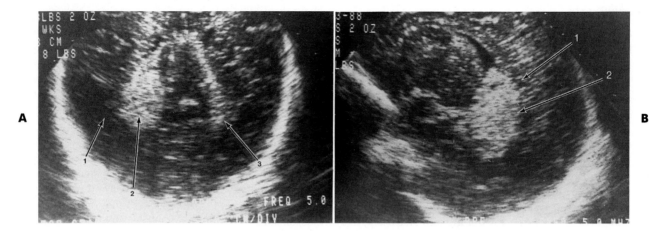

Fig. 30-36. A, Coronal sonogram (C4) in a term infant with choroid plexus papilloma: *1,* edematous white matter; *2,* irregular echogenic pattern of choroid plexus papilloma; *3,* normal choroid plexus. **B,** Sagittal sonogram (SR2) in the same infant: *1,* edematous periventricular white matter; *2,* irregular echogenic pattern of choroid plexus papilloma.

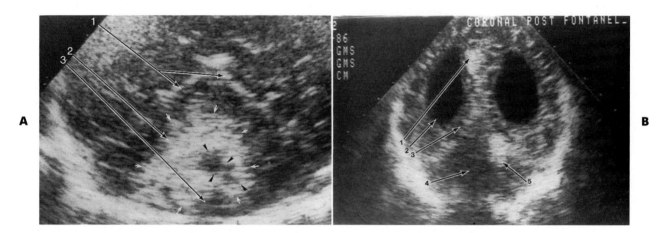

Fig. 30-37. A, Posterior fontanelle coronal sonogram (PF-C1) in a 2-month-old term infant with medulloblastoma: *1,* tentorium; *2,* medulloblastoma (*outlined by white arrows*) containing a hypoechoic cyst (*outlined by black arrowheads*); *3,* medulla. **B,** Posterior fontanelle coronal sonogram (PF-C1) in a 32-week-gestational infant with Goldenhar's syndrome and interhemispheric and posterior fossa lipomas: *1,* interhemispheric lipoma; *2,* large occipital horn; *3,* tentorium; *4,* cerebellum; *5,* posterior fossa lipoma.

components. Occasionally, calcifications produce acoustic shadowing.[19] Choroid plexus tumors tend to occur primarily in the lateral ventricles and rarely arise from the tela choroidea.[38] Most are unilateral, and approximately 17% are carcinomatous. They are highly echogenic and may contain foci of calcification and necrosis. Benign choroid plexus papillomas may grow through the ependyma into the surrounding white matter, causing surrounding edema (Fig. 30-36). Increased vascular shunting has been previously shown by color flow Doppler imaging.[7] Differentiation of the histologic type is usually not possible by ultrasound.

Infratentorial tumors

The most common infratentorial tumors are teratomas, medulloblastomas, and ependymomas. Teratomas are midline masses posterior to the vermis. They have a mixed echogenic pattern due to their soft tissue, fatty, and calcific content. Medulloblastomas arise from the roof of the fourth ventricle and always invade the cerebellar vermis before extending to one cerebellar hemisphere. These tumors are echogenic, may contain hypoechogenic cystic regions, are well defined, and are surrounded by mild to moderate edema. Calcifications are seen in 20% of the cases.[19] Ependymomas arise from the floor of the fourth ventricle (or from ependymal rests within the cerebellopontine angle). These tumors push the cerebellar vermis posteriorly and extend down toward the cisterna magna and foramen magnum. They are frequently echogenic with punctuated calcification and hypoechoic cysts. Posterior fossa tumors are best assessed through the posterior fontanelle (Fig. 30-37).

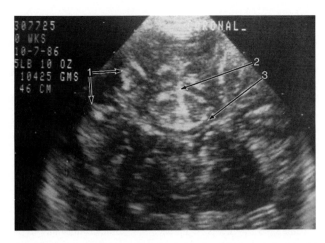

Fig. 30-38. Coronal sonogram (C2) in a term infant with Sturge-Weber syndrome: *1,* calcifications with shadowing along cortical surface of the right hemisphere; *2,* interhemispheric fissure; *3,* corpus callosum.

DISORDERS OF HISTOGENESIS

Defects of histogenesis give rise to the Sturge-Weber syndrome, to vein of Galen malformations, and to tuberous sclerosis.

Sturge-Weber syndrome

Sturge-Weber syndrome (encephalofacial angiomatosis) is a combination of facial and pial angiomatosis that is believed to result from persistence of primordial sinusoidal vascular channels that are present between the fourth and eighth week of gestation.[3] Sonography shows the pial and cortical calcifications with shadowing along the calvaria in the temporoparietooccipital region (Fig. 30-38). The ipsilateral cerebral hemisphere may be atrophic, and the choroid plexus is frequently enlarged.

Vein of Galen malformation

The vein of Galen malformation is an arteriovenous malformation resulting from the persistence of primordial arteriovenous shunts between branches of the carotid or vertebral circulations and the vein of Galen.[23] On coronal sonography, the dilated vein appears as a mildly echogenic midline mass posterior to the third ventricle and inferior to the corpus callosum. On sagittal views, the dilated vein of Galen is in continuity with a persistent falcial sinus. Doppler imaging confirms the markedly increased flow.[44] Hydrocephalus and/or parenchymal brain lesions (stroke, edema, hemorrhage, atrophy) are frequently associated with vein of Galen malformations. Intraventricular hemorrhage may occur.

Tuberous sclerosis

Tuberous sclerosis is an autosomal dominant condition characterized by hamartomas in a variety of organs and systems. On sonography, the subependymal hamar-tomas appear as small echogenic nodules protruding into the lateral ventricles. They tend to be calcified and produce acoustic shadowing.[27,29] Ventricular dilatation secondary to obstruction of the foramen of Monro by a giant-cell astrocytoma may be present. Cortical hamartomas or "tubers" are difficult to see on ultrasound unless they are calcified.

REFERENCES

1. Alasdair G, Hunter W: *Brain.* In Stevenson RE, Hall JO, Goodman R, editors: *Human malformation and related anomalies,* vol 2, New York, 1993, Oxford University Press.
2. Aleksic SN, Budzilovich GN, Greco MA, et al: Iniencephaly: a neuropathological study, *Clin Neuropathol* 2:55-61, 1983.
3. Alexander GL: *Sturge-Weber syndrome.* In Vinken PJ, Bruyn GW, editors: *Handbook of clinical neurology: the phakomatosis,* vol 14, Amsterdam, 1972, North Holland.
4. Babcock DS: Sonographic demonstration of lissencephaly (agyria), *J Ultrasound Med* 2:456-466, 1983.
5. Babcock DS: *Sonography of congenital malformation of the brain.* In Naidich TP, Quencer RM, editors: *Clinical neurosonography,* Berlin, 1987, Springer-Verlag.
6. Barth PG, Mullaart R, Stam FC, et al: Familial lissencephaly with extreme neopallial hypoplasia, *Brain Dev* 4:145-151, 1982.
7. Chow PP, Horgan JG, Burns P, et al: Choroid plexus papilloma detection by real-time and Doppler sonography, *AJR Am J Roentgenol* 7:168-170, 1986.
8. Chuang S, Harwood-Nash DC: *Tumors and cysts.* In Naidich TP, Quencer RM, editors: *Clinical neurosonography,* Berlin, 1987, Springer-Verlag.
9. Cohen MM, Lemire RJ: Syndromes with cephaloceles, *Teratology* 25:161-172, 1982.
10. Diebler C, Dulac O: Cephaloceles: clinical and neuroradiological appearance: associated cerebral malformations, *Neuroradiology* 25:199-216, 1983.
11. Diebler C, Dulac O: *Pediatric neurology and neurosonology,* Berlin, 1987, Springer-Verlag.
12. Dobyns WB, Reiner O, Carrozzo R, Ledbetter DH: Lissencephaly: a human brain malformation associated with deletion of the *LISL* gene located at chromosome 17p13, *JAMA* 270:2838-2842, 1993.
13. Filly RA, Chinn DH, Callen PW: Alobar holoprosencephaly: ultrasonographic prenatal diagnosis, *Radiology* 151;455-459, 1984.
14. Fiske CE, Filly RA: Ultrasound evaluation of the normal and abnormal fetal neural axis, *Radiol Clin North Am* 2:283-296, 1982.
15. Fraser FC, Lytwyn A: Spectrum of anomalies in the Meckel syndrome, *Am J Med Genet* 9:67-73, 1981.
16. Fried K, Liban E, Lurie M, et al: Polycystic kidney associated with malformations of brain, polydactyly, and other birth defects in newborn sibs, *J Med Genet* 8:285-290, 1971.
17. Goldstein RB, Filly RA: Prenatal diagnosis of anencephaly: spectrum of sonographic appearance and distinction from amniotic band syndrome, *AJR Am J Roentgenol* 151:547-550, 1988.
18. Grant EG, Williams AL, Schellinger D, Slovis TL: Intracranial calcification in infant and neonate: evaluation by sonography and CT, *Radiology* 157:63-68, 1985.
19. Han BK, Babcock DS, Ostreich AE: Sonography of brain tumors in infants, *Am J Roentgenol AJR* 143:31-36, 1984.
20. Hendricks SK, Cyr DR, Nyberg DA, et al: Exencephaly: clinical and ultrasonic correlation to anencephaly, *Obstet Gynecol* 72:898-901, 1988.
21. Hilpert PL, Kurtz AB: Prenatal diagnosis of agenesis of corpus callosum using endovaginal ultrasound, *J Ultrasound Med* 9:363-365, 1990.
22. Hoffman-Tretin JC, Horoupian DS, Koeningsbery M, et al: Lobar

holoprosencephaly with hydrocephalus: antenatal demonstration and differential diagnosis, *J Ultrasound Med* 5:691-697, 1986.

23. Horowitz MB, Jungreis CA, Quisling RG, Pollack I: Vein of Galen aneurysms: a review and current perspective, *AJNR Am J Neuroradiol* 15:1480-1496, 1994.

24. Imaizumi SO, Pleasure JR, Zubrow AB: Lesion mistaken for hemorrhage in premature infant: lipoma of corpus callosum, *Pediatr Neurol* 4:313-316, 1988.

25. Joubert M, Eisenring JJ, Robb JP, Andermann F: Familial agenesis of the cerebellar vermis: a syndrome of episodic hyperpnea, abnormal eye movements, ataxia, and retardation, *Neurology* 19:813-825, 1969.

26. Lam AH, Villanueva AC, de Silva M: Hemimegalencephaly cranial sonographic findings, *J Ultrasound Med* 11:241-244, 1992.

27. Lebowitz RL: Tuberous sclerosis, *Society for Pediatric Urology Newsletter* 109-110, 1984.

28. Lee TG, Warren BH: Antenatal diagnosis of hydranencephaly by ultrasound: correlation with ventriculography and computed tomography, *J Clin Ultrasound* 5:271-273, 1977.

29. Legge M, Sauerbrei E, MacDonald A: Intracranial tuberous sclerosis in infancy, *Radiology* 153:667-668, 1984.

30. DeMyer W: Classification of cerebral malformations, *Birth Defects* 7:78-93, 1971.

31. DeMyer W: *Holoprosencephaly.* In Vinken PH, Bruyn GW, editors: *Handbook of clinical neurology,* vol 30, Amsterdam, 1977, North Holland.

32. Nicolaides KH, Campbell S, Gabbe SG, et al: Ultrasound screening for spina bifida: cranial and cerebellar signs, *Lancet* 2:72-74, 1986.

33. Nyberg DA, Mack LA, Hirsch J, Nahony BS: Abnormalities of cranial contour in sonographic detection of spina bifida: evaluation of the "lemon," *Radiology* 167:387-392, 1988.

34. Pilu G, Romero R, Rizzo N, et al: Criteria for the prenatal diagnosis of holoprosencephaly, *Am J Perinatol* 4:41-49, 1987.

35. Probst FP: Congenital defects of the corpus callosum, *Acta Radiol Suppl* 331:1-152, 1974.

36. Rakic P, Yakovlev PI: Development of the corpus callosum and cavum septi in man, *J Comp Neurol* 132:45-72, 1968.

37. Roland EG, Flodmark O, Hill A: Neurosonographic features of Aicardi syndrome, *J Child Neurol* 4:307-310, 1988.

38. Schelhas KP, Siebert RC, Heithoff KB, et al: Congenital choroid plexus papilloma of the third ventricle: diagnosis with real-time sonography and MR imaging, *AJNR Am J Neuroradiol* 9:797-798, 1988.

39. Schinzel A: *Catalogue of unbalanced aberrations in man,* Berlin, 1984, Walker de Gruyter.

40. Sessions RB: Nasal dermal sinuses: new concepts and explanations, *Laryngoscope* 92(suppl 29):1-28, 1982.

41. Simpson DA, David DJ, White J: Cephaloceles: treatment, outcome and antenatal diagnosis, *Neurosurgery* 15:14-21, 1984.

42. Smith WL, Menezes A, Franken EA: Cranial ultrasound in the diagnosis of malignant brain tumors, *J Clin Ultrasound* 11:97-100, 1983.

43. Stannard MW, Jimenez JF: Sonographic recognition of multiple cystic encephalomalacia, *AJR Am J Roentgenol* 141:1321-1324, 1983.

44. Tessler FN, Dion J, Vinuela F, et al: Cranial arteriovenous malformations in neonates: color Doppler imaging with angiographic correlation, *AJR Am J Roentgenol* 153:1027-1030, 1989.

45. Vanlieferinghen P, Lemery D, Sevely A, et al: Prenatal diagnosis of congenital cerebral tumors: a propos of three cases, *Arch Fr Pediatr* 50:39-41, 1993.

46. Yokota A, Matsukado, Y, Fuwa I, et al: Anterior basal encephalocele of the neonatal and infantile period, *Neurosurgery* 19:468-478, 1986.

Transcranial Doppler Sonography: Technique, Normals, and Variants

Edward J. Truemper
Asma Fischer

Transcranial Doppler (TCD) ultrasonography has only recently been systematically used to study vascular injury and cerebral autoregulation in neonatal and pediatric populations. Hindrance to its clinical application in the study of children has come from three directions: First, neurologists, radiologists, and neonatologists have been able to measure cerebral blood flow velocity (CBFV) in infants and children with open anterior and posterior fontanelles with continuous and duplex Doppler equipment. Much published material describes changes in CBFVs in infants as a result of a variety of disorders and normal physiologic conditions; however, the work has remained largely descriptive and difficult for most clinicians to apply in relevant circumstances. Second, the knowledge base concerning interpretation of CBFV parameters in the brain-injured child in incomplete. Factors such as age, level of consciousness, hematocrit, arterial blood gases, and hemodynamic parameters including blood pressure, vascular resistance and impedance, heart rate, and cardiac output, which are known to influence CBFV, have been either incompletely described, contradictory, or not extensively studied. Third, understanding the relationship that vascular pathology may have with producing cerebral parenchymal damage is poorly understood by most pediatricians. As an example, for more than 50 years numerous case reports, retrospective studies, and postmortem series have consistently documented cerebral vascular injury and cerebral infarction within the vascular territories of vessels affected by bacterial meningitis.* Despite the volume of published clinical data, minimal attention has been focused on the pathogenesis of cerebral vascular injury as a cause of infarction using experimental animal models.

Despite these limitations, TCD is gaining a foothold in pediatric ambulatory and critical care practice, primarily driven by the lack of suitable techniques to study cerebral blood flow during dynamic clinical conditions. Its suitability as a relevant clinical tool should be determined within the next few years, as the database of

*References 1, 7, 11, 13, 26-29, 45, 52, 57, 60, 61, 85, 87, 92, 100, 105, 118, 134, 136-138, 140, 143, 147, 149, 150.

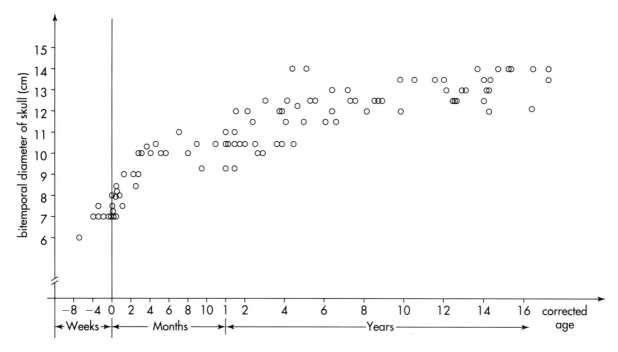

Fig. 31-1. Influence of age on the bitemporal diameter of the head.

TCD literature concerning pediatric patients continues to expand.

This chapter focuses on two subjects: (1) the application of TCD in pediatric practice coupled with practical information from our experience involving the examination of 300 pediatric patients and 2500 studies and (2) the discussion of normal physiologic factors that influence interpretation of CBFV parameters in neonates and children.

CEREBRAL BLOOD FLOW VELOCITY PARAMETERS, EXAMINATION TECHNIQUE, AND SPECIAL PREPARATIONS

The principles and physics of Doppler have been explained in preceding chapters. Physicians who routinely care for children can employ several Doppler methods including range-gated, continuous-wave, color flow duplex, and TCD, based on the available acoustic windows for a particular patient. The most commonly measured and calculated CBFV indices in pediatric practice are noted here. Direct measurements include peak systolic flow velocity (PV), mean flow velocity (MV), and end-diastolic flow velocity (EDV). Calculated variables include the following:

Pulsatility index:

$$PI = \frac{PV - EDV}{MV}$$

Systolic-diastolic ratio:

$$S{:}D = \frac{PV}{EDV}$$

Systolic mean ratio:

$$S{:}M = \frac{PV}{MV}$$

Area under the Doppler curve (AUC) envelope:

$$AUC = MV\,(t2 - t1)$$

Almost all studies use PV, MV, EDV, and PI in some combination for their analyses.

To perform a TCD examination properly, the operator must have a good working knowledge of cerebrovascular anatomy relative to the skull's surface. Technical factors important in obtaining accurate Doppler information include knowledge of the vessels that comprise the circle of Willis, direction of vessel blood flow, depth of individual vessels relative to the insonation sites, characteristic waveforms, and cerebral blood flow patterns relative to age. In infants and children, these factors are particularly important because with increasing age, the hemispheres also increase substantially in size, altering the anatomic course of the basal cerebral arteries, principally the middle (MCAs) and anterior cerebral arteries (ACAs). Also, increasing head circumference changes the bitemporal diameter, which influences the depths of insonation relative to the basal cerebral arteries (Fig. 31-1). Technicians should also be familiar with the expected ranges for each basal cerebral artery (BCA) because age is a principal determinant of CBFV amplitude and morphology. When examining a child with suspected cerebrovascular pathology, the observer must have an understanding of the possible effects that various disease states have on cerebral blood flow (CBF), CBFVs, and waveform envelope characteristics.

Prior to performing a TCD study, the blood pressure (ABP), heart rate (HR), respiratory rate (RR), and temperature should be measured. These parameters are helpful in interpreting Doppler-derived indices because these factors either directly affect CBFV parameters or indirectly indicate changes in hemodynamics or alterations in partial pressure of arterial carbon dioxide ($Paco_2$). This is particularly true in the normal preterm and term infant and the brain-injured child. A review of the medical history is important to identify pathologic processes that can influence CBFVs, including traumatic head injury, asphyxiation injuries, hydrocephalus, intracranial masses (e.g., hematomas or tumor), patent ductus arteriosus, systemic-to-pulmonary shunts, cyanotic congenital heart disease, aortic insufficiency or stenosis, severe anemia (hematocrit less than 25%), sickle cell disease (SSD), or other hemoglobinopathies. In critically ill children, a careful review of all drug therapies should be done, including all sedatives, barbiturates, opiates, diuretics (especially mannitol and acetozolamide), cardiotonic, pressor, and afterload-reducing agents because all of these drugs can potentially affect CBF and hemodynamics. Under normal circumstances, blood drawing for laboratory studies such as arterial blood gases (ABGs) and a complete blood count panel are unwarranted and may preclude a representative TCD examination due to the pain engendered by the child.

In the critically ill child with brain injury treated with mechanical ventilation, blood should be drawn for ABG testing at the time of the TCD study from a previously placed arterial catheter. If the child is heavily sedated, a capillary blood gas (CBG) is an acceptable alternative for $Paco_2$ analysis when proper technique is followed in obtaining an arterialized blood sample. Other acceptable methods for measuring carbon dioxide levels (CO_2) include the noninvasive transcutaneous ($Tcco_2$) and end-tidal CO_2 ($ETco_2$) monitors.* When properly calibrated, $Tcco_2$ monitors measurements are 2 to 5 torr above comparable $Paco_2$ values. The $ETco_2$ monitor values, however, show a wider (between 5 and 14 torr) variation below comparable $Paco_2$ values. Except for

extreme conditions (i.e., Pao_2 less than 45 torr or above 150 torr), measurement of the partial pressure of arterial oxygen (Pao_2) is not necessary. If hypoxia is suspected, oximetry is a reliable monitor when oxygen saturation is greater than 60%.[15,36,130] Newer invasive instrumentation that measures pH, $Paco_2$, Pao_2 continually via an indwelling arterial sensor have been recently validated.† The choice of the analysis technique for CO_2 determination should be used consistently whenever feasible, and documentation of the analysis technique should be made on the TCD record to aid interpretation.

Hematocrit should be measured initially and reexamined prior to each TCD study, especially if a blood transfusion has been given or if changes in hematocrit have occurred as a result of blood loss or sudden expansion of the circulatory volume secondary to intravenous fluid administration.

If an intracranial monitor is being used, the intracranial pressure (ICP) should be recorded simultaneously with the mean arterial pressure (MAP) to determine cerebral perfusion pressure (CPP). This is especially important in the child at risk for increased ICP because alterations in cerebral perfusion profoundly influence CBFV parameters, cerebral pulsatility indices (PI and resistance index [RI]), and the shape of the waveform envelope. When possible, a permanent recording of ICP waveforms should be made for the reviewer to assess the relative accuracy in the ICP value.

Transcranial Doppler in the pediatric ambulatory setting

In the ambulatory setting, the child should be brought into the examination room several minutes before the procedure to reduce anxiety and allay fear. If the child is insufficiently aware of the circumstances surrounding the TCD procedure, the child should be given the opportunity to examine the probe and mimic probe placement on the examiner or parent. Sufficient time should be made available to answer both the parent's and the child's questions. Parental participation is mandatory in order to maintain a child's trust. The procedure should never be "rushed," which generally leads to agitation, loss of cooperation, and poor results. Similarly, the routine physical examination should be performed after the TCD examination is completed. Laboratory tests requiring blood drawing or other neuroimaging procedures such as computed tomography or magnetic resonance imaging should always follow the TCD examination to avoid frightening the child.

Once suitable trust has been gained, the child should

---

*References 20, 65, 125, 129, 143, 147.

†References 14, 33, 39, 56, 81, 144, 150.

be placed in a comfortable supine position. When the child is in position, the TCD examination can initially proceed by examining the BCAs through the transtemporal window, the best-tolerated portion of the procedure. Insonation through the transtemporal window is easier in infants and children than in adults because the temporal bone exhibits a thinner cortical matrix and is significantly less ossified, resulting in less attenuation of the Doppler signal. The child can then be turned to the lateral recumbent position for insonation through the suboccipital window. Insonation through this window requires a significant decrease in gain prior to insonation, especially in the infant.

Initial Doppler settings should employ the least gain necessary to obtain a consistent waveform envelope. In the preterm infant, 5% to 10% gain is usually sufficient to obtain an adequate signal. In older infants and toddlers, the gain may need to be adjusted to 10% to 50%. In the school-age child up to late preadolescence, 50% to 75% is frequently required. In the adolescent, 50% to 100% gain is required in most cases. We have encountered only one adolescent subject in which satisfactory insonation could not be achieved at 100% gain through the transtemporal window. Children who suffer hyperostosis as a consequence of SSD anemia are frequently more difficult to insonate because of increased temporal cortical bone density, and gains higher than 100% may be required. Although there is no clinical or experimental evidence that ultrasound in the currently used power ratings on commercial TCD instruments poses a risk, gain above the minimum necessary to record consistent waveform envelopes should be avoided.[6,19,77,79,111,119] Depending upon the instrument used, these settings are documented as part of the printed copy and should be used consistently if serial studies are planned.

Sample volume should be adjusted to the minimum required to obtain a stable visual signal. Despite this adjustment, sample volume is always larger than the insonated vessel, and arterial tributaries in close proximity may be insonated as well, thus affecting the averaged signal output. These findings are confirmed if two signals can be visually discerned within the waveform envelope or if flow is detected in both antegrade and retrograde directions, such as witnessed at the MCA-ACA bifurcation.

Examination of each vessel requires adjustment of the insonation beam depth to evaluate the length of the vessel. At least two stable recordings at different points along the length of the artery should be obtained. Recordings should demonstrate minimal noise and be as free as possible of collateral circulation. In infants and toddlers, this is sometimes difficult because the BCAs and their branches are in close proximity to each other. If video recording is available, musical murmurs or bruits detected during the exam should be videotaped.

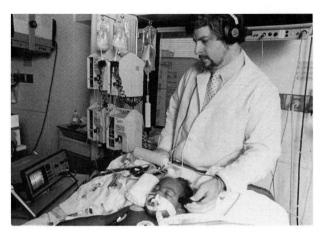

Fig. 31-2. Illustration of the most suitable location for the observer and transcranial Doppler (TCD) instrument to perform a TCD examination in a critically ill child.

Transcranial Doppler in the pediatric and neonatal intensive care unit

In the critically ill infant or child, TCD examination may be hampered by the physical environment because mechanical ventilators, cardiac monitors, fluid infusion pumps, and noninvasive BP, CO_2, and oxygen saturation monitors are often located at the head of the bed. The best position for the observer is behind the bed's head so that easy access to both temporal windows can be made in one location (Fig. 31-2). Insonation through the transtemporal window may be difficult if a head-injured child has associated cranial, facial, or zygomatic arch fractures that produce significant facial and temporal swelling, altering the shape of the window, the angle of insonation, and the insonation depth (Fig. 31-3). Wound dressings and wrappings anchoring ICP monitors can also cover the window, necessitating their manipulation or removal under physician guidance (Fig. 31-4).

Throughout the insonation procedure, careful attention should be made to evaluate the stability of the vital signs. Significant fluctuations in ABP, HR, and ICP can produce CBFV changes that could be misinterpreted. If hemodynamic changes occur, the study should be terminated until the patient regains hemodynamic and ICP stability. Occasionally, continuous recording of the MCA may prove beneficial to monitor the effects of drug therapy or $Paco_2$ manipulation following or during induced hypocapnia. Severely head-injured patients, especially those who exhibit mass effect from cerebral edema, hydrocephalus, or intracranial hemorrhage, may prove difficult to examine because of arterial displacement. The inability to insonate one or more vessels, especially the ACA or posterior cerebral artery (PCA), most frequently occurs under these conditions. Displacement of the MCA can also occur from mass effect;

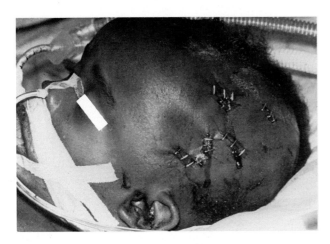

Fig. 31-3. Side view of a 10-month-old following severe closed-head injury. Significant edema is noted over the transtemporal window.

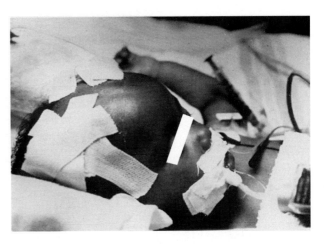

Fig. 31-4. Side view of an 8-month-old child following bilateral drainage of chronic subdural hematomas and placement of an interventricular pressure monitor. Transtemporal windows are obscured bilaterally by dressings and cotton buttresses for the ICP monitor.

however, it is generally less of a problem except for its impact on the angle of incidence.

Examination of the basilar artery (BA) and vertebral arteries (VAs) requires turning the patient to the lateral recumbent position. This maneuver should be strenuously avoided in patients with possible spinal fractures. It should also be avoided in children with cerebral swelling because it may precipitate intracranial hypertension.

In neonatal and pediatric patients with suspected communicable diseases, it is mandatory that isolation policies be rigidly followed. No particular preparation of the TCD system is needed beforehand. The external chassis of the TCD device, including all flat surfaces and the probe, should be cleaned with disinfectant.

Insonation sites in the infant and child

Transcranial Doppler is technically easier to perform in the infant and child because the temporal bone requires less power to penetrate in order to obtain an adequate signal. Additionally, the BCAs are shallower than their adult counterparts with reference to the insonation sites. Potential insonation sites include the transtemporal, high frontal, anterior fontanelle, and suboccipital approaches (Fig. 31-5). The orbital approach is avoided in routine pediatric clinical examinations because reference data from this approach is scant and there is a potential risk of developing structural eye damage. In the transtemporal approach, the probe is placed over the transtemporal window, which encompasses a variably defined area and is bordered posteriorly by the external auditory meatus, with an inferior boundary 1 to 2 cm above the zygomatic arch. In infants, the high frontal approach can be employed in that the frontal bone is sufficiently thin to allow penetration of the ultrasound beam. This

insonation site is located in the sagittal plane in front of the anterior fontanelle. The probe is directed caudally and posteriorly to the midline. If the anterior fontanelle is present, the transfontanelle approach can be used. The probe is placed midline directly over the anterior fontanelle and directed slightly caudally and laterally. The suboccipital approach requires placement of the probe at the base of the occiput, with the head flexed moderately forward. The probe is aimed superiorly and anteriorly in order for the insonation beam to pass through the foramen magnum. When the transfontanelle or suboccipital approaches are used, Doppler gain should be reduced because there are no osseous structures to dampen beam intensity. Reference depths indexed to age are published for some but not all windows and major BCAs.[23]

The insonation technique for individual basal cerebral arteries

Middle cerebral artery. Insonation of the MCA is performed from the transtemporal approach. The probe is placed over the insonation site and is directed horizontally. Frequently, the probe may need to be tilted superiorly because of the steep angle of the vessel in infants and young children. Gain should be initially set at the anticipated power level; it should be adjusted based on the strength and appearance of the waveform envelope. In infants the most distal portion of the M1 segment is generally identified at a relatively shallow depth of 25 to 30 mm. In older children, the initial MCA signal is identified at progressively deeper depths, reaching an average adult depth of 50 mm by the age of 10 years.[23] Reference depths for the MCA are listed in Table 31-1.

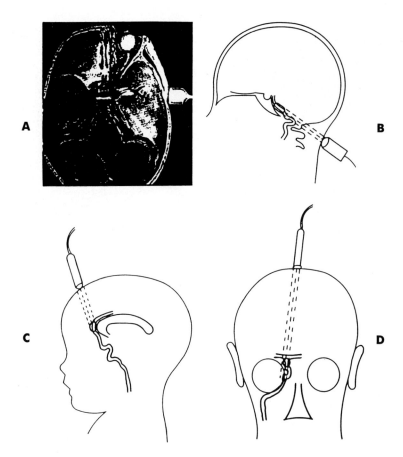

Fig. 31-5. Demonstration of potential insonation sites in the infant and child. **A,** Transtemporal approach (examination of MCA, ICA, A1 segment of the ACA, PCA); **B,** suboccipital approach (examination of the BA and VA); **C,** high frontal approach (examination of the A2 segment of the ACA); **D,** anterior fontanelle approach (examination of the ICA, infants only). (From Bode H: *Pediatric applications of transcranial Doppler sonography,* New York and Vienna, 1988, Springer-Verlag.)

Table 31-1. Reference depths where the middle cerebral artery is initially identified

Age	Depth (mm)
0-3 months	25
3-12 months	30
1-3 years	35-45
3-6 years	40-45
6-10 years	45-50
10-18 years	45-50

Modified from Bode H: *Pediatric applications of transcranial Doppler sonography,* New York and Vienna, 1988, Springer-Verlag.

Once the MCA is identified, some examiners elect to follow the vessel to its origin by adjusting beam depth by 2 to 5-mm increments. Other investigators prefer to confirm the vessel as the M1 segment prior to permanent recording by identifying the internal carotid artery (ICA) bifurcation. Either method is acceptable as long as the

examiner is experienced in recognizing the vessel. Attempts to insonate the inferior and superior trunks of the MCA M2 segment are often successful, but the data are difficult to interpret because the angle of insonation is too high to permit accurate measurements. At least two permanent records of the MCA at different depths should be made. Additional recordings to effectively map the vessel may be required if focal defects, as evidenced by marked changes in CBFV, are noted along different portions of the vessel. Using the transtemporal approach, the MCA blood flow is directed toward the probe and appears as an antegrade signal.

Anterior cerebral artery. Once the MCA has been satisfactorily examined, beam depth is adjusted to bring the ICA bifurcation into view. This is characterized by Doppler signals in both antegrade and retrograde directions. The antegrade CBFV signal represents the MCA blood flow, whereas the retrograde CBFV signal is derived from flow in the ACA. Sometimes the probe requires increased superior and anterior angulation to

Table 31-2. Reference depths where the anterior cerebral artery is initially identified

Age	Depth (mm)
0-3 months	25-30*
3-12 months	30*
1-3 years	55-60
3-6 years	60-65
6-10 years	60-70
10-18 years	65-70

*High frontal approach.
Modified from Bode H: *Pediatric applications of transcranial Doppler sonography,* New York and Vienna, 1988, Springer-Verlag.

Table 31-3. Reference depths where the internal carotid artery is initially identified

Age	Depth (mm)
0-3 months	55-65*
3-12 months	60-70*
1-3 years	40-50
3-6 years	45-55
6-10 years	50-55
10-18 years	55

*Anterior fontanelle approach.
Modified from Bode H: *Pediatric applications of transcranial Doppler sonography,* New York and Vienna, 1988, Springer-Verlag.

Table 31-4. Reference depths where the carotid siphon is initially identified

Age	Depth (mm)
0-3 months	—
3-12 months	—
1-3 years	50-60
3-6 years	55-60
6-10 years	55-60
10-18 years	60

Modified from Bode H: *Pediatric applications of transcranial Doppler sonography,* New York and Vienna, 1988, Springer-Verlag.

achieve adequate ACA insonation. This maneuver is sometimes necessary because of the incomplete migration of the ACA to its final adult location. The retrograde ACA flow signal is derived from the proximal or A1 segment. Reference depths for identification of the ACA are found in Table 31-2.

The frontal approach can also be used to insonate the distal or A2 segment of the ACA. From this approach the flow is directed toward the probe and the ACA CBFV appears antegrade on screen. The difficulty with angulating the probe to insonate the ACA from the transtemporal window is not encountered using the high frontal approach. Recordings of the ACA free of the stronger MCA signal should be obtained at least at two different depths of insonation.

Internal carotid artery. Following insonation of the ACA from the transtemporal approach, tilting the probe caudally and ventrally brings the CBFV signal from the intracranial internal carotid artery (ICA) into view. In this position, blood flow through the ICA is directed toward the probe and appears antegrade on the monitor. Angling the probe toward the midline brings the carotid siphon into view, where CBFVs are bidirectional. Reference depths for initial insonation of the ICA and carotid siphon are found in Tables 31-3 and 31-4, respectively.

In young infants, the transfontanelle approach can also be used to insonate the ICA. Placing the probe over the midline and aiming the beam caudally and slightly laterally brings the ICA into the beam path. In this location the ICA flow is directed toward the probe and the CBFV signal is displayed on screen in an antegrade direction. Inspection of ICA flow velocities is difficult in children because the increased tortuosity of the intracranial ICA causes wide variations in the angle of insonation.

Posterior cerebral artery. Insonation of the proximal or P1 segment of the PCA can be accomplished easily from the transtemporal approach by shifting the probe caudally and posteriorly and by increasing the beam

depth by 1 to 2 cm from that of the ICA. Probe angulation is similar in infants, children, and adults. Another approach is to place the probe immediately in front of or over the ear. In both positions, the insonation depth to the PCA is similar to the transtemporal window. In all three windows, the ipsilateral PCA blood flow is directed toward the probe and appears antegrade on the screen. By increasing beam depth by an additional 5 to 10 mm, blood flow is identified in both directions; this represents the ipsilateral (antegrade flow) and contralateral (retrograde flow) PCAs.

Occasionally, the examiner may experience difficulty in differentiating ICA and PCA flow velocity envelopes. Several methods can be easily employed to differentiate these two vessels. First, by reidentifying the MCA-ICA bifurcation, a standard reference point is reestablished. By directing the ultrasound beam caudally and posteriorly and by slightly increasing the beam depth, the PCA signal should come into view. Another method used in adult subjects is to perform unilateral carotid compression for several seconds. Ipsilateral ICA CBFVs are ablated or severely attenuated with this maneuver, whereas PCA blow undergo little, if any, change. This technique has not been routinely applied in children. Recently published evidence of cerebral ischemia and neurologic deficits following carotid compression in adult patients has been reported.[74,76,95,98] For this

Table 31-5. Reference depths where the posterior cerebral artery is initially identified

Age	Depth (mm)	
	P1	**P2**
0-3 months	—	—
3-12 months	—	—
1-3 years	55	50-55
3-6 years	55-60	50-60
6-10 years	60-70	55-65
10-18 years	60-70	60-65

Modified from Bode H: *Pediatric applications of transcranial Doppler sonography,* New York and Vienna, 1988, Springer-Verlag.

Table 31-6. Reference depths where the basilar artery is initially identified

Age	Depth (mm)
0-3 months	—
3-12 months	—
1-3 years	50-60
3-6 years	55-70
6-10 years	55-75
10-18 years	60-80

Modified from Bode H: *Pediatric applications of transcranial Doppler sonography,* New York and Vienna, 1988, Springer-Verlag.

reason, this maneuver should be avoided in routine clinical practice until further data are available in children. Reference depths for the PCA are given in Table 31-5.

Basilar and vertebral arteries. Using the suboccipital approach, the Doppler beam is directed superiorly and anteriorly, passing the foramen magnum between the cervical vertebrae and occiput. At short depths, angulation of the probe laterally to the right or left brings the VA CBFVs into view. At greater depths the BA can be identified when the probe direction is parallel to the midline. Blood flow is away from the ultrasound beam for the BA and VAs, and CBFV signals for all three arteries appear retrograde on the screen. Reference depths for the BA are listed in Table 31-6. Reference depths for the VAs in infants and children are not available.

Reproducibility

The accuracy of CBFVs is highly dependent upon the skill of the individual performing the study. Given that in TCD the technician is unable to visualize artery orientation in relation to the probe, considerable variation can occur in CBFVs obtained by the same technician (intraobserver) or between studies performed by different technicians (interobserver). Factors such as beam intensity, beam width, variations in insonation

Table 31-7. Reproducibility of the CBFV measurements for the MCA, ICA, and ACA in healthy infants

	MCA	ICA	ACA
PV			
M (cm/sec)	61-74	54-86	46-59
SD (cm/sec)	1.0-3.0	1.4-4.3	1.2-2.1
V (%)	1.6-4.1	2.1-7.8	2.2-4.6
MV			
M (cm/sec)	33-39	31-41	25-33
SD (cm/sec)	1.0-2.6	0.8-2.6	1.1-1.9
V (%)	2.9-6.5	2.2-8.1	3.2-6.5
EDV			
M (cm/sec)	10-23	15-17	10-19
SD (cm/sec)	0.4-2.2	0.5-1.6	0.5-1.6
V (%)	3.4-12.0	3.1-9.3	4.1-11.2
S:D			
M	3.0-7.7	3.3-5.1	2.9-5.4
SD	0.1-0.4	0.2-0.3	0.2
V (%)	2.6-6.6	3.9-6.1	3.7-6.9
RI			
M	0.67-0.87	0.69-0.80	0.66-0.82
SD	0.01-0.02	0.01-0.03	0.01-0.02
V (%)	0.8-2.2	1.2-3.6	0.9-3.4

CBFV, Cerebral blood flow velocity; *MCA,* middle cerebral artery; *ICA,* internal carotid artery; *ACA,* anterior cerebral artery; *PV,* systolic peak flow velocity; *MV,* mean flow velocity; *EDV,* end-diastolic peak velocity; *S:D,* systolic : diastolic ratio; *RI,* resistance index; *M,* highest and lowest mean value; *SD,* standard deviation; *V,* coefficient of variation (V = SD × 100/M).

From Bode H: *Pediatric applications of transcranial Doppler sonography,* New York and Vienna, 1988, Springer-Verlag.

windows, and angulation of the probe can potentially produce dissimilarities that can lead to erroneous interpretation of CBFV alterations.

Surprisingly, few studies have examined interobserver and intraobserver differences. Maeda and colleagues examined intraobserver differences for the MCA and BA in studies performed on the same day and on different days (mean interval, 22 days).[93] Reproducibility was considered good (r = 0.69 − 0.95), and the correlation coefficient was better for the BA than the MCA, which authors presumed was due to the larger insonation window for the BA. In another study, Totaro and associates demonstrated good correlation (r = 0.78 − 0.97) in interobserver measurements obtained over three time periods within 24 hours for the MCA, ACA, PCA, and BA.[141] Bode has performed the only published study in the neonatal population.[22] In a small population of infants, he examined the MCA, ICA, and ACA CBFV indices in 5-minute intervals over 30 minutes (Table 31-7). The coefficient of variation (V = S × 100/M)

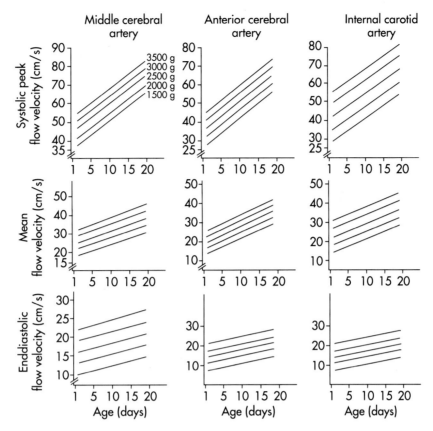

Fig. 31-6. Mean reference values of cerebral blood flow velocities in the middle cerebral artery, anterior cerebral artery and interior carotid artery for different birth weights during the first 20 days of life. (From Bode H: *Pediatric applications of transcranial Doppler sonography,* New York and Vienna, 1988, Springer-Verlag.)

increased in the order of MCA as higher than ACA, which is higher than ICA. The maximum coefficient of variation was seen in the MV for all three vessels. The smallest difference was seen in the RI.

In practical terms, because of the potentially large variation that can occur under clinical circumstances, CBFVs should not be used as absolute values to be acted upon except where published documentation exists as to their usefulness, such as in the diagnosis of brain death or vasospasm. Rather, CBFVs should be employed to show the magnitude of change over time in reference to cerebrovascular injury and response to treatment.

PHYSIOLOGIC FACTORS AFFECTING TRANSCRANIAL DOPPLER INTERPRETATION AND REFERENCE
Values

Age. Gestational and chronologic age exerts a powerful effect on CBFVs, especially in the newborn, toddler, and preadolescent, but is poorly understood. CBFV data indexed to age have been obtained by numerous groups using continuous-wave Doppler, du-

plex Doppler, and TCD.* This information is presented according to chronologic age in the subsequent paragraphs.

Birth to 21 days. In preterm infants (gestational age, 25-32 weeks), the PV, MV, and EDV nearly double during the first 6 hours of life. The PI falls from a mean value of 0.9 to 0.7. Presumably these wide variations are due to closure of the ductus arteriosus, which reduces the total body vascular resistance and thereby increases systemic blood flow to the cerebral circulation. In preterm and term infants, PV, MV, and EDV increase in a linear manner; however, the magnitude of change differs from one of these parameters to the other. In both populations, mean PV, MV, and EDV increase by 1.5, 0.8, and 0.4 cm/s (Fig. 31-6). Paralleling these changes, there is a slight increase in the PI from 0.69 to 0.72. These CBFV changes are not uniform; individual infants demonstrate wide variations from the group and from themselves on different days. The most marked difference is seen in the EDV value. Side-to-side

*References 2, 3, 10, 16, 22-25, 30, 58, 63, 68, 73, 79, 90.

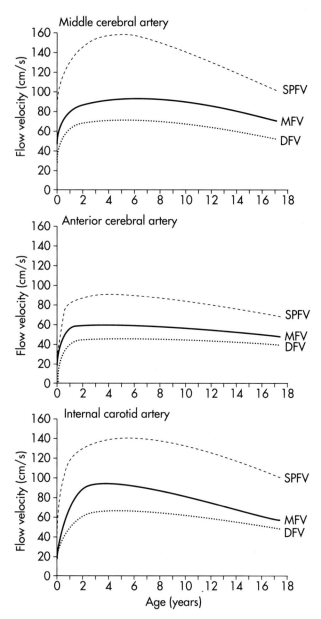

Fig. 31-7. Influence of age on mean reference values from birth to 18 years of age for the middle cerebral, internal carotid, and anterior cerebral arteries. (*SPFV*, Systolic peak flow velocity; *MFV*, mean flow velocity; *DFV*, end-diastolic peak flow velocity.) (From Bode H, Wais U: Age dependence of flow velocities in basal cerebral arteries, *Arch Dis Child* 63:606-611, 1988.)

variability is no more than 3% for the PV, 4% for the MV, and 2% to 5% for the EDV.[22]

Infancy, childhood, and adolescence. By the fourth week of life, CBFVs rise at a substantially lower rate (Fig. 31-7). The greatest magnitude of change is in the MCA and ICA. The ACA flow velocities also increase, but their amplitude of change is substantially less than that seen in either of the other vessels. Peak values for all CBFVs are seen from 4 to 8 years of age. They are up

to four times the flow velocity observed at birth and up to 50% greater than normal adult values. Beyond this period, CBFVs gradually decline at a rate of 1 to 1.5 cm/s annually, reaching adult values in late adolescence. Normative CBFV data relative to age are listed in Table 31-8.

Interrelationship between cerebral blood flow velocities, age, and other factors

Several factors appear to influence of ablate the influence of age on CBFV. In a population of children with sickle cell disease (SSD) and normal hematocrits, Adams and co-workers found that age correlated best with MCA, ACA, and CBFV changes.[2] In a later study, Adams and colleagues investigated a pediatric population with SSD and without stroke and found that the correlation of severe anemia with CBFV changes was stronger than that of age.[3] The values of correlation coefficients for the MCA (r = -0.41), ACA (-0.38), and BA (-0.56) indicate that unknown factors may be involved as well. Grolimund and Seiler have observed higher CBFV values in females than in males and have speculated that the relatively lower hematocrits in women may account for this phenomenon.[58] Adams and co-workers[2] and Brouwers and associates[25] have also identified higher CBFV values in adolescent females than in males; however, a significant difference in hematocrit between the two sexes was not found. The etiology for this gender difference has not been elucidated. The interrelationship of age and other physiologic variables has not been systematically examined. Given that cardiac output and blood pressure increase with age, it would seem that these variables should be systematically investigated in order to determine their influence on normal CBFV ranges.

Hematocrit. In determining CBFVs, hematocrit plays a large or larger role than age. Hematocrit and CBFVs have an inverse relationship in which polycythemia results in a variable decrease in CBFVs and anemia produces the opposite effect. The potential influence of hematocrit on CBFVs varies to some degree with age-related factors. In adults, the normal hematocrit range is narrow (42% to 48%) and remains relatively constant. In the developing child, profound changes in red cell volume and hematocrit occur over a short period of time. In infants, hematocrit ranges between 55% and 60% and within 2 months drops sharply to 30% to 35%. From the age of 6 months to adulthood the hematocrit increases slowly toward adult values, which are reached by adolescence. The impact of hematocrit on CBFVs relates to its effect on blood viscosity. Blood viscosity is affected by erythrocyte number (hematocrit), size, shape, and deformability, body temperature, shear rate, and hematocrit, the last two being the most important variables. Shear rate is

Table 31-8. Basal cerebral arteries CBFV (cm/s) in a cross-sectional study of 112 infants and children

Age	n	Middle cerebral artery	Internal carotid artery	Anterior cerebral artery	Posterior cerebral artery P1*	P2†	Basilar artery
Systolic peak flow velocity:							
0-10 days	18	46 (10)	47 (9)	35 (8)	—	—	—
11-90 days	14	75 (15)	77 (19)	58 (15)	—	—	—
3-11.9 months	13	114 (20)	104 (12)	77 (15)	—	—	—
1-2.9 years	9	124 (10)	118 (24)	81 (19)	67 (18)	69 (9)	71 (6)
3-5.9 years	18	147 (17)	144 (19)	104 (22)	84 (20)	81 (16)	88 (9)
6-9.9 years	20	143 (13)	140 (14)	100 (20)	82 (11)	75 (10)	85 (17)
10-18 years	20	129 (17)	125 (18)	92 (19)	75 (16)	66 (10)	68 (11)
Mean flow velocity‡:							
0-10 days	18	24 (7)	25 (6)	19 (6)	—	—	—
11-90 days	14	42 (10)	43 (12)	33 (11)	—	—	—
3-11.9 months	13	74 (14)	67 (10)	50 (11)	—	—	—
1-2.9 years	9	85 (10)	81 (8)	55 (13)	50 (17)	50 (12)	51 (6)
3-5.9 years	18	94 (10)	93 (9)	71 (15)	56 (13)	48 (11)	58 (6)
6-9.9 years	20	97 (9)	93 (9)	65 (13)	57 (9)	51 (9)	58 (9)
10-18 years	20	81 (11)	79 (12)	56 (14)	50 (10)	45 (9)	46 (8)
End diastolic peak flow velocity:							
0-10 days	18	12 (7)	12 (6)	10 (6)	—	—	—
11-90 days	14	24 (8)	24 (8)	19 (9)	—	—	—
3-11.9 months	13	46 (9)	40 (8)	33 (7)	—	—	—
1-2.9 years	9	65 (11)	58 (5)	40 (11)	36 (13)	35 (7)	35 (6)
3-5.9 years	18	65 (9)	66 (8)	48 (9)	40 (12)	35 (9)	41 (5)
6-9.9 years	20	72 (9)	68 (10)	51 (10)	42 (7)	38 (7)	44 (8)
10-18 years	20	60 (8)	59 (9)	46 (11)	39 (8)	33 (7)	36 (7)

*Precommunicating part of posterior cerebral artery.
†Postcommunicating part of posterior cerebral artery.
‡Mean flow velocity = time-mean of the maximal velocity envelope curve.
From Bode H, Wais U: Age dependence of the flow velocities in basal cerebarl arteries, *Arch Dis Child* 63:606-611, 1988.

considered important in the pathogenesis of some hemoglobinopathies such as SSD; however, in most clinical contexts shear rate is difficult to interpret and is often not measured. The hematocrit is easy to measure and has been studied in relation to its influence on CBFVs.

Using a PV, Bode first described an inverse relationship between hematocrit and CBFVs in the ACA[22] (Fig. 31-8). The relationship showed a significant negative correlation (r = −0.65, p < 0.001). In another descriptive study involving three populations of infants with normal hemoglobin, polycythemia, and anemia, demographic factors and MCA CBFV similarities and differences were tested between the groups.[22] In those with normal hematocrits and polycythemia, no significant differences were found for postbirth age, gestational age, and birth weight (Table 31-9). Only the MCA PV was significantly different between groups. When groups with normal hematocrit and anemia were compared, significant differences in chronologic age, gestational age, and birth weight were not found; however, there were significant CBFV and RI differences between the

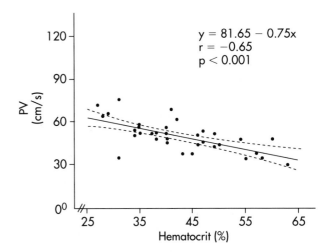

Fig. 31-8. Correlation of hematocrit and anterior cerebral artery peak systolic flow velocity in healthy premature newborns. (Regression line, ——; 95% confidence intervals, – – –.) (From Bode H: *Pediatric applications of transcranial Doppler sonography,* New York and Vienna, 1988, Springer-Verlag.)

Table 31-9. Comparison of demographics, hematocrit, and MCA CBFV indices in two populations of healthy infants with polycythemia or normal hematocrits

	Normal hematocrit	Elevated hematocrit	t-test
Age (days)	3.0	2.4	NS
Gestational age (weeks)	37.0	37.5	NS
Birth weight (g)	2707	2605	NS
Hematocrit (%)	52.6	72.0	$p < 0.0001$
PV (cm/sec)	52	40	$p < 0.01$
MV (cm/sec)	24	20	NS
EDV (cm/sec)	14	11	NS
RI	0.70	0.73	NS

CBFV, Cerebral blood flow velocity; *MCA*, middle cerebral artery; *PV*, systolic peak flow velocity; *MV*, mean flow velocity; *EDV*, end-diastolic peak velocity; *RI*, resistance index; *NS*, not significant.
From Bode H: *Pediatric applications of transcranial Doppler sonography,* New York and Vienna, 1988, Springer-Verlag.

Table 31-10. Comparison of demographics, hematocrit, and MCA CBFV indices in two populations of healthy infants with anemia or normal hematocrits

	Normal hematocrit	Decreased hematocrit	t-test
Age (days)	21	21	NS
Gestational age (weeks)	35.4	34.3	NS
Birth weight (g)	2030	1999	NS
Hematocrit (%)	51	33	$p < 0.001$
PV (cm/s)	55	68	$p < 0.06$
MV (cm/s)	28	37	$p < 0.05$
EDV (cm/s)	14	22	$p < 0.05$
RI	0.75	0.68	$p < 0.05$

CBFV, Cerebral blood flow velocity; *MCA*, middle cerebral artery; *PV*, systolic peak flow velocity; *MV*, mean flow velocity; *EDV*, end-diastolic peak velocity; *RI*, resistance index; *NS*, not significant.
From Bode H: *Pediatric applications of transcranial Doppler sonography,* New York and Vienna, 1988, Springer-Verlag.

groups (Table 31-10). Although neither study assessed the strength of the association between hematocrit and CBFV, differences between groups with normal, decreased, and increased hematocrits suggest that it is variable.

The effect of hematocrit on CBFVs has also been witnessed in other studies. Decreased CBFVs have been identified in polycythemic infants and in lambs by several groups using continuous-wave Doppler.[97,124] The increase in depressed CBFVs following partial plasma exchange transfusion (PPET) provides further, indirect evidence regarding the influence of hematocrit on CBFVs.[12,94,95,123] Using continuous wave Doppler, Bada

and associates studied term infants with the hyperviscocity syndrome.[12] Symptomatic infants showed the highest PI and lowest MV values; the asymptomatic group demonstrated PI and MV values within the normal range. Additionally, in symptomatic infants, correction of the polycythemia fully reversed hemodynamic changes detected before PPET, whereas there was no significant effect witnessed in the asymptomatic polycythemic group. These findings suggest that additional factors, presumably vascular in origin, affect CBFVs. More recently, Maertzdorf and others, using continuous-wave Doppler, investigated peripheral arterial and cerebral BFV indices and red cell transport in three polycythemic infant populations composed of preterm, small for gestational age (SGA), and appropriate for gestational age (AGA) infants pre- and post-PPET treatment.[95] Their results suggest that cerebral autoregulation with respect to viscosity-induced changes is variably influenced by gestational age.

In older children, Adams and colleagues identified age as the principal determinant of CBFVs; however, the simultaneous effect of hematocrit on CBFVs could not be studied because age and hematocrit were directly related.[2] In a later study of older children (ages 3 to 17 years) with SSD and without stroke, Adams and associates studied the relationship of CBFVs to age and to varying levels of anemia.[3] Interestingly, they found that CBFVs correlated better to the level of anemia than to age in all three vessels examined. The correlation was highest for the BA ($r = -0.58$) followed by the MCA ($r = -0.44$) and ACA ($r = -0.38$). The latter study suggests that hematocrit profoundly influences CBFVs and must be taken into account regardless of patient age when interpreting CBFV indices.

Partial pressure of arterial oxygen (Pao$_2$). An increase in Pao$_2$ (hyperoxia) causes mild vasoconstriction and increased cerebral arterial resistance, with a concomitant reduction in CBF.[74,80,113] In premature infants who are breathing pure oxygen, the mean fall in CBF is approximately 15%.[83] Other studies have documented similar but less pronounced changes in normal adult volunteers[80] and in animal models.[74] Niijima and colleagues[107] examined the response to hyperoxia in premature and term infants. A nearly uniform response to hyperoxia was marked by a fall in MV of the ACA in 30 of 32 infants. The median reduction in CBFV was calculated as 0.06 and 0.18 cm/s for each 1 KPa rise in Pao$_2$ for premature and term neonates, respectively. These data indicate that vascular maturation is important in determining the cerebrovascular response to arterial oxygenation.

A decrease in Pao$_2$ to a critical threshold (hypoxia) results in a rapid, marked vasodilatation, a reduction in cerebral vascular resistance, and a dramatic increase in CBF. This response is universally uniform in both humans and animals.[113,115,122,132,133] The combined effect of hypercapnia and hypoxia appears to be additive increasing cerebral blood flow.[115,132] To our knowledge, no pediatric or neonatal studies have employed TCD in examining the relationship between CBFVs and Pao_2.

Partial pressure of arterial carbon dioxide ($Paco_2$). One of the most powerful modulators of CBF and CBFV is $Paco_2$.[38,59,75] Increasing $Paco_2$ causes vasodilatation and a linear rise in CBF, whereas a fall in $Paco_2$ produces vasoconstriction and a linear decrease in CBF. In adults, mean changes in CBF are 3% to 4% per 1 torr change in $Paco_2$.[75] In infants and young children, changes in CBF are more pronounced than in adults.[83] In neonates, when $Paco_2$ acutely increases from 20 to 70 torr, CBF increases exponentially.[38,75] In contrast, fetal animal models tend to show less CO_2 vasoreactivity than adults.[62,121] The effect of $Paco_2$ is variably transient and does not produce a sustained effect on CBF. For example, in lambs, acute hypocapnia produces a mean decrease in CBF of $36 \pm 13\%$; if the hypocapnia is sustained for more than several hours, CBF gradually returns to baseline levels. A sudden restoration of $Paco_2$ to normocapniac levels produces a surge in CBF change up to $110 \pm 71\%$ above baseline.[55]

The effect of $Paco_2$ in various clinical and experimental settings is relatively uniform, but the amplitude of the change is variable. As expected, progressive hypocapnia causes an increase in cerebral resistance manifested by increasing PI and RI values, whereas the opposite effect is seen with rising $Paco_2$ levels.[9,37] In one study involving premature infants with hyaline membrane disease without intracranial pathology, an average increase in mean CBFV of 5.9% per 1 torr rise in $Paco_2$ was seen initially, although considerable variation existed within the group.[87] Within several days the average CBFV increase per 1 torr rise in $Paco_2$ was 7%, indicating a maturational influence with respect to CO_2 vasoreactivity. In a more recent study of premature newborns, Menke and colleagues[105] found an average change of 32.7% per 1 KPa rise in $Paco_2$,[105] a value consistent with the magnitude seen in normal premature newborns[111,112] and adults.[59] In premature infants, Fenton and associates determined that the level of CO_2 reactivity increased during the first 24 hours of life from 1.1 cm/s to 2.1 cm/s per 1 KPa rise in $Paco_2$.[43] For infants of no more than 30 weeks gestation and less than 24 hours of age, regardless of gestational age, and in infants of more than 31 weeks of gestation these data suggest that a maturational influence exists for CO_2 vasoreactivity.

Several drugs have been shown to alter the relationship between CBFV and the CO_2 response. Indomethacin attenuates the response of CBFV to CO_2 in preterm infants,[87] suggesting that prostaglandins may play a role in regulating cerebral vasomotor tone, but this, as yet,

has not been proven. Administration of pancuronium profoundly influences the CO_2 response, in which changes in CBFV in response to CO_2 modulation are closely correlated to the change in mean ABP regardless of gestational age or maturation.[43] The mechanism of action by which pancuronium influences the relationships among CBFV, mean ABP, and CO_2 vasoreactivity remains unknown. In a study of hydrocephalic infants treated with acetozolaminde, Cowan and Whitelaw found that CBFV increased by a median of 86% three times the expected rise for the slight elevation in $Paco_2$.[35]

To date, only one published study uses TCD to evaluate CO_2 reactivity in neonates and children. Bode investigated the response of premature infants to hypocapnia and hypercapnia.[22] The average MV response was 1.6 cm/s per 1 torr change in $Paco_2$, a value similar to that seen in Levene's group of preterm infants examined with duplex instruments.[87] Mild hypocapnia resulted in a decrease in EDV. Further decreases in CO_2 resulted in a more marked depression of EDV and a variable decrease in PV. Patients with either an interventricular hemorrhage or a patent ductus arteriosus did not demonstrate CO_2 reactivity, suggesting that pathophysiologic or hemodynamic factors can paralyze the cerebrovascular response to CO_2. Examples of the effect of progressive CO_2 elevation and hypocapnia are shown in Figures 31-9 and 31-10, respectively.

Body posture, activity level, and dynamic exercise

Several published studies describe the effect of body posture on CBFV indices measured by TCD. In one study involving 10 normal infants, subjects were examined in a variety of body positions, and none of the positions produced a discernible effect on CBFV.[22]

In another TCD study involving children 6 to 17 years of age, sudden changes in posture, such as moving from supine to standing positions, were used to study MCA hemodynamics.[21] In all but one child, the characteristic change was a variable drop in CBFVs. The PV remained relatively unchanged compared to supine values, whereas the MV and EDV decreased respectively to 66% and 39% of average supine values. The RI increased from an average of 0.51 to 0.83. Prolonging the duration of standing to 7 minutes maintained the reduction in CBFVs.

Using a pulsed Doppler instrument and sudden changes in body position to test cerebral autoregulation, Anthony and colleagues examined the effect of posture on CBFVs in preterm and term neonates.[8] The body position was tilted from the horizontal to a 20° head-up or a 20° head-down position. Four responses were noted and consisted of the following: no response, an equivocal or cycling response characterized by large cyclical or beat-to-beat variations in CBFV, a uniphasic response

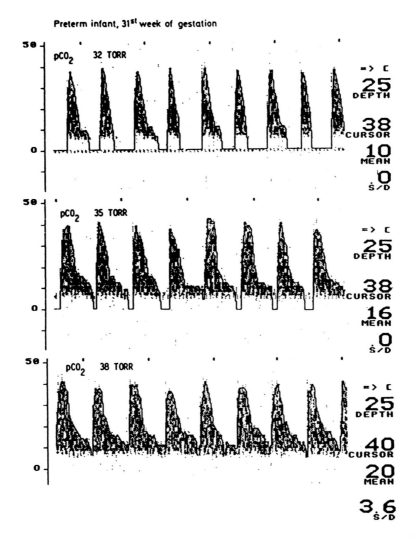

Fig. 31-9. Effect of increased CO_2 from hypocapnic to normocapneic levels on cerebral blood flow velocities amplitude and waveform envelopes in a healthy premature infant.
(From Bode H: *Pediatric applications of transcranial Doppler sonography,* New York and Vienna, 1988, Springer-Verlag.)

characterized by a sudden unidirectional change in CBFV following head tilt, and a biphasic response characterized by shift in CBFVs in one direction, followed by a second change the other direction within 20 seconds. Biphasic responses, which indicate intact cerebral autoregulation, were seen with increasing frequency with increasing gestational age.

Previous studies examining CBFV parameters during exercise show a variable increase in CBFVs that depend on the amplitude, type and duration of exercise.[64,69,70] Exercise in healthy children increases mean PV to 115%, MV to 115%, and EDV to 113%.[21] The effect of exercise on cerebral metabolic and flow parameters was investigated by Madsen and co-workers, who found that during 50% of maximal exercise the CBF decreased 7 ± 12% from baseline values, the cerebral metabolic rate of oxygen remained identical and the MCA MV increased 14 ± 10% from baseline values.[92] This study contradicts a previously held notion indicating that the increase in CBFVs observed during exertion is a result of a proportionate increase in CBF.

Sleep, arousal, and cognition

The sleep cycle has a variable influence on CBF and CBFVs. In preterm newborns, no appreciable differences in CBF have been identified between rapid eye movement (REM) and other NREM) sleep; however, CBF values are lower than those of adults, suggesting a reduced baseline metabolic activity.[57] In term infants the CBF is significantly lower during quiet (NREM) sleep than during active (REM) sleep. In both preterm and term infants, CBFVs are reduced during quiet sleep when compared to values obtained during active sleep.[66,67] Similar findings have been identified in earlier studies as well.[106,116] Using continuous-wave Doppler, Ferrari and associates examined the frequency, pattern

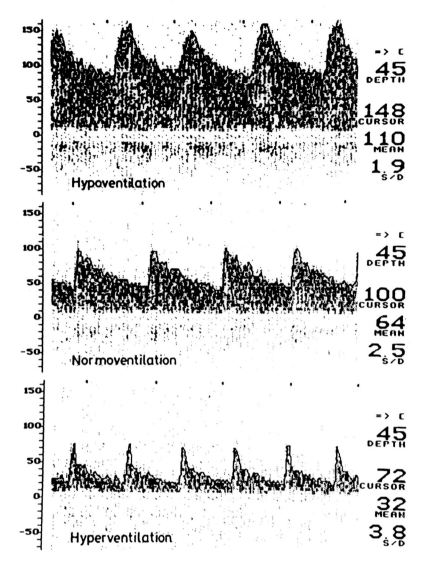

Fig. 31-10. Effect of spontaneous ventilation at different rates on cerebral blood flow velocities amplitudes and waveforms in a healthy child. (From Bode H: *Pediatric applications of transcranial Doppler sonography,* New York and Vienna, 1988, Springer-Verlag.)

characteristics, and amplitude changes in CBFV cyclic variations during active and quiet sleep.[44] They found that CBFV cyclic variations are more common in active than in quiet sleep; CBFV amplitude changes of up to 24% were detected during REM sleep and 16% in NREM sleep. Between the two stages of sleep, significant changes were seen in cycle frequency, median cycle amplitude, and median amplitude. The clinical relevance of sleep on CBFVs is twofold. First, comparison of studies between patients must take into account their specific levels of arousal. Second, cyclic variations in CBFVs should be recorded via video recorder to avoid errors of omission in obtaining randomly selected CBFV windows that do not illustrate the cyclic pattern. The origin of cyclical CBFV variations remains unknown, but the latter has been associated with autoregulatory

phenomena that influence the pial artery diameter[128] and with cyclical variations in cerebral blood volume.[89]

Relatively few studies have been published examining TCD-derived CBFVs in relation to the sleep cycle or the state of arousal in children. Fischer and others identified lower CBFVs during NREM sleep compared to presleep values in older children (ages 4 to 13 years).[49] Bode examined the effect of the state of arousal on CBFV parameters.[22] Although no data were offered, he remarked that there was a considerable variation in CBFVs and waveform envelopes in premature, term, and older infants. Bode also noted higher CBFVs at the beginning of the TCD study and ascribed the increase to apprehension or hypoventilation. These observations highlight the importance of recording the level of activity of the infant or child.

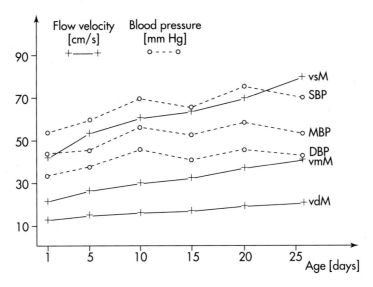

Fig. 31-11. Effect of age on blood pressure and cerebral blood flow velocities in healthy infants during the first 25 days of life. SBP = systolic blood pressure; MBP = mean blood pressure; DBP = diastolic blood pressure; VmM = mean flow velocity; VdM = diastolic flow velocity; VsM = systolic flow velocity. (From Bode H: *Pediatric applications of transcranial Doppler sonography,* New York and Vienna, 1988, Springer-Verlag.)

Several studies using TCD have documented that simple mental tasks can affect CBFVs in adults. Conrad and Klingelhofer examined the effects of visual stimulation on PCA CBFVs.[32] A sequential increase in the complexity of a simple picture resulted in a corresponding increase in PCA MV amplitude from $14.5 \pm 2.6\%$ to $38.8 \pm 6.5\%$. When the picture was withdrawn, CBFVs returned to baseline values within 10 to 15 seconds. Droste and colleagues found that special tasks that induce an asymmetric level of cerebral hemispheric activity produce a more pronounced increase in right MCA CBFVs than in left MCA CBFVs when the right hemispheric was stimulated.[41] Left hemispheric activities produced no significant asymmetry in CBFVs. This observation has been ascribed to the predominant role of the right hemisphere in attention and arousal. More recently, similar findings have also been reported by other groups using a variety of spatial and cognitive tasks.[40,71,96,140] At present, there are no published studies employing these methods in pediatric patients.

Hemodynamics

The relationship of cardiac-related variables such as HR, ABP, and cardiac output to CBFV indices is incompletely understood in the neonatal and pediatric populations. Maturational hemodymanics are pronounced during childhood, especially the first 2 years of life.[51] In infancy, stroke volume averages 1.5 ml/kg. Myocardial function at this age is characterized by poor diastolic compliance, which limits increased stroke volume efficiency, thereby limiting significant improvements in cardiac output following increases in HR. The

decrease in myocardial compliance is due to a relatively higher portion of noncontractile tissue to elastic myocardial fiber mass compared to adult hearts. With increasing age, the contractile myocardial mass increases in mass, and the chamber size grows in volume. These changes produce an increase in stroke volume and a gradual reflex decrease in HR. Between infancy and adulthood, HR decreases in a curvilinear fashion from an average of 130 ± 15 to 70 to 80 beats per minute.[109]

Bode has examined the relationship between ABP and CBFVs in normal neonates.[22] As shown in Figure 31-11, there is a steady, near-linear increase in PV, MV, and EDV. To date, there are no other published studies using TCD to examine this relationship. A later study of large for gestational age (LGA) infants of diabetic mothers found no correlation between the mean ABP and CBFVs.[17]

Bode also described the effects of HR on CBFVs in preterm and term neonates.[22] In only 7 of 216 instances was a significant relationship between HR and CBFV indices identified. This was considered by the author to be due to a "chance effect." Infants manifesting the most pronounced bradycardia showed a significant decrease in EDV, whereas older children with the same degree of bradycardia did not experience the same magnitude of CBFV changes. The circumstances surrounding the changes in HR witnessed in this population were not described. This precludes elimination of confounding variables such as alterations in $Paco_2$ or blood pressure as the culprits for the CBFV changes. It is also possible that older children can better tolerate HR changes with continued preservation of cardiac output through improved myocardial contractility or stroke volume.

The relationship of CBFVs and cardiac output has been studied in neonatal populations at risk for myocardial dysfunction. In one study, van Bel and colleagues examined CBFVs in the ACA and ICA of eight term infants of diabetic mothers using pulsed Doppler sonography.[17] Cardiac output was estimated from pulsed Doppler measurements obtained from the ascending aorta and the internal aortic root diameter. At the 84-hour postnatal examination period, the cardiac output fell by an average of 20% and the stroke volume fell by 25%. The CBFV indices during the same time interval increased variably, with PV increasing 12%, MV 14%, and EDV 50%. The PI fell from 0.8 to 0.65. These data have led to the suggestion that mild to moderate cardiac dysfunction does not produce significant CBFV changes in the neonatal population. In a later study, Saha and colleagues examined the relationship between cardiac function and CBFV indices in adults undergoing right heart catheterization.[127] A modest correlation (r = 0.45) between MCA MV and the cardiac index (CI) was found for CI values ranging between 2 and 4.5 L/minute. This suggests that low cardiac output states may influence CBFVs in adults.

Recently, van Bel and co-workers examined the relationship between cardiac output, ABP, ICA and ACA, and CBFVs in neonates with (N = 8) and without (N = 12) myocardial dysfunction following perinatal asphyxia.[18] In the myocardial dysfunction group, a modest positive correlation between mean ABP and MV (r = 0.45) and an inverse correlation for PI (r = −0.68) were found. In this population, cardiac output was significantly depressed during the first 2 days following the asphyxial event but promptly rebounded to near normal values thereafter. The mean ABP did not significantly change during this period; however, a rise in blood pressure on the second day did parallel the same findings with respect to cardiac output. In six of the eight infants with myocardial dysfunction, MV increased and PI decreased with increasing ABP, indicating pressure-passive CBF and loss of autoregulation. All six infants showed cerebral parenchymal abnormalities by computed tomography and subsequently developed the stigmata of ischemic encephalopathy. In contrast, infants without myocardial dysfunction showed stable MV, EDV, and PI values. A cardiac output increase of 11% during this time period was not statistically significant. Although in 4 of 12 patients transient neurologic abnormalities were noted, only 1 infant developed hypoxic-ischemic encephalopathy.

In summary, these findings suggest that changes in cardiac variables within the normal physiologic range have only a minimal effect on CBFV indices in normal subjects. Subjects with moderate hemodynamic dysfunction may not manifest significant changes in CBFVs.

However, in patients with significant myocardial dysfunction and concomitant cerebral autoregulatory abnormalities, changes in cardiac indices can potentially produce significantly larger changes in CBFVs. Further research is needed to understand the clinical significance of these complex interrelationships.

Basal cerebral artery variation and malformation

Because TCD techniques cannot image the basal cerebral arteries, abnormal CBFVs and waveforms can be misinterpreted as indicating either acquired stenosis or occlusion. Another potential confounding situation can arise if abnormal collateral circulatory patterns arise as result of vascular insufficiency in one or more of the BCAs. Anatomic deviation from the classic description of the circle of Willis is very common. In some series less than 20% of patients exhibit appropriately sized BCA tributaries, origins, and terminations.[50,82] For practical purposes, vascular variants can be divided into two types: (1) arteries that should exist following full development of the cerebral arterial system but are abnormal in their dimensions or attachment to other vessels and (2) persistent carotid-basilar embryonic remnants. A comprehensive review of cerebral vascular malformations is beyond the scope of this chapter in that there are more than 3000 references in the world literature related to this subject; however, a brief outline of typically encountered malformations is listed for each BCA.

Internal carotid artery

The most common anatomic variant is unilateral or bilateral hypoplasia.[85] Frequently this variant is accompanied by abnormalities in the anterior circle of Willis such as unilateral or bilateral absence or hypoplasia of the proximal ACA.[134] Increased coiling, tortuosity, and kinking have been described, involving the extracranial segment in both pediatric and adult patients.[53,114,145] Unilateral or bilateral absence of the ICA is extremely rare.[47,82]

Middle cerebral artery

In most anatomic and radiographic case series, the MCA exhibits the least incidence of anatomic variation.[101] The most common anomaly is duplication of the MCA at the proximal segment. Asymmetry between MCAs has been found in up to 4.5% of anatomic specimens in one series; however, the clinical significance of this finding must be questioned because distinct hypoplasia was not found in any of the specimens.[131] An example of duplication of the proximal MCA is shown in Figure 31-12.

Anterior cerebral artery

Varying degrees of hypoplasia and atresia are often found in both the proximal and distal ACA segments.[4] Severe hypoplasia or absence of one ACA is frequently

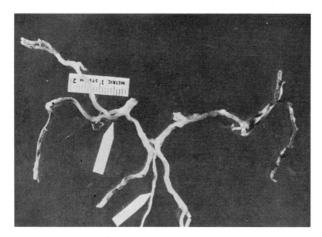

Fig. 31-12. View of the dissected anterior circulation of the circle of Willis illustrating duplication of the M1 segment *(lower arrow)* of the middle cerebral artery 3 mm from its origin and an anomalous artery arising from the anterior communicating artery *(upper arrow)*. (From McCormick WF, Schochet SS: *Atlas of cerebrovascular disease,* Philadelphia, 1976, WB Saunders.)

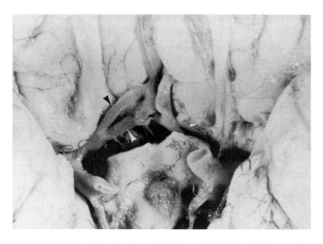

Fig. 31-13. View in situ from the base of the brain illustrating duplication of the left proximal anterior cerebral artery *(arrowheads)*. (From McCormick WF, Schochet SS: *Atlas of cerebrovascular disease,* Philadelphia, 1976, WB Saunders.)

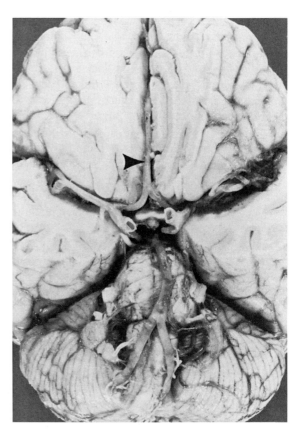

Fig. 31-14. View in situ from the base of the brain illustrating complete fusion of the distal anterior cerebral artery *(arrowhead)*. (From McCormick WF, Schochet SS: *Atlas of cerebrovascular disease,* Philadelphia, 1976, WB Saunders.)

associated with a concomitant increase in the caliber of the contralateral ACA.[77,88] Examples of duplication of the proximal ACA and fusion of the distal segment of the ACA are shown in Figures 31-13 and 31-14.

Anterior communicating artery

The anterior communicating artery (AcomA) exhibits the second highest incidence of vascular malformation.[4,42,131] The most common anomalies involve duplication and fenestration with plexiform formation.[4,42,131] Although not routinely examined with TCD, the AcomA represents one of the two collateral circulation channels at the level of the circle of Willis.

Posterior cerebral artery

The PCA demonstrates a higher incidence of vascular anomalies than the MCA, BA, or ACA, presumably by virtue of its fetal origin from the ICA.[5,46,131] The most common anomaly is the persistence of a large embryonic channel to the ICA, which fails to involute by the eighth week after gestation. Occasionally, hypoplasia or atresia of the proximal PCA stem is seen.[131]

Posterior communicating artery

The posterior communicating artery (PcomA) is rarely examined during routine TCD testing. Its importance is related to its role as a collateral channel within the circle of Willis. In normal circumstances, however, the PcomA is a vestigial vessel. Persistence as a large embryonic channel is seen in conjunction with the same anomaly involving the PCA.[77] In most anatomic series, the PcomA has the highest incidence of vascular malformation.[5,46,131] Severe unilateral or bilateral hypoplasia is the most frequently seen anomaly, often in

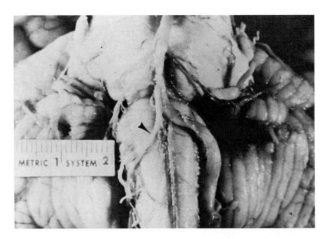

Fig. 31-15. View in situ from the base of the brainstem demonstrating hypoplasia of the left vertebral artery (VA) *(arrowhead)* with compensatory growth in the right VA. (From McCormick WF, Schochet SS: *Atlas of cerebrovascular disease*, Philadelphia, 1976, WB Saunders.)

association with anomalies in the anterior portion of the circle of Willis.[5,46,131]

Basilar artery

The BA, like the MCA, appears relatively resistant to malformation. The most common anomaly is variable duplication.[102,119,120,126] This phenomenon is understandable because the BA arises embryonically from a pair of neural arteries located along dorsal surface of the brain. These primitive arteries then completely fuse by the sixth week after gestation.[108] Other vascular abnormalities of the BA, such as complete duplication, failure to anastomose to one or both PCAs, and hypoplasia, appear to be of little clinical consequence.[100]

Vertebral artery

In most patients, the VAs show variable anatomic asymmetry.[100] Anatomic dominance is more commonly seen in the right VA. A representative example of VA asymmetry with unilateral VA hypoplasia is shown in Figure 31-15.

Persistent embryonic remnants

Numerous case reports have described abnormal collateral channels that persist beyond the embryonic period. The majority of these cases represent collateral circulation between the extracranial and intracranial circulations prior to the ossification of the skull. These anatomic remnants are often curious anomalies that bear little clinical significance. Occasionally, severe stenosis of one or both carotid vessels produces significant collateral circulation through one or more of these channels.[34,48,103,138] Several primitive carotid-basilar anastomoses can persist beyond the normal involution period to form collateral channels between the anterior

and posterior circulations caudal to the circle of Willis. The most important of these vessels include the persistent trigeminal, hypoglossal, otic, and proatlantal arteries. In normal circumstances these vessels are vestigial remnants that represent innocent findings either at autopsy or during cerebral angiography. Occasionally they can provide significant collateral circulation, compress cranial nerve roots, or provide a nidus for aneurysm formation.[31,54,72]

REFERENCES

1. Adams RD, Kubik CS, Bonner FJ: The clinical and pathological aspects of influenza meningitis, *Arch Pediatr* 65:354-376, 1948.
2. Adams R, Nichols FT, Stephens S, et al: Transcranial Doppler: influence of hematocrit in children with sickle cell anemia without stroke, *J Cardiovasc Ultrasonogr* 7:20-205, 1988.
3. Adams RJ, Nichols FT, McKie VC, et al: Transcranial Doppler: influence of hematocrit in children with sickle cell anemia without stroke, *J Cardiovasc Ultrasonogr* 8:97-101, 1989.
4. Alpers BJ, Berry RG: Circle of Willis in cerebral vascular disorders, *Arch Neurol* 8:398-402, 1963.
5. Alpers BJ, Berry RG, Paddison RM: Anatomical studies of the circle of Willis in normal brain, *Arch Neurol Neurosurg Psychiatry* 81:408-418, 1959.
6. American Institute of Ultrasound in Medicine, Bioeffects Committee: Bioeffects consideration for the safety of diagnostic ultrasound, *J Ultrasound Med* (suppl) 53-56, 1989.
7. Amith JF, Landing BH: Mechanisms of brain damage in *H. influenzae* meningitis, *J Neuropathol Exp Neurol* 19:248-265, 1960.
8. Anthony MY, Evans DH, Levene MI: Neonatal cerebral blood flow velocity responses to changes in posture, *Arch Dis Child* 69:304-308, 1993.
9. Archer LNJ, Evans DH, Paton JY, Levene J: Controlled hypercapnia and neonatal cerebral artery Doppler ultrasound waveforms, *Pediatr Res* 20:218-221, 1986.
10. Arnolds BJ, von Reutern GM: Transcranial Doppler sonography: examination technique and normal reference values, *Ultrasound Med Biol* 12:115-123, 1986.
11. Artopoulos J, Artopoulos J, Chalemis Z, et al: Sequential computed tomography in tuberculous meningitis in infants and children, *Comput Radiol* 8:271-277, 1984.
12. Bada HS, Korones SB, Pourcyrous M, et al: Asymptomatic syndrome of polycythemic hyperviscosity: effect of partial exchange transfusion, *J Pediatr* 120:579-585, 1992.
13. Baker CJ, Barrett FF, Gordon RC, YOW MD: Supparative meningitis due to streptococci of Lancefield group B: a study of 33 infants, *J Pediatr* 82:724-729, 1973.
14. Barker SJ, Hyatt J: Continuous measurement of intraarterial pHa, PaCO2, PaO2 in the operating room, *Anesth Analg* 73:43-48, 1991.
15. Barker SJ, Tremper KK: Pulse oximetry: applications and limitations, *Int Anesthesiol Clin* 25:155-164, 1987.
16. van Bel F, Den Ouden L, van de Bor M, et al: Cerebral blood-flow velocity during the first week of life of preterm infants and neurodevelopment at two years, *Dev Med Child Neurol* 31:320-328, 1989.
17. van Bel F, van der Bor M, Walther FJ: Cerebral blood flow velocity and cardiac output in infants on insulin-dependent diabetic mothers, *Acta Paediatr Scand* 80:905-910, 1991.
18. van Bel F, Walther FJ: Myocardial dysfunction and cerebral blood flow velocity following birth asphyxia, *Acta Paediatr Scand* 79:756-762, 1990.
19. Bergman I: Questions concerning the safety and use of cranial ultrasonography in the neonate, *J Pediatr* 103:853-858, 1983.

20. Blanton HM: Transcutaneous gas monitoring, *Probl Crit Care* 5:69-75, 1991.

21. Bode H: Cerebral blood flow velocities during orthostatis and physical exercise, *Eur J Pediatr* 150:738-743, 1991.

22. Bode H: *Pediatric applications of transcranial Doppler sonography,* New York and Vienna, 1988, Springer-Verlag.

23. Bode H, Wais U: Age dependence of flow velocities in basal cerebral arteries, *Arch Dis Child* 63:606-611, 1988.

24. van de Bor, M, Walther FJ: Cerebral blood flow velocity regulation in preterm infants, *Biol Neonate* 59:329-335, 1991.

25. Brouwers P, Vriens EM, Musback M, et al: Transcranial pulsed Doppler measurements of blood flow velocity in the middle cerebral artery: reference values at rest and during hyperventilation in healthy children and adolescents in relation to age and sex, *Ultrasound Med Biol* 16:1-8, 1990.

26. Brown LW, Zimmermann RA, Bilaniuk LT: Polycystic brain disease complicating neonatal meningitis: documentation of evolution by computed tomography, *J Pediatr* 94:757-759, 1979.

27. Buchan GC, Alword EC: Diffuse necrosis of subcortical white matter associated with bacterial meningitis, *Neurology* 19:1-9, 1969.

28. Bullock MRR, Wellchman JM: Diagnostic and prognostic features of tuberculous meningitis on CT scanning, *J Neurol Neurosurg Psychiatry* 45:1098-1101, 1982.

29. Cairna H, Russell DS: Cerebral arteritis and phlebitis in pneumococcal meningitis, *J Pathol Bacteriol* 58:649-663, 1946.

30. Calvert SA, Ohlsson A, Hosking MC, et al: Serial measurements of cerebral blood flow velocity in preterm infants during the first 72 hours of life, *Acta Paediatr Scand* 77:625-631, 1988.

31. Campbell RL, Dyken ML: Four cases of carotid-basilar anastomosis associated with central nervous dysfunction, *J Neurol Neurosurg Psychiatry* 24:250-253, 1961.

32. Conrad B, Klingelhofer J: Dynamics of regional cerebral blood flow for various visual stimuli, *Exp Brain Res* 77:437-441, 1989.

33. Conway M, Durbin GM, Ingram D, et al: Continuous monitoring of arterial oxygen tension using a catheter-tip polarographic electrode in infants, *Pediatrics* 57:244-250, 1976.

34. Coutree RW, Vijayanathan T: External carotid artery in internal carotid artery occlusion angiographic, therapeutic, and prognostic considerations, *Stroke* 10:450-460, 1979.

35. Cowan F, Whitelaw A: Acute changes of acetozolamide on cerebral blood flow velocity and PCO2 in the newborn infant, *Acta Paediatr Scand* 80:22-27, 1991.

36. Craig KC: Clinical application of pulse oximetry, *Prob Resp Care* 2:255-263, 1989.

37. Daven JR, Milstein JM, Guthrie RD: Cerebral vascular resistance in premature infants, *Am J Dis Child* 137:328-331, 1983.

38. Davis SM, Ackerman RH, Correia JA, et al: Cerebral blood flow and cerebrovascular CO_2 reactivity in stroke-age normal controls, *Neurology* 33:391-399, 1983.

39. Dodd KL: Continuous monitoring of arterial oxygen tension in the newborn, *Br J Hosp Equipment* May 76:35-48, 1975.

40. Droste DW, Harders AG, Rastogi E: Two transcranial Doppler studies on blood flow velocity in both middle cerebral arteries during rest and the performance of cognitive tasks, *Neuropsychologia* 27:1221-1230, 1989.

41. Droste DW, Harders AG, Rastogi E: A transcranial Doppler study of blood flow velocity in the middle cerebral arteries performed at rest and during mental activities, *Stroke* 20:1005-1011, 1989.

42. Fawcett F, Blachford JV: The circle of Willis, an examination of 700 specimens, *J Anat Physiol* 40:63-70, 1906.

43. Fenton AC, Woods KL, Evans DH, Levene MI: Cerebrovascular carbon dioxide reactivity and failure of autoregulation in preterm infants, *Arch Dis Child* 67:835-839, 1992.

44. Ferrari F, Kelsall AWR, Rennie JM, Evans DH: The relationship between cerebral blood flow and velocity fluctuations and sleep state in normal newborns, *Pediatr Res* 35:50-54, 1994.

45. Ferris EJ, Rudikoff JC, Shapiro JH: Cerebral angiography of bacterial meningitis, *Radiology* 90:727-734, 1968.

46. Fetterman GH, Moran TJ: Anomalies of the circle of Willis in relation to cerebral softening, *Arch Pathol* 32:251-257, 1941.

47. Fischer AG: A case of complete absence of both internal carotid arteries, with a preliminary report on the development of the stapedial artery, *J Anat Physiol* 8:37-49, 1914.

48. Fischer AQ, Anderson JC, Shuman RM: The ultrasound appearance or early periventricular leukomalacia with neuropathologic correlates, *J Islamic Med Assoc* 17:34-37, 1985.

49. Fischer AQ, Taormina MA, Aktar B, Chaudhary BA: The effect of sleep on intracranial hemodynamics: a transcranial Doppler study, *J Child Neurol* 6:155-158, 1991.

50. Fischer CM: The circle of Willis: anatomic variations, *Vasc Dis* 2:99-105, 1965.

51. Friedman WF: The intrinsic properties of the developing heart, *Prog Cardiovasc Dis* 15:87-111, 1972.

52. Gado M, Axley J, Appleton DB, Prensky AL: Angiography in the acute and post-treatment phases of *Haemophilus influenzae* meningitis, *Radiology* 110:439-444, 1974.

53. Gass HH: Kinks and coils of the cervical carotid artery, *Surg Forum* 8:721-731, 1958.

54. George AE, Lin JP, Moranz RA: Intracranial aneurysm on a persistent primitive trigeminal artery, *J Neurosurg* 35:601-604, 1971.

55. Gleisen CA, Short BL, Jones MD: Cerebral blood flow and metabolism during and after prolonged hypocapnia in newborn lambs, *J Pediatr* 115:309-314, 1989.

56. Goddard PJ, Keith I, Marcovitch IJ, et al: A catheter-tip oxygen electrode; experience in newborn infants with respiratory distress, *Arch Dis Child* 47:675, 1972.

57. Gosling RG, King DH: *Continous wave ultrasound as an alternative and complement to x-rays in vascular examination.* In Reneman RE, editor: *Cardiovascular applications in ultrasound,* Amsterdam, 1974, North-Holland.

58. Greisen G, Hellstrom-Vestas L, Lou L, et al: Sleep-waking shifts and cerebral blood flow in stable preterm infants, *Pediatr Res* 19:1156-1159.

59. Grolimund P, Seiler RW: Age dependence of the flow velocity in the basal cerebral arteries: transcranial Doppler ultrasound study, *Ultrasound Med Biol* 4:191-198, 1988.

60. Hauge A, Thoresen M, Walloe L: Changes in cerebral blood flow during hyperventilation and CO_2-breathing measured transcutaneously in humans by a bi-directional pulsed, ultrasound Doppler blood flow velocity meter, *Acta Physiol Scand* 110:167-173, 1980.

61. Haupt HM, Kurlinski JP, Barnett NK, Epstein M: Infarction of the spinal cord as a complication of pneumococcal meningitis, *J Neurosurg* 55:121-123, 1981.

62. Headings DL, Glasgow LA: Occlusion of the internal carotid artery complicating *Haemophilus influenzae* meningitis, *Am J Dis Child* 131:854-856, 1977.

63. Henandez MJ, Brennan RW, Vannucci RC, et al: Cerebral blood flow and oxygen consumption in the newborn dog, *Am J Physiol* 234:R209-R215, 1978.

64. Horiuchi I, Sanada S, Ohtahara S: Developmental and physiological changes in cerebral blood flow velocity, *Pediatr Res* 34:385-388, 1993.

65. Huang SY, Tawney KW, Bender PR, et al: Internal carotid flow velocity with exercise before and after acclimatization to 4,300 m, *J Appl Physiol* 71:1469-1476, 1991.

66. Huch R, Huch A, Albani M, et al. Transcutaneous PO_2 monitoring in routine management of infants and children with cardiorespiratory problems, *Pediatrics* 57:681-688, 1976.

67. Jorch G, Huster T: State dependent changes of blood flow

velocity in the anterior cerebral artery of neonates measured by pulsed Doppler investigations, *Eur J Pediatr* 144:530A, 1986.

68. Jorch G, Huster T, Rabe H: Dependency of Doppler parameters in the anterior cerebral artery on behavioral states in preterm and term neonates, *Biol Neonate* 58:79-86, 1990.

69. Jorch G, Rabe H, Michel E, et al: Resuscitation of the very immature infant: cerebral Doppler flow velocities in the first 20 minutes of life, *Biol Neonate* 64:215-220, 1993.

70. Jorgensen LG, Perko G, Hanel B, et al: Middle cerebral artery flow velocity and blood flow during dynamic exercise in humans, *J Appl Physiol* 72:1123-1132, 1992.

71. Jorgensen LG, Perko G, Secher NH: Regional cerebral artery mean velocity and blood flow during dynamic exercise in humans, *J Appl Physiol* 73:1825-1830, 1992.

72. Kelley RE, Chang JY, Suzuki S, et al: Selective increase in the right hemisphere transcranial Doppler velocity during a spatial task, *Cortex* 29:45-52, 1993.

73. Kempe LG, Smith DR: Trigeminal neuralagia, facial spasm intermedius trigeminal artery presenting with osterior fossa transient ischemic attacks: report of two cases, *J Neurosurg* 49:614-619, 1978.

74. Kempley ST, Gamsu HR, Nicolaides K: Effects of intrauterine growth retardation on postnatal visceral and cerebral blood flow velocity, *Arch Dis Child* 66:1115-1118, 1991.

75. Kennedy C, Grave D, Jehle JW: Effect of hyperoxia on the cerebral circulation of the newborn puppy, *Pediatr Res* 5:659-667, 1971.

76. Kety SS, Schmidt CF: The effects of altered arterial tensions of carbon dioxide and oxygen on cerebral blood flow and cerebral oxygen consumption in young men, *J Clin Invest* 27:484-492, 1948.

77. Khaffaf N, Karnik R, Winkler W-B, et al: Embolic stroke by compression maneuver during transcranial Doppler sonography, *Stroke* 25:1056-1057, 1994.

78. Kirgis HD, Llewellyn RC, Peebles EM: Functional trifurcation of the internal carotid artery and its potential clinical significance, *J Neurosurg* 17:1062-1072, 1960.

79. Kremkau FW: *Biologic effects and safety*. In Rumack CN, Wilson SR, Charboneau JW, editors: *Diagnostic ultrasound*, St Louis, 1992, Mosby–Year Book.

80. Kurmanavichius J, Karrer G, Hebisch G: Fetal and preterm newborn cerebral blood flow velocity, *Early Hum Dev* 26:113-120, 1991.

81. Lambertsen CJ, Kough RH, Cooper DY, et al: Oxygen toxicity: effect in man of oxygen inhalation at 1 and 3.5 atmospheres upon blood gas transport, cerebral circulation, and cerebral metabolism, *J Appl Physiol* 5:471-486, 1953.

82. Larson CP, Divers GA, Riccitelli SD: Continuous monitoring of PaO2 and PaCO2 in surgical patients, *Crit Care Med* 19:S25, 1991.

83. Le T: *Congenital anomalies of the carotid arteries,* Amsterdam, 1968, Excerpta Medica.

84. Leahy FA, Cates D, MacCallum M, Rigatto H: Effect of CO_2 and 100% O_2 on cerebral blood flow in preterm infants, *J Appl Physiol* 48:468-472, 1980.

85. Leeds NE, Goldberg HI: Angiographic manifestations in cerebral inflammatory disease, *Radiology* 98:595-604, 1971.

86. Lehrer HZ: Relative caliber of the cervical internal carotid artery: normal variation within the circle of Willis, *Brain* 91:339-348, 1968.

87. Leiguarda R, Barthier M, Starstein S, et al: Ischemic infarction in 25 children with tuberculous meningitis, *Stroke* 19:200-204, 1988.

88. Levene DH, Shortland D, Gibson N, Evans DH: Carbon dioxide reactivity of the cerebral circulation in extremely premature infants: effects of post-natal age and indomethacin, *Pediatr Res* 24:175-179, 1988.

89. Lie TA, Abnormale congenitale arteriele verbindingen aan de schedel basis, *Ned Tijdschr Geneeskd* 110:787-791, 1966.

90. Liever LN, Wickramasinghe YABD, Spencer SA, et al: Cyclical variations in cerebral blood volume, *Arch Dis Child* 67:62-63, 1992.

91. Low JA, Froese AB, Galbrith, et al: Middle cerebral artery blood flow velocity in the newborn following delivery, *Clin Invest Med* 16:29-37, 1993.

92. Lyons EL, Leeds NE: The angiographic demonstration of arterial vascular disease in purulent meningitis, *Radiology* 88:935-938, 1967.

93. Madsen PL, Sperling BK, Torsten W, et al: Middle cerebral artery flow velocity and cerebral blood flow and O_2 uptake during dynamic exercise, *J Appl Physiol* 74:245-250, 1993.

94. Maeda H, Etani H, Handa NA: A validation study on the reproducibility of transcranial Doppler sonography, *Clin Investig* 71:46-48, 1993.

95. Maertzdorff WJ, Tangelder GJ, Slaaf DW, Blanco CE: Effects of partial exchange transfusion on cerebral blood flow velocity in polycythemic preterm, term and small for dates newborn infants, *Eur J Pediatr* 148:774-778, 1989.

96. Maertzdorf WJ, Tangelder GJ, Slaaf DW, Blanco CE: Effects of partial plasma exchange transfusion on blood velocity in large arteries of arm and leg, and in cerebral arteries in polycythemic newborn infants, *Acta Paediatr* 82:12-18, 1993.

97. Markus HS, Boland M: "Cognitive activity" monitored by noninvasive measurement of cerebral blood flow velocity and its application to the investigation of cerebral dominance, *Cortex* 28:575-581, 1992.

98. Massik J, Tang Y, Hudak ML, et al: Effect of hematocrit on cerebral blood flow with induced polycythemia, *J Appl Physiol* 62:1090-1096, 1987.

99. Mast H, Ecker S, Marx P: Cerebral ischemia induced by compression tests during transcranial Doppler sonography, *Clin Investig* 71:46-48, 1993.

100. Maurette P, Maurett P, Dabadie P, et al: 2 cases of intracerebral arteritis, a rare complication of acute bacterial meningitis, *Agressologie* 24:191-192, 1983.

101. McCormick WF: *Vascular disorders of nervous tissue: anomalies, malformations, and aneurysms*. In Bourne GH, editor: *The structure and function of nervous tissue*, vol 3, New York, 1969, Academic Press.

102. McCormick WF, Shochet SS Jr: *Atlas of cerebrovascular disease*, Philadelphia, 1976, WB Saunders.

103. McCullough AW: Some anomalies of the cerebral arterial circle (of Willis) and related vessels, *J Anat Physiol* 168:537-542, 1947.

104. McDowell FH, Potes J, Groch J: The natural history of internal carotid and vertebro-basilar artery occlusions, *Neurology* 11:153-157, 1961.

105. McMenamin JB: Internal carotid artery occlusion in *Haemophilus influenzae* meningitis, *J Pediatr* 101:723-725, 1982.

106. Menke J, Michel E, Rabe H, et al: Simultaneous influence of blood pressure of blood pressure, PCO_2 and PO_2 on cerebral blood flow velocity in preterm infants of less than 33 weeks' gestation, *Pediatr Res* 34:173-177, 1993.

107. Muktar AI, Cowan FM, Stothers JK: Cranial blood flow and blood pressure changes during sleep in the human neonate, *Early Hum Dev* 6:59-64, 1982.

108. Niijima S, Shortland DB, Lebvene MI, Evans DH: Transient hyperoxia and cerebral blood flow velocity in infants born prematurely and at full term, *Arch Dis Child* 63:1126-1130, 1988.

109. Padgett DH: The development of the cranial arteries in the vascular system of the human embryo, *Contrib Embryol* 32:205-261, 1948.

110. Perloff WH: *Physiology of the heart and circulation*. In Swedlow

DB, Raphaely RC, editors: *Cardiovascular problems in pediatric critical care,* New York, 1986, Churchill Livingstone.

111. Pourcelot L: *Applications cliniques de l'examnen Doppler transcutane.* In Peronneau P, editor: *Velocimetre ultrasonore par Doppler,* Paris, 1975, INSERM.

112. Pryds O, Andersen GE, Friis-Hansen B: Cerebral blood flow reactivity in spontaneously breathing, preterm infants shortly after birth, *Acta Paediatr Scand* 79:391-396, 1990.

113. Pryds O, Greisen G, Lou H, Friis-Hansen B: Heterogenicity of cerebral vasoreactivity in preterm infants supported by mechanical ventilation, *J Pediatr* 115:638-645, 1989.

114. Purvis MJ, James IM: Observations on the control of cerebral blood flow in the sheep fetus and newborn lamb, *Circ Res* 25:651-657, 1969.

115. Quattlebaum JK, Upson ET, Neville RL: Stroke associated with elongation and kinking of the internal carotid artery, *Ann Surg* 150:824-836, 1959.

116. Quint SR, Scremin OU, Sonnenschein RR, et al: Enhancement of cerebrovascular effect of CO2 by hypoxia, *Stroke* 11:286-289, 1980.

117. Rahilly PM: Effects of sleep state and feeding on cranial blood flow of the human neonate, *Arch Dis Child* 55:265-270, 1980.

118. Raimondi AJ, Di Rocco C: The physiopathological basis for the diagnosis of bacterial infections of the brain and its coverings in children, *Childs Brain* 5:1-13, 1979.

119. Reece EA, Assimakopoulos E, Zheng XZ, et al: The safety of obstetric ultrasonography: concern for the fetus, *Obstet Gynecol* 75:139, 1990.

120. Rendall SM: Unusual abnormality of the arteries at the base of the brain, *J Anat Physiol* 13:397-405, 1879.

121. Riggs H, Griffith JO: Anomalies of the circle of Willis in persons with nervous and mental disorders, *Arch Neurol Neurosurg Psychiatry* 39:1353-1356, 1938.

122. Rosenberg AA, Jones MD Jr, Traystman RJ, et al: Response to cerebral blood flow changes in PaCO$_2$ in fetal, newborn, and adult sheep, *Am J Physiol* 242:H862-H868, 1982.

123. Rosenberg AA, Narayanan V, Jones MD: Comparison of anterior cerebral artery blood flow velocity and cerebral blood flow during hypoxia, *Pediatr Res* 19:67-70, 1985.

124. Rosenkrantz RS, Oh W: Cerebral blood flow velocity in infants with polycythemia and hyperviscocity: effects of partial exchange transfusion with plasmanate, *J Pediatr* 101:94-98, 1982.

125. Rosenkrantz TS, Stonestreet BS, Hansen NB, et al: Cerebral blood flow in the newborn lamb with hyperviscocity and polycythemia, *J Pediatr* 104:276-280, 1984.

126. Rowe MI, Weinberg G: Transcutaneous oxygen monitoring in shock and resuscitation, *J Pediatr Surg* 14:773-778, 1979.

127. Saeki N, Rhoton AL Jr: Microsurgical anatomy of the upper basilar artery and the posterior circle of Willis, *J Neurosurg* 46:563-578, 1977.

128. Saha M, Muppala MR, Castaldo JE, et al: The impact of cardiac index on cerebral hemodynamics, *Stroke* 24:1686-1690, 1993.

129. Sayama I, Auer LM: *Oscillating cerebral blood volume the origin of B waves.* In Ishii S, Nagai H, Brock M, editors: *Intracranial pressure* 5, Berlin, 1983, Springer-Verlag.

130. Schieber RA, Nmnoum A, Sugden A, et al: Accuracy of expiratory carbon dioxide measurements using the coaxial and circle breathing circuits in small subjects, *J Clin Monit* 1:149-154, 1985.

131. Severinghaus JW, Astrup PB: History of blood gas analysis, VI: oximetry, *J Clin Monit* 2:270-278, 1986.

132. Seydel HG: The diameters of the cerebral arteries of the human fetus, *Anat Rec* 150:79-88, 1965.

133. Shapiro W, Wassermann AJ, Patterson JL: Human cerebrovascular response to combined hypoxia and hypercapnia, *Circ Res* 19:903-909, 1966.

134. Snyder RD, Stovring J, Cushing AH, et al: Cerebral infarction in childhood bacterial meningitis, *J Neurol Neurosurg Psychiatry* 44:581-585, 1981.

135. Stebhens WE: Aneurysms and anatomical variation of the cerebral arteries, *Arch Pathol* 75:45-76, 1963.

136. Stovring J, Snyder RD: Computed tomography in childhood bacterial meningitis, *J Pediatr* 96:820-823, 1980.

137. Taft TA, Chusid MJ, Sty JR: Cerebral infarction in *Haemophilus influenzae* type B meningitis, *Clin Pediatr (Phila)* 25:177-179, 1986.

138. Takeda N, Matsuoka N, Kurihara E: A case of cerebral arteritis secondary to bacterial meningitis, *Brain Nerve* 40:647-650, 1988.

139. Taveras JM, Mount LA, Freidenberg RM: Angiographic demonstration of external-internal carotid anastomosis through the ophthalmic artery, *Radiology* 63:525-530, 1964.

140. Teoh R, Humphries MJ, Hoare RD, O'Mahony RC: Clinical correlations of CT changes in 64 Chinese patients with tuberculous meningitis, *J Neurol* 236:48-51, 1989.

141. Thomas C, Harer C: Simultaneous bihemispheric assessment of cerebral blood flow velocity changes during a mental arithmetic task, *Stroke* 23:614-615, 1992.

142. Totaro R, Marini C, Cannarsa C, Prencipe M: Reproducibility of transcranial Doppler sonography: a validation study, *Ultrasound Med Biol* 18:173-177, 1992.

143. Truemper EJ, Smith KG, Krishnamurphy SC: Group B streptococcal infarction presenting with massive cerebral necrosis, *J Perinatol* 7:267-269, 1987.

144. Trumper KC, Shoemaker WC: Transcutaneous oxygen monitoring of critically ill adults, with and without low flow shock, *Crit Care Med* 9:706-709, 1981.

145. Venkatesh B, Brock THC, Hendry SP: A multiparameter sensor the continuous intra-arterial blood gas monitoring: a prospective evaluation, *Crit Care Med* 22:588-594, 1994.

146. Weibel J, Field WS: Tortuosity, coiling and kinking of the internal carotid artery: I, etiology and radiographic anatomy, *Neurology* 15:7-18, 1965.

147. Wertman F: The cerebral lesions in purulent meningitis, *Arch Neurol* 26:549-582, 1931.

148. Whitesall R, Assidao C, Gollman D, Jablonski J: Relationship between arterial and peak expired carbon dioxide pressure during anesthesia and factors influencing the difference, *Anesth Analg* 60:508-512, 1981.

149. Yamashima T, Kashihara K, Ikeda K, et al: Three phases of cerebral arteriography in meningitis: vasospasm and vasodilation followed by organic stenosis, *Neurosurgery* 16:546-553, 1985.

150. Yoshioka K, Yoshioka K: Arterial occlusion in purulent meningitis and multicystic encephalomalacia, *Eur J Pediatr* 139:303-305, 1982.

151. Zimmerman JL, Dellinger RP: Initial evaluations of a new intra-arterial blood gas system in humans, *Crit Care Med* 21:495-500, 1993.

Transcranial Doppler Sonography: Diagnosis and Pathology

Edward J. Truemper
Asma Fischer

Information related to the application of transcranial Doppler (TCD) in the evaluation and treatment of cerebrovascular disease in the brain-injured pediatric population is limited when compared to the volume of data compiled in the study of adults with cerebrovascular disease. This chapter covers the available information discovered from its application to a wide range of clinical conditions that afflict children. Each section briefly outlines the clinical problem, its effect on cerebral blood flow (CBF), and Doppler-derived indices measured by continuous-wave, duplex, and transcranial Doppler. Clinical recommendations are offered where TCD can be used in routine clinical management.

BRAIN DEATH
Background

The diagnosis of brain death is based on the demonstration of the absence of all cortical and brainstem activity and absence of neurodepressants such as sedatives, anticovulsants, muscle relaxants, or significant hypothermia.* The addition of ancillary tests to confirm

brain death is frequently based on many legal and ethical issues dictated by local policies developed by hospital ethics committees and by the personal preferences of clinicians.[9,88,215,301] Supplemental laboratory procedures can be divided into those that determine absence of cerebral blood flow (four-vessel cerebral angiography, contrast computed tomography [CT], xenon CT, radionucleotide angiography with technetium-99 D-L-hexamethylene propyleneamine)† and those that determine absence of cerebral electrical activity (electroencephalogram, auditory, visual, and brainstem evoked potentials).[11,108,159,260] These supplemental tests exhibit a variable number of false positives and false negatives and can be limited by the patient's condition.‡ Additionally, application of a number of these techniques can be problematic because of the need to transport the patient from the intensive care unit (ICU) to an imaging site. In an effort to find a simple bedside test to serve as a confirmatory study and to guide the timing of other ancillary confirmatory tests

*References 31, 51, 194, 226, 233, 270, 290.

†References 15, 16, 19, 23, 93, 100, 120, 140, 142, 197, 199, 209, 216, 242, 253.
‡References 17, 34, 42, 65, 128, 136, 148, 214.

such as an electroencephalogram (EEG), a number of investigators have evaluated TCD and other Doppler methods to determine their reliability in this specific circumstance.

Rationale

The rationale in using TCD in confirming cerebral circulatory arrest results from the effect of cerebral swelling and compression of intracranial vessels, which are almost universal in brain-damaged patients. Hassler and colleagues have written an excellent qualitative description of the interrelationships among intracranial pressure (ICP), mean arterial pressure (MAP), and cerebral blood flow velocities (CBFVs) and waveform characteristics that define key features that determine progressive decline and eventual arrest of the cerebral circulation.[114] Increasing ICP produces a progressive decline in end-diastolic CBFV coupled with narrowing of the systolic peak waveform. Also, mean CBFV falls, but not to the same magnitude as end-diastolic CBFV, while peak CBFV amplitude remains relatively preserved. In turn, the cerebral resistive indices (PI and RI) progressively increase. When ICP equals the diastolic blood pressure, the end-diastolic blood flow stops and the corresponding CBFV becomes zero. As ICP increases above diastolic pressure, the end-systolic cerebral intraarterial blood volume is propelled retrogradely during diastole, presumably because of a markedly diminished volume capacitance of compressed small muscular arteries distal to the basal cerebral arteries (BCAs). As ICP continues to increase, diminishing the systolic blood pressure–ICP difference, the systolic flow velocity continues to lose amplitude gradually. Once ICP increases to match the systolic blood pressure, all net flow into the intracranial compartment ceases and no detectable CBFV can be identified in the BCAs.

Doppler investigations in children

A number of Doppler devices have been used to investigate intracranial and extracranial blood flow during brain death. McMenamin and Volpe, using duplex Doppler from the transfontanelle approach, identified a characteristic sequence of changes in the ACA CBFV in six brain-dead infants: (1) loss of diastolic CBFV, (2) diminution of systolic CBFV, (3) retrograde diastolic CBFV, and (4) complete loss of all discernible CBFV.[170] Using pulsed Doppler, Ahmann and colleagues studied the extracranial ICA CBFV indices in 44 children who met clinical brain death criteria.[10] In children older than 4 months of age, 19 of 23 cases were found to have ICA CBFV waveforms characterized by short systolic peaks followed by a retrograde diastolic flow signal. In children younger than 4 months of age, the same waveform did not occur. All younger patients manifested some degree of antegrade diastolic CBFV. In

a smaller study, Yoneda and co-workers, using duplex Doppler, examined the common carotid arteries in eight brain-dead adults and one child.[299] Their study identified a CBFV waveform pattern consisting of low-amplitude systolic spikes and end-diastolic flow reversal in all patients. From this diverse group of Doppler studies, it is apparent that CBFV waveform patterns are very similar regardless of the cerebral vessel. However, infants appear to be different from older children and adults for unknown reasons.

Transcranial Doppler investigations

Petty and associates identified waveform patterns associated with brain death that included absent or reversed diastolic CBFV and short systolic spikes in at least two basal cerebral arteries.[204] In their population of 57 subjects, 23 of whom met brain death criteria, application of these CBFV criteria established a sensitivity of 91.3% and specificity of 100%. In 24 brain-dead adults, Roper and colleagues investigated the flow velocities from the middle cerebral artery and found short, sharp systolic spikes with reversed diastolic flow (14 subjects), bifid systolic peaks (3 subjects), low-amplitude systolic spikes with antegrade diastolic flow (2 subjects), and low-amplitude antegrade envelope reaching zero velocity at the end of diastole (2 subjects).[225] In a mixed population of children and adults, Newell and co-workers identified Doppler waveform patterns consisting of forward systolic flow and retrograde diastolic flow in all cases in which brain death criteria were met.[186] More recent investigations performed primarily in adults have largely supported these findings.[208,213,279]

Three studies have investigated TCD as a confirmatory test of brain death in pediatric patients. In a large series of comatose children, Kirkham and colleagues found in all cases who met clinical brain death criteria a CBFV pattern characterized by mean flow velocities less than 10 cm/s, retrograde diastolic flow, and an index of flow (1 − antegrade/retrograde flow) of 0.8 or less.[130] Bode and associates found in eight of nine brain-dead children a reverberating flow pattern of systolic antegrade flow and diastolic retrograde flow.[37] Fischer and co-workers studied 20 comatose children manifesting a Glasgow coma scale score of 8 or less to evaluate the level of agreement between TCD criteria of cerebral blood flow cessation (reverberating flow pattern, low-amplitude systolic CBFV without diastolic CBFV, short systolic spikes or middle cerebral artery [MCA] flow velocity less than 10 cm/s) and the clinical brain death examination.[86] Examples of representative CBFV waveforms consistent with cerebral circulatory arrest are shown in Figures 32-1 and 32-2. In all 17 patients older than 2 months of age, agreement was found between the TCD and clinical brain death examinations. In the 3 patients younger than 2 months of age, the TCD and

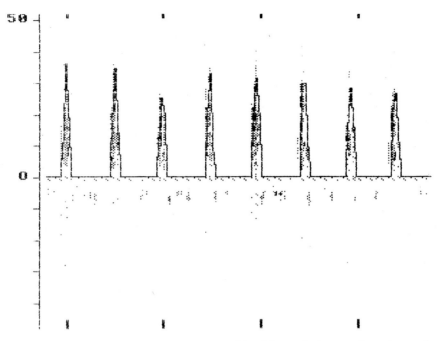

Fig. 32-1. Classic middle cerebral artery cerebral blood flow velocity waveform pattern found at brain death. It shows low-amplitude systolic spikes and absence of retrograde diastolic flow.

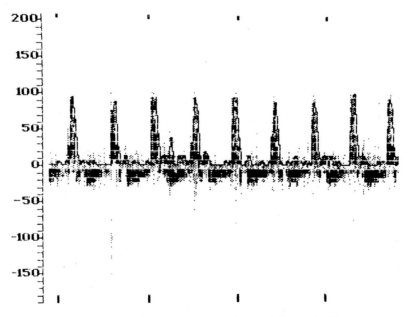

Fig. 32-2. Classic internal carotid artery cerebral blood flow velocity waveform with a reverberating pattern in a 20-month-old toddler following severe traumatic head injury. Clinical examination was consistent with brain death. Antegrade systolic and retrograde diastolic flow indicating complete cerebral circulatory arrest is seen. (From Fischer AQ, Truemper EJ: *Pediatric applications II: cerebrovascular control and applications to specific disease processes.* In Newell DW, Aaslid R, editors: *Transcranial Doppler,* New York, 1992, Raven Press.)

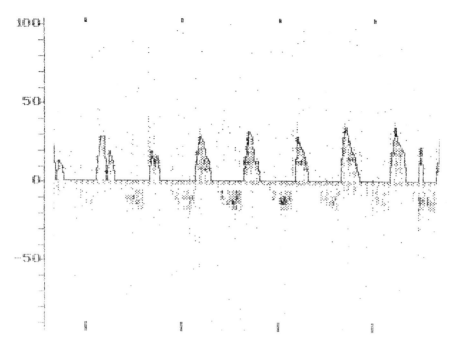

Fig. 32-3. Example of a false-positive Transcranial Doppler study in a 2-week-old neonate following severe perinatal asphyxia complicated by severe cerebral edema. The cerebral blood flow velocity waveform is from the left middle cerebral artery (MCA) and is consistent with complete circulatory arrest. Similar waveform patterns were identified in the contralateral MCA and bilateral internal carotid and anterior cerebral arteries. Neurologic examination revealed agonal respirations, positive pupillary light response, suck reflex, and decerebrate posturing to deep pain stimulus.

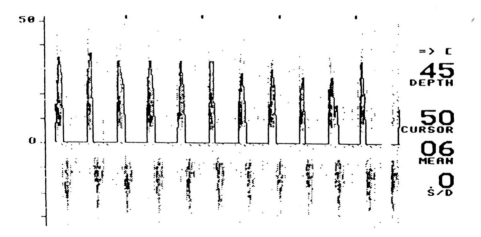

Fig. 32-4. Example of a false-positive transcranial Doppler study in a 2-month-old infant with near-miss sudden infant death syndrome and a clinical course complicated by severe cerebral edema and recurrent generalized tonic seizures. The cerebral blood flow velocity waveform is from the right internal carotid artery (ICA) and is consistent with the diagnosis of complete circulatory arrest. Similar waveforms were identified in the contralateral ICA and bilateral middle cerebral arteries; however, anterior cerebral artery flow could not be identified. Clinical examination revealed preservation of the pupillary light reflex, gag and corneal reflexes, and extensor posturing with deep pain stimulus.

brain death examinations did not have agreement. Representative examples of false-positive and false-negative TCD studies are shown in Figures 32-3 to 32-5.

These findings are not unique to the neonatal population, in that Petty and colleagues[204] and Ropper and associates[225] identified in their brain-dead adult populations patients who exhibited normal CBFVs and had clinical examinations consistent with brain death (false negative). It has been suggested that cerebral hyperfusion may coexist with clinical brain death.[239] The

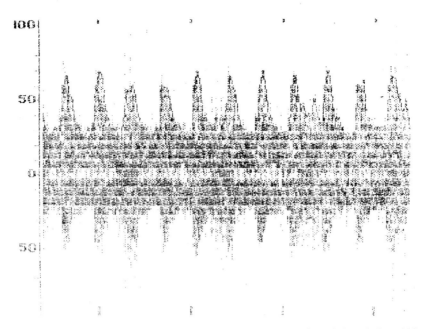

Fig. 32-5. Example of a false-negative transcranial Doppler (TCD) study in a 3-day-old infant 2 days following unexplained cardiopulmonary arrest. The TCD tracing was obtained from the right middle cerebral–anterior cerebral artery bifurcation and shows a normal waveform pattern and indices consistent with the age of the child. Serial neurologic examinations before and after the TCD study were consistent with brain death. (From Fischer AQ, Truemper EJ: *Pediatric applications II: cerebrovascular control and applications to specific disease processes.* In Newell DW, Aaslid R, editors: *Transcranial Doppler,* New York, 1992, Raven Press.)

observation of false-positive TCD findings has been ascribed to examination limited to the anterior circle of Willis, whereas the posterior circulation is not studied. Additionally, because the false-positive cases were infants less than 4 months of age, a lower cerebral perfusion threshold may be needed to maintain a modicum of neurologic function. In both cases, however, the infants remained in a chronic vegetative state until their deaths 15 and 22 months later. These data suggest that although TCD criteria for confirming cerebral circulatory arrest may prove inadequate in the pediatric population, identification of these parameters may prove useful as a prognostic tool in determining poor outcome. The small incidence of false-negative cases has led some authors to advocate that both the anterior and posterior circulations of the circle of Willis be examined.[293]

The "brain death" transcranial Doppler examination

Practical and special considerations. The TCD examination of a potentially brain-dead patient poses several potential problems that should be addressed to reduce the possibility of unsatisfactory examinations. First, the TCD examination, as in other ancillary tests, should never be used in isolation to supplant the clinical neurologic findings. Second, TCD testing should always be performed at the bedside in the ICU. This can sometimes pose special challenges because the amount of medical equipment at the bedside can inhibit effective maneuvering of the technician and the TCD instrument. Third, the examination should ideally be performed for a minimum of 30 minutes to document complete cessation of blood flow. Fourth, serial TCD examination sampling each vessel in the anterior and posterior circulation at set intervals should be obtained to avoid CBFV patterns consistent with transient cerebral circulatory arrest.[99,246]

Several factors can influence TCD recordings during the study. Respiratory variability has been witnessed by most investigators.[86,204,213] This sinusoidal rise and fall in peak systolic CBFVs, in synchrony with the mechanical ventilator, arises from the effect of positive intrathoracic pressure on the arterial pulse-pressure waveform. With inspiration, as the intrathoracic pressure increases, there is a corresponding increase in peak systolic CBFVs. During expiration, the intrathoracic positive pressure falls, and the peak systolic CBFVs decrease in amplitude.

The absence of CBFVs does not automatically imply absence of circulation. This is particularly true in the case of space-occupying lesions, which can displace vessels from their normal location. If no signal can be identified from a transtemporal window, the submandibular window can be used to insonate the internal carotid artery (ICA). Other alternatives include portable duplex Doppler examinations and radionucleotide brain imaging.

Insonation of the suboccipital window can prove difficult. In some cases insonation of the posterior circulation is precluded (e.g., unstable neck fractures, cervical collar) or instability of the patient (increased ICP with manipulation). Assistance should be obtained in order to maneuver the patient into the lateral recumbent position and avoid autoextubation. Insonation of the basilar artery (BA) is usually sufficient to determine posterior cerebral circulatory arrest. Monitoring should be performed for at least 5 to 10 minutes, although no published criteria exist concerning the adequate length of study time.

Transcranial Doppler can be used as an adjunct to the diagnosis of pediatric brain death and to provide data indicating the degree of cerebrovascular compromise rather than an absolute criterion for brain death. A normal TCD examination in a child who is deeply comatose may prevent the performance of other supplemental tests for confirming brain death.

ANOXIC-ISCHEMIC ENCEPHALOPATHY
Background

Over the past 15 years considerable efforts have been devoted to understanding the biochemical and cellular mechanisms that contribute to the injury witnessed during global brain ischemia.* Children differ from adults in that they more commonly experience respiratory arrest, whereas adult patients experience cardiac arrest.[154,193,273] In children, the primary mechanism leading to cardiac standstill is asphyxiation, whereas in adults the etiology is predominantly electromechanical dissociation brought about by a malignant cardiac dysrhythmia. This difference contributes significantly to the poorer outcome in both survival and worse morbidity seen in out-of-hospital arrests involving children.[150,154,193,273,302] The most common causes of asphyxial arrest in children are perinatal asphyxia, apnea syndromes, aspiration, submersion, and upper airway obstruction.

Current therapeutic options

Current management of the successfully resuscitated pediatric patient following asphyxial arrest are limited to the symptomatic treatment and prevention of anticipated complications, which, in broad terms, mirror the management strategy used in treating traumatically head-injured patients and Reye's syndrome victims.[132] Current management options include hyperventilation to reduce $Paco_2$ and thereby reduce cerebral blood volume and ICP.[234] This method of ICP control has not been studied in a randomized fashion, and its utility is

*References 32, 44, 55, 133-135, 168, 174, 189, 191, 229, 251, 252, 304.

increasingly coming under question. A number of animal studies have demonstrated reduced CBF during sustained hypocapnia in areas already receiving reduced CBF.[179,181,272] The capability of reducing CBF by decreasing $Paco_2$ in patients who manifest hyperemia is limited at best because many of these patients have decreased CO_2 vasoreactivity.[33,60,223]

The use of controlled hypothermia (less than 32° C) has been investigated and found to be nonbeneficial.[38] Similarly, although osmotic diuretics are frequently used,[234] their effectiveness remains unknown; no randomized clinical trial investigating their effect on outcome has been completed. The use of ICP monitoring is also not routinely advocated in that multiple studies have failed to document improvement with ICP control.[67,89,190,240] Other therapeutic measures such as sedation and muscle relaxation are used for the theoretical reduction of cerebral metabolic activity or for prevention of sharp changes in cerebral blood volume, which are potentially deleterious to the patient. Treatment of seizures, which occur with some frequency, is intravenous anticonvulsants. Hyperpyrexia is treated with external cooling systems and antipyretics. In summary, clinical management other than life-support measures has not been shown to influence outcome.

Cerebral blood flow studies

Almost all animal models used to investigate postarrest cerebral ischemia show a remarkably similar set of CBF changes.[121,178,228,294] Following restoration of central circulation, CBF rapidly increases beyond baseline (hyperemic phase) for 15 to 30 minutes. This is followed by a rapid decline in flow to levels below baseline for many hours. The magnitude and duration of the hyperemia and hypoperfusion sequence are influenced by the duration of the precipitating insult. This response, however, is not uniform in that some cerebral region may demonstrate a heterogeneous pattern of increased and decreased perfusion simultaneously.[294] Cerebral metabolic rate of oxygen ($CMRO_2$) is globally depressed during the immediate period following reperfusion, but it increases to baseline over a variable period of time. In areas where CBF remains diminished, the potential exists for a second ischemic insult.[180]

In human studies, coupling of CBF and $CMRO_2$ was noted 2 and 6 hours after injury.[26] Within 2 days, however, an uncoupling of these two components was seen, with global CBF increasing to normal or above baseline values compared to relatively depressed $CMRO_2$ values. Additional studies have documented delayed hyperemia and associated this finding with a poor neurologic outcome.[60,223] Loss of $Paco_2$ vasoreactivity in adults is nearly uniformly associated with a poor outcome.[60]

Studies performed in children have also investigated

the relationship of CBF and $Paco_2$ reactivity with eventual outcome. In seven children with strangulation injury, Ashwal and colleagues found either an impaired or a paradoxical response to $Paco_2$ changes 24 hours after injury.[18] All patients who manifested this finding had a poor outcome. Beyda observed in near-drowning victims depressed CBF at 24 hours after injury, with recovery to baseline levels at the 48-hour interval.[33] Carbon dioxide vasoreactivity was also preserved in these patients. In contrast, children who either died or remained vegetative following submersion demonstrated either reduced or absent $Paco_2$ vasoreactivity and hyperemia within 24 hours. This was followed by a gradual decline of CBF values to baseline over the next 12 hours to 3 days in children who remained vegetative, whereas children who died had markedly decreased CBF values.

In summary, it is apparent that alterations in CBF following postasphyxial injury may be helpful in prognostication. Development of hyperemia and loss or attenuation of $Paco_2$ vasoreactivity appear to be associated with poor outcome.

Doppler studies

Using range-gated and continuous-wave Doppler, van Bel and associates[277] studied infants suffering from asphyxiation shortly after birth and demonstrated a marked increase in peak systolic and end-diastolic CBFVs with a concomitant decrease in the resistivity index, suggesting the presence of vasodilation within the cerebral vessels.[277] Ando and co-workers, using continuous Doppler, examined 15 infants following perinatal asphyxiation and found that infants with mild asphyxia had normal PIs, whereas severely asphyxiated infants manifested either significantly increased or decreased PIs.[14] Infants who manifested low PIs also had severe neurologic sequelae or died. Levene and colleagues, utilizing duplex Doppler, examined the anterior cerebral artery (ACA) in asphyxiated neonates and found two flow patterns; one pattern consisted of abnormally high flow velocities, which were typically found within 24 hours of birth.[149] The second consisted of abnormally low CBFVs. The authors speculated that these findings were the result of either "luxury perfusion" or the "no reflow phenomenon."[13,141] Infants with markedly increased or decreased CBFV either died or were neurologically devastated. Raemakers and Casaer examined the ACA CBFVs and PI with pulsed Doppler and found in normal infants a significant decrease in PI and a rise in mean CBFV following red cell transfusions.[218] Infants with severe asphyxiation showed no change in PI following blood transfusion. These data suggested that impaired or absent autoregulation must have been present in the asphyxiated infants. Bode, using TCD, investigated an asphyxiated neonatal population.[35] Ini-tially, all CBFVs were above normal, and lower than normal resistivity indices were seen. Hyperventilation failed to alter the waveform and the CBFV indices, indicating vasomotor paralysis. By the third day of life, CBFVs increased to twice normal for age. When coupled with other Doppler studies, this report suggests that TCD testing could detect the presence of hyperemia, permit the assessment of CO_2 vasoreactivity at bedside, and be potentially useful in prognostication. In a more recent study, Gray examined the relationship of CBFV parameters and outcome in 26 term infants with hypoxic-ischemic brain injury.[106] Abnormal CBFVs in the anterior cerebrovasculature and a low resistivity indices were significantly associated with an adverse neurologic outcome.

TRAUMATIC BRAIN INJURY
Demographics

Trauma is the leading cause of death in children older than 1 year of age, and head trauma is the major factor influencing mortality in pediatric trauma victims.[161] Mortality in severely head-injured children ranges as high as 35%.* Between 7% and 20% of physically abused children have associated neurologic injuries.[110]

Mechanisms of injury

Cerebral injuries can be divided into primary and secondary categories. Primary cerebral injuries result either from a physical blow to the head or from acceleration-deceleration forces that are applied to the brain. Secondary injury results from perturbations in cerebral blood flow, which can produce ischemia. Primary injuries produce brain damage by a number of different mechanisms, such as fractures, direct vascular trauma, hemorrhage, or diffuse axonal injury. Cranial fractures can also result in tearing of blood vessels, such as the middle meningeal artery or the sagittal sinus. Another mechanism is direct vascular trauma, which tears the vessel completely, creates intimal injury, or produces arteriovenous fistulae. Mass lesions can arise from subdural, epidural, subarachnoid, or intracerebral hemorrhage.

Diffuse axonal injury results from the shearing of cerebral tissues. It is caused by a sudden impact to the skull, which creates shearing and stretching of the axonal fibers.[3] Pathologically, this is seen as focal lesions within the corpus callosum and brainstem adjacent to the cerebellar peduncle.[123] This form of injury is dependent upon the direction, amount, and duration of the applied force. In experimental studies, short bursts of acceleration produce frontal and occipital lobe contusions. By increasing the force of acceleration, the bridging veins are torn, thereby creating a subdural hematoma. Further

---

*References 41, 45, 46, 110, 161, 167, 280, 306.

increases in the duration of acceleration produce the pattern of cerebral damage seen in diffuse axonal injury. The direction of the acceleration also appears to play a role in the pathogenesis of this lesion.[95] Acceleration in the lateral direction in reference to the skull consistently produces a higher incidence of diffuse axonal injury as compared to acceleration in the sagittal or oblique directions.[95] Falls do not routinely produce this type of injury because the burst of acceleration at impact is short.

Children are more susceptible to cerebral injury than adults for several anatomic reasons, including malleability of the skull, increased gelatinous consistency of the brain secondary to increased water content, and large basal cisterns relative to the brain parenchymal volume.[220] The head is appreciably larger with less supporting neck musculature, which predisposes to increased acceleration on impact. These differences translate into a larger percentage of young children who manifest severe craniocerebral trauma. Another factor that potentially increases the risk of brain injury is that children's cerebral vasoreactivity and metabolic activity are higher than those of adults.[176,305] This may lead to increased hyperemia and cerebral swelling.

Secondary injury arises from both local cerebral and systemic responses to cerebral injury. Ischemia as a result of apnea or hypoventilation is an often unappreciated consequence of traumatic head injury.[103] Common causes include airway obstruction, pneumothorax, hemothorax, pulmonary edema, aspiration pneumonia, and bronchospasm. Disruption of normal brainstem respiratory centers or cervical injury can also occur. This results in systemic hypoxia and cerebral hypoxemia. Hypoxia and hypercapnia act as a potent vasodilator and increase cerebral blood volume and ICP.[222]

Hypotension is often overlooked as a contributor to significant changes in cerebral perfusion.[78,284] It occurs commonly after a major cerebral injury. Following the injury, a massive outpouring of catecholamines initially raises blood pressure; however, this is frequently followed by hypotension. Other potential contributors include direct myocardial injury, hypovolemic shock secondary to blood loss, and cardiac dysrhythmias as a result of myocardial contusion or hypoxemia. Children tolerate blood loss very poorly.[285] Loss of vasomotor tone leads to a decrease in systemic vascular resistance.

Cerebral arterial vasospasm is a more recently recognized problem that is thought to be a major contributor to late ischemic change following head injury.* It appears between 2 and 7 days postinjury and may last for 10 to 24 days. Animal studies have shown that cell-free hemoglobin, when placed in situ, produces profound, sustained cerebral vasoconstriction.[112,166] At present,

little information is available concerning the time of onset, amplitude, duration, and clinical significance of cerebral vasospasm in pediatric head-injured victims.

Current management options

The present strategy for managing pediatric head injury victims is focused on maintaining cerebral perfusion pressure (CPP) by manipulating the systemic arterial pressure (SAP) and the ICP. Adequate volume replacement and close hemodynamic monitoring are accomplished with central venous pressure and SAP catheters placed at the outset in the emergency room or the ICU.[152] Hypothermia, which occurs frequently, is treated aggressively with external warming systems. In severely head-injured children, intubation and manual ventilation are performed to prevent hypercapnia and hypoxia. A CT scan is performed as soon as possible to rule out significant space-occupying lesions that require emergency evacuation. Intracranial pressure monitoring is determined by the severity of the neurologic injury and has been shown to be useful in reducing mortality when intracranial hypertension is treated successfully.[248] A currently accepted clinical threshold for ICP monitoring is a Glasgow coma scale score of 8 or less. The type of monitoring is dictated by the degree of brain swelling, clotting abnormalities, and the experience of the neurosurgeon. Initial ICP management typically includes sustained hypocapnia using mechanical hyperventilation, strict control of intravascular volume, and drainage of ventricular cerebrospinal fluid.

Loop diuretics, mannitol, or glycerol is often used to reduce cerebral swelling with variable effects.[69] Sedation with benzodiazepines and opiates is frequently used to reduce agitation. Although barbiturate coma has not been shown to be beneficial in improving neurologic recovery, some centers still utilize this maneuver if other measures fail.[25,47] Late sequelae including communication hydrocephalus, early and late seizures, late-onset cerebral hemorrhage, and cerebral infarction are monitored by repeated clinical examinations and appropriate neurodiagnostic procedures.[303]

**Transcranial Doppler applications
in adult head trauma**

Transcranial Doppler studies performed with the freehand technique have documented marked changes in intracranial hemodynamics-related hyperperfusion, subdural hematoma, increased ICP, cerebral infarction, and intracranial hemorrhage.† Newell and colleagues investigated the pressure autoregulatory response in 20 adults with severe head trauma and compared it to that of normals;[187] as expected, pressure autoregulation was diminished in most patients with trauma.[2] They also

---

*References 160, 198, 222, 231, 263, 292.

†References 1, 47, 62, 101, 152, 184, 241, 288, 303.

tested CO_2 vasoreactivity in this same population and identified good response.[187] The effect of a pulsed dose of barbiturate was also examined. Following intravenous infusion of thiopentone, three responses were observed: A good response was identified by a significant fall in MCA mean CBFV and in ICP, with preservation of the SAP and a concomitant rise in CPP. A poor response was defined as a transient fall in MCA mean CBFV, with minimal or no fall in ICP; the SAP exhibited a small decrease. The unfavorable response was defined as a marked drop in MCA mean CBFV and SAP, without a change in ICP. This resulted in a concomitant deterioration in CPP. The findings of this study indicated that it is possible to monitor the effect of therapeutic measures on CPP and neurologic outcome.

Vasospasm is a recognized sequela of cerebral trauma. It is usually first detected 2 days after head trauma and reaches peak incidence 2 weeks later. Its severity gradually declines during the subsequent 3 weeks.* A similar pattern has been witnessed in nontraumatic subarachnoid hemorrhage.[244,245] Increases in CBFVs in this context can be caused by either increased CBF or vasospasm. A recently described method based on the MCA–extracranial ICA mean CBFV ratio has aimed at correcting the effects of CBF changes.[288] Normal values in adults are in the range of 1.7 ± 0.4. During cerebral vasospasm, the average MCA-ICA ratio increases to 3, and values exceeding 5 have been reported in patients with severe vasospasm.[288]

Although the findings of the preceding studies can be judiciously used to take care of children, the response of the infant brain may be unique, and outcomes can be markedly different in the pediatric population. Even though large studies have not been published, vasospasm has been detected in pediatric patients with traumatic head injury and has been associated with cerebral infarction.[274]

EPILEPSY

It has been estimated that 6% to 7% of children manifest seizures during the first 7 years of age, an incidence far higher than that witnessed in adults.[192] Seizures are frequently accompanied by pronounced cerebral metabolic effects as well as changes in CBF.† During the interictal phase, varying degrees of regional hypoperfusion and hypometabolism have been noted.[39,79,235,271] Using TCD to study the relation of CBFVs and seizure variety, Murikami and colleagues investigated a small pediatric population manifesting a variety of seizure disorders.[182] In patients with typical absence seizures, MCA CBFVs decreased 7 to 12 seconds after seizure onset. The rate and magnitude of

*References 1, 52-54, 62, 152, 184, 288.
†References 61, 124, 172, 192, 211, 212, 287.

CBFV changes correlated with the presence of clinical seizures. Rapid recovery was witnessed within 30 seconds in all cases, with a rebound effect that lasted for more than a minute prior to recovery to baseline. Infants with infantile spasms showed a dramatic rise in CBFVs immediately after the onset of seizure activity; their peak CBFVs lasted 10 to 20 seconds. Approximately 1 minute transpired before these MCA CBFVs returned to normal. Sanada and associates studied in two patients the effect of absence seizures on MCA CBFVs during the ictal and postictal phase.[238] The CBFVs decreased within 9 seconds, recovered within a short period, and had a rebound phenomenon. These results are consistent with the findings of the previous study. In contrast, Shimizu and co-workers found an increase in CBFVs with the onset of spike and wave epileptiform activity in one patient, whereas in a second no change in CBFVs was detected with the onset of petit mal EEG activity.[249] In a larger study, Bode investigated 51 children with various forms of epilepsy.[36] In five children manifesting absence seizures, a decrease in mean CBFVs was noted within 2 seconds of the onset of epileptic EEG activity. The decrease in mean CBFV varied from 46% to 82%. No alterations in pulse or respiratory rate were noted. In four children manifesting tonic seizures, CBFVs increased from 132% to 191%. The rapid rise in CBFV occurred at the onset of epileptic activity. Fischer and Truemper monitored pediatric patients after status epilepticus and found flow disturbances in all. A 30% to 80% reduction in ICA mean CBFVs was present in three of seven patients; in addition, vasospasm was detected in six of seven patients studied during the first 24 hours.[85] The effect of ACTH treatment on CBFVs in infants with infantile spasms has also been reported in two studies. Futagi and colleagues[91] and Futagi and Abe[90] identified a fall in CBFVs within 30 minutes from ACTH injection; the CBFVs continued to decline gradually during the first week of treatment, after which they began to recover to baseline.

HYDROCEPHALUS
Demographics and clinical management

Hydrocephalus is a common disorder characterized by progressive enlargement of the ventricular system; it can result from a variety of pathophysiologic mechanisms. Neonatal hydrocephalus occurs in approximately 3% to 4% of live births.[196,289] Nearly 50% of these infants manifest varying degrees of neurologic impairment, including mental retardation and cerebral palsy.[298] In infants, primary stenosis or absence of the aqueduct of Sylvius can occasionally cause hydrocephalus. More commonly, hydrocephalus results from a variety of secondary insults, including interventricular hemorrhage or meningitis. In older children, secondary etiologies are by far the most common and include head trauma, bacterial meningitis, and infratentorial tumors. In infants and children with open fontanelles, real-time cranial sonography can be used to measure ventricular size.[82] In older children, the ventricular size is most commonly monitored with CT. In neither case can neuroimaging techniques determine the physiologic impact of increasing ventricular size on the cerebrovascular system.

Doppler studies

Almost all studies evaluating the consequences of hydrocephalus have been performed in infants suffering predominantly from intracerebral or intraventricular hemorrhage. Bada and colleagues identified decreases in end-diastolic CBFV and increases in PI during progressive hydrocephaly.[22] In contrast, Grant and others found no significant differences in CBFV or PI between normal children and those with hydrocephaly.[104]

Fischer and Livingstone examined normal and hydrocephalic infants using real-time cranial ultrasonography and transcranial Doppler.[83] Three groups were identified: group 1 consisted of infants without hydrocephalus, group 2 consisted of infants with progressive hydrocephalus, and group 3 consisted of infants with hydrocephalus treated with interventricular-peritoneal (V-P) shunts. In the normal control population, the mean PI was 1.23. In the hydrocephalic population with increasing ventricular size (group 2), the PI was 1.71, whereas in the shunted hydrocephalic population (group 3) the PI was 0.93. The differences in PI values was related to changes in the end-diastolic CBFV. An inverse correlation was witnessed between end-diastolic CBFV and increasing ventricular size obtained from the mid-sagittal plane of the third ventricle. In a later study, Norelle and associates using TCD examined 47 pediatric patients with ventriculomegally secondary to a variety of causes.[188] Three groups were identified in this study as well: one population (group 1) children manifested stable hydrocephalus by clinical and radiographic parameters, the second population (group 2) manifested changes in ventricular size, and the third population (group 3) was monitored following placement of a V-P shunt. In groups 1 and 3 the mean PIs for the left MCA were found to be 1.06 and 1.02, respectively, whereas in group 2 the mean PI was 1.72. Similar findings were reported for the right MCAs. Mean CBFVs for the right and left MCAs of group 1 were 121 and 123 cm/s, respectively. In group 2, mean CBFV values in the right and left MCAs were 84 cm/s and 91 cm/s, respectively. Although group 3 patients had mean CBFV values 20% higher than individuals in group 2, the difference was not statistically significant. Based on these observations, Fischer has advocated the use of TCD in hydrocephalic children when the etiology of neurologic deterioration is unclear and a decision regarding placement of a ventricular drain or shunt revision is needed. The threshold MCA PI value suggested by Fischer for shunt consideration revision is 1.5. In another study of hydrocephalic children, Goh and co-workers examined the relationship between CBFVs and ICP during sleep.[98] Two responses were observed when the ICP increased: the type 1 response was characterized by a significant decrease in mean CBFV, a fall in CPP, and a rise in the RI; a type 2 response was characterized by increases in mean CBFV and RI and a drop in CPP. As reported in earlier studies, the rise in RI found in both responses best correlated with a decrease in end-diastolic CBFV. Based on these data, the authors have suggested that monitoring CPP alone may not be adequate when reduced intracranial compliance is found.

It is extremely difficult to determine how infant brains accommodate growing ventricles. In some patients, the parenchyma is compressed to some extent, but in other instances the ventricles enlarge to a moderate degree and then appear to undergo no further enlargement. It is unclear whether the pressure exerted by hydrocephalus is arrested or the intracranial vascular compartment is compromised. Fischer and Livingstone have shown that compromise of the cerebrovascular compartment is not necessarily related to the rate of ventricular system enlargement, particularly in posthemorrhagic hydrocephaly.[83]

A simplistic explanation of events noted on TCD can be summarized as follows: As the ventricles increase in size and the brain allows for their growth by compression of the parenchyma, a point is reached when the parenchyma begins to resist the ventricular pressure, and further pressure is exerted on the cerebrovascular system. As the cerebral resistance increases, passive forward flow in diastole immediately decreases and finally disappears. The systolic upstroke becomes sharp in its upswing, and the pulsatility rises. For the physician, the gradual decrease in end-diastolic CBFV and the steady increase in PI indicate a window of opportunity for an elective and well-planned shunt procedure.[188]

In a patient who already has a ventriculoperitoneal shunt in place, a clinical dilemma occurs when the patient presents with headache, vomiting, and lethargy, and the differential diagnosis lies between a "shunt infection" and a shunt malfunction. In our experience, in the presence of a shunt malfunction, the TCD abnormalities described previously occur relatively rapidly. In shunt infection, the TCD parameters usually do not significantly change unless neurovascular complications from the infection have set in. Thus, the management of hydrocephalus should include serial TCD testing to detect the early signs of compromise, to plan for the optimal time of intervention, and, in patients with V-P shunts who present with new neurologic signs and symptoms, to differentiate between shunt malfunction and shunt infection.

CARDIAC LESIONS
Background

The incidence of congenital heart disease (CHD) in the neonatal and pediatric population ranges between 4.1 and 10.2 per 1000 live births.[73,81,143,177,232] The effects of CHD on cerebral oxygen transport can be loosely grouped into five categories based on the perturbations in aortic blood flow: (1) potential reduction in CBF due to cardiac or vascular obstruction (mitral and aortic stenosis or atresia, hypoplastic left heart syndrome), (2) potential reduction in cerebral blood oxygenation (truncus arteriosus, transposition of the great vessels, tetralogy of Fallot, tricuspid atresia, pulmonary atresia), (3) reduction in CBF secondary to systemic-to-pulmonary artery steal (patent ductus arteriosus [PDA], ventricular septal defect, pulmonary arteriovenous malformation), (4) critical reduction in cardiac output secondary to physiologic dysfunction (congenital cardiomyopathy, myocarditis, anomalous left coronary artery syndrome, congenital complete atrioventricular block), and (5) potential hyperaugmentation in CBF (coarctation of the aorta). Moreover, CBF and CBFV change as a result of surgical palliative or corrective procedures (systemic-to-pulmonary shunts, bidirectional venacaval-pulmonary shunt, and right atrial-pulmonary shunt) and numerous pharmacologic and other interventions used to treat myocardial dysfunction, such as mechanical ventilation, sustained hypocapnia, diuretics, antihypertensives, vasopressors, and cardiotonic agents. These maneuvers may have considerable effect on CBF and autoregulation but have received minimal attention thus far.

Doppler investigations

Five areas examining cerebral circulatory function in patients with cardiac disease have been studied with Doppler technology: (1) the effect of hypothermia, (2) the effect of cardiopulmonary bypass (CPB) and profound hypothermic circulatory arrest (PHCA), (3) $Paco_2$ vasoreactivity response during CPB, (4) detection of intercardiac shunts, and (5) the effect of systemic-to-pulmonary shunts.

Lundar and colleagues and others found in adult patients an increase in MCA mean CBFVs with the institution of CPB.[155] The increase appeared to be pressure passive, with linear increases in CBFV corresponding to increasing CPP. Buijs and associates examined pressure autoregulation during hypothermia and CPB in infants and children undergoing cardiac repair for cyanotic and acyanotic congenital heart defects.[49] Two populations were identified. The first demonstrated loss of pressure autoregulation during hypothermic CPB, and the second manifested intact CPB. No relationship

was identified between mean SAP and core temperature (Tc); however, a strong relation was identified between mean CBFV and Tc. A significant relationship was also identified between mean SAP and mean CBFV. The relationship of Tc and mean SAP defined in the mathematical expression Tc × mean SAP demonstrated a significant inverse relation with CBFV. To the authors, this suggested that hypothermia contributed to the development of vasoparesis.

In children younger than 9 months of age, Burrows and Bissonnette examined the effects of CPB versus PHCA (nasopharyngeal temp less than 20° C) on cerebral hemodynamics.[50] Five groups of children were identified: group A received normal flow CPB, group B received low-flow CPB with detectable CBFV, group C received PHCA, and Groups D1 and D2 received low-flow CPB with CBFVs less than 3 to 4 cm/s. Parameters measured at 15-minute intervals during the procedure included anterior fontanelle pressure (AFP), SAP, CPP, and MCA mean flow velocity. Calculation of the ΔV/ΔP using CBFV and CPP was performed at each interval. In group A, patients manifested a normal ΔV/ΔP relationship within the normal range of CPB. Group B children manifested a higher ΔV/ΔP during the recovery phase of CPB than during the induction of low-flow CPB. Additionally, detectable CBFVs were identified throughout the CPB when the CPP value was 13 ± 2 mm Hg. In this group it was also noted that CBFVs normalized to baseline values once CPP returned to normal. In group C, patients treated with PHCA, detectable CBFVs disappeared at a CPP of 9 ± 2 mm Hg; CBFVs returned with resumption of CPB when the CPP was 13 ± 2 mm Hg. The ΔV/ΔP relationship was also significantly reduced, and the CBFVs did not return to normal after termination of CBP. In group D, following induction of CBP, CBFVs disappeared at a CPP of 9 mm Hg. During the period following low-flow CPB, two responses were noted. One response was similar to that of group B, whereas the other response was similar to that of group C. The D1 group patients required a significantly higher CPP to achieve detectable CBFV when compared to D subjects.

The findings in group A patients were thought to be the result cold-induced vasoparesis. In group B patients, the disparity in changes between pre- and post-CBP was postulated to result from vascular hysteresis. In group C patients, the low ΔV/ΔP prior to PHCA was thought to be due to prolonged reduction in CBF, cerebral hypoxia, consequent rise in ICP, and a fall in the critical closing pressure of cerebral vessels. In group D patients, the observed differences were felt to be due to the same phenomenon as in group C, whereas individuals who manifested the pattern typical for low-flow CPB appeared similar to group B patients. Based on the findings of this complex study, the authors speculated that the primary determining factor was the critical closing pressure. They noted that when the CPP was greater than the critical closing pressure, the cerebral perfusion was maintained. However, when the CPP was lower than this threshold, cerebral perfusion was ablated. It would thus appear that PHCA may potentially produce a higher level of cerebral ischemia than CPP. This view is supported by other studies in which cerebral lactate release was significantly higher following PHCA than in CPP.[119,278] The development of cerebral edema during PHCA could also explain some of the changes witnessed in group C. This is supported by the work of others as well.[21,107] In an earlier investigation, Hillier and co-workers used continuous TCD and SAP monitoring and calculated a modified cerebrovascular resistance index (MCVR).[119]

$$\text{MCVR (mm Hg} \times \text{cm/s)} = \frac{(\text{MAP} - \text{CVP})}{\text{CBFV}}$$

Hillier and co-workers found a higher cerebrovascular resistance index post-PHCA than pre-PHCA. Because CPP did not change, they assumed changes in cerebrovascular resistance were not due to increased ICP but rather to a decrease in $CMRO_2$ following PHCA.[119,139]

Lundar and others have investigated cerebral $Paco_2$ vasoreactivity during moderate hypothermia (28 to 32° C) and nonpulsatile CPB.[155] Cerebral perfusion pressure was maintained within the range 17 to 75 mm Hg by adjusting CPB flow. The CO_2 vasoreactivity was found to decrease with decreasing CPP and was particularly impaired when the CPP was less than 35 mm Hg.

The capability of detecting right-to-left intracardiac shunts has been studied by Nemec and colleagues, who compared contrast TCD, transesophageal echocardiography (TEE), and transthoracic echocardiography (TTE) in adult patients.[185] Intracardiac shunting was identified by both contrast TCD and TEE in 13 of 13 patients, and intrapulmonary shunting was detected by TEE and contrast TCD in 3 of 6 and 6 of 6 patients, respectively. The sensitivity, specificity, and accuracy of contrast TCD in predicting interatrial shunting were reported as 100%, whereas the contrast TTE sensitivity was 54%, specificity 94%, and accuracy 77%. These limited data suggest that TCD may be more accurate than TTE in detecting interatrial shunts.

Finally, a limited number of studies have investigated the effect of cardiac lesions on CBFV. Illustrations of this effect are presented in Figures 32-6 and 32-7. Virtually all studies have been performed in infants with PDA, an extracardiac anomaly characterized by a system-to-pulmonary shunt that allows for free communication between the two circulations. This cardiac abnormality is most commonly noted in infants with birth weights less than 1500 g and is more common in infants

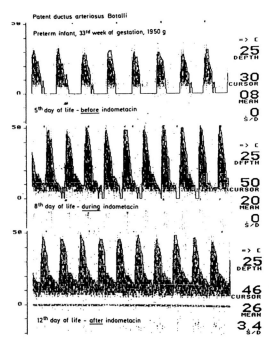

Fig. 32-6. Middle cerebral artery cerebral blood flow velocity waveforms in a premature infant with a patent ductus arteriosus before, during, and after treatment with indomethacin to induce ductal closure. (From Bode H: *Pediatric applications of transcranial Doppler sonography,* New York and Vienna, 1988, Springer-Verlag.)

with prematurity, hyaline membrane disease, and metabolic acidosis.[58,64,96,131] The consequences of PDA on systemic circulation are variable and often dramatic. Measurements of aortic blood flow by duplex echocardiography have shown a mean flow decrease of 40% following PDA closure.[12] Ductal closure also causes a significant improvement in systemic arterial oxygenation and an increase in mean systolic blood pressure.[162] In infants with varying size PDAs, Serwer and associates documented a linear correlation between the descending aortic resistance index and intrapulmonary shunting.[247] They also showed that, following PDA ligation, the aortic resistance decreased significantly.

Several investigators have described the perturbations in CBFV associated with PDA. Batton and co-workers demonstrated that in full-term newborns increases in ACA and MCA CBFVs during the first 2 days postdelivery are not due to ductal closure.[24] Lipman and colleagues examined the ACA in infants with large PDAs and high PIs when compared to values obtained following ductal closure.[153] Martin and associates studied the ACA CBFV in preterm infants with large PDAs and reported retrograde diastolic flow in 43% of patients and significantly reduced end-diastolic CBFVs in 57%.[163] The PIs were correspondingly elevated. These abnormalities resolved after PDA ligation. Bode identi-

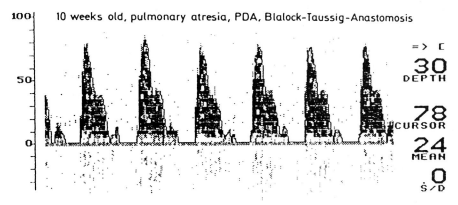

Fig. 32-7. Example of the effect of congenital heart disease on the middle cerebral artery cerebral blood flow velocity waveform in a 10-month-old child with pulmonary atresia, patent ductus arteriosus (PDA), and a surgically placed systemic-to-pulmonary shunt. Note the almost complete absence of diastolic flow. From Bode H: *Pediatric applications of transcranial Doppler sonography,* New York and Vienna, 1988, Springer-Verlag.)

fied the cerebrovascular effects of different-sized PDAs preablation and postablation with either indomethacin or surgical closure.[35] Large PDAs produced pansuppression of all CBFVs and a marked increase in PIs. Ductal closure, regardless of method, produced a significant increase in CBFVs and a reduction in cerebrovascular resistance. Small PDAs produced no significant effect on cerebral hemodynamics. Wilcox and associates examined three groups of premature infants with and without PDAs and with or without diastolic flow reversal.[291] In the group without diastolic flow reversal, normal hemodynamic indices were noted in all cases. In the group with late diastolic flow reversal, significant abnormalities in pulse pressure and echocardiographic indices were found. In the group with pandiastolic flow reversal, there was no difference in the echocardiographic indices, but systemic pressure indices were relatively increased. These data suggested that increased ductal shunting may produce sequential alterations in CBFVs and SAP. Mellander and co-workers examined the effect of mechanical ventilation and PDA on systemic and cerebral hemodynamics in a premature infant population.[173] In the mechanically ventilated infants, the presence of a hemodynamically significant PDA (HsPDA) was associated with lower values for CBFV parameters and diastolic and mean blood pressures when compared to the non-HsPDA infants. In the spontaneously breathing group, the presence or absence of a HsPDA did not have a significant effect on CBFV parameters and systemic blood pressure. The investigators suggested that the sick preterm infant requiring significant support was impaired in its ability to support systemic perfusion. Perlman and colleagues examined the ACA CBFV in 55 premature infants, 10 of whom developed a PDA.[201] Before ductal opening, the mean PI was 0.67 ± 0.05, whereas following PDA development the mean PI sig-

nificantly increased to 0.91 ± 0.03. Following ductal closure, the mean PI fell to 0.66 ± 0.03. These changes appeared to be due to fluctuations in the end-diastolic CBFV, which in turn were closely correlated with the diastolic blood pressure. The changes in CBFV are thought to correlate with alterations in SAP.[295]

The relationship between abnormal cerebral hemodynamics and intracranial hemorrhage or ischemia has also been investigated. An association between intracranial hemorrhage (IVH) and the presence of PDAs has been suggested, based on clinical data.[63,75,153] Dykes and associates reported a close association between the presence of a PDA and grade IV IVH.[75] New or enlarged IVHs have been noted in infants with PDAs following surgical closure of the ductus or following aortograms.[27-29,162] Ductal closure with indomethacin, however, does not produce this result.[27,162] Additional supporting evidence is offered in the Saliba and co-workers study, in which the RI significantly fell following ductal closure and an increase in the mean CBFV was witnessed.[236] In addition, a significant correlation between end-diastolic CBFV and diastolic SAP was identified before and after ductal closure. Interestingly, no changes in systolic CBFV or systolic SAP were detected either before or after ductal closure. The authors concluded that CBFV changes were not related to alterations in cerebral vessels and that the risk of IVH was not increased. Shortland and associates studied the relationship between PDA and periventricular leukomalacia (PVL) in preterm infants.[250] Although an association between the presence of a PDA and PVL was found, no significant differences in mean and end-diastolic CBFVs could be found in PDA patients with or without PVL. The observations of this study support the view that changes in cerebral hemodynamics cannot fully explain the relationship between PDA and PVL.

MOYAMOYA DISEASE
Demographics

Moyamoya disease is a chronic vasoocclusive disorder of obscure etiology that primarily affects the ICAs and the anterior cerebral circulation. Initially, this disorder was thought to be exclusive to the Japanese; however, it has been reported in most ethnic groups.[126,137] Its incidence is biphasic, with the larger population presenting in the early adolescent years. Children typically present with acute hemiplegia secondary to acute ischemia, whereas adults present with a variable symptom complex related to site of intracranial hemorrhage.[127,164,165,264,268] The clinical course is dependent on the presence of collateral circulation and the extent of vascular occlusion. Angiography is the definitive method for diagnosis. It typically shows stenosis or occlusion of the distal ICA or its main branches and extensive collateralization involving the dural, leptomeningeal, and pial arteries giving the classic "puff of smoke" appearance.[126] Aneurysm formation is more commonly found in the vertebrobasilar system, especially at the basilar bifurcation.[281,296] This observation has been ascribed to higher wall stress associated with high CBFVs in the PCAs.[183] Parenchymal defects within the vascular territories of the anterior circle of Willis are found in almost 80% of symptomatic cases. Ischemic changes, large arterial occlusions, and vascular and collateral circulation can be demonstrated with a combination of magnetic resonance imaging and angiography.[70] The vascular pattern seen in moyamoya has also been observed in patients with sickle cell disease[68] and other conditions.

Cerebral blood flow and Doppler investigations

Hanada, using xenon-133 CT to measure CBF, identified a global flow decrease in patients with moyamoya disease.[111] Similar observations have also been made in other studies.[269,276] The CBF and $CMRO_2$ values have varied according to the degree of occlusion or stenosis and the presence of neurologic sequelae.[76] In subjects with complete occlusion of the circle of Willis, both CBF and $CMRO_2$ values were markedly reduced. Individuals manifesting partial occlusion had variable CBF and $CMRO_2$ values that were higher than those of patients with complete occlusion. When compared to patients without neurologic impairment, patients with hemiparesis and other neurologic deficits manifested lower CBF and $CMRO_2$ values. Cerebral pressure autoregulation and $Paco_2$ reactivity were preserved in all patients. Application of TCD to the management of moyamoya disease has been limited to a handful of anecdotal reports and one case study. Bode studied two adolescents and found significant elevations in ICA, MCA, and ACA CBFVs consistent with vascular stenosis.[35] However, in one of his patients, reduced CBFVs were identified in the MCAs following documentation of carotid stenosis by angiography. Muttaqin and co-workers examined four adults and four children with moyamoya disease by using angiography and TCD.[183] Low CBFVs were identified in all ICAs. In adults, the MCA CBFVs were significantly lower than the corresponding ICA values, whereas in children the decrease in MCA CBFVs was slightly lower, but not clinically significant. The angiographic demonstration of mild to severe stenosis, coupled with reduced CBFVs on TCD testing, is contrary to previous experience with atherosclerotic lesions or vasospasm[72,151] and has not been explained satisfactorily.[151,258]

SICKLE CELL DISEASE
Demographics

The most common hemopoietic disorder that causes cerebrovascular pathology is sickle cell disease (SCD).[175,261] Ischemic stroke is SCD's most common devastating abnormality and has an incidence of 6% to 9%. Hemorrhagic stroke is considered rare. Although several etiologies have been considered, the cause of this high incidence of stroke remains unknown.[129,195,286] The anterior circulation is more often affected than the posterior, and stenotic lesions can be found in the ICAs, ACAs, and MCAs.[175,261] Intracranial aneurysms have also been reported.[195]

Doppler investigations

Anemia causes CBFV elevations beyond the normal values.[6,43,117,129] Investigators aiming at a CBFV criterion that identifies SCD patients at an increased risk for stroke have had to take this effect into consideration. Adams and colleagues, in a first study of a large SCD population, determined that the mean MCA mean CBFV was 115 ± 31 cm/s.[6] In their subsequent study,[7] Adams and associates examined the predictive capability of TCD compared to cerebral angiography in detecting vascular abnormalities in 33 neurologically symptomatic children with SCD. In 25 of 29 instances, TCD correctly identified significant cerebral vasculopathy (more than 50% narrowing of the vascular lumen). Sensitivity and specificity values were reported as 89% and 100%, respectively. In a recently published 5-year trial, 190 asymptomatic children with SCD were longitudinally monitored to assess the predictive value of TCD indices regarding the subsequent development of stroke.[8] Children were classified as TCD positive if ACA or MCA CBFVs were greater than 170 cm/s at any time during the trial prior to development of symptoms; they were TCD negative if mean CBFVs never exceeded this threshold. Six of 23 TCD-positive patients and 1 of 167 TCD-negative patients developed an ischemic stroke during follow-up. The difference between the two groups was highly significant. Additionally, the presence of positive

TCD criteria significantly correlated with the risk of future infarction. Based on these observations, Adams and co-workers have suggested that a threshold of 170 cm/s differentiated between high- and low-risk groups.[5] Other indicators of cerebrovascular abnormality included an ACA-MCA ratio of 0.8, a CBFV exceeding 200 cm/s, and an ACA-MCA ratio exceeding 1.2. It should be noted that more recent studies have used other indicators.[243]

These findings suggest that TCD may be useful in defining the subset of patients with SCD at risk for cerebrovascular pathology.

CENTRAL NERVOUS SYSTEM INFECTIONS
Background

Bacterial meningitis represents a potentially devastating central nervous system disorder. Although the variety of organisms reported to produce meningitis in humans is very large, the most common organisms in children are coliform bacteria, *Streptococcus agalactiae*, *S. pneumoniae*, *Neisseria meningitidis*, *Mycobacterium tuberculosis*, and *Haemophilus influenzae*.[224,254] Numerous postmeningitic complications have been described.* Mortality in neonatal suppurative meningitis is as high as 20%, whereas in adults mortality rates varying from 15% to 40% have been observed.[48,94,138,206,256] Numerous clinical reports have described a wide variety of cerebrovascular complications in patients with meningitis.†

Neuroimaging and histologic correlates

Angiography during the acute infectious stage has identified obstruction of bridging veins, transmural extravasation of contrast medium, vasodilatation and delayed filling of cortical branches, and retrograde flow.‡ Postmortem histopathologic examinations have consistently found intimal thickening, vasodilation, stenosis and thrombosis of cerebral arteries and arterioles, mycotic aneurysms of cortical arteries, and bridging veins. These findings have almost invariably been associated with infarction in the affected vascular territories.§

Cerebral blood flow investigations

Paulsen and colleagues examined $PaCO_2$ vasoreactivity and pressure autoregulation using xenon CBF imaging in 15 adults manifesting either encephalitis or meningitis.[200] They found a large number of patients who exhibited impaired or absent pressure autoregulation and preserved CO_2 vasoreactivity. Pneumococcal

meningitis was found to produce a 30% to 40% decrease in global CBF. In a later study of patients with bacterial meningitis, Ashwal and associates detected a marked CBF reduction in 30% of cases.[20] In this subgroup, gray and white matter CBF were, respectively, reduced by 50% and 55% from reference normal values. Pressure autoregulation was maintained in the normal range. Although global $PaCO_2$ vasoreactivity was preserved in all but one case, considerable heterogenicity was observed within different brain regions.

Doppler studies

McMenamin and Volpe initially examined ACA CBFV indices using duplex Doppler, and estimated ICP by way of transfontanelle pressure recording in infants with uncomplicated acute bacterial meningitis.[171] In newborn infants, no correlation between ICP and mean CBFV was observed; however, in older infants (mean age 5.75 months) a significant inverse correlation was found between decreasing ICP and rising CBFV. It was postulated that the increased ICP was a result of cerebral edema because no space-occupying lesions were identified by sonography. In a later report, Fischer and colleagues examined CBFVs in the ACAs, ICAs, and BAs of infants with uncomplicated viral or bacterial meningitis.[84] Elevation of end-diastolic CBFVs was found at 12 hours. This observation is in keeping with the observations by McMenamin and Volpe, who also identified sequential increases in CBFVs during the first 3 days following presentation. The increases plateaued by the time of discharge at day 10.[171] Goh and associates used TCD to examine children with acute suppurative meningitis.[97] The most dramatic changes in MCA PIs were witnessed during the first 2 days following presentation; in all survivors the PIs were normal at the time of discharge. Mannitol was used in four cases in which ICP monitoring was performed. In all cases the ICP decreased, the PI fell 8%, and the end-diastolic CBFV rose 18% following mannitol infusion. In another study, Haring and co-workers examined CBFV indices in patients with a variety of viral, bacterial or unspecified central nervous system infections.[113] In 77% of patients with bacterial meningitis, MCA CBFVs were significantly increased during the early course of the illness, whereas none of the patients with viral or unspecified CNS infection manifested significant elevations in MCA CBFVs. Patients with uncomplicated purulent meningitis manifested a return to normal values within 14 to 21 days of illness. An example from Bode's treatise demonstrating the evolution of CBFVs during acute meningitis is shown in Figure 32-8.[35]

In summary, although the incidence of bacterial meningitis is decreasing in most nations where widespread *Haemophilus influenzae* vaccination is performed, bacterial meningitis remains an endemic problem in

---

*References 30, 56, 57, 59, 71, 74, 77, 105, 118, 122, 125, 144-146, 157, 202, 203, 205-207, 210, 217, 227, 230, 255, 262, 265, 266, 282, 283.
†References 30, 57, 59, 77, 87, 92, 102, 109, 115, 116, 122, 125, 156, 158, 169, 202, 205, 206, 219, 230, 237, 259, 262, 267, 275, 297, 300.
‡References 92, 116, 125, 145, 156, 169, 219, 297, 300.
§References 4, 66, 145, 147, 219, 257.

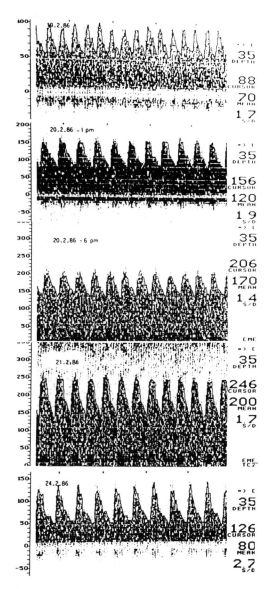

Fig. 32-8. Example of serial Doppler recordings from a 6-month-old infant with meningitis caused by *Streptococcus pneumoniae*. Transcranial Doppler tracings are from days of hospitalization 3, 4, 5, and 8. (From Bode H: *Pediatric applications of transcranial Doppler sonography,* New York and Vienna, 1988, Springer-Verlag.)

much of the world. From these initial observations it would appear that TCD may be useful in examining cerebral hemodynamics during the acute phase of the illness and during the late stages of the clinical course, when complications such as hydrocephalus may occur.

FUTURE DIRECTIONS IN RESEARCH AND CLINICAL PRACTICE

The primary and extremely effective role of TCD in pediatric neurologic disease is in the prevention of brain injury by providing timely information to assist the physician in making decisions. There is, at present, a considerable lag in the application of TCD information to the management of neurologic disease by pediatric care clinicians. The reasons may be many and varied, but the outcome is a loss for brain-injured children and their parents. The criteria for the diagnosis of cerebral vasospasm have been well established in traumatic brain diseases as well as in other clinical scenarios; however, in pediatric ICUs throughout the country, the available TCD information is underutilized. Children arriving in emergency rooms and pediatric ICUs with traumatic head injury, subarachnoid hemorrhage, and decompensating hydrocephalus can benefit immeasurably from the judicious use of the results of TCD, which is one of the few clinician-friendly techniques that can provide an ongoing picture of the hemodynamically changing pediatric brain. It is unlike other traditional anatomic neuroimaging techniques, such as CT and MRI, in which the radiographic information is recorded after the damage has already occurred.

Transcranial Doppler is a challenge to the clinician. Although inexpensive, it is labor-intensive, and its ideal application depends on evaluating CBFV indices in real time. The data it generates do not have much meaning if they are not analyzed in the context of the clinical scenario. Successful use of TCD requires an understanding of cerebrovascular anatomy and physiology and of the biomechanics of the developing brain. The future use of TCD in pediatric practice depends upon clinicians incorporating relevant information from TCD with other accepted standards of medical care to protect the brains of injured patients.

REFERENCES

1. Aaslid R, Huber P, Nornes H: Evaluation of cerebral vasospasm with transcranial Doppler ultrasound, *J Neurosurg* 60:37-41, 1984.
2. Aaslid R, Lindegaard K-F, Sorteberg, W, Nornes H: Cerebral autoregulation dynamics in humans, *Stroke* 20:45-52, 1989.
3. Adams JH, Graham DI, Murray LS, Scott G: Diffuse axonal injury due to nonmissle head injury in humans: an analysis of 45 cases, *Ann Neurol* 12:557-563, 1981.
4. Adams RD, Kubic CS, Bonner FJ: The clinical and pathologic aspects of influenzae meningitis, *Arch Pediatr* 65:354-358, 1984.
5. Adams RJ, Litaker M, Nichols FT: *Anemia and sickle cell disease.* In Babikian VL, Wechsler LR, editors, *Transcranial Doppler ultrasonography,* St Louis, 1993, Mosby–Year Book.
6. Adams RJ, Nichols FT, McKie VC, et al: Transcranial Doppler: influence of hematocrit in children with sickle cell anemia without stroke, *J Cardiovasc Technol* 8:97-101, 1989.
7. Adams RJ, Nihols FT, Figuroa R, et al: Transcranial Doppler correlation with cerebral angiography in sickle disease, *Stroke* 23:1073-1077, 1992.
8. Adams RJ, McKie V, Nichols F, et al: The use of transcranial ultrasonography to predict stroke in sickle cell disease, *N Engl J Med* 326:605-610, 1992.
9. Ad Hoc Committee of the Harvard Medical School: A definition of irreversible coma: report of the Ad Hoc Committee of the Harvard Medical School to examine the definition of brain death, *JAMA* 205:337-340, 1968.
10. Ahmann PA, Carrigan TA, Carlton D, et al: Brain death in children: characteristic common carotid arterial velocity patterns

measured with pulsed Doppler ultrasound, *J Pediatr* 110:723-728, 1987.

11. Alvarez LA, Moshe SL, Belman MD: EEG and brain death determination in children, *Neurology* 38:227-230, 1988.

12. Alverson D, Eldridge MW, Johnson JD, et al: Effect of patent ductus arteriosus on left ventricular output in premature infants, *J Pediatr* 102:754-757, 1983.

13. Ames A, Wright RL, Kowada M: *Cerebral insult: II, the no reflow phenomenon, Am J Pathol* 52:437-453, 1968.

14. Ando Y, Takashima S, Takeshita K: Cerebral blood flow velocities in postasphyxial term neonates, *Brain Dev* 5:529-532, 1983.

15. Arnold H, Kuhne D, Rohr W: Contrast bolus technique with rapid CT scanning: a reliable diagnostic tool for the determination of brain death, *Neuroradiology* 22:129-132, 1981.

16. Ashwal S: Xenon computed tomography measuring cerebral blood flow in the determination of brain death in children, *Ann Neurol* 25:539-546, 1989.

17. Ashwal S, Schneider S: Failure of electroencephalography to diagnose brain death in comatose children, *Ann Neurol* 6:512-517, 1979.

18. Ashwal S, Schneider S, Tomasi L, Thompson J: Prognostication implications of hyperglycemia and reduced cerebral blood flow in childhood neardrowning, *Neurology* 40:820-823, 1990.

19. Ashwal S, Smith AJK, Torres F: Radionucleotide bolus angiography: a technique for verification of brain death in infants and children, *J Pediatr* 91:722-728, 1977.

20. Ashwal S, Stringer W, Tomasi L, et al: Cerebral blood flow and carbon dioxide reactivity in children with bacterial meningitis, *J Pediatr* 117:523-530, 1990.

21. Astudillo R, van der Linden J, Ekroth R, et al: Absent diastolic cerebral blood flow velocity after circulatory arrest but not after low flow in infants, *Ann Thorac Surg* 56:515-519, 1993.

22. Bada HS, Hajjar W, Chua C, Sumner DS: Non-invasive diagnosis of neonatal asphyxia and intraventricular hemorrhage by Doppler ultrasound, *J Pediatr* 95:775-779, 1979.

23. Balslev-Jorgensen P, Heilbrun MP, Boysen G: Cerebral perfusion pressure correlated with regional cerebral blood flow and aortocervical anteriography in patients with severe brain disorders progressing to brain death, *Eur Neurol* 8:207-212, 1972.

24. Batton DC, Riordan S, Riggs T: Cerebral blood flow velocity in normal, full term newborns is not related to ductal closure, *Am J Dis Child* 146:737-740, 1992.

25. Becker DP, Gardner S: *Intensive management of head injury.* In Wilkins RH, Rengachary SS, editors: *Neurosurgery,* New York, 1985, McGraw-Hill.

26. Beckstead JE, Tweed WA, Lee J, Mackeen WL: Cerebral blood flow and metabolism in man following cardiac arrest, *Stroke* 9:569-573, 1978.

27. Bejar R, Culbelo V, Schneider H, et al: Early PDA treatment with indomethacin and intraventricular hemorrhage, *Pediatr Res* 15:649, 1981.

28. Bejar R, Meritt TA, Coen RW, et al: Pulsatility index, patent ductus arteriosus, and brain damage, *Pediatrics* 69:818-821, 1982.

29. Bejar R, Schneider H, Edwards C, et al: Association of early aortogram and PDA ligation with intraventricular hemorrhage, *Pediatr Res* 15:650, 1981.

30. Bell WE, McCormick WF: *Neurologic infections in children.* In Bell WE, editor: *Major problems in clinical pediatrics,* vol 13, Philadelphia, 1975, WB Saunders.

31. Belsh JM, Blatt R, Schiffman PL: Apnea testing in brain death, *Arch Intern Med* 146:2385-2388, 1986.

32. Benveniste H, Diemer NH: Early postischemic ^{45}Ca accumulation in rat dentate hilus, *J Cereb Blood Flow Metab* 8:713-718, 1988.

33. Beyda DH, Wade J, Knezevic S, et al: *The prognostic value of measuring regional cerebral blood flow in the neuro-compromised paediatric patient.* In Wade J, Knezevic S, Maximillian VA, et al, editors: *Current problems in neurology: impact of functional imaging in neurology and psychiatry,* London, 1987, J Libbey Co.

34. Blend MJ, Pavel DG, Hughes JR: Normal cerebral radionucleotide angiogram in a child with electrocerebral silence, *Neuropediatrics* 17:S170, 1986.

35. Bode H: *Pediatric applications of transcranial Doppler sonography,* New York and Vienna, 1988, Springer-Verlag.

36. Bode H: Intracranial blood flow velocities during seizures and generalized epileptic discharges, *Eur J Pediatr* 151:706-709, 1992.

37. Bode H, Sauer M, Pringsheim W: Diagnosis of brain death by transcranial Doppler in confirming brain death, *Arch Dis Child* 63:1474-1478, 1988.

38. Bohn DJ, Biggar WD, Smith CR, et al: Influence of hypothermia, barbiturate therapy, and intracranial pressure monitoring on morbidity and mortality after near drowning, *Crit Care Med* 14:529-534, 1986.

39. Bonte FJ, Stokely EM, Devons MD, Homan RW: Single-photon tomographic study of regional cerebral blood flow in epilepsy, *Arch Neurol* 40:267-270, 1983.

40. Boros L, Thomas C, Weiner WJ: Large cerebral vessel disease in sickle cell disease, *J Neurol Neurosurg Psychiatry* 39:1236-1239, 1976.

41. Bowers SA, Marshall LF: Outcome in 200 consecutive cases of severe head injury in San Diego county: a prospective analysis, *Neurosurgery* 6:237-242, 1980.

42. Boyd SG, Harden A: Neonatal auditory brainstem response cannot reliably diagnose brainstem death, *Arch Dis Child* 60:396, 1985.

43. Brass L, Pavakis SG, De Vivo D, et al: Transcranial Doppler measurements of the middle cerebral artery: effect of hematocrit, *Stroke* 19:1466-1469, 1988.

44. Bromont C, Marie C, Bralet J: Increased lipid peroxidation in vulnerable brain regions after transient forebrain ischemia in rats, *Stroke* 20:918-924, 1989.

45. Bruce DA, Raphaely RC, Goldberg AI, et al: Pathophysiology, treatment and outcome following severe head injury in children, *Childs Brain* 5:174-191, 1979.

46. Bruce DA, Schut L, Bruno L, et al: Outcome following severe head injuries in children, *J Neurosurg* 48:675-688, 1978.

47. Bruce DA, Schut L, Sutton LN: *Pediatric head injury.* In Wilkins RH, Rengachary SS, editors: *Neurosurgery,* New York, 1985, McGraw-Hill.

48. Bruyn GAW, Kremer HPH, deMarie S, et al: Clinical evaluation of pneumococcal meningitis in adults over a twelve-year period, *Eur J Clin Microbiol Infect Dis* 8:695-700, 1989.

49. Buijs J, van Bel F, Nandorff A, et al: Cerebral blood flow pattern and autoregulation during open-heart surgery in infants and young children: a transcranial, Doppler ultrasound study, *Crit Care Med* 20:771-777, 1992.

50. Burrows FA, Bissonnette B: Cerebral blood flow velocity patterns during cardiac surgery utilizing profound hypothermia with low-flow cardiopulmonary bypass or circulatory arrest in neonates and infants, *Can J Anaesthes* 40:298-307, 1993.

51. Casino GD: Neurophysiological monitoring in the intensive care unit, *J Intensive Care Med* 3:215-223, 1988.

52. Chan K-H, Dearden NM, Miller JD: The significance of posttraumatic increase in cerebral blood flow velocity: a transcranial Doppler ultrasound study, *Neurosurgery* 30:697-700, 1992.

53. Chan K-H, Dearden NM, Miller JD: Transcranial Doppler-sonography in severe head injury, *Acta Neurochir Suppl (Wien)* 59:81-85, 1993.

54. Chan K-H, Dearden M, Miller JD, et al: Transcranial Doppler waveform difference in hyperemic and nonhyperemic patients after severe head injury, *Surg Neurol* 38:433-436, 1992.

55. Chemtob S, Beharry K, Rex J, et al: Prostanoids determine the range of cerebral blood flow in newborn piglets, *Stroke* 21:777-784, 1990.

56. Chequer RS, Tharp BR, Dreimane D, et al: Prognostic value of EEG in neonatal meningitis: retrospective study of 29 infants, *Pediatr Neurol* 8:417-422, 1992.

57. Chu N-S: Tuberculous meningitis: computerized tomographic manifestations, *Arch Neurol* 37:458-460, 1980.

58. Clyman RI, Jobe A, Heymann M, et al: Increased shunt through the patient ductus arteriosus after surfactant replacement therapy, *J Pediatr* 100:100-107, 1982.

59. Cockrill HH, Dreisbach J, Lowe B, Yamauchi T: Computed tomography in leptomeningeal infections, *AJR Am J Roentgenol* 130:511-515, 1978.

60. Cohan SL, Mun SK, Petite J, et al: Cerebral blood flow in humans following resuscitation from cardiac arrest, *Stroke* 20:761-765, 1989.

61. Collins R, Kennedy C, Sokoloff L, Plum F: Metabolic anatomy of focal motor seizures, *Arch Neurol* 33:536-542, 1976.

62. Compton JS, Teddy PJ: Cerebral arterial vasospasm following severe head injury: a transcranial Doppler study, *Br J Neurosurg* 1:435-439, 1987.

63. Crawford CS: Incidence and risk factor analysis of subependymal/intraventricular hemorrhages in <1500 gram infants born at a perinatal center, *Pediatr Res* 16:284A, 1982.

64. Danilowiez D, Rudolph AM, Hoffman JIE: Delayed closure of the ductus arteriosus in premature infants, *Pediatrics* 73:56-58, 1984.

65. Dar PRF, Godfrey DJ: Neonatal auditory brainstem response cannot reliably diagnose brainstem death, *Arch Dis Child* 60:17-19, 1985.

66. Davis DO, Dilenge D, Schlaepfer W: Arterial dilatation in purulent meningitis: case report, *J Neurosurg* 32:112-115, 1970.

67. Dean JM, McComb JG: Intracranial pressure monitoring in severe pediatric near-drowning, *Neurosurgery* 9:627-630, 1981.

68. Debrun G, Sauvegrain J, Aicardi J, Goutieres F: Moyamoya, a nonspecific radiologic syndrome, *Neuroradiology* 8:241-244, 1975.

69. De Los Reyes RA, Ausman JI, Diaz FG: Agents for cerebral edema, *Clin Neurosurg* 28:98-107, 1981.

70. Demaerel P, Casaer P, Casteels I, et al: Moyamoya disease: MRI and MR angiography, *Neuroradiology* 33(suppl):50-52, 1991.

71. DeSousa AL, Kleiman MB, Mealy J Jr: Quadriplegia and cortical blindness in *Haemophilus influenzae* meningitis, *J Pediatr* 93:253-254, 1978.

72. De Witt LD, Wechsler LR: Transcranial Doppler, *Stroke* 19:915-921, 1988.

73. Dickerson DF, Arnold R, Wilkerson JL: Congenital heart disease among 160,480 liveborn children in Liverpool 1960-1969: implications for surgical treatment, *Br Heart J* 46:55-62, 1981.

74. Dodge PR, Swartz MN: Bacterial meningitis—a review of selected aspects: II, special neurologic problems, postmeningitic complications and clinicopathological correlation, *N Engl J Med* 272:954-960, 1965.

75. Dykes FD, Lazzara A, Ahmann P, et al: Intraventricular hemorrhage: a prospective evaluation of etiopathogenesis, *Pediatrics* 66:42-49, 1980.

76. Ebihara S-I, Gotoh E, Kanda T, et al: Cerebral blood flow and metabolism in moyamoya disease (occlusion of the circle of Willis), *Neurochirurgie* 22:404-405, 1989.

77. Edwards MK, Brown DL, Chua GT: Complicated infantile meningitis: evaluation by real-time sonography, *AJNR Am J Neuroradiol* 3:431-434, 1982.

78. Eisenberg HM, Levin HS: The devastated head injury patient, *Clin Neurosurg* 34:572-586, 1988.

79. Engel J, Kuhl DE, Phelps ME: Patterns of human local cerebral glucose metabolism during epileptic seizures, *Science* 218:684-690, 1985.

80. Faraci FM, Brian JE: Nitric oxide and the cerebral circulation, *Stroke* 25:692-703, 1994.

81. Ferencz C, Rubin JD, McCarter RJ, Cardiac and noncardiac malformations: observations in a population-based study, *Teratology* 35:367-378, 1987.

82. Fischer AQ: Pediatric applications of clinical ultrasound, *Neurol Clin North Am* 8:759-774, 1990.

83. Fischer AQ, Livingstone JN: Transcranial Doppler and real-time cranial sonography in neonatal hydrocephalus, *J Child Neurol* 4:64-69, 1989.

84. Fischer AQ, Sheffield MV, Truemper EJ: Evolutionary changes in cerebral blood flow velocity in infants with uncomplicated meningitis, *Ann Neurol* 28:427A, 1990.

85. Fischer AQ, Truemper EJ: Vasoreactivity of cerebral vessels pediatric status epilepticus: a hemodynamic study, *Ann Neurol* 36:460, 1993.

86. Fischer AQ, Truemper EJ, Hartlage PL, Flannery AM: Transcranial Doppler findings in infants and children with suspected brain death, *Ann Neurol* 5:75A, 1990.

87. Floret D, Delmas MC, Cochat P: Cerebellar infarction as a complication of pneumococcal meningitis, *Pediatr Infect Dis J* 8:57-58, 1989.

88. Fost N: What does a hospital ethics committee do for you? *Contemp Pediatr* 3:119-129, 1986.

89. Frewen TC, Sumabat WO, Han VK, et al: Cerebral resuscitation therapy in pediatric near-drowning, *J Pediatr* 106:615-617, 1985.

90. Futagi Y, Abe J, Ohtani K, Okamoto N: Cerebral blood flow during ACTH therapy: especially diurnal changes during the first week of therapy, *Brain Dev* 10:164-168, 1988.

91. Futagi Y, Abe J: The effect of ACTH on cerebral blood flow in children with intractable epilepsy, *Brain Dev* 7:53-55, 1985.

92. Gado M, Axley J, Appleton B, Prensky AL: Angiography in the acute and post-traumatic phases of *Haemophilus influenzae* meningitis, *Radiology* 110:439-444, 1974.

93. Galaske RG, Schober O, Hyer R: Determination of brain death in children with (123) I-IMP and Tc99m HMPAO, *Psychiatry Res* 29:343-345, 1989.

94. Geiseler PI, Nelson KE, Levin S, et al: Community-acquired purulent meningitis: a review of 1316 cases during the antibiotic era 1954-1976, *Rev Infect Dis* 2:725-745, 1980.

95. Gennarelli TA, Thibault LE, Adams JH, et al: Diffuse axonal injury and traumatic coma in the primate, *Ann Neurol* 12:564-574, 1982.

96. Girling DJ, Hallidie-Smith KA: Persistent ductus arteriosus in ill and premature babies, *Arch Dis Child* 46:177-181, 1971.

97. Goh D, Minns RA: Cerebral blood flow velocity monitoring in pyogenic meningitis, *Arch Dis Child* 68:111-119, 1993.

98. Goh D, Minns RA, Pye SD, Steers AJW: Cerebral blood-flow velocity and intermittent intracranial pressure elevation during sleep in hydrocephalic children, *Dev Med Child Neurol* 34:676-689, 1992.

99. Gomez CR, McLaughlin JR, Njemanzi PC, et al: Effect of cardiac dysfunction upon diastolic cerebral blood flow, *Angiology* 43:625-630, 1992.

100. Goodman JM, Hek LL, Moore BD: Confirmation of brain death with protable isotope angiography: a review of 204 consecutive cases, *Neurosurgery* 16:492-497, 1985.

101. Goraj B, Rifkinson-Mann S, Leslie DR, et al: Cerebral blood flow velocity after head injury: transcranial Doppler evaluation, *Radiology* 188:137-141, 1993.

102. Gotshall RA: Conus medullaris syndrome after meningococcal meningitis, *N Engl J Med* 286:882-883, 1972.

103. Graham DI, Adamas JH, Doyle D: Ischemic brain damage in non-missile head injuries, *J Neurol Sci* 39:213-234, 1978.

104. Grant EG, White EM, Schellinger P, et al: Cranial duplex sonography of the infant, *Radiology* 163:177-185, 1987.

105. Gray PH, O'Reilley C: Neonatal *Proteus mirabilis* meningitis and cerebral abscess: diagnosis by real-time ultrasound, *J Clin Ultrasound* 12:441-443, 1984.

106. Gray PH, Tudehope DI, Masel JP, et al: Perinatal hypoxic-ischaemic brain injury: prediction of outcome, *Dev Med Child Neurol* 35:965-973, 1993.

107. Greeley WJ, Kern FH, Ungerleider RM, et al: Cardiopulmonary-bypass and total circulatory arrest alters cerebral metabolism in infants and children, *Anesthesiology* 73:A91, 1990.

108. Grigg MM, Kelly MA, Celestia GG, et al: Electroencephalographic activity after brain death, *Arch Neurol* 44:948-954, 1987.

109. Gupta RK, Pant CS, Sharma A, Khalilullah A: Ultrasound diagnosis of multiple cysticencephalomalacia, *Pediatr Radiol* 18:6-8, 1988.

110. Hahn YS, Raimondi AJ, McLone DG, Yamanouchi Y: Traumatic mechanisms of head injury in child abuse, *Childs Brain* 10:229-241, 1983.

111. Hanada J: Computerized tomography in moya-moya syndrome, *Surg Neurol* 7:315-322, 1967.

112. Harada T, Suzuki Y, Satoh S, et al: Blood component induction of cerebral vasospasm, *Neurosurgery* 27:252-256, 1990.

113. Haring H-P, Rotzer H-K, Reindl H, et al: Time course of cerebral blood flow velocity in central nervous system infections, *Arch Neurol* 50:98-101, 1993.

114. Hassler W, Steinmetz H, Gawlowski J: Transcranial Doppler ultrasonography in raised pressure and in intracranial circulatory arrest, *J Neurosurg* 68:745-751, 1988.

115. Haupt HM, Kurlinski JP, Barnett NK, Epstein M: Infarction of the spinal cord as a complication of pneumococcal meningitis, *J Neurosurg* 55:121-123, 1981.

116. Headings DL, Glasgow LA: Occlusion of the internal carotid artery complicating *Haemophilus* meningitis, *Am J Dis Child* 131:854-856, 1977.

117. Henriksen L, Paulson OB, Smith RJ: Cerebral blood flow following normovolemic hemodilution in patients with high hematocrit, *Ann Neurol* 24:454-457, 1981.

118. Herson VC, Todd JK: Prediction of morbidity in *Haemophilus influenzae* meningitis, *Pediatrics* 59:35-39, 1977.

119. Hillier SC, Burrows FA, Bissonette B, Taylor RH: Cerebral hemodynamics in neonates and infants undergoing cardiopulmonary by-pass and profound hypothermic circulatory arrest: assessment by transcranial Doppler sonography, *Anesth Analg* 72:723-728, 1991.

120. Holzman B, Curless R, Sfakianakis G: Radionuclide cerebral perfusion scintigraphy in determination of brain death in children, *Neurology* 33:1027-1031, 1983.

121. Hossman KA: Treatment of experimental cerebral ischemia, *J Cereb Blood Flow Metab* 2:275-281, 1982.

122. Hung K-L: Cranial ultrasound in the detection of post-meningitic complications in the neonates, *Brain Dev* 8:31-36, 1986.

123. Imajo T, Roessman U: Diffuse axonal injury, *Am J Forensic Med Pathol* 5:217-222, 1984.

124. Ingvar DH: rCBF in focal cortical epilepsy, *Stroke* 4:359-360, 1973.

125. James AE, Hodges FJ, Jordan CE, et al: Angiography and cisternography in acute meningitis due to *Haemophilus influenzae*, *Radiology* 103:601-606, 1972.

126. Jayakumar PN, Arya BYT, Vasudev MK, et al: Moyamoya disease: computed tomography and angiographic correlation in 10 caucasoid patients, *Acta Neurol Scand* 84:339-343, 1991.

127. Karasawa J, Touho H, Onishi H, et al: Long-term follow-up study after extracranial-intracranial bypass surgery for anterior circulation ischemia in childhood moyamoya disease, *J Neurosurg* 77:84-89, 1992.

128. Kaufman HH, Geisler FH, Kopitnik T, et al: Detection of brain death in barbiturate coma: the dilemma of an intracranial pulse, *Neurosurgery* 25:275-278, 1989.

129. Kaul DK, Fabry ME, Nagel RL: *Erythrocytic and vascular factors influencing the microcirculatory behavior of blood in sickle cell anemia.* In Whitten CF, Bertles JF, editors, *Sickle cell disease,* New York, 1989, New York National Academy of Sciences.

130. Kirkham FJ, Levin SD, Padayachee KMC, et al: Transcranial Doppler ultrasound findings in brain stem death, *J Neurol Neurosurg Psychiatry* 50:1504-1513, 1987.

131. Kitterman JA, Edmunds IH Jr, Gregory GA, et al: Patent ductus arteriosus in premature infants: incidence, relation to pulmonary disease and management, *N Engl J Med* 287:473-477, 1972.

132. Kochanek PM, Uhl MW, Schoettle RJ: *Hypoxic-ischemic encephalopathy: pathobiology and therapy of the post-resuscitation syndrome in children.* In Fuhrman BP, Zimmerman JJ, editors: *Pediatric critical care,* St Louis, 1991, Mosby–Year Book.

133. Kontos HA: Oxygen radicals from arachidonate metabolism in abnormal vascular responses, *Am Rev Resp Dis* 136:474-477, 1987.

134. Kontos HA: Oxygen radicals in CNS damage, *Chem Biol Interact* 72:229-255, 1989.

135. Kontos HA, Wei EP, Ellis EF, et al: Appearance of superoxide anion radical in cerebral extracellular space during increased prostaglandin synthesis in cats, *Circ Res* 57:142-153, 1985.

136. Kostteljanetz M, Ohrstrom JK, Skjodt S, Teglbjaerg PS: Clinical brain death with preserved cerebral circulation, *Acta Neurol Scand* 78:418-421, 1988.

137. Krayenbuhl HA: The moya moya syndrome and the neurosurgeon, *Surg Neurol* 4:353-360, 1975.

138. Kresky B, Buchbinder S, Greenberg IW: The incidence of neurologic residua in children after recovery from bacterial meningitis in children, *Pediatr Clin North Am* 8:1177-1192, 1961.

139. Kurth CD, Steven JM, Nicolsen SC, et al: Changes in brain oxygenation during cardiopulmonary by-pass and circulatory arrest (CA) in neonates, *Anesthesiology* 71:A1035, 1989.

140. Langfitt TW, Kassell NF: Non-filling of cerebral vessels during angiography: correlation with intracranial pressure, *Acta Neurochir (Wien)* 14:96-104, 1966.

141. Lassen NA: The luxury perfusion syndrome and its possible relation to acute metabolic acidosis localized within the brain, *Lancet* 2:1113-1115, 1966.

142. Laurin NR, Driedger AA, Hurwitz GA: Cerebral perfusion imaging ith technetium-99m HMPAO in brain death and severe central nervous system injury, *J Nucl Med* 30:1627-1635, 1989.

143. Laursen HB: Some epidemiologic aspects of congenital heart disease in Denmark, *Acta Paediatr Scand* 69:619-624, 1980.

144. Laxar RM, Marks MI: Pneumococcal meningitis in children, *Am J Dis Child* 131:850-853, 1977.

145. Leeds NE, Goldberg HI: Angiographic manifestations in cerebral inflammatory disease, *Radiology* 98:595-604, 1971.

146. Legido A, Clancy RR, Berman PH: Neurologic outcome after electroencephalographically proven neonatal seizure, *Pediatrics* 88:583-596, 1991.

147. Lehrer H: The angiographic triad in tuberculous meningitis: a radiographic and clinico-pathologic correlation, *Radiology* 87:829-835, 1966.

148. LeMancusa J, Cooper R, Vieth R: The effects of the falling therapeutic and subtherapeutic barbiturate blood levels on electrocerebral silence in clinically brain dead children, *Clin Electroencephalogr* 22:112-117, 1991.

149. Levene MI, Fenton AC, Evans DH, et al: Severe birth asphyxia and abnormal cerebral blood-flow velocity, *Dev Med Child Neurol* 31:427-434, 1989.

150. Lewis JK, Minter MG, Eschelman SJ, Witte MK: Outcome of pediatric resuscitation, *Ann Emerg Med* 12:297-299, 1983.

151. Lindegaard K-F, Bakke SJ, Aaslid R, Nornes H: Doppler

diagnosis of intracranial artery occlusive disorders, *J Neurol Neurosurg Psychiatry* 49:510-518, 1986.

152. Lindegaard KF, Lundar T, Wiberg J, et al: Variations in the middle cerebral artery blood flow investigated with noninvasive transcranial blood flow velocity measurements, *Stroke* 18:1025-1030, 1987.

153. Lipman B, Serwer GA, Brazy JE: Abnormal cerebral hemodynamics in preterm infants with patent ductus arteriosus, *Pediatrics* 69:778-791, 1982.

154. Love T, Darby J, Yonas H: CO₂ reactivity and CBF in comatose survivors of cardiac arrest, *Crit Care Med* 17:346-350, 1989.

155. Lundar T, Lindegaard KF, Froysaker T, et al: Cerebral carbon dioxide reactivity during nonpulsatile cardiopulmonary bypass, *Ann Thorac Surg* 41:525-530, 1986.

156. Lyons EL, Leeds NE: The angiographic demonstration of arterial disease in purulent meningitis, *Radiology* 88:935-938, 1967.

157. Maccabe JJ: Hydrocephalus secondary to meningitis; developmental, *Dev Med Child Neurol* 4:268-269, 1962.

158. MacDonald RL, Findlay JM, Tator CH: Sphenoethmoidal sinusitis complicated by cavernous sinus thrombosis and pontocerebellar infarction, *Can J Neurol Sci* 15:310-313, 1988.

159. Machado C, Valdes P, Garcia-Tigera J, et al: Brain-stem auditory evoked potentials and brain death, *Electroencephalogr Clin Neurophysiol* 80:392-398, 1991.

160. MacPherson P, Graham DI: Correlation between angiographic findings and ischaemia of head injury, *J Neurol Neurosurg Psychiatry* 41:122-127, 1978.

161. Mahoney WJ, D'Souza BJ, Haller JA, et al: Long-term outcome of children with severe head trauma and prolonged coma, *Pediatrics* 71:756-762, 1983.

162. Marshall TA, Marshall F II, Reddy PP: Physiologic changes associated with ligation of the ductus arteriosus in preterm infants, *J Pediatr* 101:749-753, 1982.

163. Martin CG, Snider AR, Katz SM, et al: Abnormal cerebral blood flow patterns in preterm infants with a large patent ductus arteriosus, *J Pediatr* 101:587-593, 1982.

164. Matsushima Y, Aoyagi M, Suzuki R, et al: Perioperative complications of encephalo-duro-arterio-synangiosis: prevention and treatment, *Surg Neurol* 36:343-353, 1991.

165. Matsushima Y, Inabe Y: Moyamoya disease in children and its surgical treatment: introduction of a new surgical procedure in children and its follow-up angiograms, *Childs Brain* 11:155-170, 1984.

166. Mayberg MR, Okada T, Bark DH: Morphologic changes in cerebral arteries after subarachnoid hemorrhage, *Neurosurg Clin N Am* 1:417-432, 1990.

167. Mayer T, Walker MI, Shasha I, et al: Effect of multiple trauma on outcome of pediatric patients with neurologic injuries, *Childs Brain* 8:189-197, 1981.

168. McCord JM: Oxygen derived free radicals in postischemic tissue injury, *N Engl J Med* 312:159-163, 1985.

169. McMenamin JB: Internal carotid artery occlusion in *Haemophilus influenzae* meningitis, *J Pediatr* 101:723-725, 1982.

170. McMenamin JB, Volpe JJ: Doppler ultrasonography in the determination of neonatal brain death, *Ann Neurol* 14:302-307, 1983.

171. McMenamin JB, Volpe JJ: Bacterial meningitis in infancy: effects on intracranial pressure and cerebral blood flow velocity, *Neurology* 34:500-504, 1984.

172. Meldrum BS, Brierley JB: Prolonged epileptic seizures in primates, *Arch Neurol* 28:10-17, 1973.

173. Mellander M, Larsson LE: Effects of left-to-right ductus shunting on left ventricular output and cerebral blood flow velocity in 3-day-old preterm infants with and without severe lung disease, *J Pediatr* 113:101-109, 1988.

174. Ment LR, Stewart WB, Duncan CC, et al: Beagle puppy model

of brain injury: regional cerebral blood flow and cerebral prostaglandins, *J Neurosurg* 67:278-283, 1978.

175. Merkell KHH, Ginsberg PL, Parker JC Jr, Post MJD: Cerebrovascular disease in sickle cell anemia: a clinical and pathological and radiologic correlates, *Stroke* 9:45-52, 1978.

176. Merten DF, Osborne DRS: Craniocerebral trauma in the child abuse syndrome, *Pediatr Ann* 12:882-887, 1983.

177. Meszaros M, Nagy A, Czeizel A: Incidence of congenital heart disease in Hungary, *Hum Hered* 25:513-519, 1975.

178. Michenfelder JD, Milde JH: Postischemic canine cerebral blood flow appears to be determined by cerebral metabolic needs, *J Cereb Blood Flow Metab* 10:71-76, 1990.

179. Michenfelder JD, Sundt TM: The effect of PaCO₂ on the metabolism of ischaemic brain in squirrel monkeys, *Anesthesiology* 38:445-453, 1973.

180. Milde LN, Milde JH, Michenfelder JD: Delayed treatment with nimodipine improves cerebral blood flow after complete ischemia in the dog, *J Cereb Blood Flow Metab* 6:332-337, 1986.

181. Miller C, Alexander K, Lampard D, et al: Local cerebral ischemia: II, effect of arterial PCO₂ on reperfusion following global ischemia, *Stroke* 11:542-548, 1980.

182. Murikami N, Sanada S, Horiuchi I, Ohtahara S: Relation of cerebral blood flow in patients with various types of childhood epilepsies, *Jpn J Psychiatry Neurol* 44:407-409, 1990.

183. Muttaqin Z, Ohba S, Arita K, et al: Cerebral circulation in Moya-moya disease: a clinical study using transcranial Doppler study, *Surg Neurol* 40:306-313, 1993.

184. Muttaqin Z, Uozumi T, Kuwabara S, et al: Hyperaemia prior to acute cerebral swelling in severe head injuries: the role of transcranial Doppler monitoring, *Acta Neurochir (Wien)* 123:76-81, 1993.

185. Nemec JJ, Marwick TH, Lorig RJ, et al: Comparison of transcranial Doppler ultrasound and transesophageal contrast echocardiography in the detection of interatrial right-to-left shunts, *Am J Cardiol* 68:1498-1502, 1991.

186. Newell DW, Grady MS, Sirotta P, Winn HR: Evaluation of brain death using transcranial Doppler, *Neurosurgery* 24:509-513, 1989.

187. Newell DW, Seiler RW, Aaslid R: *Head injury and cerebral circulatory arrest.* In Newell DW, Aaslid R, editors: *Transcranial Doppler,* New York, 1992, Raven Press.

188. Norelle A, Fischer AQ, Flannery AM: Transcranial Doppler: a noninvasive method to monitor hydrocephalus, *J Child Neurol* 4:S87-S90, 1989.

189. Nowichi JP, Duval D, Poignet H, Scatton B: Nitric oxide mediates neuronal cell death after focal cerebral ischemia in the mouse, *Eur J Pharmacol* 209:339-340, 1991.

190. Nussbaum E, Galant SP: Intracranial pressure monitoring as a guide to prognosis in the nearly drowned, severely comatose child, *J Pediatr* 102:215-218, 1983.

191. Oliver CN, Starke-Reed PE, Stadman ER, et al: Oxidative damage to brain proteins, loss of glutamine synthetase activity, and production of free radicals during ischemia/reperfusion-induced injury to gerbil brain, *Proc Natl Acad Sci U S A* 87:5144-5149, 1990.

192. Oppenheimer EY, Rosman NP: Seizures in childhood: an approach to emergency management, *Pediatr Clin North Am* 26:837-855, 1979.

193. O'Rourke PP: Outcome of children who are apneic and pulseless in the emergency room, *Crit Care Med* 14:466-468, 1986.

194. Outwater KM, Rockoff MA: Apnea testing to confirm brain death in children, *Crit Care Med* 12:357-358, 1984.

195. Oyesiku N, Barrows DL, Eckman JR, et al: Intracranial aneurysms in sickle-cell anemia: clinical features and pathogenesis, *J Neurosurg* 75:356-363, 1991.

196. Palmer P, Dubowitz LM, Levene MI, et al: Developmental and neurological progress of preterm infants with intraventricular

hemorrhage and ventricular dilation, *Arch Dis Child* 57:748-752, 1982.

197. Parvey LS, Geral A: Arteriographic diagnosis of brain death in children, *Pediatr Radiol* 4:79-82, 1976.

198. Pasqualin A, Vivenza C, Rosta L, et al: Cerebral vasospasm after head injury, *Neurosurgery* 15:855-858, 1984.

199. Patel YP, Gupta SM, Batson R, Herrera NE: Brain death: confirmation by radionucleotide cerebral angiography, *Clin Nucl Med* 13:438-442, 1988.

200. Paulsen OB, Brodersen P, Hansen EL, Kristensen HS: Regional cerebral blood flow: cerebral metabolic rate of oxygen, and cerebrospinal fluid acid-base variables in patients with acute meningitis and with acute encephalitis, *Acta Med Scand* 196:191-198, 1974.

201. Perlman JM, Hill A, Volpe JJ: The effect of patent ductus arteriosus on flow velocity in the anterior cerebral arteries: ductal steal in the premature newborn infant, *J Pediatr* 99:767-771, 1981.

202. Perrin C, Lecacheux C, Bazin C, et al: Hydrocephalie aigue drainee en urgence: Consequence d'un infarctus du cervelet au cours d'une meningite a Haemophilus, *Arch Fr Pediatr* 44:875-877, 1987.

203. Pesso JL, Floret D, Cochat P, Dumont C: Meningite suppuree a pneumocoque chez le nourrisson et l'enfant: complications et facteurs pronostiques, *Pediatrie* 43:263-267, 1988.

204. Petty GW, Mohr JP, Pedley TA, et al: The role of transcranial Doppler in confirming brain death: sensitivity, specificity, and suggestions for performance and interpretation, *Neurology* 40:300-303, 1990.

205. Pfister H-W, Borasio GD, Dirnagl U, et al: Cerebrovascular complications of bacterial meningitis in adults, *Neurology* 42:1497-1504, 1992.

206. Pfister H-W, Feiden W, Einhaupt K-M: Spectrum of complications during bacterial meningitis in adults, *Arch Neurol* 50:575-581, 1993.

207. Pike G, Wong K, Bencivenga R, et al: electrophysiologic studies, computed tomography, and neurologic outcome in acute bacterial meningitis, *J Pediatr* 116:702-706, 1990.

208. Pillay PK, Wilberger J: Transcranial Doppler evaluation of brain death, *Neurosurgery* 25:481-482, 1989.

209. Pistoia F, Johnson DW, Darby JM: The role of xenon CT measurements of cerebral blood flow in the clinical determination of brain death, *Am J Neuroradiol* 12:97-103, 1991.

210. Platau RV, Rinkar A, Derrick J: Acute subdural effusions and late sequalae of meningitis, *Pediatrics* 23:962-971, 1959.

211. Plum F, Posner JB, Troy B: Cerebral metabolic and circulatory responses to induced convulsions in animals, *Arch Neurol* 18:1-13, 1968.

212. Posner JB, Plum F, Van Poznak A: Cerebral metabolism in induced seizures in man, *Arch Neurol* 20:388-395, 1969.

213. Powers AD, Graeber MC, Smith RR: Transcranial Doppler ultrasonography in the determination of brain death, *Neurosurgery* 24:884-889, 1989.

214. Powner D: Drug-associated isoelectric EEG's: a hazard in brain death certification, *JAMA* 236:1123, 1976.

215. President's Commission for the Study of Ethical Problems in Medicine and Biomedical and Behavioral Research: *Defining death: medical, legal, and ethical issues in the determination of death,* Washington, DC, 1981, US Government Printing Office.

216. Pribham HFW: Angiographic appearances in acute intracranial hypertension, *Neurology* 11:10-12, 1961.

217. Rabe EF, Flynn RE, Dodge PR: A study of subdural effusions and late sequalae in meningitis, *Neurology* 12:79-92, 1962.

218. Raemakers VH, Casaer P: Defective regulation of cerebral oxygen transport after severe birth asphyxia, *Dev Med Child Neurol* 32:56-62, 1990.

219. Raimondi AJ, Di Rocco C: The physiopathogenetic basis for the

220. Raimondi AJ, Hirschauer J: *Clinical criteria – children's coma score and outcome scale – for decision making in managing head injured infants and toddlers.* In Raimondi AJ, Choux M, Di Rocco C, editors: *Head injuries in the newborn and infant,* New York, 1986, Springer-Verlag.

221. Reimer H, Burrows FA, Bissonette B: Cerebral metabolism during low-flow cardiopulmonary by-pass and profound hypothermic circulatory arrest, *Anesthesiology* 77:A1135, 1992.

222. Reivich M: Regulation of the cerebral circulation, *Clin Neurosurg* 16:378-418, 1969.

223. Roine RO, Somer H, Kaste M: Neurological outcome after out-of-hospital cardiac arrest, *Arch Neurol* 46:753-756, 1989.

224. Roos KL, Tunkel AR, Scheld WM: *Acute bacterial meningitis in children and adults.* In Scheld WM, Whitley RJ, Durack DT, editors, *Infections of the central nervous system,* New York, 1991, Raven Press.

225. Ropper AH, Kehne SM, Wechsler L: Transcranial Doppler in brain death, *Neurology* 37:1733-1735, 1987.

226. Ropper AH, Kennedy SK, Russell L: Apnea testing in the diagnosis of brain death, *J Neurosurg* 55:942-946, 1981.

227. Rorke LB, Pitts FW: Purulent meningitis: the pathologic basis of clinical manifestations, *Clin Pediatr (Phila)* 2:64-71, 1963.

228. Rosenberg AA: Cerebral blood flow and O2 metabolism after asphyxia in newborn lambs, *Pediatr Res* 20:778-782, 1986.

229. Rosenberg AA, Murdaugh E, White CW: The role of oxygen free radicals in post-asphyxia cerebral hypoperfusion in newborn lambs, *Pediatr Res* 26:215-219, 1989.

230. Rosenberg HK, Levine RS, Stoltz K, Smith DR: Bacterial meningitis in infants: sonographic features, *AJNR Am J Neuroradiol* 4:822-825, 1983

231. Rosza L: Vasospasm after head injury studied by transcranial Doppler sonography, *Radiol Diagn* 30:151-157, 1989.

232. Roth MP, Dott B, Alembik Y, Stoll C: Malformations congenitales dans une serie de 66,068 naissances consecutives, *Arch Fr Pediatr* 44:173-176, 1987.

233. Rowland TW, Donnelly JH, Jackson AH: Apnea documentation for determination of brain death in children, *Pediatrics* 74:505-508, 1984.

234. Safar P: Cerebral resuscitation after cardiac arrest: a review, *Circulation* 74:138-153, 1986.

235. Sakai S, Meyer JS, Naritomi H, Hsu M: Regional cerebral blood flow and EEG in patient with epilepsy, *Arch Neurol* 35:648-657, 1978.

236. Saliba EM, Chantepie A, Gold F, et al: Intraoperative measurements of cerebral hemodynamics during ductus arteriosus ligation in preterm infants, *Eur J Pediatr* 150:362-365, 1991.

237. Samuel AM, Vidvans AS: Radionuclide scintigraphy of the brain and ultrasound studies in tuberculous meningitis, *Clin Nucl Med* 12:298-302, 1987.

238. Sanada S, Murakami N, Ohtahara: Changes in blood flow velocity of the middle cerebral artery during absence seizures, *Pediatr Neurol* 4:158-161, 1988.

239. Sanker P, Roth B, Frowein RA, Firsching R: Cerebral reperfusion in brain death of a newborn: a case report, *Neurosurg Rev* 15:315-317, 1992.

240. Sarnaik AP, Preston G, Lieh-Lai M, Eisenbrey AB: Intracranial pressure and cerebral perfusion pressure in near-drowning, *Crit Care Med* 13:224-227, 1985.

241. Saunders FW, Cledgett P: Intracranial blood velocity in head injury, *Surg Neurol* 29:401-409, 1988.

242. Schwartz JA, Baxter J, Brill DR: Diagnosis of brain death in children by radionucleotide cerebral imaging, *Pediatrics* 73:14-18, 1984.

243. Seibert JJ, Miller SF, Kirby RE, et al: Cerebrovascular disease in

symptomatic and asymptomatic patients with sickle cell anemia; screening with duplex transcranial Doppler ultrasound, correlation with MR and MR angiography, *Radiology* 189:457-466, 1993.

244. Seiler RW, Grolimund P, Aaslid R, Nornes H: Cerebral vasospasm evaluated by transcranial ultrasound correlated to clinical grade and CT-visualized subarachnoid hemorrhage, *J Neurosurg* 64:594-600, 1986.

245. Seiler RW, Newell DW: *Subarachnoid hemorrhage and vasospasm.* In Newell DW, Aaslid R, editors: *Transcranial Doppler,* New York, 1992, Raven Press.

246. Serra VS, Chandram R, Redman CWG: Abnormal transcranial Doppler pattern in a pregnant woman during orthostatic hypotension, *Lancet* 337:1296-1297, 1991.

247. Serwer GA, Armstrong BE, Anderson PAW: Continuous wave Doppler ultrasonographic quantitation of patent ductus arteriosus flow, *J Pediatr* 100:297-299, 1982.

248. Shapiro K, Marmarou A: Clinical applications of the pressure-volume index in the treatment of pediatric head injuries, *J Neurosurg* 56:819-825, 1982.

249. Shimizu H, Futagi Y, Mimaki T: Cerebral blood flow measured by Doppler flow meter during petit mal seizure, *Brain Dev* 5:58-61, 1983.

250. Shortland DB, Gibson NA, Levene MI, Patent ductus arteriosus and cerebral circulation in preterm infants, *Dev Med Child Neurol* 32:386-393, 1990.

251. Siesjo BK: Mechanisms of ischemic brain damage, *Crit Care Med* 16:954-963, 1988.

252. Siesjo BK, Wieloch T: Cerebral metabolism in ischaemia: neurochemical basis for therapy, *Br J Anaesth* 57:47-67, 1985.

253. Smith AJK, Walker AE: Cerebral blood flow and brain metabolism as indicators of cerebral death: a review, *Hopkins Med J* 133:107-119, 1973.

254. Smith AL, Haas J: *Neonatal bacterial meningitis.* In Scheld WM, Whitley RJ, Durack DT, editors: *Infections of the central nervous system,* New York, 1991, Raven Press.

255. Smith DH, Ingram DL, Smith AL, et al: Bacterial meningitis: a symposium, *Pediatrics* 52:586-600, 1973.

256. Smith ES: Purulent meningitis in infants and children, *J Pediatrics* 45:425-436, 1954.

257. Smith JF, Landing BH: Mechanisms of brain damage in *H. influenzae* meningitis, *J Neuropath Exp Neurol* 19:248-265, 1960.

258. Spencer MP, Whistler D: Transorbital Doppler diagnosis of intracranial arterial stenosis, *Stroke* 17:916-921, 1986.

259. Stannard MW, Jimenez JF: Sonographic recognition of multicystic encephalomalacia, *AJR Am J Roentgenol* 141:1321-1324, 1983.

260. Steinhart CM, Weiss IP: Use of brainstem auditory evoked potentials in pediatric brain death, *Crit Care Med* 13:560-562, 1985.

261. Stockman JA, Nigro MA, Mishkin MM, Oski FA: Occlusion of large cerebral vessels in sickle cell anemia, *N Engl J Med* 287:846-849, 1972.

262. Stovring J, Snyder RD: Computed tomography in childhood bacterial meningitis, *J Pediatr* 96:820-823, 1980.

263. Suwanwela C, Suwanwela N: Intracranial arterial narrowing and spasm in acute head injury, *J Neurosurg* 36:314-323, 1972.

264. Suzuki J, Kodama N: Moyamoya disease: a review, *Stroke* 14:104-109, 1983.

265. Swartz MN, Dodge PR: General clinical features: a review of selected aspects. I. General clinical features, special problems and unusual meningeal reactions mimicking bacterial meningitis, *N Engl J Med* 272:725-731, 1965.

266. Synder RD, Stovring J, Cushing AH, et al: Cerebral infarction in childhood bacterial meningitis, *J Neurol Neurosurg Psychiatry* 44:581-585, 1981.

267. Syrjanen J: Central nervous system complications in patients with bacteremia, *Scand J Infect Dis* 21:285-296, 1989.

268. Takanashi J, Sugita K, Ishii M, et al: Moyamoya syndrome in young children: MR comparison with adult onset, *AJNR Am J Neuroradiol* 14:1139-1143, 1993.

269. Takeuchi S, Tanaka R, Ishii R, et al: Cerebral hemodynamics in patients with moyamoya disease: a study of regional cerebral blood flow by the [133]Xenon inhalation method, *Surg Neurol* 23:468-474, 1985.

270. Task Force on Brain Death in Children: Guidelines for the determination of brain death in children, *Pediatrics* 80:298-300, 1987.

271. Theodore WH, Brooks R, Margolin R: Positron emission tomography in generalized seizures, *Neurology* 25:684-690, 1985.

272. Todd MM, Tommasino C, Shapiro HM: Cerebrovascular effects of prolonged hypocarbia and hypercarbia after experimental global ischemia in cats, *Crit Care Med* 13:720-723, 1985.

273. Torphy DE, Minter MG, Thompson BM: Cardiorespiratory arrest and resuscitation in children, *Am J Dis Child* 138:1099-1102, 1984.

274. Truemper EJ, Fischer AQ: Application of TCD in the detection of cerebral vasospasm in children following traumatic closed head injury (work in progress).

275. Truemper EJ, Smith KG, Sekar KC: Group B streptococcal infection and cerebral necrosis, *J Perinatol* 7:267-269, 1987.

276. Uemura K, Yamaguchi K, Kojimal S, et al: Regional cerebral blood flow on cerebrovascular moyamoya disease. Study by ^{133}Xe clearance method and cerebral angiography, *No To Shinkei* 27:385-393, 1975.

277. Van Bel F, Van De Bor M: Cerebral edema caused by perinatal asphyxia: detection and followup, *Helv Paediatr Acta* 40:361-366, 1985.

278. Van der Linden J, Astudillo R, Ekroth R, et al: Cerebral lactate release after circulatory arrest but not after low flow in pediatric heart operations, *Ann Thorac Surg* 56:1485-1489, 1993.

279. Van Velthoven V, Calliauw L: Diagnosis of brain death: transcranial Doppler sonography as an additional method, *Acta Neurochir (Wien)* 95:57-60, 1988.

280. Vapalahi M, Luukkonen M, Puranen M, et al: Early clinical signs and prognosis in children with brain injuries, *Ann Clin Res* 47:37-42, 1986.

281. Waga S, Tochio H: Intracranial aneurysm associated with moyamoya disease in childhood, *Surg Neurol* 23:237-243, 1985.

282. Waggener JD. *The pathophysiology of bacterial meningitis and cerebral abscesses: an anatomical interpretation.* In Thompson RA, Green JR, editors, *Advances in neurology,* vol 6, New York, 1974, Raven Press.

283. Wald E, Berbman I, Taylor H, et al: Long-term outcome of group B streptococcal meningitis, *Pediatrics* 77:217-221, 1986.

284. Walker ML, Storrs BB, Mayer T: Factors affecting outcome in the pediatric patient with multiple trauma, *Childs Brain* 11:387-397, 1984.

285. Walker ML, Storrs BB, Mayer TA: *Head injuries.* In Mayer TA, editor: *Emergency management of pediatric trauma,* Philadelphia, 1985, WB Saunders.

286. Wang Z, Bogdan AR, Zimmerman RA, et al: Investigation of stroke in sickle cell disease by ^{1}H nuclear magnetic resonance spectroscopy, *Neuroradiology* 35:57-65, 1991.

287. Wasterlain CG: Effects of neonatal status epilepticus on rat brain development, *Neurology* 26:975-986, 1976.

288. Weber M, Grolimund P, Seiler RW: Evaluation of posttraumatic cerebral blood flow velocities by transcranial Doppler ultrasonography, *Neurosurgery* 27:106-112, 1990.

289. Weller RO, Shulman K: Infantile hydrocephalus: clinical, histological and ultrastructural study of brain damage, *J Neurosurg* 36:255-265, 1972.

290. Wickler DI, Weisbard AJ: Appropriate confusion over "brain death," *JAMA* 261:2246-2248, 1989.

291. Wilcox WD, Carrigan TA, Dooley KJ, et al: Range-gated pulsed Doppler ultrasonographic evaluation of carotid arterial blood flow in small preterm infants with patent ductus arteriosus, *J Pediatr* 102:294-298, 1983.

292. Wilkins RH: *Trauma-induced cerebral vasospasm.* In Wilkins RH, editor: *Cerebral arterial spasm,* Baltimore, 1980, Wilkins & Wilkins.

293. Williams MA, Razumovsky AY, Diringer M, Hanley DF: *Transcranial Doppler ultrasonography in the intensive care unit.* In Babikian VL, Wechsler LR, editors: *Transcranial Doppler ultrasonography,* St Louis, 1993, Mosby–Year Book.

294. Wolfson SK, Safar P, Reidi H, et al: Multifocal, dynamic cerebral hypoperfusion after prolonged cardiac arrest in dogs, measured by the stable xenon-CT technique, *Crit Care Med* 16:390, 1988.

295. Wright LL, Baker KR, Hollander DI, et al: Cerebral blood flow velocity in term infants: changes associated with ductal flow, *J Pediatr* 112:768-773, 1988.

296. Yabumoto M, Funahashi K, Fujii T, et al: Moyamoya disease associated with intracranial aneurysm, *Surg Neurol* 20:20-24, 1983.

297. Yamashima T, Kashihhara K, Ikeda K, Three phases of cerebral arteriopathy in meningitis: vasospasm and vasodilatation followed by organic stenosis, *Neurosurgery* 16:546-553, 1985.

298. Yashon D, Jane JA, Sugar D: The course of severe untreated hydrocephalus: prognostic significance of the cerebral mantle, *J Neurosurg* 23:509-515, 1965.

299. Yoneda S, Nishimoto A, Nukada T, et al: To-and-fro movement and external escape of carotid arterial blood in brain death assessment: a Doppler ultrasonic study, *Stroke* 5:707-713, 1974.

300. Yoshioda H, Yoshioda H: Arterial occlusion in purulent meningitis and multicystic encephalomalacia, *Eur J Pediatr* 139:303-305, 1982.

301. Youngner SJ: Brain death and organ retrieval: a cross-sectional survey of knowledge and concepts among health care professionals, *JAMA* 261:2205-2210, 1989.

302. Zaritsky A, Nadkarni V, Getson P, Kuehl K: CPR in children, *Ann Emerg Med* 16:1107-1111, 1987.

303. Zee S, Segall HD, Ahmandi J, et al: *Computed tomography in head trauma.* In Wilkins RH, Rengachary SS, editors: *Neurosurgery,* New York, 1985, McGraw-Hill.

304. Zhang ZG, Chopp M, Zaloga C, et al: Cerebral endothelial nitric oxide synthetase expression after focal cerebral ischemia in rats, *Stroke* 24:2016-2022, 1993.

305. Zimmerman RA, Bilanik LT, Bruce DA, et al: Computed tomography of pediatric head trauma: acute general cerebral swelling, *Radiology* 126:403-408, 1978.

306. Zucarello EF, Facco E, Zampieri P, et al: Severe head injury in children: early prognosis and outcome, *Childs Nerv Syst* 23:158-162, 1985.

Real-Time Neuromuscular Sonography: Technique, Normals, and Pathology

Asma Fischer

Neuromuscular sonography has been successfully used for imaging muscles and nerves in the evaluation of diseases of the muscles and nerves in children and adults.[1-3,13,16,20]

METHOD

The standardized method for examining muscles has been well described.[9,11] By adherence to the standardized method, the intertest and interpatient variability is kept at a minimum. Because muscle size, depth, and characteristics change with age and maturity, each ultrasound laboratory should have its own reference set of sonographic norms of several subjects who have no evidence of neuromuscular disease in the three major age groups: newborn to 12 months, 12 months to 5 years, and 5 years to adult.

Any standard high-resolution real-time ultrasound equipment can be used. At the time of the sonogram, a muscle group, the depth gain compensation (DGC), overall gain, preprocessing and postprocessing, and persistence should be optimized for age and thick-ness of muscles being examined. The optimized technical combinations for each age group are then stored in the equipment memory for use in the sonography of patients with neuromuscular diseases.

For obtaining a successful examination of the muscles free of contraction and movement artifact, it is essential to relax the muscle being examined. Muscle sonography is best performed with the patient supine and in a comfortable position. Children can usually be reassured by sliding the transducer on the examiner's or the parent's arm, which demonstrates the benign nature of the test. Sonographic images in the transverse and longitudinal planes of all four limbs are documented at approximately the midsection of the imaged limb. This enables clarification of the anatomy and pathology and allows measurement of muscle, subcutaneous fat, and the ratio of skin to muscle and muscle to bone. Minor instrumental adjustments may occasionally be needed to optimize the image in patients with neuromuscular diseases, but major departures from the standardized methods can obscure subtle findings. In patients with

Table 33-1. Standard terms used for interpretation of sonographic variables in muscle disease

Sonographic variable	Descriptive terms
Echogenicity	
Intensity	Euechoic, hyperechoic, hypoechoic
Distribution	Homogenous, heterogeneous
Bone edge	Normal, diminished, indeterminate, absent
Bone shadow	Normal, diminished, indeterminate, absent
Fascial interfaces	Normal, diminished, indeterminate, absent

Adapted from *Neuromuscular diseases*. In Fornage B, editor: Fischer AQ: *Musculoskeletal ultrasound,* New York, 1995, Churchill Livingstone.

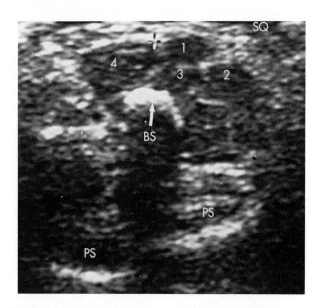

Fig. 33-1. Transverse sonogram of an infant with no muscle disease. *1,* Rectus femoris; *2,* vastus lateralis; *3,* vastus intermedius; *4,* vastus medialis; *arrow,* bone edge; *BS,* bone shadow; *SQ,* subcutaneous tissue/fat; *PS,* posterior surface of the thigh.

generalized neuromuscular disease in which the disease affects all the muscles, the sonographic evaluation can be done by sampling the muscles using the aforementioned method. However, in patchy muscle disease or cases of focal muscle involvement associated with localized peripheral neuropathy, it is advisable to sonogram the affected muscles in the distribution of the affected peripheral nerve. At the same time, a similar unaffected muscle of the opposite or same limb should be sonogrammed for comparison. Patients can be followed over time by using neuromuscular sonography to evaluate the natural history of a particular disease and/or the effect of therapy.

INTERPRETATION

An objective, consistent interpretation of the sonograms is desirable, especially if the patient is being followed linearly. A standardized method has been devised and successfully used clinically as it provides inter-interpreter reliability.

Each sonogram is described by using a standardized method. In any one neuromuscular sonogram, five major findings are described (Table 33-1). Subcutaneous fat and muscle thickness measurements are made. In normal muscle, fascial planes and bone edges appear hyperechoic; the bone edge is hyperechoic but casts a crisp shadow. Normal muscle parenchyma gives a somewhat less intense signal, termed *euechoic.* The exact signal intensity corresponding to the term *euechoic* differs slightly between age groups[9,11] (Figs. 33-1 and 33-2).

DISEASES PRIMARILY INVOLVING MUSCLES (MYOPATHIC)

For myopathic diseases in which almost all skeletal muscles are involved in the disease process, insonating the nondominant midarm and midthigh is sufficient; however, for patients with an inflammatory myopathy in

which the distribution of pathology is patchy, it is advisable to sonogram the clinically weak muscles first and then compare them to the clinically unaffected muscles. The major sonographic abnormality observed in myopathic disease is an alteration in the degree, site, and distribution of the echogenicity. An increase in muscle parenchymal echogenicity is the hallmark abnormality in these diseases.

Progressive muscular dystrophies

In the progressive muscular dystrophies such as Duchenne's muscular dystrophy, limb-girdle dystrophy, and Emery-Dreifuss dystrophy, the primary sonographic abnormality is characterized by a general increase in echogenicity in muscle parenchyma. The degree of abnormality on the sonogram often reflects the advancement of the disease; thus, the more the abnormal collection of fibrous tissue and the degeneration and replacement of the muscle with other tissue are apparent, the more abnormal the sonogram.

Early in disease, the muscle is mildly affected, and an increase in the muscle parenchymal echogenicity is noted without major loss of anatomic landmarks. As the disease ravages the muscle parenchyma, these changes are reflected in the sonogram as loss of anatomic landmarks and marked increase in granular echogenicity, in the muscle parenchyma reminiscent of a snowstorm. In the most advanced disease, this blizzard like echogenic haze obliterates almost all the usual anatomic landmarks and, in mild cases, causes diminution of the landmarks (Fig. 33-3). The hallmark of myopathies is a

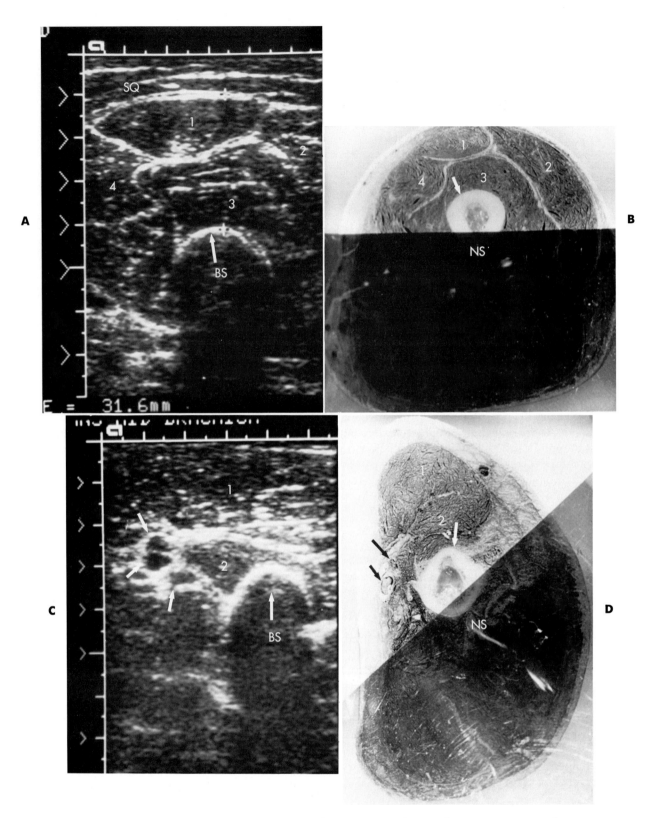

Fig. 33-2. A, Transverse sonogram midthigh in a normal adult. *Area between cursors,* muscle thickness; *1,* rectus femoris; *2,* vastus lateralis; *3,* vastus intermedius; *4,* vastus medialis; *arrow,* bone edge; *BS,* bone shadow; *SQ,* subcutaneous tissue/fat. **B,** Transverse anatomic section of midthigh in an adult without muscle disease. *1,* Rectus femoris; *2,* vastus lateralis; *3,* vastus intermedius; *4,* vastus medialis; *arrow,* bone edge; *NS,* areas not visualized by sonography. **C,** Transverse sonogram midarm in a normal adult. *1,* Biceps; *2,* brachialis; *thin arrows,* brachial vessels; *arrow,* bone edge; *BS,* bone shadow. **D,** Transverse anatomic section of the midarm in an adult without muscle disease. *1,* Biceps; *2,* brachialis; thin arrows, brachial vessels; *arrow,* bone edge; *NS,* areas not visualized by sonography.

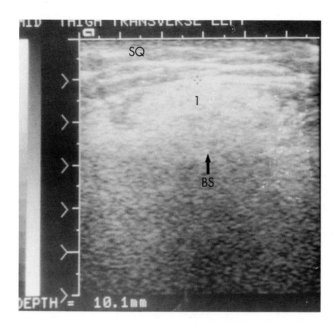

Fig. 33-3. Transverse sonogram midthigh in a child with advanced Duchenne's muscular dystrophy. *Cursor,* muscle, subcutaneous interface; *SQ,* subcutaneous fat; *I,* hyperechoic muscle parenchyma, obliterating the myofascial interfaces; *arrow,* diminished bone edge; *BS,* bone shadow is no longer crisp.

generalized increase in muscle parenchymal echogenecity and decreased clarity of the the myofascial planes, bone edge, and boneshadow.[4,15]

The sonographic findings on myotonic dystrophies are varied. Some reports indicate abnormalities with increased echogenicity, but at other times the sonograms may be normal. Therefore, a normal sonogram on a patient suspected of having myotonic dystrophy does not rule out the disease.[17]

Congenital muscular dystrophies

Both Fukuyama and occidental type of congenital muscular dystrophies (CMD) present in early infancy with hypotonia.[12,17] Sonographic findings in patients with CMD are characterized by a generalized increase of muscle parenchymal echogenecity in selected muscles, such as the quadriceps vasti, and may spare the rectus femoris.[19] This pattern of selective muscle involvement may also occur in inflammatory myopathies, but inflammatory myopathies seldom occur in infants.

Congenital myopathies

Infants with congenital myopathies usually present clinically as floppy infants. Early in diseases such as nemaline body myopathy, central core disease, and myotubular myopathy, the sonogram may appear normal. As the disease progresses, a mild to moderate increase in echogenicity is noted.[17]

Metabolic myopathies

In those metabolic myopathies in which the material deposited in the muscles is a normal component of the muscle, such as glycogen, and the muscle architecture is not disturbed significantly, the sonographic picture is not abnormal; patients with glycogen storage disease and Kearns-Sayre disease usually have unaffected sonograms. Increased echogenicity may be seen in the muscles of patients with mitochondrial myopathies, but the findings are variable.[15]

Inflammatory myopathies

Polymyositis and dermatomyositis are characterized by a patchy distribution of muscle pathology. The individual muscles affected by the disease in inflammatory myopathies (IMD) demonstrate increased echogenicity. A patchy distribution of hyperechoic muscles in the extremities is seen on sonography, along with a relative decrease in bone edge and myofascial planes (Figs. 33-4 and 33-5). With regression of disease, the muscles do not usually return to their completely normal state but retain a mild increase in echogenicity or reflect signs of denervation, particularly if the disease has been severe and of long duration (Table 33-2).[19]

Sonography is particularly helpful to the clinician in patients with IMD. Early in the disease, the distribution of the echogenicity correlates with the affected group of muscles. As the disease advances, all muscles of the group become affected, and hyperechogenicity spreads to all the muscles.[5,6] In a study correlating muscle biopsy findings with sonographic findings in IMD patients, a significant correlation was found between abnormal bone edge and perivascular inflammation, abnormal bone shadow and fat replacement, and abnormal myofascial interfaces and necrosis. In the same study, the ratio of the distance between skin to muscle and muscle to bone correlated best with the presence of fat replacement and presence of vacuoles[8] (Table 33-3). At the time of biopsy site selection, ideally the sample should be taken from an area of the diseased muscle, but because the disease is patchy, a blind site selection may miss the pathologic muscle and give an erroneous diagnostic result. Visualization of the diseased muscle by ultrasound is recommended, as it gives optimum site selection for biopsy material.[14]

NEUROPATHIES

The main sonographic abnormality associated with neuropathies is hyperechogenicity of the muscle parenchyma, but the differentiation of this increase in echogenicity from myopathies is in the characteristic distribution of the echogenicity. This particular type of distribution is termed *heterogeneous,* which means that within a single muscle, areas of increased echogenicity, as

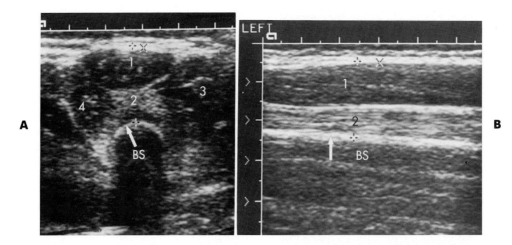

Fig. 33-4. A, Transverse sonogram midthigh of a child with moderately severe polymyositis. *Cursor,* muscle thickness; *1,* rectus femoris, which is normal in echogenicity or relatively hypoechoic; *2,* hyperechoic vastus intermedius; *3,* vastus lateralis; *4,* vastus medialis; *arrow,* bone edge; *BS,* bone shadow. **B,** Longitudinal sonogram midthigh of a child with moderately severe polymyositis. *Cursors,* muscle thickness; *1,* rectus femoris, which is normal in echogenicity or relatively hypoechoic; *2,* hyperechoic vastus intermedius; *arrow,* bone edge; *BS,* bone shadow.

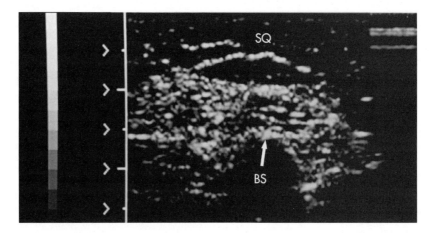

Fig. 33-5. Transverse sonogram midarm of the patient in Fig. 33-4, with now advanced polymyositis and severe weakness. All muscles of the midarm are hyperechoic with loss of distinction of the myofascial planes. *Arrow,* Bone edge has diminished clarity; *BS,* bone shadow; *SQ,* subcutaneous fat.

well as low or normal echogenicity, are found (Table 33-4).[4]

Peripheral and focal neuropathies

The best approach for imaging the muscles of a patient with peripheral neuropathy is to be cognizant of the muscles supplied by the abnormal nerve. In the path of the affected peripheral nerve, signs of denervation manifest reflected as areas of low echogenicity alternating with areas of normal echogenicity within a muscle[4] (Figs. 33-6 and 33-7; Table 33-5).

Hereditary sensorimotor neuropathy

Sonography of the distal muscles in patients with hereditary sensorimotor neuropathy (HSMN) reveals an increase in muscle echogenicity and a loss of muscle mass due to atrophy. It has been reported that in HSMN the distribution of the sonographic abnormality may be proximal in some cases, and the lower extremities may be more involved than the upper. In some cases of HSMN type 1, the muscles may be sonographically normal.[15]

Spinal muscular atrophy

The classical pattern of early but established disease findings in floppy babies with spinal muscular atrophy (SMA) is a heterogeneous increase in muscle parenchymal echogenicity, found within the muscle parenchyma of each muscle, giving it a "moth eaten" appearance, that is, areas of increased echogenicity with islands of hypoechoic or normal echogenicity within one muscle.

Table 33-2. Sonography of myopathies: comparison of sonographic characteristics of progressive dystrophies and inflammatory myopathies

Sonogram findings	Progressive dystrophies	Inflammatory myopathies
Echo degree	Increased	Increased
Site	All muscles	Individual muscles
Type	Homogeneous	Homogeneous
Bone edge	Diminished	Preserved or diminished
Bone shadow	Diminished	Usually preserved or diminished
Affected muscles	All	Patchy
Muscle thickness	Increased/ unaffected	Decreased or unchanged

Adapted from *Neuromuscular diseases.* In Fornage B, editor: Fischer AQ: *Musculoskeletal ultrasound,* New York, 1995, Churchill Livingstone.

Table 33-3. Summary of muscle biopsy and sonography correlates in inflammatory myopathy

Ultrasound	Biopsy
Inc echogenicity	Necrosis
	Perifascicular atrophy
Dec bone edge	Fat replacement
	Perivascular inflammation
	Conn tissue replacement
Dec bone shadow	Fat replacement
Dec fascial interfaces	Conn tissue replacement
	Necrosis
	Perivascular inflammation
Inc stm/mtb ratio	Conn tissue replacement
	Fat replacement
Dec stm/mtb	Vacuoles

Inc, Increased; *dec,* decreased; *conn,* connective; *stm,* skin to muscle distance; *mtb,* muscle to bone.[8]

The changes in echogenicity of muscle parenchyma may also be associated with decreases in the echogenicity of the bone edge and indistinguishable or diminished myofascial interfaces. The bone shadow is preserved until late in the disease process. The moth eaten appearance of the muscle parenchyma is the earliest diagnostic change detected by ultrasound[4,7] (Fig. 33-8). In patients with SMA, sonographic abnormalities may be found in all muscle groups. In peripheral neuropathies, only the muscles supplied by the affected nerve are sonographically abnormal.

DIFFERENTIAL DIAGNOSIS

The clinical presenting symptom of hypotonia in floppy infants is not always due to a neuromuscular disorder, and differentiating the nonneuromuscular etiologies from neuromuscular disease is a challenge to the diagnostician. Even though floppy infants with

Table 33-4. Sonographic characteristics in myopathies and neuropathies

Sonogram findings	Myopathies	Neuropathies
Echogenicity	Increased	Increased
Type of echo	Homogeneous	Heterogeneous
Site of echo	Entire muscle	Part within a muscle
Bone edge	Moderately decreased	Mildly decreased
Bone shadow	Diminished	Relatively preserved
Affected muscles	Proximal or all	Distal or focal
Muscle thickness	Increased or unchanged	Decreased

Adapted from *Neuromuscular diseases.* In Fornage B, editor: Fischer AQ: *Musculoskeletal ultrasound,* New York, 1995, Churchill Livingstone.

cerebral palsy, Prader-Willi syndrome, or lax ligaments may mimic some of the symptoms of neuromuscular disease, on sonography the muscles of these patients are usually normal.[4,15] The features of muscle masses are noted in Table 33-6.[10]

SUMMARY

Most progressive myopathies demonstrate muscle parenchymal abnormalities by sonography. The intensity and extent of findings depend on the degree and type of the disease. Even though increased echogenicity, which is a hallmark abnormality of muscle disease, is a nonspecific change, the site, distribution, and intensity of the echogenicity may guide the clinician to the diagnosis and assist in choosing specific tests for making a definite pathologic diagnosis. The majority of metabolic or storage myopathies are not easily identifiable on ultrasound unless significant architectural distortion has taken place.[4] The best use of sonography for the clinician is in the management of IMD, initially for biopsy site selection and then as an objective method of evaluating the affected muscles while therapy is being instituted. In some cases of IMD, the ultrasound abnormalities at the onset of disease may precede the clinical changes and give the clinician a window of time to plan treatment before the patient becomes significantly weak. Sonographic recovery of muscle architecture after a prolonged bout of IMD may succeed apparent clinical recovery, and in some cases, even though the patient may regain strength, the muscle may never return to complete normality on sonography.

Most neuropathies are evident on sonography. The abnormal muscles can be searched out and identified if the distribution of the affected nerve is known to the examiner. Other neuropathies, such as SMA, can be identified by their classical pattern, which is widespread in most of the arm and thigh muscles. Neuromuscular disease affecting the neuromuscular junction, such as

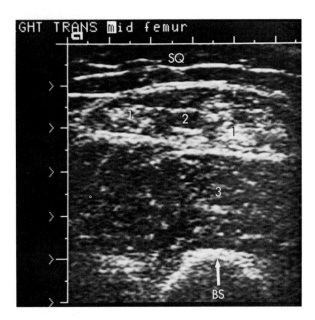

Fig. 33-6. Transverse sonogram midthigh in an adult patient with focal neuropathy leading to atrophy of the rectus femoris. *SQ,* Subcutaneous tissue; *1,* hyperechoic areas within the rectus femoris; *2,* hypoechoic areas within the rectus femoris; *3,* vastus intermedius with normal echogenicity; *arrow,* bone edge; *BS,* normal bone shadow. (From Fischer AQ: *Neuromuscular diseases.* In Fornage B, editor: *Musculoskeletal ultrasound,* New York, 1995, Churchill Livingstone.)

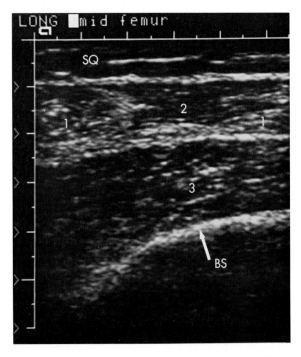

Fig. 33-7. Longitudinal sonogram of the patient in Fig. 33-6. SQ, Subcutaneous tissue; *1,* hyperechoic areas within the rectus femoris; *2,* hypoechoic area within the rectus femoris; *3,* vastus intermedius with normal echogenecity; *arrow,* bone edge; *BS,* normal bone shadow. (From Fischer AQ: *Neuromuscular diseases.* In Fornage B, editor: *Musculoskeletal ultrasound,* New York, 1995, Churchill Livingstone.)

Table 33-5. Sonography of neuropathies: sonographic characteristics of focal neuropathies and spinal muscular atrophy

Sonogram findings	Peripheral neuropathies	Spinal muscular atrophy
Echo	Mild increase	Moderate increase
Site	Focal	Multiple muscles
Type	Heterogeneous	Heterogeneous
Atrophy	Focal	General/late

Adapted from *Neuromuscular diseases.* In Fornage B, editor: Fischer AQ: *Musculoskeletal ultrasound,* New York, 1995, Churchill Livingstone.

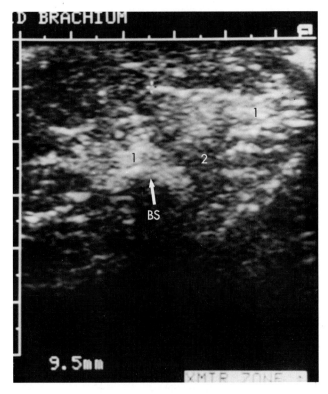

Fig. 33-8. Transverse sonogram of the midarm of a child with spinal muscular atrophy. *1,* hyperechoic areas within the arm muscles; *2,* hypoechoic or relatively normal areas of echogenicity within the arm muscles; *Arrow,* smeared bone edge; *BS,* bone shadow. (From Fischer AQ: *Neuromuscular diseases.* In Fornage B, editor: *Musculoskeletal ultrasound,* New York, 1995, Churchill Livingstone.)

myasthenia gravis, is not visualized with current methods of ultrasonography and remains a challenge for future ultrasound researchers (Table 33-7).

Most neuromuscular diseases are progressive, and an initial normal sonogram may not rule out disease. Serial muscle sonograms on patients who demonstrate progressive symptomatology are indicated for diagnostic purposes, as well as for timely and appropriate planning of

Table 33-6. Ultrasound findings in muscle masses

Diagnosis	Ultrasound finding	Adjacent muscle
Abscess	Anechoic with echoic core	Hyperechoic
Hematoma	Anechoic	Normal
Neoplasm	Hyperechoic	Variable
Contraction	Myofascial planes compressed	Normal
Pyomyositis (early)	Hyperechoic, swollen muscle	Normal

Table 33-7. Comparison of computerized neuromuscular sonography (CRS) and electromyography (EMG) in the recognition of patterns associated with neuromuscular conditions

Characteristics	CRS	EMG
1. Dx neuropathy	yes	yes
2. Type of neuropathy	no	yes
3. Dx myopathy	yes	yes
4. Type of myopathy	occ.	no
5. Floppy infants	yes	?
6. Motor neuron disease	yes	yes
7. Progression of disease	yes	?
8. Biopsy site selection	yes	no
9. Punch biopsy under vision	yes	no
10. NM transmission defects	?	yes

Dx, Diagnosis; *?,* uncertain or nonspecific findings; *NM,* neuromuscular.

Advantages of neuromuscular sonography

1. High resolution of normal anatomy
2. Minimum patient preparation
3. Maximum patient cooperation
4. Ready availability
5. No known risk factors
6. Reliably reproducible
7. Objective data for longitudinal studies
8. Less expensive than CT or MRI

CT, Computed tomography: *MRI,* magnetic resonance imaging. Modified from Fischer AQ, Stephens S: Computerized real-time neuromuscular sonography: a new application, techniques, and methods, *J Child Neurol* 3:69-74, 1988.

further investigations such as muscle biopsy and electromyography. In this day and age of fiscal consciousness, it is best to identify the abnormal muscles on the sonogram prior to launching an expensive and extensive investigation. This statement holds true only for those patients whose sonographic findings are well established and have been well correlated with biopsy findings,

---

Limitations of neuromuscular ultrasound

1. Normals for age
2. Standardization of settings
3. Not diagnostic for all types of neuromuscular disease
4. Operator-dependent

---

which include most of the progressive muscular dystrophies, spinal muscular atrophies, and inflammatory myopathies.[8,14,17] The advantages and limitations of neuromuscular sonography are noted in the accompanying boxes.

REFERENCES

1. Bowen PA II, Wynn JJ, Fischer AQ, et al: Nontropical pyomyositis in renal allograft recipient, *Transplantation* 47:539-541, 1989.
2. Fischer AQ: Pediatric applications of clinical ultrasound, *Neurosurg Clin N Am* 8:759-774, 1990.
3. Fischer AQ: *Neuromuscular diseases.* In Fornage B, editor: *Musculoskeletal ultrasound,* New York, 1995, Churchill Livingstone.
4. Fischer AQ, Carpenter DW, Hartlage PL, et al: Muscle imaging in neuromuscular disease using computerized real-time sonography, *Muscle Nerve* 11:270-275, 1988.
5. Fischer AQ, Hartlage PL, Carroll J: Inflammatory myopathies of childhood: diagnosis and follow-up by computerized realtime sonography, *Ann Neurol* 22:451, 1987.
6. Fischer AQ, Longenecker E: Muscle sonography in inflammatory myopathic disease, *Ann Neurol* 30:502, 1991.
7. Fischer AQ, Longenecker E: *Spinal muscular atrophy* In Fleckenstein JL, Crues JV, Reimers CD, editors: *Imaging skeletal muscle in health and disease,* Springer-Verlag, New York (in press).
8. Fischer AQ, Longenecker E, Trefz J: Muscle sonography and biopsy correlates in inflammatory myopathic disease, *Ann Neurol* 32:438, 1992.
9. Fischer AQ, Stephens S: Computerized real-time neuromuscular sonography: a new application, techniques, and methods, *J Child Neurol* 3:69-74, 1988.
10. Fincher RME, Jackson MJ, Fischer AQ: Pyomyositis caused by *Citrobacter Freundii:* a case and analysis of the diagnostic utility of neuromuscular ultrasound in two additional cases, *Am J Med Sci* 299:331-333, 1990.
11. Fornage BD: *Ultrasonography of muscles and tendons: examination technique and atlas of normal anatomy of the extremities,* New York, 1989, Springer-Verlag.
12. Fukuyama Y, Osawa M, Suzuki H: Congenital progressive muscular dystrophy of the Fukuyama type: clinical genetic and pathological considerations, *Brain Dev* 3:1-29, 1981.
13. Heckmatt JZ, Dubowitz V: *Diagnosis of spinal muscular atrophy with pulse echo ultrasound imaging.* In Gamstorp I, Sarnat HB, editors: *Progressive spinal muscular atrophies,* New York, 1984, Raven Press.
14. Heckmatt JZ, Dubowitz V: Diagnostic advantage of needle biopsy in the diagnosis of selective involvement in muscle disease, *J Child Neurol* 2:205-213, 1987.
15. Heckmatt JZ, Dubowitz V: Realtime ultrasound imaging of muscles, *Muscle Nerve* 11:56-65, 1988.
16. Hicks JE, Shawker TH, Jones BL, et al: Diagnostic ultrasound: its use in the evaluation of muscle, *Arch Phys Med Rehabil* 65:129-131, 1984.
17. Lamminen A, Jaaskelainen, J, Juhani R, Suramo I: High-frequency

ultrasonography of skeletal muscle in children with neuromuscular disease, *J Ultrasound Med* 7:505, 1988.

18. McMenamin JB, Becker LE, Murphy EG: Congenital muscular dystrophy: a clinicopathologic report of 24 cases, *J Pediatr* 100:692-697, 1982.

19. Topaloglu H, Gucuyener K, Yalaz K, et al: Selective involvement of quadriceps muscle in congenital muscular dystrophies: an ultrasonic study, *Brain Dev* 14:84-87, 1992.

20. Young A, Hughes I, Russel P, et al: Measurements if quadriceps muscle wasting by ultrasonography, *Rheumatol Rehabil* 19:141-148, 1980.

34

Neuromuscular Sonography: Anatomic Basis and Dynamic Approach

Francis O. Walker

NORMAL MUSCLE ANATOMY

Muscle tissue, the system that enables humans to interact with the environment, comprises approximately 45% of human body weight. Its actions range from delicate expressive movements of the face to feats of athletic skill and power. A variety of disorders can affect muscles directly, as in the case of the inflammatory myopathies and muscular dystrophies, or indirectly, as in the case of peripheral nerve damage or vasculitis.

Of nervous system tissues, the muscles are the easiest for clinicians to study. They can be examined not only by inspection, palpation, and strength testing but also by a variety of accepted laboratory techniques, including serum enzyme measurement, electromyography, and biopsy. Imaging modalities, including computed tomography (CT), magnetic resonance imaging (MRI), and radionucleide scans, are not as well established but offer unique information. Proper appreciation of all available techniques for investigating the neuromuscular system helps place the role of sonography in perspective as a clinical and research tool.

Applications of sonography to the study of skeletal muscle are relatively new. This chapter reviews aspects of muscle anatomy and physiology relevant to sonography and then describes muscle imaging techniques and normal findings.

Types of muscle

Of the three types of muscle, ultrasound has been used to study smooth muscles (arterial walls and myometrium) and cardiac muscle (echocardiography) more than skeletal muscle.

The microanatomy of cardiac muscle differs from that of striated muscle in several ways. Cardiac muscle cells branch and anastomose in a semiirregular pattern, presumably enhancing the ability to constrict their vascular chambers. In contrast, skeletal muscle fibers stack neatly in linear rows and columns. The fibrous tissue and bone insertions necessary for skeletal attachments are absent in cardiac muscle.[25]

Although, in the past, sonographic evaluation of the heart has primarily looked at dynamic and vascular aspects of cardiac function (e.g., valvular movement, wall movement, embolus detection), recent studies have also indicated that imaging of the muscle itself can be clinically informative.[5,19,20]

Skeletal or striated muscle. At its most fundamental level, muscle is organized into highly redundant patterns of actin and myosin filaments.[25] These combine to form the banding patterns of muscle visible by light microscopy. The muscle fibers themselves are grouped as tightly packed cylinders, with flattened but longitudinally oriented nuclei at their periphery. Each myocyte is sheathed with thin layers of connective tissue.

Interspersed within the muscle matrix are nerves and blood vessels. They typically enter the muscle closer to its origin (the more fixed attachment point of the muscle) than to its insertion, in the form of a neurovascular bundle,[25] and these entry points are fairly consistent across different individuals. The nerve fibers divide, and each motor nerve typically innervates multiple noncontiguous muscle fibers. The sum of all the muscle fibers innervated by a single motor nerve comprises a motor unit, and it represents the basic functional unit of muscle.

After branching out, the vasculature of the muscle tends to run longitudinally with the fibers, with interspersed transverse anastomoses. The blood supply of the muscle can be divided into nutritive and nonnutritive pathways. The nutritive pathway, as described previously, supplies the muscle fibers along their length in capillary form. The nonnutritive pathway consists of arterioles that pass directly into draining veins without capillaries. These vessels are typically located at the periphery of muscle and presumably act as shunts when intense muscle contraction interferes with the nutritive supply. Under such conditions, the muscle functions anaerobically.

Muscle supporting structures

Muscles vary considerably in shape, size, and form; to what extent this variation relates to differential involvement of muscles in different disease states (e.g., eye muscle sparing in motor neuron disease, proximal involvement in inflammatory myopathy) is unknown. However, general patterns of muscle structure are relevant to imaging and are addressed later in this chapter.

Muscles take a variety of forms and generally can be classified as parallel, oblique, or spiralized, according to the orientation of their fibers. Strap muscles are typical of the parallel group with fibers parallel to the primary direction of muscle contraction; the sternocleidomastoid is a representative example. The dorsal interossei are typical of oblique muscles with bipennate or featherlike muscle fibers attaching to a central linear aponeurosis. Other muscles, such as latissimus dorsi, have a spiralized attachment, rotating fully 180° between origin and insertion. The insertion, origin, and function of individual muscles determine their fiber orientation.[25]

Collagen is the major component of tendons, apo-neuroses, and fasciae. The irregular and coarse disposition of collagen fibrils in these tissues gives these structures their iridescent glow. The relatively sparse vasculature is associated with their whitish color. Tendons and aponeuroses are relatively flexible in shape but invariant in length because of their substantive collagen component.

MUSCLE PHYSIOLOGY

The central control of movement involves a complex and incompletely understood interaction of brain and spinal cord nuclei. Nonetheless, after central processing is complete, final common pathway of movement is contraction of a motor unit. Each muscle possesses multiple different sizes of motor units, ranging from several muscle fibers to hundreds. With the slightest activation of muscle, the smallest motor unit begins to discharge first, at a frequency of approximately 5 Hz. With increasing force, this unit increases its firing frequency up to 8 to 12 Hz, and then it is joined by a slightly larger motor unit. This process repeats itself until multiple motor units recruit at frequencies as high as 50 Hz.[3,4,12,24]

The end result of this preprogrammed sequence of motor unit recruitment is exquisite control of the force of contraction. Such control is not brought about by the conscious selection of individual motor units but rather by control only of increments of motor unit firing rates and motor unit recruitment.[3]

The scattered distribution of different-sized motor units in muscle and the recruitment of new motor units at different firing frequencies than their predecessors ensure temporal and anatomic desynchronization of motor unit firing in muscle. This diffuse and asynchronous activation of muscle fibers within a muscle is critical for the maintenance of smooth contraction. Even slight degrees of motor unit firing synchrony can disturb contraction. Central programming errors that lead to such synchrony are thought to underlie essential tremor disorders.[26]

Muscles contract by an active process of shortening. Using ATP, actin and myosin filaments climb each other, shortening the muscle and expanding its girth. In addition to performing mechanical work, contracting muscle generates vibration. By cupping the hands over one's ears and intermittently tightening the palms, the vibrations in the audible dimension can be heard in the form of a low-pitched rumbling.[2]

ELECTROMYOGRAPHY

Electromyography is a technique for evaluating muscle that involves sampling small areas with a recording electrode needle. The electrical signals recorded by muscle in this technique prove to be of considerable diagnostic value. The electrical activity of

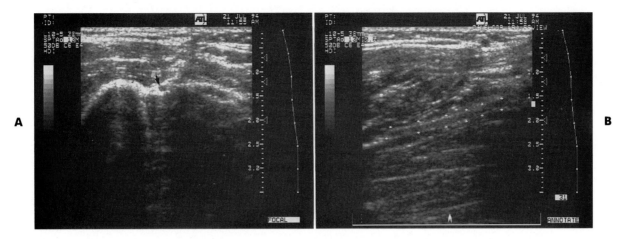

Fig. 34-1. A transverse (**A**) and longitudinal (**B**) image of the ulnar nerve (*arrow, asterisks*) proximal to the cubital tunnel.

muscle, although it often correlates with its mechanical activity,[2] differs in certain substantive ways. For example, the duration of the electrical component of a motor unit action potential is approximately 5 ms, but the duration of its actual mechanical contraction is approximately 300 ms.[12,23]

Electromyographic study of muscle is particularly relevant to ultrasound in that both techniques involve real-time evaluation. Both techniques can therefore be used to study static and dynamic properties of muscle, including muscle contraction, recruitment, fasciculations, cramp, myotonia, and myokymia. Further, sonography can demonstrate needle movement in muscle.

One useful location for an ultrasound instrument, in fact, is in the electromyography laboratory. Clinical examination, electrodiagnostic studies, and neuromuscular sonography may all provide valuable diagnostic information.

When imaging muscle, vascular structures are readily identified by either compressibility (veins) or pulsatile behavior. If necessary, M-mode can be used to verify their synchrony with a palpable pulse.

Imaging normal peripheral nerves is difficult, in part because of their small size, and in part because their echogenic properties often do not distinguish them clearly from surrounding tissues. The vascular component of the neurovascular bundle can be used to approximate the location of some nerves, even where the nerve itself does not stand out clearly. In areas where peripheral nerves are palpable, they can be imaged in some subjects (Fig. 34-1). Pathologically enlarged nerves, as in Charcot-Marie-Tooth disease, can be relatively easy to image.[14]

MICROANATOMIC CORRELATIONS OF STATIC IMAGES OF MUSCLE

Sonographic echoes in muscle arise at reflection points between tissues of different acoustic conduc-

tance. Muscle itself, in view of its highly organized and homogeneous structure, therefore presents no significant areas of reflectivity. However, where it abuts fibrous tissue, with its highly disorganized matrix, reflections occur. Muscles, therefore, have a distinctly heterogeneous appearance. Areas of hypoechoic tissue contrast with punctate linear areas, which correspond to the fibrous supporting matrix (Figs. 34-2 and 34-3).[23]

Proper understanding of the relationship of microanatomic features and imaging is critical because, in pathologic conditions, the normal reflecting pattern is distorted. Where muscle tissue is replaced by fat or fibrous tissue, acoustic conductance becomes more homogeneous in muscle, and the image becomes not only more echogenic but also more uniform.[7,15,16] The distinction between muscle and more echogenic structures such as bone becomes less clear.

DYNAMIC BEHAVIOR OF MUSCLE

Perhaps one of the least explored but most intriguing sonographic aspects of muscle is its dynamic behavior. During active muscle contraction, sonography reveals shortening and bulging of the muscle, information useful for kinesiologic assessment (Figs. 34-4 and 34-5). However, this is not a completely gradual and uniform process; rather, as muscle fibers bulge, they compete for space and, at irregular intervals, slip over one another to accommodate the volume change. In longitudinal section, the movements are much less apparent, but the extent and shape of the muscle bulging become grossly apparent.

Tendons, because of their more fibrous character, have a more echogenic and homogeneous appearance than muscle. They arise from the muscle tissue, and this area of gradual transition can be imaged.[6] Their movement, particularly, for example, at the wrist, is readily apparent when imaged in a longitudinal plane.

Benign fasciculations, a normal variant of healthy,

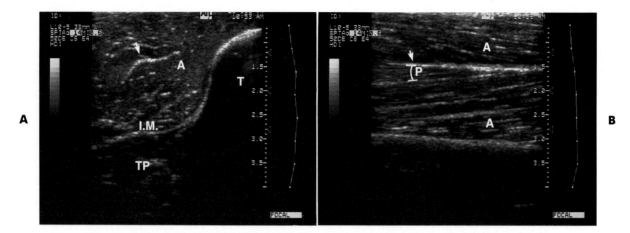

Fig. 34-2. Transverse (**A**) and sagittal (**B**) images of anterior tibialis. On the cross-section, note the centrally placed aponeurosis (*arrow*) at a depth of 1.3 to 1.7 cm. The bone edge of the tibia (*T*) provides sharp contrast. On the sagittal image, the aponeurosis (*arrow*) is seen at its mid-depth (1.5 cm), demonstrating the angle of pennation (*P*) of the muscle fibers. (*A,* Anterior tibialis; *IM,* interosseus membrane.)

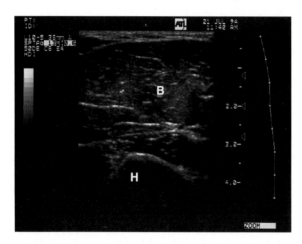

Fig. 34-3. The biceps (*B*) in the transverse plane. The humerus (*H*) is present at the bottom of the figure. Note the multiple fibrous tissue structures in the muscle.

dynamic muscle, occur sporadically in the population, sometimes in the gastrocnemius muscle after exercise.[12] Fasciculations represent the isolated contraction of individual motor units, scattered randomly throughout muscle. When they shorten, they create a local disturbance in muscle, apparent on the transverse image, where one area selectively thickens.[23] Although the thickening is not always apparent, fasciculations are often associated with a rotational twist that makes them easy to image.

In a muscle at rest, the slack elastic elements surrounding the contracting element allow for its movement to become apparent. Using M-mode imaging (or frame-by-frame counting), the duration of this type of muscle contraction can be easily measured, and typically such contractions are on the order of hundreds of milliseconds. Both the contraction and the relaxation

phase are apparent (Fig. 34-6). Fasciculations can be distinguished from pulses in muscle because they are random and not synchronous with the heart rate. Usually, fasciculations are distributed randomly throughout the muscle itself. They are readily distinguished from voluntary activation of muscle or central nervous system movements (e.g., tics, myoclonus, chorea) because only fasciculations are focal, scattered, and random.[12]

The behavior of muscle in isometric contraction is likewise of interest. Although such activity involves the contraction of hundreds of motor units, no motor unit movement can be resolved.[23] This relates to two phenomena. First, motor units recruit at frequencies of 5 Hz or greater. At this rate, there is considerable fusion of their mechanical contractions, without complete cycles of contraction and relaxation in between, as seen in fasciculations. The majority of units in actively contracting muscle fire much faster than 5 Hz, so many of the motor units show very little thickening and relaxing over time, and the variations so induced occur at frequencies beyond the resolution of ultrasound. Second, motor units are interspersed and fire asynchronously. As such, when looked at in the aggregate, the movement of individual motor units in muscle tissue blend together imperceptibly. From a mechanical perspective, such lack of gross or jerky synchrony is probably advantageous, for it maximizes control.[23]

Unlike electromyography, which demonstrates the activity of isometrically contracted muscle, ultrasound shows a relatively quiescent fixed image during such activity. Here, acoustic myography proves to be a useful corollary technique for measuring the work output of a seemingly fixed muscle. As each motor unit contracts and relaxes against the relatively elastic resistance of

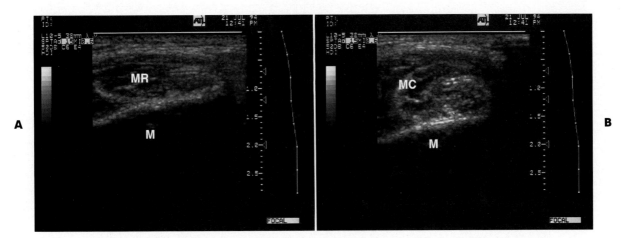

Fig. 34-4. These transverse figures demonstrate the masseter muscle at rest (**A**) and with voluntary isometric contraction (**B**). Note the 150% increase in cross sectional diameter. (*MR,* Masseter relaxed; *MC,* masseter contracted; *M,* mandible.)

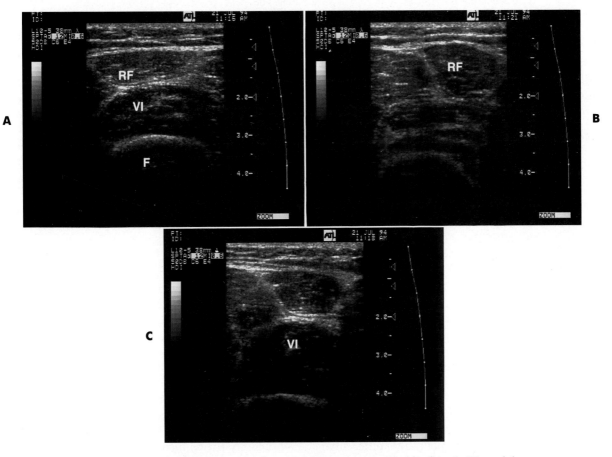

Fig. 34-5. These figures represent the quadriceps at rest (**A**) hip flexed (**B**) and knee hyperextended (**C**). The image is taken through the rectus femoris and vastus intermedius. Note that, with hip flexion, the rectus femoris thickens more than vastus intermedius, yet the reverse occurs with hyperextension of the knee. (*S,* Subcutaneous fat; *RF,* rectus femoris; *VI,* vastus intermedius; *F,* femur.)

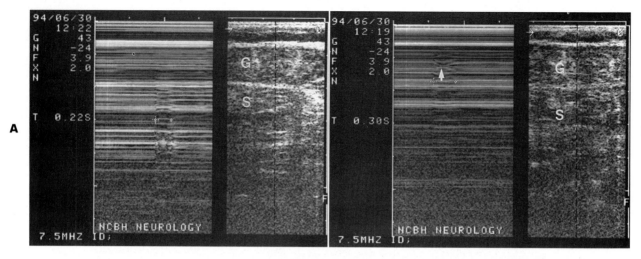

Fig. 34-6. Combined B-mode and M-mode images of fasciculations (*asterisks*) in a patient with the syndrome of benign fasciculations. **A,** The fasciculation localizes to soleus (*S*), sparing the medial gastrocnemius (*G*). The duration of the fasciculation is 220 ms. **B,** The fasciculation occurs in the gastrocnemius, and the soleus shows no contraction (although some shadow changes are present on the M-mode image). Also note that the most superficial portion of the gastrocnemius is uninvolved by the fasciculation. The peak contraction (arrows) of this fasciculation occurs at approximately 100 ms. The scan line on the B-mode images are indicated by the dashed lines.

muscle and tendon, it sets up vibrations. The sound of these vibrations (much of it below audible frequencies) is measurable and correlates fairly well with the force output of muscle.[2]

INDIVIDUAL MUSCLES

The study of muscle is complicated by their sheer number and anatomic diversity. However, several principles can be used to identify subsets of muscles particularly useful for the study of specific clinical disorders. From a sonographic standpoint, the most informative muscles should be of significant size, be close to an imaging surface, and have well-defined fascial boundaries. A number of such muscles are described in this chapter.

From a pathologic standpoint, distal muscles, such as the gastrocnemius and tibialis anterior, are most likely to be involved in peripheral neuropathies. Proximal muscles, such as deltoid, biceps, iliopsoas, and quadriceps femoris, are more likely to be involved in myopathic diseases. Screening for systemic disorders, then, at a minimum should involve a proximal and distal muscle pair, such as biceps and anterior tibialis. As in electromyography, however, the more that is known about the clinical features of the patient, the differential diagnoses, and the distribution of findings common to the diagnoses entertained, the better the physician can select appropriate muscles for sonographic study.

Anterior tibialis

The anterior tibialis, a pennate muscle, has a characteristic aponeurosis apparent on transverse image in its center. Deep to it, across the interosseus membrane, lies the tibialis posterior. At the edge of the tibia, just above the interosseus fascia, is the neurovascular complex. The tibia itself lies alongside the muscle and provides a bright reflective surface for reference. The tibialis anterior presents a relatively flat surface that makes imaging relatively simple; furthermore, because of its tight compartment, it is not particularly subject to compression artifact (Figs. 34-2 and 34-7). Reliable cross-sectional measurements can be made of this muscle by using a standardized protocol.[13]

Abductor hallucis and extensor digitorum brevis

The abductor hallucis and extensor digitorum brevis are small muscles surrounded by the small bones of the foot. Like other superficial small muscles, a standoff pad is helpful for imaging. Unlike the massive tibia, these bones may have no clear bone edge. The muscle itself tends to be highly echolucent. Fasciculations are common in this muscle, either as benign fasciculations or as a result of the chronic repetitive trauma to this muscle from walking and running. The extensor digitorum brevis is somewhat less likely to be traumatized and is readily imaged (Fig. 34-8). Following injections of botulinum toxin, measurable atrophy occurs in this muscle.[9]

Gastrocnemius

Sonography reveals the distinct medial and lateral heads of the gastrocnemius muscle superficial to and distinct from the soleus (Fig. 34-6). Because the fibula is small and without distinct bone edge on ultrasound, this

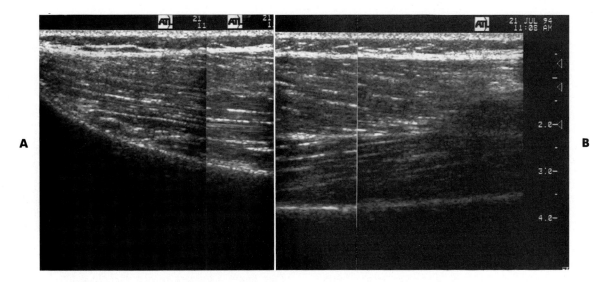

Fig. 34-7. A composite sagittal image spanning proximal (**A**) and distal (**B**) portions of the anterior tibialis. Sequential scans can be used to study entire muscles in detail.

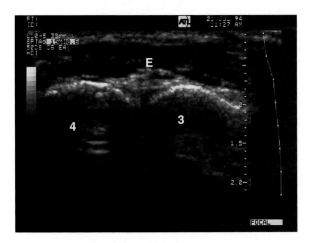

Fig. 34-8. An image of extensor digitorum brevis (*E*). This muscle overlies the third (*3*) and fourth (*4*) metatarsal bones at its greatest bulk, here shown in transverse section. It can sometimes be atrophied in otherwise healthy individuals.

muscle, although sometimes apparent in the studies, provides relatively poor referential bone material in the images obtained.

Quadriceps

The quadriceps group of four muscles—the vastus medialis, vastus lateralis, vastus intermedius, and rectus femoris—represents an ideal proximal group of muscles for study (Fig. 34-5). They are relatively susceptible to compression artifact but otherwise are anatomically consistent and large, and they have the femur for contrast.

A striking example of kinesiologic variation is evident in these muscles, which are considered an agonist group. With attempted fixing of the knee (i.e., forcible extension at the knee joint), the vastus intermedius bulges considerably, with relatively little bulging in rectus femoris. With forcible flexion of the hip, the rectus femoris bulges with little change in vastus intermedius.

It is difficult to incorporate a complete image of all the muscles in this group, but, for standard purposes, a single image through the bellies of the rectus femoris and vastus intermedius is informative. Pennate angles can be readily measured in these muscles.[17]

Iliopsoas

The iliopsoas is a proximal muscle that is somewhat more difficult to image than the quadriceps complex. Fat and fibrous tissue at the inguinal ligament may obscure it somewhat. It acts to flex at the hip.

First dorsal interosseus and abductor pollicis

The first dorsal interosseus and abductor pollicis represent two hand muscles commonly involved in peripheral neuropathy, mononeuropathy (carpal tunnel syndrome and tardy ulnar palsy), lower trunk brachial plexopathies, and C8 radiculopathies. Because of their size and immediately superficial location, they can be difficult to image. This is further complicated by difficulties getting the transducer to line up in the hollows presented by the hand and by the angular directions of their pennate fibers. The small bones in the area do not present a sharp bone edge (Fig. 34-9).

Fortunately, simple inspection is usually quite sufficient to identify atrophy or disease within these muscles, and they are readily tested clinically and with neurophysiologic techniques. A standoff agar gel may improve images, particularly if the muscle is atrophic.

Flexor digitorum profundus

Because of their number, close proximity, faintness of separating fascial planes, and agonistic activation pat-

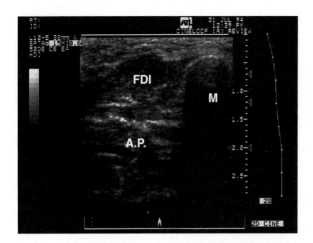

Fig. 34-9. First dorsal interosseous (*FDI*) shown in a transverse plane. This image is magnified somewhat more than those of larger muscles. Note the relatively faint bone edge of the second metacarpal (*M*) and the fascial plane separating first dorsal interosseus from the adductor pollicis (*AP*).

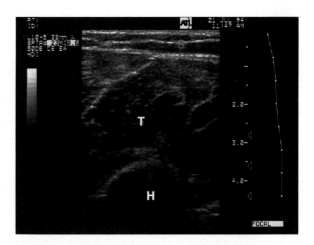

Fig. 34-10. A transverse image of the triceps (*T*) showing its relatively hypoechoic nature; the humerus (*H*) is at the bottom of the figure. Compare to Fig. 34-7. In general, the thickest layer of subcutaneous fat (*S*) in the upper extremity overlies this muscle.

terns, forearm muscles can be taxing to identify by ultrasound. Nonetheless, they can be important. One recent study suggests that inclusion body myositis selectively involves flexor digitorum profundus.[18] A cross-sectional atlas of forearm muscles is recommended for any detailed investigation.

Biceps

The biceps contains a prominent neurovascular bundle. It is an easy muscle to image with the humerus as a bony reference. Because of its length and range of shortening, contractile behavior is easy to study in this muscle (Fig. 34-3).

Deltoid

The compact deltoid muscle overlies the humerus and has relatively little superficial fat above it. Its striations are particularly easy to image.

Triceps

The triceps muscle (Fig. 34-10) tends to be less echoic than the biceps. In general, more body fat overlies the triceps than other upper extremity muscles, a finding that may relate to its echoic properties.[8]

Posterior paracervical muscles

The paracervical muscles comprise a group of overlapping muscles of different orientation and action. They include the trapezius, splenius capitis, semispinalis capitis, and levator scapulae. Much of their clinical importance derives from the use of botulinum toxin for the treatment of cervical dystonia. The multilayered structure of these muscles is apparent from an image made in a transverse plane to the spine in left and right paracervical areas.

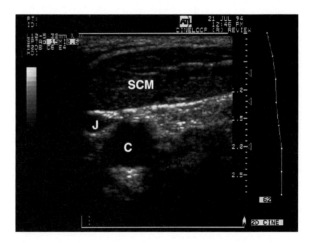

Fig. 34-11. Sternocleidomastoid in cross-section. Note the large carotid artery and slightly smaller jugular vein just below the muscle. This structure is informative in imaging patients with cervical dystonia. (*SCM,* Sternocleidomastoid; *C,* carotid artery; *J,* internal jugular vein.)

Sternocleidomastoid

The sternocleidomastoid muscle is also important in cervical dystonia and shares useful parallel relations with carotid structures. As a result, it is probably the most frequently imaged skeletal muscle in the body (Fig. 34-11), but only recently has it been studied systematically.[21,22]

Multifidus and other paraspinal muscles

Paraspinal muscles can be imaged the entire extent of the spinal column. The most midline muscles constitute multifidus, and its relationship to surrounding muscles can be easily delineated with sonography. In patients with scoliosis, focal atrophy can be imaged along the convex curvature.[10]

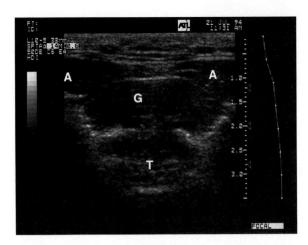

Fig. 34-12. A transverse image of the tongue (with water held passively in the mouth), imaged from below the mandible. At the top of the figure, the laterally placed anterior bellies of the digastric (*A*) are apparent. The thick midline structure is the genioglossus (*G*) and, below that, the mobile intraoral portion of the tongue (*T*).

Tongue

The architecture of the tongue, unlike other skeletal muscles, involves randomly interweaving patterns of muscle fibers. Further, it lacks tendons or aponeuroses, a property it shares with cardiac muscle. The tissue has a more echogenic and less heterogeneous appearance than other skeletal muscles (Fig. 34-12). Although the tongue can be imaged directly with standoff water baths, it also proves simple to image it from below the mandible. Water held in the mouth can enhance the image.

Masseter, facial, and temporalis muscles

The masseter is readily imaged and represents an excellent muscle for studying isometric muscle contraction (Fig. 34-4).[1,11] The temporalis muscle, although not as thick, behaves similarly. Muscles innervated by the facial nerve are thin and tax the imaging capacity of most instruments. In certain pathologic conditions, imaging can be helpful. For example, in some patients with anterocollis, platysma hypertrophy is apparent.

SUMMARY

Sonography provides unique information about the structure and function of normal skeletal muscle. The technique entails minimal discomfort, expense, or risk, making it ideal for use in clinical studies. As instrumentation develops and as additional experience is gained, neuromuscular sonography can be expected to become an increasingly informative diagnostic and research tool.

REFERENCES

1. Bakke M, et al: Ultrasound image of human masseter muscle related to bite force, electromyography, facial morphology, and occlusal factors, *Scand J Dent Res* 100:164-171, 1992.

2. Barry DT, Geringer SR, Ball RD: Acoustic myography: a noninvasive monitor of motor unit fatigue, *Muscle Nerve* 8:189-194, 1985.
3. Brooks VB: *The neural basis of motor control,* New York, 1986, Oxford University Press.
4. Cespedes I, et al: Elastography: elasticity imaging using ultrasound with application to muscle and breast in vivo, *Ultrason Imaging* 15:73-88, 1993.
5. Chandrasekaran K, et al: Feasibility of identifying amyloid and hypertrophic cardiomyopathy with the use of computerized quantitative texture analysis of clinical echocardiographic data, *J Am Coll Cardiol* 13:832-840, 1989.
6. Fornage BD: *Ultrasonography of muscles and tendons: examination technique and atlas of normal anatomy of the extremities,* New York, 1989, Springer-Verlag.
7. Gunreben G, Bogdahn U: Real-time sonography of acute and chronic muscle denervation, *Muscle Nerve* 14:654-664, 1991.
8. Haberkorn U, et al: Ultrasound image properties influenced by abdominal wall thickness and composition, *J Clin Ultrasound* 21:423-429, 1993.
9. Hamjian JA, Walker FO: Neurophysiological studies of intramuscular botulinum-A toxin in man, *Muscle Nerve* 17:1385-1392, 1994.
10. Kennelly KP, Stokes MJ: Pattern of asymmetry of paraspinal muscle size in adolescent idiopathic scoliosis examined by real-time ultrasound imaging: a preliminary study, *Spine* 18:913-917, 1993.
11. Kiliardis S, Kalebo P: Masseter muscle thickness measured by ultrasonography and its relation to facial morphology, *J Dent Res* 70:1262-1265, 1991.
12. Kimura J: *Electrodiagnosis in diseases of nerve and muscle: principles and practice,* Philadelphia, 1983, FA Davis.
13. Martinson H, Stokes MJ: Measurement of anterior tibial muscle size using real-time ultrasound imaging, *Eur J Appl Physiol* 63:250-254, 1991.
14. Naganuma M, et al: MR imaging of nerve hypertrophy in chronic demyelinating polyneuropathy, *Muscle Nerve* 17(suppl):237, 1994.
15. Reimers K, et al: Muscular ultrasound in idiopathic inflammatory myopathies of adults, *J Neurol Sci* 116:82-92, 1993.
16. Reimers K, et al: Skeletal muscle sonography: a correlative study of echogenicity and morphology, *J Ultrasound Med* 12:73-77, 1993.
17. Rutherford OM, Jones DA: Measurement of fibre pennation using ultrasound in the human quadriceps in vivo, *Eur J Appl Physiol* 65:433-437, 1992.
18. Sekul E, Chow C, Dalakas MD: Magnetic resonance imaging (MRI) of the forearm as a diagnostic aid in patients with inclusion body myositis (IBM), *Neurology* 44(suppl 2):A130, 1994.
19. Stuhlmuller JE, et al: Effects of instrument adjustments on quantitative echocardiographic gray level texture measures, *J Am Soc Echocardiogr* 4:533-540, 1991.
20. Vandenberg BF: Diagnosis of recent myocardial infarction with quantitative backscatter imaging: preliminary studies, *J Am Soc Echocardiogr* 4:10-18, 1991.
21. Walker F: Ultrasound imaging of muscle, *Muscle Nerve* (suppl 1)17:68, 1994.
22. Walker F, Hunt V: Sonographic imaging of cervical muscles following botulinum toxin injections, *Muscle Nerve* (suppl 1)17:112, 1994.
23. Walker FO, et al: Sonographic imaging of muscle contraction and fasciculations: a comparison with electromyography, *Muscle Nerve* 13:33-39, 1990.
24. Walsh EG: *Muscles, masses & motion: the physiology of normality, hypotonicity, spasticity & rigidity,* London, 1992, MacKeith Press.
25. Warwick R, Williams PL: *Gray's anatomy, 35th British edition,* Philadelphia, 1973, WB Saunders.
26. Weiner WJ, Lang AE: *Movement disorders: a comprehensive survey,* Mt Kisco, NY, 1989, Futura.

35

Transfontanelle Duplex Doppler Sonography

Jeffrey M. Perlman

The fontanelles of the newborn have been utilized as windows through which it is possible to measure cerebral blood flow velocities (CBFV) in the anterior and middle cerebral arteries using Doppler techniques.[22,32,39] These measurements have provoked considerable interest and study because the techniques that allow their acquisition are noninvasive and readily applicable at the bedside. Thus, it is possible to detect and follow derangements of the cerebral circulation and to assess their role in the pathogenesis of numerous pathologic processes that involve the developing neonatal brain. This chapter deals with the application of Doppler techniques to the assessment of the neonatal cerebral circulation, including a review of the background, methodology, and existing clinical experience.

METHODOLOGY
Basic principles

Ultrasonic techniques that allow measurement of the CBFV are based upon the Doppler principle: When a sound wave of a given frequency transverses a blood vessel, it is reflected by a moving target (i.e., red blood cells) and the reflected wave has a different frequency (i.e., undergoes a frequency shift) than that of the original wave.[35] Several factors may influence the measured Doppler frequency shift, including the velocity of red blood cells, the angle of the transmitting probe relative to the axis of the vessel, the effect of broad-frequency spectrum shift, and the effect of mixed arterial and venous signals. The frequency of the reflected wave, when compared to that of the emitted wave, relates to it by the Doppler equation:

$$\Delta f = \frac{2foV\, Cos\phi}{c}$$

where Δf indicates the Doppler frequency shift; fo indicates the transmitted frequency; V, the velocity of the red blood cells; $Cos\, \phi$, the angle of incidence of the ultrasound beam and the axis of blood flow; and c, the velocity of ultrasound in tissues.

For practical purposes, fo (the transmitted frequency) and c (velocity of ultrasound in the tissues) are constant in any one determination. Thus, the velocity of the red blood cell and the angle of the transducer are the major determinants of Δf. In regard to the latter, when the transducer angle is no more than

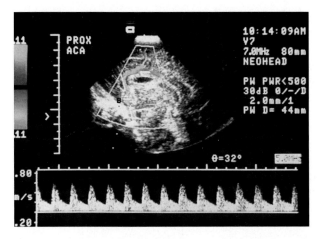

Fig. 35-1. Typical flow image of the pericallosal branch of the anterior cerebral artery as it courses around the corpus callosum (parasagittal view).

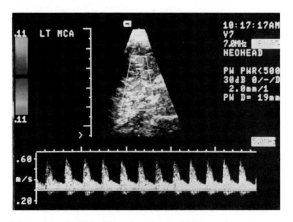

Fig. 35-2. Axial view of the middle cerebral artery. Note the nearly zero degree of insonation achieved for the Doppler measurement.

15°, the error of estimation of the blood flow velocity is less than 5%.[6]

Instrumentation

The instruments utilized to study the cerebral circulation in the newborn are based upon one of two types of Doppler systems: continuous-wave Doppler or pulsed-wave Doppler.

Continuous wave Doppler ultrasound. These systems comprise three major components: (1) a bidirectional Doppler flow velocity meter, (2) a transducer, and (3) a two-channel chart recorder. The Doppler signal is obtained by placing a transducer over the blood vessel of interest. The Doppler signals are continuously transmitted, and the probe is adjusted to obtain maximum pulsations from the specific vessel insonated.[22]

Pulsed wave Doppler ultrasound. These systems were developed because of the need to measure blood flow velocities selectively from points located at specific distances from the probe. The velocity can be determined from a small area within a vessel by adjusting the time between the pulses and by gating the reception of the signal. This enhances the quality of the Doppler recordings obtained. A variant of this method is color Doppler imaging.

Color Doppler imaging. These instruments provide information with regard to the Doppler frequency shift at different points within the vessel. The Doppler sampling volume displays the flow direction relative to the transducer in either blue or red (Figs. 35-1 and 35-2; see also Plates 103 and 104). Shades of color reflect relative velocities at different points in the vessel. The most distinctive benefit of these instruments is the precision with which an anatomic delineation can be achieved. A disadvantage is that it provides only qualitative velocity data,[44] making it necessary to use pulsed-wave Doppler to measure velocities.

Scanning method

The anterior cerebral artery is visualized in a parasagittal plane through the anterior fontanelle. Specifically, the pericallosal artery is insonated as it courses around the anterior part of the corpus callosum (Fig. 35-1). In this plane the directed ultrasound beam is tangential to the vessel, and the Doppler angle is close to zero. The middle cerebral artery is insonated in the axial plane, with the transducer placed in front of the ear. In this plane the Doppler angle is also close to zero (Fig. 35-2).

Parameters measured

In addition to directly measuring CBFV, two other parameters have been utilized to attempt to quantitate abnormalities of the cerebral circulation. These calculations, originally intended to improve the sensitivity and specificity of the measurements, must be clearly understood in order to avoid diagnostic pitfalls (Fig. 35-3).

Pulsatility index. In their original study, Bada and colleagues utilized a pulsatility index (PI) as a measure of cerebrovascular resistance,[3] having adapted it from the Pourcelot resistant index.[31] The PI is calculated with the formula:

$$PI = \frac{V_s - V_d}{V_s}$$

where PI = pulsatility index; V_s = systolic velocity, and V_d = diastolic velocity. It was originally thought that the PI would minimize the effects of probe position because changes in probe angle affect the values for V_s and V_d simultaneously. However, although it can be useful in the comparison of serially acquired measurements, its use as an isolated variable may provide ambiguous data. Theoretically, serial measurements of PI may reflect changes in cerebral perfusion as well as cerebrovascular resistance. But if both V_s and V_d change proportionately,

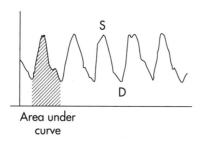

Fig. 35-3. Typical cerebral blood flow velocity tracing. (*S,* Peak systolic velocity, *D,* end-diastolic velocity; *shaded area,* area under the velocity curve; pulsatility index = S − D/S.)

serial determinations of PI result in similar values and do not reveal changes in perfusion or resistance (Fig. 35-4).

Area under the velocity curve. A second method for assessing cerebral hemodynamic abnormalities with Doppler measurements involves the determination of the area under the velocity curve (AUVC). Rosenkrantz and Oh tested the validity of this method in vitro by circulating blood through a system of tubes by means of a pulsatile pump.[34] The actual flow rate of the pump was compared to the AUVC, and a linear correlation was found ($r = 0.99$). The AUVC can be measured by means of a manual planimeter, or it can be

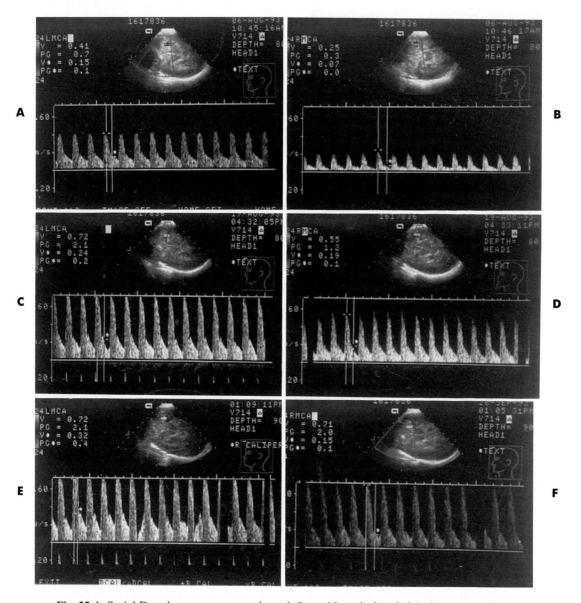

Fig. 35-4. Serial Doppler measurements in an infant with an isolated right intraparenchymal echodensity **(A, B)** that progressed to cystic formation **(C, D).** Note the ipsilateral decrease in the middle cerebral blood flow velocity at initial diagnosis, and the gradual increase in cerebral blood flow velocity with subsequent measurements **(E, F).** The area under the velocity curve increased from 50 to 150 planimeter units/3 seconds. However, the pulsatility index remained greater than 0.90.

determined electronically by certain ultrasound instruments.

Relationship between cerebral flow velocities and cerebral blood flow

The degree to which the CBFV reflects the volume of cerebral blood flow (CBF) is of considerable importance because direct measurements of CBF can be performed only with techniques that are complex, expensive, and invasive. Conversely, CBV measurements are performed using readily available and noninvasive bedside techniques. Conventionally, regional CBF is measured as the volume of blood perfusing a mass of brain tissue per unit of time. The magnitude of CBF in a particular vessel, however, is expressed as units of volume per unit of time. Vascular blood flow is directly related to the blood flow velocity and to the cross-sectional area of the vessel as follows:

$$CBF = CBFV \times area$$

Thus, as long as the cross-sectional area of the vessel remains constant, CBFV is the major determinant of CBF. However, the vessel diameter, and the volume of tissue that constitutes the vascular territory may change under normal physiologic circumstances or as the result of pathologic processes. Indeed, even the proximal cerebral arteries, i.e., Circle of Willis, have vasoconstrictor properties of their own and are not simply conducting systems.[11,14] Several reports, in fact, suggest that large cerebral arteries (e.g., middle cerebral artery) may be involved in the cerebrovascular response to hypercapnia and hypocapnia.[1]

EXPERIENCE USING TRANSFONTANELLE DOPPLER SONOGRAPHY
Experimental studies

Several studies have examined the relationship of CBFV to CBF in both newborn animals and the human newborn. In animal studies, CBF is changed by altering the $Paco_2$ or Cao_2[4,10,33] Measurements of CBFV were performed in the anterior cerebral artery, whereas CBF was determined by radioactively labeled microspheres or by autoradiography. Changes in CBFV, PI, and AUVC correlated with changes in CBF, but the degree of correlation varied among the various parameters studied, with the lowest value being that of the PI ($r = 0.3$) and the highest, that of the AUVC ($r = 0.9$). Because the correlation coefficient (r) is only a measure of the intensity of the association between the two variables,[43] coefficients of determination (r^2) were also calculated. These are a measure of the amount of variability of one variable (e.g., CBF) that is accounted for by the second variable (e.g., CBFV). In the examples previously described, a variation of the PI ($r^2 = 0.09$) accounts only for about 10% of the variation in CBF, whereas variation

of AUVC ($r^2 = 0.81$) accounts for approximately 80% of the variability of CBF. Thus, changes in CBF produced experimentally are associated with a significant change in CBFV, and the changes in CBFV may account for up to 80% of the variability in CBF. Because the PI accounts for only about 10% of the variability of CBF, at least under the conditions studied, it is not prudent to use this index as a general indicator of CBF. Moreover, as noted before, changes in CBFV do not necessarily indicate changes in CBF. For example, during autoregulation, CBFV and blood vessel caliber change, while CBF remains constant.

Studies in the human newborn

Attempts to correlate CBFV with CBF have been carried out in newborn infants. Griesen and colleagues compared CBF, measured by the xenon inhalation technique, with anterior cerebral artery and common carotid artery blood flow velocities.[9] All CBFV variables measured were significantly related to CBF; however, the correlation coefficients (r) varied from 0.4 to 0.8 with V_d exhibiting the highest correlation. We have observed a similar relationship in the newborn infant, comparing CBFV in the anterior cerebral arteries and CBF in the frontal region, as measured with positron emission tomography (PET).[30] In 25 premature infants with a variety of neurologic disorders, CBF measured with PET was significantly related to CBFV with a correlation of 0.70 ($p < 0.001$) (Fig. 35-5). This relationship can be best described as curvilinear. Thus, at lower CBF values, the correlation with CBFV is high, whereas at higher CBF values the relationship with CBFV is poor.

Evaluation of the neonatal cerebral circulation

Since the initial report of Bada and colleagues demonstrating the feasibility of assessing the cerebral circulation noninvasively by using Doppler,[3] numerous studies have demonstrated changes in CBFV with different clinical conditions. Prior to discussing some of these observations, it is important to understand that several factors may influence the cerebral Doppler signal independent of pathology. These include the specific insonated vessel (e.g., anterior versus middle cerebral artery), the site of the vessel insonated (proximal versus distal), the gestational age of the infant, the postnatal age of the infant, the systemic blood pressure, and the sleep state of the infant.

Insonated vessel. The CBFV measurements obtained from the anterior cerebral artery differ from those obtained from the middle cerebral artery in healthy newborn infants. Thus, AUVC measurements from the middle cerebral artery are approximately 1.5-fold to twofold of those from the pericallosal branch of the anterior cerebral artery.

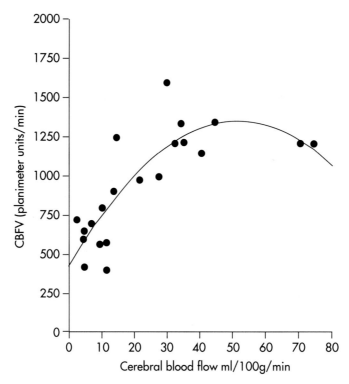

Fig. 35-5. Relationship of cerebral blood flow velocity as determined by area under the velocity curve and cerebral blood flow as determined by positron emission tomography (r = 0.70; p < 0.001).

Location of Doppler sample volume. Doppler measurements vary within the distribution of a major cerebral vessel. For example, AUVC measurements from the distal segment of the anterior cerebral artery are consistently lower than the AUVC measurements from its more proximal segment. In fact, in a study of 14 very low birth weight infants with normal cranial sonograms, AUVC measurements on day 14 from the proximal segment of the anterior cerebral artery were 32% of AUVC measures from the distal segment of the anterior cerebral artery.[20]

Postnatal age. Doppler measurements increase as a function of postnatal age.[21,40] In a longitudinal study of healthy and sick premature infants, AUVC measurements obtained from the distal anterior cerebral artery increased significantly as a function of postnatal age. This increase was observed in infants irrespective of gestational age.[21]

Arterial blood pressure. The cerebral circulation of the premature infant, particularly the sick premature infant, is considered to be "pressure passive" (i.e., changes in CBF directly reflect changes in systemic blood pressure).[39] For example, transient increases in systemic blood pressure, such as may occur with a standard neonatal procedure like suctioning of an infant, are associated with increases in CBFV.[28] Thus, when obtaining serial Doppler measurement, simultaneous blood pressure measurements are critical.

Sleep state of the infant. Insonation of the anterior and middle cerebral arteries varies according to the behavioral state of the infant, CBFV increasing during rapid eye movement (REM) sleep and decreasing during deep sleep.[13]

Doppler measurements in sick infants

Because derangements of CBF are considered to be of paramount importance in the genesis of many neurologic disorders noted in the newborn period (e.g., periventricular-intraventricular hemorrhage [PV-IVH] in the premature infant and hypoxic ischemic cerebral injury in term infant), serial Doppler studies of the cerebral circulation have been performed in sick infants to determine the relationship between changes in CBFV and subsequent brain injury (Table 35-1). It has been possible to document Doppler changes in the brain arteries of infants with interventricular hemorrhage,[26] patent ductus arteriosus,[17,23] neonatal seizures,[27] respiratory distress syndrome,[24,25] apnea and bradycardia,[29] asphyxia,[2] theophylline,[8] cocaine,[38] surfactant administration,[36,38] infantile hydrocephalus,[12] brain death,[18] meningitis,[19] polycythemia,[34] indomethacin,[7] and carbon dioxide reactivity.[16] To illustrate the useful role of Doppler measurements in defining the pathogenesis of brain injury in the neonatal period, examples of some studies are presented next.

Table 35-1. Cerebral Doppler changes in neonates

Condition	Cerebral blood flow velocity measurements	
	Area under the velocity curve	Pulsatility index
Intraventricular hemorrhage[27]	Fluctuating	↑ or ↓
Seizures[28]	↑	↓
Asphyxia[3]	↑	↓
Patent ductus arteriosus[18,24]	↓	↑
Pneumothorax[23]	↑	↓
Brain death[19]	↓ to absent	↑
Hydrocephalus[20]	↓	↑
Polycythemia[35]	↓	↑
Surfactant[38,39]	↑	?
Indomethacin[8]	↓	↑
Cocaine[40]	↓	↑
CO_2 reactivity[17]	↑	?

Infants with respiratory distress syndrome. Because of the strong association that exists between respiratory distress syndrome (RDS) and intraventricular hemorrhage (IVH),[6,15] we prospectively evaluated 50 mechanically ventilated preterm infants in the first days of life with RDS.[25] To determine whether perturbations in CBFV are important in the pathogenesis of PV-IVH, serial Doppler determinations were recorded, together with simultaneous arterial blood pressure recordings. We noted two patterns of CBFV in the first days of life in these 50 premature infants, that is, a *stable* and *fluctuating* pattern (Fig. 35-6). The stable pattern is characterized by equal peaks and troughs of peak systolic and end-diastolic flow velocity. In contrast, the fluctuating pattern is characterized by continuous alterations in both systolic and diastolic flow velocity. The CBFV patterns closely reflect similar patterns of arterial blood pressure. A striking relationship of the fluctuating CBFV pattern to the subsequent development of IVH was noted (Table 35-2). Also noted in this study was the dramatic effect of pharmacologic paralysis on CBFV. By eliminating the infant's own respiratory effort, the fluctuating pattern was immediately converted to a stable pattern (Fig. 35-7). In a subsequent study, we demonstrated that elimination of the fluctuating pattern by muscle paralysis was associated with a significant reduction in IVH.

Neonatal seizures. Neonatal seizures also represent an important clinical problem for the neurologist and neonatologist. We studied the relationship of neonatal seizures and changes in CBFV in the premature infant.[27] At the time of seizures, a marked increase in CBFV was observed in every infant. The changes in CBFV appeared principally to reflect changes in diastolic flow velocity. The changes in CBFV returned to the values observed prior to the onset of the convulsive phenomena within 5 minutes. The increase in CBFV with seizures, while an adaptive response in older individuals, may be maladaptive in the newborn infant with vulnerable capillary beds (e.g., the germinal matrix in the premature infants or margins of infarction in the asphyxiated infant). Indeed, we have observed the subsequent development of PV-IVH in at least one infant with seizures.

Infants with patent ductus arteriosus. Patent ductus arteriosus (PDA) is another important clinical problem in the sick premature infant; it occurs in up to 30% of such infants. Because symptomatic PDA is associated with left-to-right ductal shunting, the potential for cerebral circulatory changes to occur secondary to ductal steal is high. To address this important issue, we and others have studied CBFV in infants with symptomatic PDA.[17,30] Striking changes in CBFV (e.g., the pulsatility index increased significantly) were noted with symptomatic PDA. This increase in PI was principally as a consequence of a decrease in diastolic flow velocity (Fig. 35-8). The changes in the cerebral circulation appeared to reflect directly similar changes in systemic blood pressure, with lower diastolic blood pressures occurring with symptomatic PDA consistent with a pressure-passive circulation. Closure of the ductus either medically or surgically was associated with a striking decrease in PI. These data suggest that in infants with symptomatic PDA and left-to-right shunting, diastolic flow velocity reflects relatively low CBF. The latter may be important in the genesis of ischemic infarction in the germinal matrix, periventricular white matter, or both. Moreover, these data indicate that a decrease in diastolic flow velocity resulting in an increase in PI is not solely indicative of change in resistance but influenced by proximal factors as well.

Potential applications in neonatology

Determination of neonatal brain death. The Doppler technique may serve as an important clinical tool in the evaluation of neonates who meet other criteria for brain death. McMenamin and Volpe defined a characteristic sequence of flow velocity pattern deterioration in these patients.[18] Thus, the sequence consisted of (1) loss of diastolic flow, (2) the appearance of retrograde flow during diastole, (3) diminution in systolic flow in the pericallosal artery, and (4) no detectable flow in the pericallosal artery. These findings suggest a progressive increase in cerebral vascular resistance and a progressive decrease in cerebral perfusion pressure, compatible with diffuse cerebral necrosis.

Infants with hydrocephalus. A second condition in which Doppler measurements may serve as useful clinical adjuncts is hydrocephalus in an infant. With increasing ventriculomegaly, there is a progressive decrease in diastolic flow velocity and an increase in the

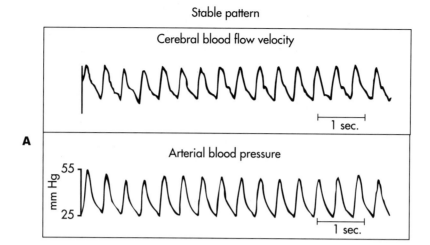

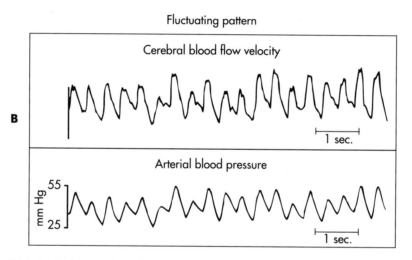

Fig. 35-6. A, Stable and **B,** fluctuating patterns of cerebral blood flow velocity and simultaneously recorded arterial blood pressure. The stable pattern has equal peaks and troughs in systolic and diastolic flow velocity and arterial pressure, whereas the fluctuating pattern has marked fluctuations. (From Perlman JM, McMenamin JB, Volpe JJ: Fluctuating cerebral blood flow velocity in respiratory distress syndrome: relationship to the development of intraventricular hemorrhage, *N Engl J Med* 309:204-209, 1983.)

Table 35-2. Relationship of fluctuating and stable cerebral blood flow velocity (CBFV) and the subsequent occurrence of periventricular-intraventricular hemorrhage

CBFV pattern	Intraventricular hemorrhage
Fluctuating (N = 23)	20*
Stable (N = 27)	7

*p < 0.001.

Adapted from Perlman JM, McMenamin JB, Volpe JJ: Fluctuating cerebral blood flow velocity in respiratory distress syndrome: relationship to the development of intraventricular hemorrhage, *N Engl J Med* 312:1353-1357, 1985.

PI.[19] Treatment of the hydrocephalus results in an increase in CBFV, affecting principally an increase in the diastolic component. The data suggest that changes in CBFV may be a sensitive indicator of ischemic injury with evolving ventriculomegaly, particularly following PV-IVH.

Doppler changes following asphyxia. Neonatal asphyxia is an important clinical problem. The ability to identify early the asphyxiated infant at greatest risk for irreversible cerebral injury is critical. In a study of postasphyxial infants, Archer and colleagues reported a marked decrease in PI, principally affecting an increase in diastolic flow velocity in infants with asphyxia.[2] Infants with a decrease in PI were more likely to exhibit an

Cerebral blood flow velocity

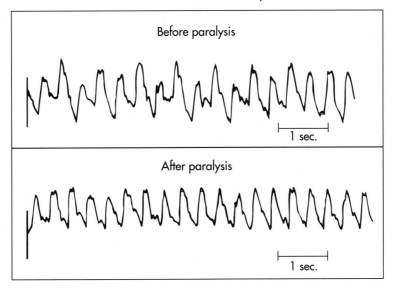

Fig. 35-7. Effect of muscle paralysis on cerebral blood flow velocity. After paralysis was induced by pancuronium bromide, the fluctuating pattern was eliminated. (From Perlman JM, McMenamin JB, Volpe JJ: Fluctuating cerebral blood flow velocity in respiratory distress syndrome: relationship to the development of intraventricular hemorrhage, *N Engl J Med* 309:204-209, 1983.)

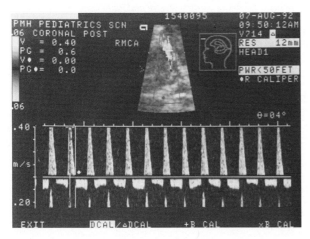

Fig. 35-8. Typical Doppler tracing in an infant with symptomatic patent ductus arteriosus. Note that retrograde flow is observed during diastole.

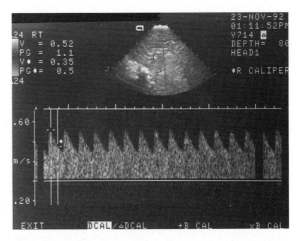

Fig. 35-9. Doppler tracing from an asphyxiated infant. Note the marked increase in diastolic flow velocity. This infant exhibited an abnormal outcome.

abnormal long-term outcome than infants with a normal PI. We have made similar Doppler observations in asphyxiated infants who subsequently exhibited a poor outcome (Fig. 35-9). These results suggest that Doppler may play a useful role in identifying the asphyxiated infant at highest risk for developing irreversible cerebral injury.

CONCLUSIONS

The Doppler technique provides a useful means of serially evaluating the cerebral circulation of the sick neonate. Because Doppler measurements may be influ-

enced by numerous variables, such as the levels of Pao_2, systemic blood pressure, sleep state, and medications, such variables need to be accounted for in any Doppler evaluation. Measurement of AUVC appears to be closely related to CBF, whereas the other indices of flow velocity are poorly related to CBF. Finally, because Doppler evaluation of the cerebral circulation in the neonate is a complex procedure requiring skill in appropriately insonating the vessel of interest, as well as an understanding of the many factors that may influence a Doppler frequency shift, its clinical use is likely to be limited, whereas it should continue to be an invaluable research tool for the serial evaluation of the cerebral circulation of the sick neonate.

REFERENCES

1. Abboud FM: Special characteristics of the cerebral circulation, *Fed Proc* 40:2296-2309, 1981.
2. Archer LNJ, Levene MI, Evans DH: Cerebral artery doppler ultrasonography for prediction of outcome after perinatal asphyxia, *Lancet* 2:1116-1118, 1986.
3. Bada HS, et al: Noninvasive diagnosis of neonatal asphyxia and intraventricular hemorrhage by Doppler ultrasound, *J Pediatr* 95:775-779, 1979.
4. Batton DG, et al: Regional cerebral blood flow, cerebral blood velocity, and pulsatile index in newborn dogs, *Pediatr Res* 17:908-912, 1983.
5. Burns PN: *Doppler flow estimations in the fetal and maternal circulations: principles, techniques, and some limitations.* In Maulik D, McNellis D, editors: *Doppler ultrasound measurement of maternal fetal hemodynamics,* Ithaca, NY, 1987, Perinatology Press.
6. Dykes FO, et al: Intraventricular hemorrhage: a prospective evaluation of etiopathogenesis, *Pediatrics* 66:42-49, 1980.
7. Edwards AD, et al: Effects of indomethacin on cerebral hemodynamics in very preterm infants, *Lancet* 335:1491-1495, 1990.
8. Ghai V, et al: Regional cerebral blood flow velocity after aminophylline therapy in premature infants, *J Pediatr* 114:870-873, 1989.
9. Griesen G, et al: Cerebral blood flow in the newborn infant: comparison of Doppler ultrasound and ^{133}Xenon clearance, *J Pediatr* 104:411-417, 1984.
10. Hansen NB, et al: Validity of doppler measurements of anterior cerebral artery blood flow velocity: correlation with brain blood flow in piglets, *Pediatrics* 72:526-530, 1983.
11. Heistad DD, Marcus MM, Abboud FM: Role of large arteries in regulation of cerebral blood flow in dogs, *J Clin Invest* 62:761-768, 1978.
12. Hill A, Volpe JJ: Decrease in pulsatile flow in the anterior cerebral arteries in infantile hydrocephalus, *Pediatrics* 69:4-6, 1982.
13. Jorch G, Huster T, Rabe H: Dependency of Doppler parameters in the anterior cerebral artery on behavioral states in preterm and term neonates, *Biol Neonate* 58:79-86, 1990.
14. Kontos HA, et al: Response of cerebral arteries and arterioles to acute hypotension and hypertension, *Am J Physiol* 234:H371-H383, 1978.
15. Levene MI, Fawer CL, Lamont RF: Risk factors in the development of intraventricular hemorrhage in the premature neonate, *Arch Dis Child* 57:410-417, 1982.
16. Levene MJ, et al: Carbon dioxide reactivity of the cerebral circulation in extremely premature infants: effects of postnatal age and indomethacin, *Pediatr Res* 24:175-179, 1988.
17. Lipman B, Server GA, Brazy JE: Abnormal cerebral hemodynamics in preterm infants with patent ductus arteriosus, *Pediatrics* 69:778-782, 1982.
18. McMenamin JB, Volpe JJ: Doppler ultrasonography in the determination of neonatal brain death, *Ann Neurol* 14:302-306, 1983.
19. McMenamin JB, Volpe JJ: Bacterial meningitis in infants, effects on intracranial pressure and cerebral blood flow velocity, *Neurology* 34:500-504, 1984.
20. Morris C, Perlman JM, Rollins NR: Regional cerebral blood flow differences at the anterior and middle cerebral arteries in sick premature infants, *Pediatr Res* 375A, 1993.
21. Perlman J, et al: Cerebral flow velocity increases in the healthy premature infant, *Pediatr Res* 357A, 1985.
22. Perlman JM: Neonatal cerebral blood flow velocity measurement, *Clin Perinatol* 12:179-193, 1985.
23. Perlman JM, Hill A, Volpe JJ: The effect of patent ductus arteriosus on flow velocity in the anterior cerebral arteries: ductal steal in the premature newborn infant, *J Pediatr* 99: 767-771, 1981.
24. Perlman JM, Kreusser KL, Volpe JJ: Eliminating fluctuating cerebral blood flow velocity in preterm infants with respiratory distress syndrome significantly reduces the incidence of intraventricular hemorrhage, *N Engl J Med* 312:1353-1357, 1985.
25. Perlman JM, McMenamin JB, Volpe JJ: Fluctuating cerebral blood flow velocity in respiratory distress syndrome: relationship to the development of intraventricular hemorrhage, *N Engl J Med* 309:204-209, 1983.
26. Perlman JM, Volpe JJ: Cerebral blood flow velocity in relation to intraventricular hemorrhage in the premature newborn infant, *J Pediatr* 100:956-958, 1982.
27. Perlman JM, Volpe JJ: The effects of seizures on cerebral blood flow velocity, intracranial pressure, and systolic blood pressure in the preterm infant, *J Pediatr* 102:288-293, 1983.
28. Perlman JM, Volpe JJ: The effects of suctioning on cerebral blood flow velocity, intracranial pressure, and systolic blood pressure in the preterm infant, *Pediatrics* 72:329-334, 1983.
29. Perlman JM, Volpe JJ: The effects of apnea and bradycardia on cerebral blood flow velocity in the preterm infant, *Pediatrics* 76:333-338, 1985.
30. Perlman JM, et al: Cerebral blood flow velocities as determined by Doppler is related to regional cerebral blood flow as determined by positron emission tomography, *Ann Neurol* 18:407, 1985.
31. Pourcelot L: *Diagnostic ultrasound for cerebrovascular disease.* In Donald J, Levi S, editors: *Present and future diagnostic ultrasound,* New York, 1976, Kooker.
32. Raju T: Cerebral Doppler studies in the fetus and newborn infant, *J Pediatr* 119:165-171, 1991.
33. Rosenberg AA, Narayanan V, Jones MD Jr: Comparison of anterior cerebral flow velocity and cerebral blood flow during hypoxia, *Pediatr Res* 19:67-70, 1985.
34. Rosenkrantz TS, Oh W: Cerebral blood flow in infants with polycythemia and hyperviscosity: effect of partial exchange transfusion with plasmanate, *J Pediatr* 101:94-98, 1982.
35. Strandness DE, Sumner DS: *Ultrasonic techniques in angiology,* Bern, 1975, Hans Huber.
36. Van Bel F, et al: Cerebral and aortic blood flow velocity patterns in preterm infants receiving prophylactic surfactant treatment, *Acta Paediatr* 81:504-510, 1992.
37. Van der Bor M, Ma EJ, Walther FJ: Cerebral blood flow velocity after surfactant instillation in preterm infants, *J Pediatr* 118:285-287, 1990.
38. Van der Bor M, Walther FJ, Sims ME: Increased cerebral blood flow velocity in infants of mothers who abuse cocaine, *Pediatrics* 85:733-736, 1990.
39. Volpe JJ: *Neurology of the newborn,* ed 3, Philadelphia, 1987, WB Saunders.
40. Winnberg P, Sonesson SE, Lundell BPW: Postnatal changes in intracranial blood flow velocity in preterm infants, *Acta Paediatr Scand* 79:1150-1155, 1990.
41. Zar JH: *Biostatistical analysis,* ed 2, Englewood Cliffs, NJ, 1984, Prentice-Hall.
42. Zwiebel WJ: Color duplex imaging and Doppler spectrum analysis: principle, capabilities and limitations, *Semin Ultrasound CT MR* 11:84-96, 1990.

Perioperative and Intraoperative Sonography

36

Intraoperative Cranial B-mode Scanning

George J. Dohrmann
Jonathan M. Rubin

Intraoperative localization of lesions within the brain has been a challenge for neurosurgeons. Techniques such as computed tomography (CT), magnetic resonance imaging (MRI), and angiography have been helpful preoperatively, but they are all somewhat inadequate for the purpose of real-time lesion definition in the operating room. This is because only a portion of the brain is exposed during neurosurgical procedures and that care is taken not to expose any more brain than is necessary. Ultrasound, however, is an ideal method for imaging the brain intraoperatively, once the highly attenuating bone has been removed. Although A-mode (*A* = amplitude) scanning has been tried in the past, its usefulness has been limited because it is unidimensional and does not produce anatomic-type images. Real-time B-mode (*B* = brightness) ultrasound imaging was first utilized during neurosurgical operative procedures in the early 1980s.[3,4,21] It is ideal for intraoperative scanning of the brain because the brain is clearly imaged, the fluid-filled ventricles are seen as anechoic structures, and solid pathologic lesions (e.g., tumors, hematomas) are generally hyperechoic.[2,7,11,14,18] Intraoperative ultrasound is, therefore, a dynamic technique that allows the neurosurgeon to use the scanner as a surgical instrument.[5]

During the intraoperative performance of ultrasound imaging (Fig. 36-1), the plane of the craniotomy should ideally be horizontal so that saline solution, the acoustic coupling agent, can be kept within the wound. The transducer is covered with a sterile plastic drape, and imaging can be performed by placing the transducer over the dura or on the brain surface. In general, exposures for neurosurgical procedures are lateral or near the vertex; therefore, ultrasonic imaging of the brain is most easily accomplished along the coronal plane. Imaging along this plane using transducers with a frequency of 3 MHz provides the standard orientation based upon the ventricular anatomy as the main anatomic landmark (Fig. 36-2). Turning the transducer 90° from the previous position allows imaging in the transaxial or sagittal planes, depending upon whether the craniotomy is in a lateral or vertex location, respectively. Imaging using transducers of higher frequencies (5 to 7.5 MHz) is possible, but higher resolution is limited by less penetration.[5,14] After the scanning plane and the frequency of the transducer are chosen, and basic standard images

417

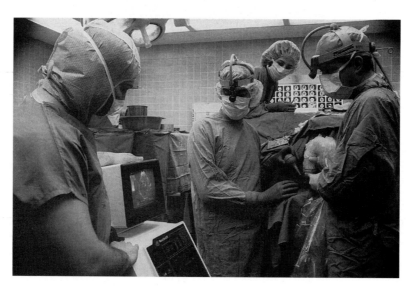

Fig. 36-1. The B-mode ultrasound scanner in the operating room. Acoustic gel is applied to the scanhead, which is then covered by a sterile plastic drape and touched to the surface of brain or dura. Saline irrigation is used to provide acoustical coupling. The image of the underlying brain is displayed on the video screen.

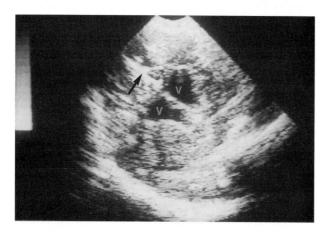

Fig. 36-2. Coronal ultrasound scan of brain. The coronal plane is a good one to use to get orientation relative to the ventricular system *(V)* and the falx *(arrow).* Frequency is 3 MHz.

have been obtained, further information may be gathered by moving the transducer from side to side to explore the extent of the lesion in all available planes. The various aspects of the brain anatomy are displayed according to a video in which bony structures appear very echogenic, while the cerebrospinal fluid is displayed as echo heat. Imaging of the brain intraoperatively allows localization of the lesion and characterization of its size and consistency (solid versus fluid). Ultrasound is inherently stereotactic because it defines a frame of reference relative to the transducer and, hence, the craniotomy site. Because scanning is a dynamic process, this imaging can be used to guide instrumentation of lesions (e.g., biopsy, drainage, shunting).[6,16] It can guide the neurosurgeon to a lesion and then gauge the extent

of the resection or the results of instrumentation. Since its application in the operating room, ultrasound scanning of the brain has become an important instrument in the armamentarium of the neurosurgeon.

TUMORS

Most brain tumors are hyperechoic and can be differentiated from the surrounding brain.[6,11,18] Small subcortical tumors, such as single metastatic lesions, are difficult to localize, and B-mode scanning demonstrates them well (Fig. 36-3). As they are very superficial, it often becomes necessary to use a large amount of saline solution over the brain surface in order to create an acoustic standoff and permit better near-field imaging of the lesion. In these cases, transducers with a frequency 7.5 MHz provide the most detail. The solid portion of the tumor, as well as any cystic components, can be clearly differentiated from any surrounding edema (Fig. 36-3). Edema is displayed as hyperechoic; therefore, it can obscure the margins of some infiltrating tumors.[14]

Small tumors located deep within the brain represent a neurosurgical challenge. For example, colloid cysts of the third ventricle without accompanying ventricular enlargement can be difficult to locate. Intraoperative ultrasound, however, allows the neurosurgeon to approach the lesion expeditiously.[13] Ideally, the tumor is imaged ultrasonically before the cortical resection is performed. Brain tissue is then removed, creating a "tunnel" that allows access to the neoplasm.[19] At various points during the operative procedure, this tunnel is filled with saline solution and ultrasound imaging is done. The distance from the bottom of the tunnel to the lesion is measured on the video screen, and resection is

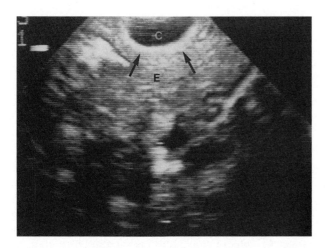

Fig. 36-3. Metastatic tumor within brain shown in this ultrasound scan. Note solid wall of tumor *(arrows),* cystic portion of tumor *(C)* and the surrounding hyperechoic edema *(E).*

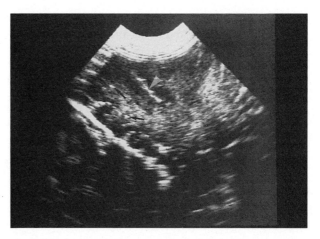

Fig. 36-5. Low-grade glioma imaged with B-mode ultrasound. The tumor is slightly more echogenic than brain and has scattered bright dots of of hyperechogenicity *(arrows)* within it. Note that the sulcus *(arrowhead)* has been preserved.

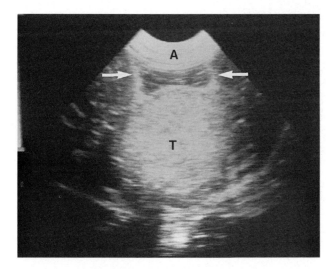

Fig. 36-4. Ultrasound scan illustrates the tunnel technique used by the neurosurgeon to approach this subcortical brain tumor. Note near-field artifact *(A)* above fluid-filled tunnel that extends to the surface of the tumor *(T).* Saline in tunnel contains some echogenic air bubbles. The walls of tunnel are identified by arrows.

progressively continued until the lesion is reached (Fig. 36-4). An operating microscope can be used to aid the neurosurgeon working through the tunnel, and the lesion is resected. The degree of resection is determined by filling the wound again with saline solution and imaging the resection site further.[19,20]

Low-grade gliomas infiltrate brain tissue and are not as echogenic as other brain tumors. Ultrasonically, they appear as areas of slightly increased echogenicity with small, bright dots of hyperechogenicity scattered within them (Fig. 36-5). They may be difficult to distinguish from edema. By contrast, high-grade gliomas (i.e.,

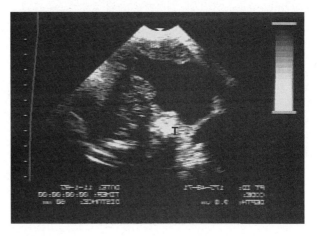

Fig. 36-6. This ultrasound scan shows a high-grade glioma within the brain. It is much more echogenic than the surrounding brain.

astrocytoma grade IV, glioblastoma multiforme) always have a hyperechoic appearance (Fig. 36-6).[1,6] They may contain cystic areas within them. The appearance of these cystic areas has diagnostic importance. If they are clearly hypoechoic, then they probably are cysts. If they have some echogenic material within them, however, especially layered out within the cystlike space, they probably represent areas of necrosis. These tumors frequently are associated with edema. Because the neurosurgical goal is to remove as much of the "tumor cell burden" as possible, intraoperative ultrasound aids the neurosurgeon in determining the presence and location of residual tumor. Whether the remaining tumor needs to be resected, however, remains a matter of neurosurgical judgment.

Although much of this section about tumors has

focused on the cerebral hemispheres, intraoperative ultrasound scanning is helpful in localizing and characterizing tumors of the cerebellum as well. Tumors beneath the brain, such as basal meningiomas, can be localized relative to the topography of the brain. This allows the neurosurgeon to plan more precisely the infracerebral approach to these base-of-skull tumors.

ABSCESSES AND CYSTS

Intracranial abscesses and cysts can also be visualized by utilizing ultrasonography in the operating room. Abscesses have hyperechoic walls containing less hyperechoic material within them. Cysts are seen as anechoic

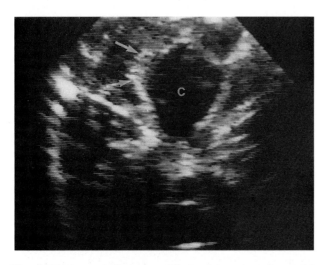

Fig. 36-7. A cerebellar cyst *(C)* is demonstrated on this ultrasound scan. The focally thickened cyst wall *(arrows)* is a mural tumor nodule. Diagnosis: cystic cerebellar astrocytoma.

regions within the brain. If the cyst wall is prominent or if the cyst wall has one or more areas of increased echogenicity, the lesion could represent a tumor cyst and the area of increased echogenicity a mural tumor nodule (Fig. 36-7).[5,14,18] These lesions can be assessed intraoperatively by ultrasound. They become smaller as the drainage procedure continues. Sometimes "daughter" abscesses are present and they can be identified and drained as well.

HEMATOMAS

When imaged with ultrasound, bleeding within the brain first appears as a dark, hypoechoic swirl that begins to develop echogenicity within the first minute. This change to hyperechogenicity is probably related to clumping of the blood cells; the area of hemorrhage then appears as quite echogenic (Fig. 36-8, *A*; see also Plate 105).[9,12] As the clot ages and breaks down, it becomes progressively more hypoechoic (Fig. 36-8, *B*; see also Plate 106). Hemorrhage into the cerebral ventricles, if not a cast of the ventricles, can appear as echogenic dots within the cerebrospinal fluid. The dots have a tendency to fall in a snowlike patterns to the dependent portion of the ventricle. Intraoperative ultrasound scanning can therefore be used to guide the neurosurgical approach to the hematoma and, as well, to assess the completeness of the hematoma removal.[20] What appears by CT or MRI to be one large hematoma is sometimes several small hematomas. Ultrasound can assure the proper identification of each of them.

VASCULAR MALFORMATIONS

Small vascular malformations (e.g., cavernous angiomas, small arteriovenous malformations) occurring in

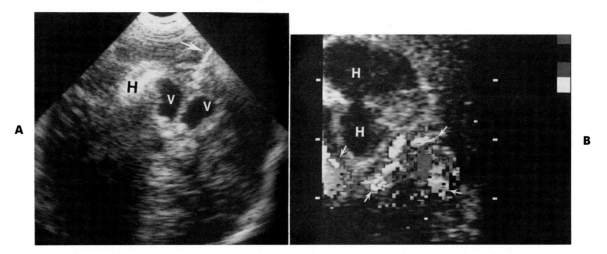

Fig. 36-8. A, Coronal ultrasound scan showing an acute hematoma *(H);* all of the hematoma is hyperechoic. (*V,* lateral ventricles; *arrow,* falx.) **B,** Color-flow Doppler image showing an arteriovenous malformation *(arrows)* and a subacute hematoma associated with it. The liquefied portions of the hematoma *(H)* are hypoechoic and are surrounded by the solid portion of the hematoma that is hyperechoic.

the brain occasionally can be located with ultrasound scanning whether or not a hematoma is associated with them. However, gray scale imaging has very little to offer for the evaluation of these lesions, and it is color Doppler that is the most helpful ultrasonic technique (Fig. 36-9; see also Plates 107 and 108).[14,20] Using the tunnel technique described previously, the vascular malformation may be approached in the same manner as a metastatic lesion (Fig. 36-10). Knowing its precise location, the surgeon can dissect around it, thereby excising the lesion in toto. Following excision, the wound can be filled with saline solution, and ultrasonography can then be performed in search of areas of hemorrhage, either in the region of the excision or in the adjacent areas. If hemorrhage occurs, its location is identified, and the neurosurgeon can deal with it promptly rather than discovering the hemorrhage once the patient's postoperative status deteriorates.

TRAUMA

Intraoperative ultrasound is also useful in the management of trauma victims, not only to locate the hematoma shown by CT or MRI preoperatively but also to image the so-called delayed hematomas that develop subsequent to the initial CT or MRI scans. This practice allows rapid identification of these delayed hematomas and their evacuation, if necessary. Indriven foreign bodies (e.g., fragments of glass or plastic) can also be located within the brain with ultrasound scanning (Fig. 36-11). They are seen as very echogenic structures relative to the surrounding brain tissue. They also produce acoustic shadows, a characteristic that absolutely distinguishes them from normal structures. Intraoperatively, ultrasound can be also used to serve as a guide to locate and remove them, if necessary.[8]

INSTRUMENTATION

Imaging of the intracranial lesions with intraoperative ultrasound also allows probes or instruments to be guided down the ultrasound plane to these lesions.[5,6,10,16] There are instrument guides designed to keep the biopsy probe or catheter in the same plane as the ultrasound (Fig. 36-12). This equipment allows imaging and biopsy of intracranial lesions (Fig. 36-13).[17]

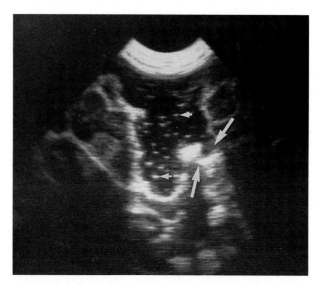

Fig. 36-10. The "tunnel" technique (see Fig. 36-4) is used in this patient to approach and then to surround and excise a small vascular malformation deep within the brain. The "tunnel" contains saline with multiple air bubbles *(small arrows);* it extends around the left side of the vascular malformation *(large arrows).* The neurosurgeon will complete the resection by dissecting around the right side as was done on the left and then resecting the tissue beneath the vascular malformation, thereby isolating it just prior to removal.

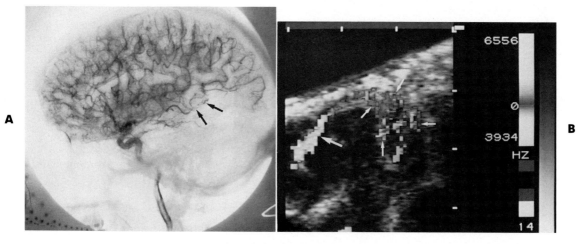

Fig. 36-9. A, Cerebral angiogram revealing a small arteriovenous malformation (AVM) *(arrows)* within the left cerebral hemisphere. **B,** Color flow Doppler scan illustrating the intracerebral AVM *(small arrows)* and the large blood vessel associated with it *(large arrow).*

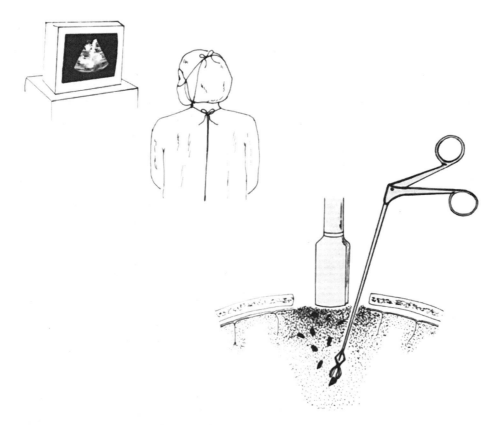

Fig. 36-11. Neurosurgeon using ultrasound to image indriven bone fragments and foreign bodies (e.g., glass or plastic fragments) within the brain and then operating under continuous ultrasound guidance.

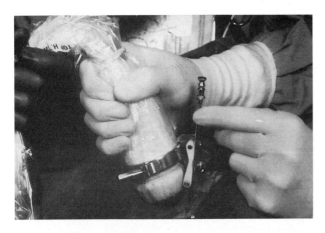

Fig. 36-12. This instrument guide attaches to the ultrasound scanhead and serves to keep the probe, catheter, or instrument within the ultrasound plane, thereby allowing it to be visualized as the neurosurgeon advances it toward the target within the brain.

Because of the dynamic nature of real-time ultrasound scanning, it is possible to assess the spatial relationship between the lesion and the probe. If the target lesion moves as the result of tissue shifts or if the probe does not enter the lesion, corrective measures can be imple-mented. The exact area of the lesion biopsied can be inspected, and, particularly after biopsy, repeat ultra-sound can help identify any hemorrhagic changes. If hemorrhage occurs, the neurosurgeon can follow the probe tract right down to the source of the hemorrhage.

Placing intraventricular catheters for intracranial pressure monitoring in patients can be a technical challenge because, following the development of cere-bral edema, the ventricles can be slitlike. Ultrasound imaging and instrument guides can be utilized to place the catheter in the optimal position. The same is true for the placement of ventricular catheters and Ommaya reservoirs in patients needing intrathecal chemotherapy. In patients with hydrocephalus, ultrasound imaging can be used to visualize the position of the tip of the catheter and to assure that it is within the ventricle and away from the choroid plexus, thereby avoiding shunt obstruction because of suboptimal positioning (Fig. 36-14).[5,6,14,16]

CONCLUSIONS

Intraoperative ultrasound imaging is very helpful to neurosurgeons in localizing, characterizing, and instru-menting lesions. It is useful in assessing what was accomplished and in evaluating the presence of hemor-

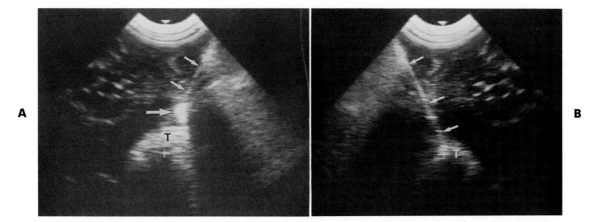

Fig. 36-13. Ultrasound scans showing biopsy of a tumor located deep within the brain. **A,** Biopsy probe *(small arrows)* with very echogenic tip *(large arrow)* being advanced to the tumor *(T)*. (Cursor is placed in the center of the tumor as the target.) **B,** Biopsy probe *(small arrows)* is now within the tumor *(T)*. The very echogenic top of the biopsy probe cannot be seen now because it is within the tumor. Real-time ultrasound imaging was very helpful to the neurosurgeon. The firm tumor kept being displaced by the biopsy probe; knowing this, the neurosurgeon could manipulate the biopsy probe until it entered the tumor. If ultrasound imaging was not used, the biopsy probe would have skimmed off to the side and given a spurious tissue specimen, one from the brain immediately surrounding the tumor.

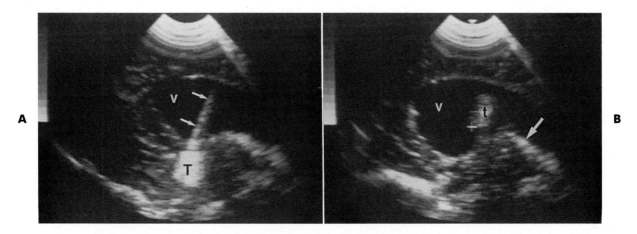

Fig. 36-14. Ultrasound scans showing incorrect placement of a ventricular catheter and correction of that placement in a patient with hydrocephalus. **A,** Sagittal ultrasound scan showing that the ventricular catheter *(arrows)* has passed through the lateral ventricle *(V)* and the hyperechoic catheter tip *(T)* is through the foramen of Monro and within the third ventricle. **B,** Recognizing the suboptimal location of the ventricular catheter with dynamic ultrasound imaging, the neurosurgeon repositioned it. Now the hyperechoic catheter tip *(t)* is within the lateral ventricle *(V)* and well away from the choroid plexus *(arrow)* located on the floor of the lateral ventricle. (Note the cursor that has been placed as the target within the lateral ventricle.)

rhage within the operative field following the procedure. Ultrasound serves as a neurosurgical "eye" within the brain, allowing the exploration of the brain without having to enter it.[15] As such, the real-time ultrasound scanner is a valued instrument in the neurosurgical operating room.

REFERENCES

1. Chandler WF, Knake JE: Intraoperative use of ultrasound in neurosurgery, *Clin Neurosurg* 31:550-563, 1984.
2. Chandler WF, Knake JE, McGillicuddy JE: Intraoperative use of real-time ultrasonography in neurosurgery, *J Neurosurg* 57:157-163, 1982.
3. Dohrmann GJ, Rubin JM: Use of ultrasound in neurosurgi-

cal operations: a preliminary report, *Surg Neurol* 16:362-366, 1981.

4. Dohrmann GJ, Rubin JM: Intraoperative ultrasound imaging of spinal cord: syringomyelia, cysts and tumors: a preliminary report, *Surg Neurol* 18:395-399, 1982.

5. Dohrmann GJ, Rubin JM: *Intraoperative real-time ultrasonography: localization, characterization and instrumentation of lesions of brain and spinal cord.* In Fasano VA, editor: *Advanced intraoperative technologies in neurosurgery,* New York, 1985, Springer-Verlag.

6. Dohrmann GJ, Rubin JM: Dynamic intraoperative imaging and instrumentation of brain and spinal cord using ultrasound, *Neurol Clin* 3:425-437, 1985.

7. Dohrmann GJ, Rubin JM: *Intraoperative diagnostic ultrasound.* In Wilkins RH, Rengachary SS, editors: *Neurosurgery,* New York, 1995, McGraw-Hill.

8. Dohrmann GJ, Rubin JM: Intraoperative ultrasound in neurotraumatology: brain, spinal cord and cauda equina, *Adv Neurotraum* 251-264, 1986.

9. Enzmann DR, Britt RH, Lyons BE: Natural history of experimental intracerebral hemorrhage: sonography, computed tomography and neuropathology, *AJNR Am J Neuroradiol* 2:517-526, 1981.

10. Knake JE, Chandler WF, Gabrielsen TO, et al: Accurate, nonsterotaxic biopsy and aspiration of subcortical brain lesions using intraoperative real-time sonography, *AJNR Am J Neuroradiol* 4:672-674, 1983.

11. Koivukangus J: Ultrasound imaging in operative neurosurgery, *Acta Univ Ouluensis* (Series D), 115:1, 1984.

12. Lillehei KO, Chandler WF, Kanke JE: Real-time ultrasound characteristics of the acute intracerebral hemorrhage: as studied in the canine model, *Neurosurgery* 14:48-51, 1984.

13. Rezvani L, Rubin JM, Dohrmann GJ: Colloid cysts with and without ventriculomegaly: role of intraoperative real-time ultrasound, *Surg Neurol* 22:515-518, 1984.

14. Rubin JM, Chandler WF: *Ultrasound in neurosurgery,* New York, 1990, Raven Press.

15. Rubin JM, Dohrmann GJ: Intraoperative neurosonography: the surgeon's eye into the brain, *Diag Imaging* 4:26-30, 1982.

16. Rubin JM, Dohrmann GJ: Use of ultrasonically guided probes and catheters in neurosurgery, *Surg Neurol* 18:143-148, 1982.

17. Rubin JM, Dohrmann GJ: A cannula for use in ultrasonically guided biopsies of the brain, *J Neurosurg* 59:905-907, 1983.

18. Rubin JM, Dohrmann GJ: Localization and characterization of intracranial masses using intraoperative ultrasonography, *Radiology* 148:519-524, 1983.

19. Rubin JM, Dohrmann GJ: Operating on inoperable lesions using intraoperative neurosurgical ultrasound, *Radiology* 157:283, 1985.

20. Rubin JM, Dohrmann GJ: Efficacy of intraoperative ultrasound for evaluation of intracranial masses, *Radiology* 157:509-511, 1985.

21. Rubin JM, Mirfakhraee M, Duda EE, et al: Intraoperative ultrasound examination of the brain, *Radiology* 137:831-832, 1980.

37

Intraoperative Spinal Ultrasound

David P. Chason

Over the past 10 years, ultrasound has developed into a useful and often invaluable adjunct to surgery of the spinal canal and its contents. Although the vast majority of spinal lesions are localized and characterized preoperatively by magnetic resonance imaging (MRI), computed tomography (CT), or myelography, real-time ultrasound is the only modality that routinely offers the capability of intraoperative assessment of surgical lesions and their relationship to the surrounding anatomy. Ultrasound can extend the surgeon's field of view through the laminectomy site and confirm the location of lesions prior to dural incision. Lesions out of view, particularly those within or ventral to the spinal cord, can be easily detected to expedite biopsy, excision, or shunting procedures, thereby minimizing potential spinal cord manipulation and trauma. Furthermore, ultrasound can monitor the progress and confirm the results of the surgical procedure.

The purpose of this chapter is to describe the techniques for intraoperative spinal ultrasound imaging and equipment considerations, as well as the normal ultrasound anatomy of the spinal cord and canal. Finally, the typical appearance of pathologic processes is discussed and demonstrated.

TECHNIQUE

Intraoperative ultrasound scanning may be performed by the sonographer or by the surgeon. It is often more efficient for the surgeon to scan, enabling the sonographer to operate the ultrasound instrument. To coordinate their efforts, an ongoing dialogue is necessary.[22] The time requirements for the performance of intraoperative spinal sonography can be significant. According to Quencer and Montalvo, the sonographer can spend an average of 1 hour in the operating room, during which only an average 10 minutes are actually needed to perform the ultrasound study.[35]

Transducer selection/consideration

Many mechanical sector and linear array transducers are available and can be used for intraoperative spinal sonography. However, only those with frequencies of 5 MHz or greater, ideally 7.5 to 10 MHz, are of clinical utility.[8] High-frequency ultrasound beams provide better near-field resolution than do those of low frequency, enabling the spinal canal and contents to be seen in much better detail.[2] Tissue absorption increases with increasing beam frequency, resulting in decreased tissue penetration. Fortunately, the shallow depth of the spinal

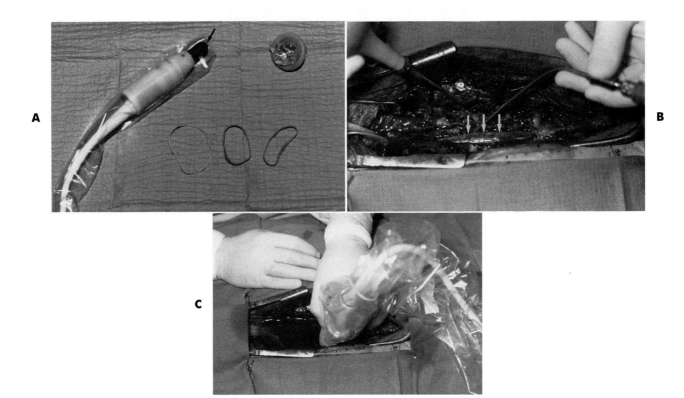

Fig. 37-1. A, Preparation of the ultrasound probe and operative site for scanning. The transducer and electrical cable are draped in sterile fashion using a plastic sheath, acoustic gel, condom, and rubber bands. It is important to keep the tip of the transducer (*arrow*) clear of the plastic sheath to ensure adequate coupling between it and the gel-filled condom. The sheath and condom are secured with rubber bands, taking care not to introduce air pockets or bubbles in the gel between the tip of the transducer and the condom. These rubber bands also serve to keep the acoustic gel near the transducer tip. If good coupling is not maintained and air and/or plastic lies between the sound beam and the region to be imaged, the resulting images will be heavily degraded by near-field artifact and inadequate penetration. **B,** Intraoperative photograph demonstrates a thoracic laminectomy with the patient prone. Note the convex upward margin of the dorsal dural sac (*arrows*). Retraction of the paraspinal muscles creates a cavity ideal to hold a water bath for scanning. When the operative site is filled with sterile saline, an attempt should be made to minimize air bubbles, debris, and blood mixing with the saline that may attenuate the sound beam. **C,** The probe tip need only be covered by saline and should be kept several centimeters above the dura or cord.

canal negates the loss of beam penetration with the high-frequency probes.

Mechanical sector scanners produce greater near-field (i.e., cap) artifact than do linear array probes. This artifact restricts their ability to image reliably in the near field. To circumvent this problem, an offset (i.e., water bath) is required to image this region effectively. If contact scanning is required, linear array probes are superior. Furthermore, focused linear array transducers restrict beam width and improve lateral resolution, providing generally higher-quality images than do mechanical scanners.[2] Efforts are underway to develop transducers of extremely small size, in order to allow scanning in tight operative fields or under the microscope.[12]

Transducer (equipment) preparation

Depending upon the probe to be used, a sterile drape is required to facilitate scanning (Fig. 37-1). A reservoir-tipped condom may be useful to cover probes with smaller scan faces. Some of the newer linear array transducers may undergo gas sterilization (i.e., ethylenetrioxide), obviating the need for a sheath. This is more convenient, and some of the potential artifact and beam attenuation are eliminated from the system. The manufacturer and equipment warranty should be consulted before trying this approach. When preparing the saline bath over the operative site, careful attention to details such as the elimination of air bubbles can markedly improve image quality.

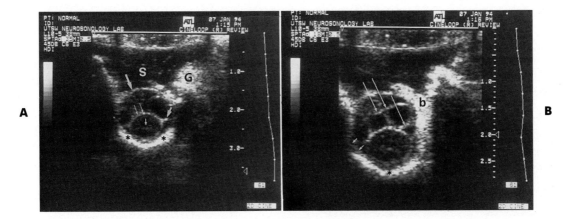

Fig. 37-2. Normal thoracic spinal cord. Transverse images through intact dura. **A,** Demonstrates the laminectomy site filled with echolucent saline (*S*). The first highly reflective structure seen is the posterior dural surface (*long arrow*). The spinal cord surface appears as an echogenic ring (*two small arrows*) about an hypoechoic underlying cord substance. The central echo complex is seen within the ventral half of the cord (*small arrow*). The thin ventral cerebrospinal fluid space separated the anterior aspect of the cord from the densely echogenic posterior vertebral body–ventral dural comple (*asterisk*). The dentate ligaments are seen connecting the lateral surface of the cord to the dura (*short arrow*). Gelfoam (*G*) appears brightly echogenic and attenuates the sound beam distally. **B,** The ventral aspect of the dura may be seen as a distinct structure laterally (*small arrows*) but is difficult to separate from the echo complex of the posterior longitudinal ligament and vertebral body medially (*asterisk*). Dorsal arachnoid bands or septae may be found normally and can be quite prominent in the region of the septum posticum (*long arrows*). Echogenic blood lies along the dorsal lateral aspect of the thecal sac (*b*). (Images courtesy of Howard Morgan, M.D., and Cole Giller, M.D.)

Acoustic window

Fortuitously, the vast majority of intraoperative sonography of the spinal canal and its contents is performed with the patient prone. In this position, the saline-filled laminectomy site becomes a suitable acoustic window for scanning (Fig. 37-2, *A*). The saline window allows the face of the transducer to be well away from the structures to be imaged, prevents physical trauma, and serves to improve image quality. Furthermore, this window places the region of interest outside the transducer's near-field artifact (more prominent on a mechanical sector scanner than a linear array), allows superficial lesions to lie within the focal zone of the transducer, and expands the field of view of the laminectomy.[3,37,38,40]

Similarly, scanning may be accomplished anteriorly through a saline bath created by a corpectomy, allowing imaging of the ventral aspect of the spinal canal first.[31] With slightly greater difficulty, patients may even be scanned in the sitting position. A Steri-drape (3M, St. Paul) is placed over the caudal and lateral aspect of the wound, forming a cavity to be filled with saline. Scanning is then achieved through the bath.[49]

In one instance, we have had occasion to scan the upper cervical spine from a posterior approach with the patient in the lateral position. Instead of the Steri-drape technique, a small, sterile, saline-filled balloon was fashioned from a latex condom. This was gently wedged into the wound and coupled to the dura with sterile acoustic gel, providing an adequate window through which to scan.

SCANNING TECHNIQUE

When the transducer and acoustic window are prepared and potential artifact is minimized, scanning is ready to proceed in a methodic, organized fashion. Initially, a survey of the region is done for general orientation and to assure that adequate surgical exposure has been obtained. This is accomplished by transverse scanning of the exposed canal from its cephalad to caudal margin, followed by longitudinal scanning from side to side. Direction of scanning and images should be labeled consistently to prevent confusion. A common convention while scanning the patient prone is, on transverse scans, the right side of the image represents the patient's right; on longitudinal scans, the cephalad end is imaged on the left.[22,39] Scanning is then focused on evaluating the lesion in question and its surrounding milieu to guide the surgical approach. The preoperative studies are often helpful for reference as well as to give an overview of the region to be scanned. Scanning can then be performed, as necessary, to monitor the progress and confirm the results of the operation.[34] While scanning in real time, the images may be recorded using

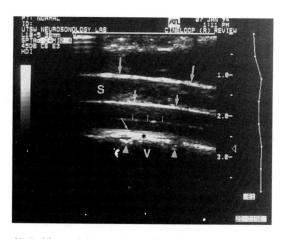

Fig. 37-3. Normal lower thoracic spinal cord. Longitudinal scan of patient in Fig. 37-2. Midline image through intact dura reveals the thoracic cord to be anteriorly placed within the thecal sac. The large echolucent posterior subarachnoid space (*S*) separates the densely echogenic posterior dura (*arrows*) and posterior margin of the cord (*short arrows*). Little subarachnoid fluid separates the ventral aspect of the cord (*thin arrow*) from the posterior margin of the vertebral bodies and ventral dura (*asterisk*). The central echo complex (*tiny arrows*) is well seen within the ventral aspect of the more echolucent cord. Notice the complete attenuation of the sound beam beyond the posterior margin of the vertebral bodies (*V*). A small amount of sound that penetrates the intervertebral disk spaces (*arrowheads*) permits assessment of vertebral body alignment. (Images courtesy of Howard Morgan, M.D., and Cole Giller, M.D.)

videotape or printed as hard copies for evaluation. The videotape recording permits hard-copy images to be made at a later time. Finally, it is necessary to monitor cautiously other parameters such as time-gain compensation and intensity settings in order to create images that are consistently of equivalent diagnostic quality.

ANATOMY

Of paramount importance to the understanding of ultrasound-generated images is the correct recognition of the transducer's orientation in relation to the anatomic plane of the region being evaluated. Furthermore, one must correlate the findings of preoperative imaging studies with the anatomy demonstrated by ultrasound, in order to make sense of the pathologic process displayed in real time.

Awareness of the anatomic differences between the different spinal levels allows for better diagnostic capability and may prevent misinterpretation. In the cervical region, the spinal cord has an elliptical appearance on transverse scans and occupies a central position within the surrounding cerebrospinal fluid (CSF).[24,25] The ventral surface of the cord is slightly flattened, the dorsal more rounded. Also, the configuration of the spinal canal is somewhat triangular, with the apex directed dorsally and the base ventrally. In the thoracic

region, transverse images demonstrate the cord to have a more rounded shape (Fig. 37-2), further enlarging at the lumbar segment. The spinal canal is round in contour, with the cord occupying the ventral aspect of the subarachnoid space.[24,25] In the lower region, the spinal cord then rapidly decreases in size to become the conus medullaris, terminating at approximately L1-L2 in the filum terminale and cauda equina (Fig. 37-3). The conus medullaris and filum terminale are surrounded by the dorsal and ventral nerve roots of the cauda equina (Figs. 37-4 and 37-5). As in the cervical region, the lumbar canal is triangular in shape, with the base oriented ventrally.[24]

The posterior dural surface is easily visualized (Fig. 37-2, *A*) after a laminectomy has been performed. The ventral dura, however, is difficult to separate from the strong echo complex of the posterior longitudinal ligament and adjacent vertebral body, particularly in the cervical and thoracic regions.[34] The inability to separately visualize the ventral dura may be due in part to the paucity of ventral epidural fat found at these levels, as the ventral dura is better appreciated in the lower lumbar spine and occasionally laterally in the cervical and thoracic spine (Fig. 37-2, *B*), where more prominent ventral epidural fat exists.[13,24,34] When the normal relationship of the dura to the ventral echo complex is disturbed in the cervical or thoracic spine, an epidural process may be suspected.[22] The lateral recesses and neural foramina are not visualized by ultrasound.[20,22]

The spinal cord substance is hypoechoic, with a brightly echogenic rim well delineated by the surrounding echolucent CSF. Gray-white differentiation cannot be made, nor can the dorsal sulci be visualized. The central echo complex is consistently seen from the cervical region to the conus. Some maintain that this echo complex represents the central canal; others have more convincingly demonstrated the source of the echo to be the interface between the end of the anterior median fissure and the ventral white commissure.[21,23,31,34,46] In the evaluation of the cord, the echo complex should be routinely sought, as its absence strongly suggests underlying intramedullary or extramedullary pathology.[22,38]

Transverse scans of the cervical and thoracic region may reveal dorsal arachnoid septations (Fig. 37-2, *B*) and the dentate ligaments laterally tethering the cord to the dura (Fig. 37-2, *A*). The ventral and dorsal nerve roots are infrequently seen except in the region of the conus medullaris and cauda equina (Fig. 37-5). Longitudinal scans are ideal for evaluating vertebral body alignment and intervertebral disk spaces (Figs. 37-3 and 37-4, *C*). The disk material allows some penetration of the sound beam as compared to the dense echo complex of the posterior vertebral body, posterior longitudinal ligament, and dura.

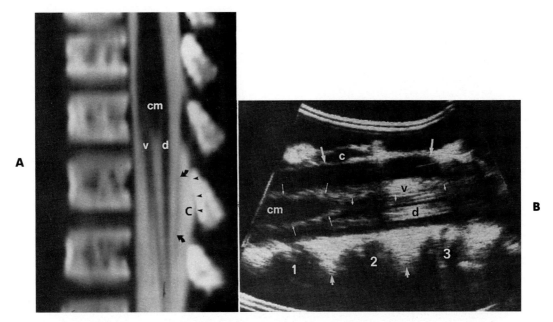

Fig. 37-4. Normal conus medullaris and filum terminale with an extradural arachnoid cyst at the level of L2. **A,** Sagittal postmyelogram computed tomography reconstruction illustrates a contrast-filled posterior extradural cystic lesion (*c*) remodeling the adjacent lamina (*arrowheads*) and mildly compressing the posterior dural margin (*curved short arrows*). Conus medullaris (*cm*), ventral (*v*), and dorsal (*d*), nerve roots of the cauda equina can be seen. **B,** Longitudinal ultrasound scan demonstrates the echolucent cystic lesion (*c*) immediately dorsal to the posterior dural margin (*long arrows*). The normal conus medullaris (*cm*) is seen as mildly echogenic with a brightly echogenic rim (*long small arrows*). The moderately echogenic filum terminale (*short small arrows*), and ventral (*v*) and dorsal (*d*) nerve roots are surrounded by echolucent cerebrospinal fluid. Note that the sound is completely attenuated by the vertebral bodies (*1, 2, 3*) but penetrates the disk spaces (*short arrows*). (Images courtesy of William P. Sanders, M.D.)

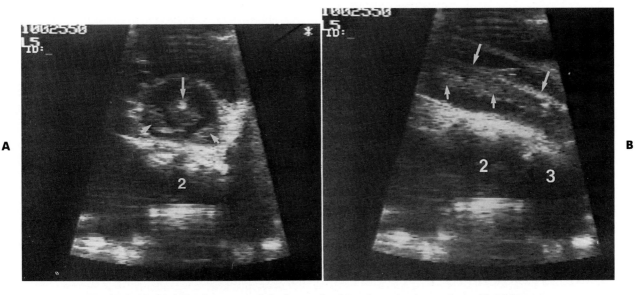

Fig. 37-5. Normal distal conus medullaris–proximal cauda equina in a patient with L2 fracture postreduction and a lipoma of the filum terminale. **A,** Transverse image reveals a brightly echogenic filum terminale (*long arrow*) infiltrated with fat, surrounded by normal, moderately echogenic nerve roots of the cauda equina (*short arrows*). The nerve roots are not significantly compressed after realignment of the posterior margin of L2 (*2*). **B,** Midline longitudinal scan. The most caudal aspect of the conus medullaris is outlined by the more echogenic nerve roots (*short arrows*) as it extends into the filum terminale and lipoma (*arrows*). Note the mild dorsal position of L2 (*2*) compared to L3 (*3*).

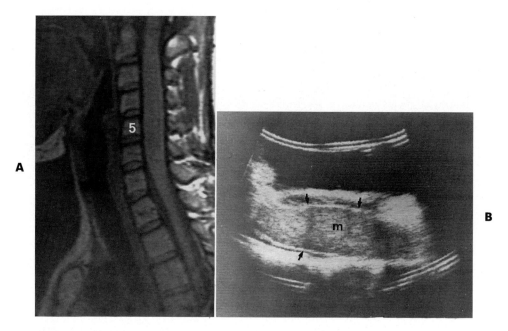

Fig. 37-6. Grade II astrocytoma of the cervical cord. **A,** Sagittal T1 of the cervical spine demonstrates expansion of the cord from C2 to C7. **B,** Longitudinal ultrasound scan shows the moderately echogenic mass (*m*) to be solid with loss of the central echo complex. The echogenic rim of the spinal cord is preserved (*arrows*). The lesion expands the spinal cord and narrows the adjacent cerebrospinal fluid spaces. Ultrasound aided in choosing the biopsy site. (Images courtesy of William P. Sanders, M.D.)

Only during real-time scanning can the anterior spinal artery and, much less frequently, the lateral spinal arteries be seen as an oscillating line or point.[38] Similarly, real-time ultrasound facilitates evaluation of spinal cord, nerve root, and dural sac motion.[11,41] Normally, when scanned through a laminectomy, the cord and nerve roots are seen to move minimally or to pulsate mildly with the frequency of the cardiac cycle.[22,38] Furthermore, spinal cord or nerve root pulsation of high amplitude may indicate underlying extrinsic compression.[11] Normally, the pulsatile force of the noncompressed anterior or lateral spinal artery is dispersed into the CSF, resulting in little cord motion. When maximally compressed between an extrinsic mass and the cord, the artery's pulsatile force may be offset by the mass and cord, resulting in little cord motion. The cord pulsation, however, may increase away from, or at the point of, less complete compression, giving rise to a rocking motion of high amplitude.[41]

LESIONS INVOLVING THE SPINAL CANAL AND ITS CONTENTS
Intradural (intramedullary) lesions

Various sonographic imaging criteria have been used to evaluate the spinal cord for the presence of pathologic processes.[22,27,33,37,38] The most reliable are the following.

1. Cord echogenicity greater or more heterogeneous than normal
2. Obliteration of the central echo complex and distortion of normal cord anatomy
3. Expansion or enlargement of the cord with narrowing of the subarachnoid space
4. Loss of the normal echogenic rind of the cord surface
5. Sonolucent region(s) suggesting cyst or syrinx
6. Abnormal pulsation of the lesion or cord

Intramedullary neoplasms may manifest with one or more of these characteristics. The vast majority of these lesions are hyperechoic as compared to the normal cord (Figs. 37-5 through 37-9, pp. 429-433).[27,33] When the region of hyperechogenicity is associated with acoustic shadowing, mineralization may be present within the lesion. Additionally, most spinal cord neoplasms result in alteration of the central echo complex as well as enlargement of the involved cord segment.[37,46] Hyperechogenicity, obscuration of the central echo complex, and cord enlargement are not seen exclusively with neoplastic lesions, however. Myelomalacia, radiation necrosis, myelitis, cord edema, and hematoma can all present as hyperechoic lesions with loss of the central echo complex.[19,27,31,38] Furthermore, expansion or enlargement of the cord with narrowing of the subarachnoid space may indicate an underlying mass lesion such as a tumor, hematoma, cyst, syrinx, or edema but would

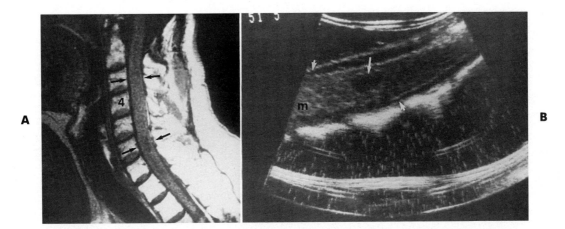

Fig. 37-7. Metastatic cervical cord lesion with associated cystic change. **A,** Sagittal T1-weighted magnetic resonance image shows expansion of the cord from C2-3 to C7-T1 with focal regions of decreased signal at C2-3 and C6-T1 (*arrows*). **B,** Longitudinal ultrasound scan through the lower aspect of the moderately echogenic metastatic lesion (*m*) shows a focal region of sonolucency along its caudal margin (*arrow*) confirming the suspected cystic change. This helped delineate the extent of the lesion. Obliteration of the central echo complex is seen. Narrowing of the ventral and dorsal subarachnoid space is seen in the region of the mass (*short arrows*). (Images courtesy of William P. Sanders, M.D.)

not be expected with myelomalacia or in the late stages of radiation necrosis. Loss of the normal echogenic margin of the cord has been described with myelomalacia and may be seen with myelitis.[19]

Edema of the cord alone can mimic a neoplastic lesion sonographically and, when present about a true lesion, can obscure its margins.[27] Interestingly, whereas most describe edema as echogenic in the spinal cord and brain, others have demonstrated edema to be hypoechoic by ultrasound and were able to differentiate metastatic cord lesions from edema.[27,29,45]

Four cases of demyelinating lesions in the spinal cord were shown to be hypoechoic by ultrasound without associated hyperechogenicity.[6] These lesions revealed little or no mass effect and preserved the central echo complex. It is possible that the hypoechoic appearance of the lesion was on the basis of edema.

Attempts have been made to correlate ultrasonic patterns of intramedullary tumors with their histology.[6,13] Ultrasound cannot, however, differentiate primary from metastatic lesions (Fig. 37-7), nor is the echoic pattern specific to the underlying histology.[27] Between 31% and 53% of spinal cord tumors are associated with cystic lesions.[27] Ultrasound can easily localize both cystic and solid components of a tumor and delineate their margins, allowing resection, biopsy, aspiration, or shunting to be more effective (Figs. 37-7 and 37-9). The ability of ultrasound to distinguish cystic from solid lesions far exceeds that of CT or MRI.[10,26,36] The ultrasonic hallmark of a cyst is sonolucency with through-transmission of the sound beam. One should bear in mind, however, that cystic lesions containing hemorrhage, debris, or pus may appear solid. Platt and colleagues described this potential pitfall in a case of an intramedullary teratoma.[26] The echogenic appearance of the lesion was felt to be due to the multiple reflective interfaces produced by thick creamy fluid and desquamated tissue found within the cyst during surgery.

Ultrasound has been invaluable in the intraoperative assessment and treatment of syringomyelia (Fig. 37-10) and posttraumatic spinal cord cysts.[1,3,31,49] Prior to shunting these cystic lesions, the portion of the cyst or syrinx closest to the dorsal cord surface can be selected for myelotomy.[3] Furthermore, intraoperative ultrasound can demonstrate internal septations and loculations within syrinx or cyst cavities and thereby improve shunt placement and ultimately drainage. After shunting, subsequent decompression of the syrinx or cyst can be confirmed prior to completion of surgery and may obviate additional procedures.[3,37,49]

The presence of vascular channels with arterial pulsation in association with a cystic and solid hyperechoic mass has been reported to be suggestive of hemangioblastoma (Fig. 37-9).[27,43] An intramedullary arteriovenous malformation (AVM) has also been described ultrasonically as a complex echogenic mass pulsating at the cardiac rate. Ultrasound is felt to be particularly helpful in evaluating those AVMs with ventral or intramedullary components.[42] Cavernous angiomas have been described as nonpulsatile hyperechoic lesions.[15] Ultrasound is particularly useful in locating those not present on the dorsal cord surface.

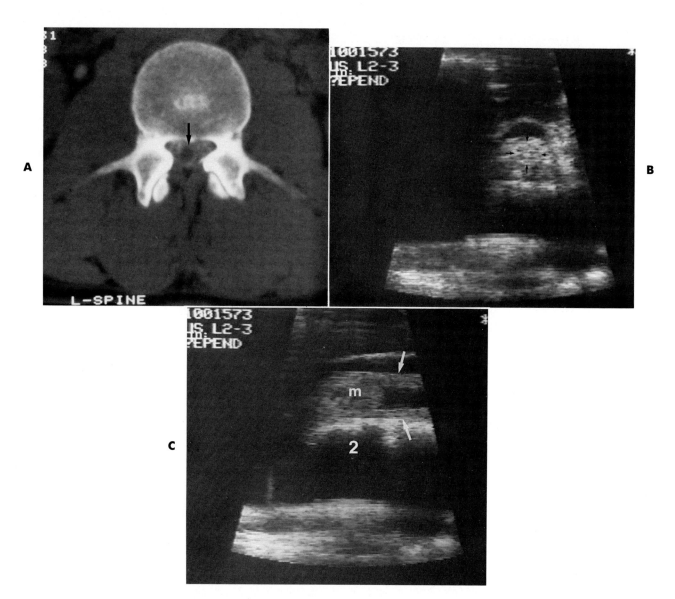

Fig. 37-8. Myxopapillary ependymoma of the filum terminale. **A,** Postmyelogram–computed tomography axial image defines the lesion (*arrow*) as low density at the L2-3 level. **B,** Transverse intraoperative sonogram confirms the location and characterizes the homogeneously echogenic lesion as a solid mass prior to opening the dura. Note how the lesion is nestled between the nerve roots (*arrows*). **C,** Longitudinal scan again illustrates the solid nature of the egg-shaped lesion (*m*), which lies between the ventral and dorsal nerve roots (*arrows*), outlined by the sonolucent cerebrospinal fluid.

Interestingly, color flow Doppler shows no evidence of flow in these angiographically occult lesions.[16]

Intradural extramedullary lesions

Lesions within the dural sac, but separate from the cord, are easily localized by ultrasound. The plane of dissection between the lesion, the cord, and the dura can be defined, as well as the position of the cord and degree of any compression. This evaluation can be accomplished prior to dural incision and is particularly useful for locating ventrally placed lesions.

Like intramedullary neoplastic lesions, noncystic extramedullary lesions are predominantly hyperechoic as compared to the spinal cord.[14,18,37] This has been demonstrated with neurilemomas, meningiomas, metastatic lesions, dermoid and epidermoid cysts, and lipomas (Fig. 37-5). With rare exceptions, extramedullary lesions do not result in obscuration of the central echo complex.[18,31,37,46] Lesions of the filum terminale, such as ependymomas, or exophytic lesions of the cord can be confusing, as they may appear extramedullary when they are, in fact, intramedullary (Fig. 37-8).

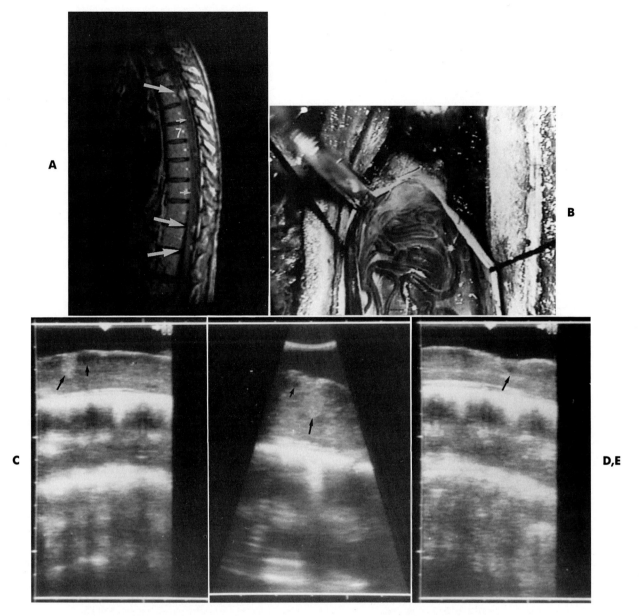

Fig. 37-9. Spinal hemangioblastoma. **A,** Sagittal T1-weighted images of the spine following the administration of gadolinium reveal three intramedullary enhancing lesions, the largest at T5 (*arrows*). Note the associated very low signal intensity of the central portion of the cord which was thought to represent syrinx (*small arrows*). **B,** Intraoperative photograph with dura reflected and cord surface exposed shows meningeal varicosities overlying the dorsal surface of the cord. The exact location of the lesion, however, was not evident grossly. **C,** Sagittal scan and (**D**) transverse scan easily identify the echogenic lesion (*arrow*) with an associated small cystic component (*small arrow*) and correctly demonstrate the overall solid nature of the cord. Note the diffusely echogenic cord substance with focal loss of the central echo complex. **E,** Sagittal postexcision scan verifies complete removal of the lesion (*arrow*). (Surgical photograph (B) courtesy of Bruce Mickey, M.D.)

Although not pathognomonic, certain sonographic characteristics may distinguish neurilemomas and meningiomas and suggest their histologic identification intraoperatively.[18] Neurilemomas are more prone to have rounded and smooth surfaces, whereas meningiomas demonstrate irregular margins. Furthermore, meningiomas tend to be more echogenic than neurilemomas and reveal dural attachment. Because of their dural involvement, the meningiomas are not observed to pulsate with the cardiac cycle as neurilemomas do.[18] Arachnoiditis may be suggested when clumping deformity of the nerve roots is visualized.[20]

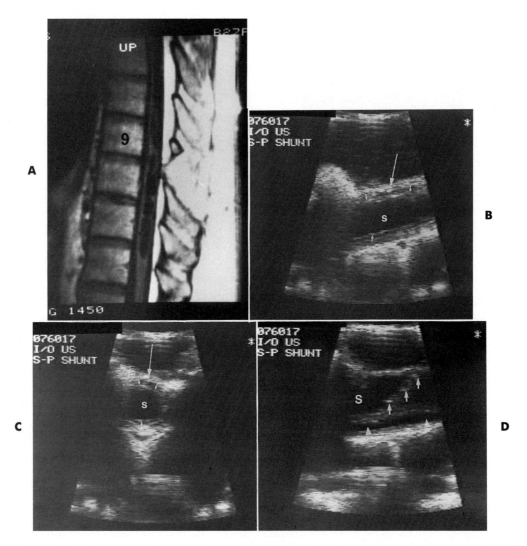

Fig. 37-10. Syringomyelia. **A,** Sagittal T1-weighted magnetic resonance image reveals multiseptated syrinx from T5-T12. **B,** Longitudinal scan and (**C,**) transverse scan of the syrinx (*s*) through intact dura (*long arrow*) in a location with few septations. Note the loss of the central echo complex and the paucity of cerebrospinal fluid surrounding the expanded spinal cord (*short arrows*). Ultrasound aided in choosing the best myelotomy site. **D,** Image as the shunt catheter was ultrasonically guided into the syrinx (*s*). Note the parallel echoes of the catheter (*arrows*). The syrinx cavity had not yet decreased in size. The increase in size of the ventral subarachnoid space (*arrowheads*) is due to the dural incision.

Ultrasound is useful in localizing extramedullary intradural cystic lesions such as arachnoid or subarachnoid cysts (Fig. 37-11) and cysticercosis.[4,44,47] Mass effect on adjacent neural structures can be readily determined. As with intramedullary cysts and syrinxes, sonography may aid in surgical planning and postoperative assessment following shunting, fenestration, or excision of these lesions. Subarachnoid cysts resulting from the sequelae of trauma or chronic inflammation are frequently associated with cord abnormalities such as myelomalacia, spinal cord cysts, hematoma, or syrinx formation at or away from the level of the injury.[44]

Ultrasound is particularly well suited to evaluate these lesions.

Extradural lesions

The ultrasound beam cannot penetrate the dense echogenic complex of the ventral dura and the posterior longitudinal ligament–vertebral body margin except at the disk space level. This limitation, however, does not prevent sonography from being a useful tool for the intraoperative evaluation of the ventral extradural space. This is particularly true in the lower thoracic and lumbar spine, where the epidural space is the largest.

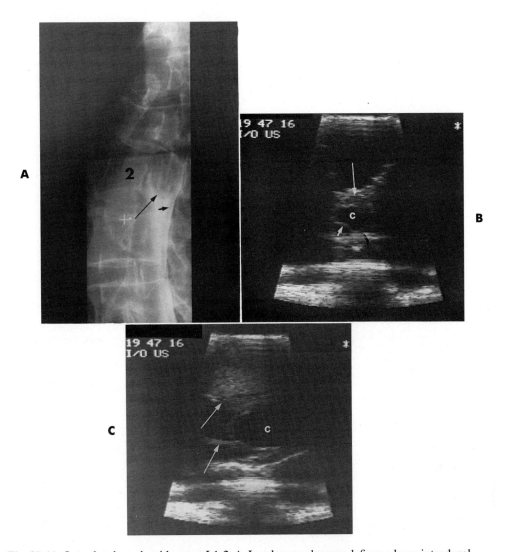

Fig. 37-11. Intradural arachnoid cyst at L1-2. **A,** Lumbar myelogram defines a large intradural extramedullary filling defect (*long arrow*) at L1-2 with deviation of the adjacent nerve roots (*short arrow*). **B,** Transverse ultrasound scan reveals the compressed distal conus and proximal cauda equina (*long arrow*) just beneath the intact dura by the ventrally placed, sonolucent cystic lesion (*c*) with anterolateral septation (*short arrow*). **C,** Longitudinal scan shows the arachnoid cyst (*c*) and surrounding subarachnoid space with deviation of the nerve roots (*arrows*).

Furthermore, the ventral extradural space may be the most difficult region for the surgeon to evaluate by direct inspection.

The benefits of intraoperative ultrasound have been established in the assessment of spinal trauma, abnormalities of vertebral body alignment, disk herniation, spinal stenosis, and epidural lesions.

Real-time intraoperative ultrasound has proven to be an effective tool for monitoring the surgical reduction of thoracic and lumbar vertebral body fractures (Fig. 37-12).[5,17,19,32,48] Prior to and during reduction, ultrasound permits the surgeon to define the severity of vertebral malalignment, demonstrate the presence and position of retropulsed bone fragments within the spinal canal, and assess the degree of neural element impingement. Following reduction, ultrasound can confirm the restoration of vertebral body alignment, relief of neural compression, and reappearance of the ventral subarachnoid space. More traditional intraoperative methods used to confirm these desired results include cross-table lateral plain films and myelography.[17] Although overall vertebral body alignment can be demonstrated and gross neural impingement can be seen by these studies, small bone fragments and subtle but clinically important neural compression may be missed. Ultrasound may be the most accurate intraoperative technique to monitor reduction of vertebral body fractures and to assess neural compression.[17,32,48] Additionally, ultrasound can

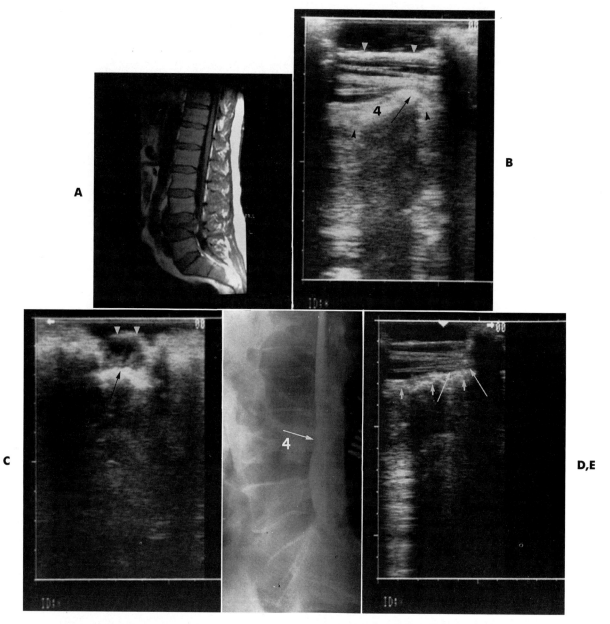

Fig. 37-12. Burst fracture of L4 vertebral body with bone fragments narrowing the spinal canal more than 50%. **A,** Sagittal T1-weighted magnetic resonance image of the lumbar spine with corresponding prereduction intraoperative ultrasound. **B,** Longitudinal scan and (**C**) transverse scan through intact dura. The abnormal alignment is well depicted on the longitudinal scan with good visualization of the intervertebral disk spaces (*arrowheads*). The retropulsed vertebral body (*arrow*) is seen to compress the adjacent ventral thecal sac and underlying nerve roots. Ultrasound demonstrates improvement of the dorsal compromise of the spinal canal as a result of the laminectomy performed prior to fracture reduction (*white arrowheads*). **D,** Postreduction intraoperative myelogram reveals improvement in vertebral body alignment and a more normal shape of the canal without apparent neural compromise (*arrow*). **E,** Postreduction longitudinal scan well demonstrates the return to a more normal vertebral alignment (*short arrows*) and relief of neural impingement and return of the ventral cerebrospinal fluid space (*long arrows*).

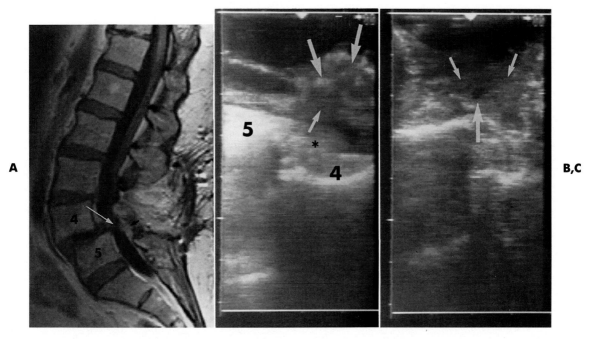

A

B,C

Fig. 37-13. Spondylolisthesis with spinal stenosis. **A,** Sagittal T1-weighted images demonstrate a grade I anterior spondylolisthesis of L4 on L5. Extensive scar tissue is seen along the dorsal aspect of the thecal sac from prior laminectomy and fusion (*short arrow*) with persistent spinal stenosis (*long arrow*). **B,** Sagittal ultrasound shows the echogenic scar tissue overlying and adherent to the distorted dorsal dura (*long arrows*) as well as defines the underlying stenosis (*short arrow*). The nerve roots of the cauda equina are difficult to isolate in the region of stenosis. The spondylolithesis of L4 on L5, widened disk space, and prominent ventral epidural space with bulging disk material of medium echogenicity are well delineated (*asterisk*). **C,** Off-angle scan displays the scar tissue (*short arrows*) surrounding a stenotic echolucent thecal sac (*long arrow*).

aid in identifying associated traumatic lesions, including spinal cord hematomas and cysts, epidural hematoma, and disk herniation, and can expedite the location of foreign bodies.[17,19] This information cannot be easily obtained by plain film or intraoperative myelography.

Although not widely used, some authors feel that intraoperative ultrasound has a place in the surgical management of disk disease and canal stenosis.[9,20] The ability of ultrasound to detect residual disk material after routine diskectomy and persistent canal stenosis following decompressive surgery was demonstrated and was felt to improve clinical outcome (Fig. 37-13).[20]

Extradural lesions, such as abscesses and arachnoid cysts (Fig. 37-4) may also be evaluated intraoperatively by ultrasound. Ultrasound was found to be helpful in defining the location and extent of epidural abscesses and monitoring their decompression.[7,30] Furthermore, ultrasound demonstrated the abscesses to be hyperechoic masses and was felt to be effective in distinguishing these lesions from the spinal cord and from adjacent meningitis, if present.[30]

REFERENCES

1. Chadduck WM, Flanigan S: Intraoperative ultrasound for spinal lesions, *Neurosurg* 16(4):477-483, 1985.
2. Curry TS, Dowdey JE, Murry RC: *Christensen's physics of diagnostic radiology,* ed 4, Baltimore, 1990, Lea & Febiger.
3. Dohrman GJ, Rubin JM: Intraoperative ultrasound imaging of the spinal cord: syringomyelia, cysts, and tumors—a preliminary report, *Surg Neurol* 18(6):395-399, 1982.
4. Duncan AW, Hoare RD: Spinal arachnoid cysts in children, *Radiology* 126:423-429, 1978.
5. Eismont FJ, et al: The role of intraoperative ultrasonography in the treatment of thoracic and lumbar spine fractures, *Spine* 9(8):782-787, 1984.
6. Epstein FJ, Farmer JP, Schneider SJ: Intraoperative ultrasonography: an important surgical adjunct for intramedullary tumors, *J Neurosurg* 74:729-733, 1991.
7. Feldenzer JA, et al: Anterior cervical epidural abscess: the use of intraoperative spinal sonography, *Surg Neurol* 25:105-108, 1986.
8. Gooding GAW, et al: Transducer frequency considerations in intraoperative use of the spine, *Radiology* 160:272-273, 1986.
9. Gooding GAW, Boggan JE, Weinstein PR: Intraoperative sonography during lumbar laminectomy: work in progress, *AJNR Am J Neuroradiol* 5:571-573, 1984.
10. Goy AM, et al: Intramedullary spinal cord tumors: MR imaging, with emphasis on associated cysts, *Radiology* 161:381, 1986.

11. Jokich PM, Rubin JM, Dohrmann GJ: Intraoperative ultrasonic evaluation of spinal cord motion, *J Neurosurg* 60:707-711, 1984.

12. Kawakami N, et al: New transducers for intraoperative spinal sonography, *J Neurosurg* 79:787-790, 1993.

13. Kawakami N, Mimatsu K, Kato F: Intraoperative sonography of intramedullary spinal cord tumóurs, *Neuroradiology* 34:436-439, 1992.

14. Knake JE, et al: Intraoperative sonography of intraspinal tumors: initial experience, *AJNR Am J Neuroradiol* 4:1199-1201, 1983.

15. Lunardi P: Comments on the role of intraoperative ultrasound imaging in the surgical removal of intramedullary cavernous angiomas, *Neurosurg* 34(3):523, 1994.

16. Lunardi P, et al: The role of intraoperative ultrasound imaging in the surgical removal of intramedullary cavernous angiomas, *Neurosurg* 34(3):520-523, 1994.

17. McGahan JP, et al: Intraoperative sonographic monitoring of reduction of thoracolumbar burst fractures, *AJR Am J Roentgenol* 145:1229-1232, 1985.

18. Mimatsu K, et al: Intraoperative ultrasonography of extramedullary spinal tumours, *Neuroradiology* 34:440-443, 1992.

19. Montalvo BM, et al: Intraoperative sonography in spinal trauma, *Radiology* 153:125-134, 1984.

20. Montalvo BM, et al: Lumbar disk herniation and canal stenosis: value of intraoperative sonography in diagnosis and surgical management, *AJNR Am J Neuroradiol* 11:31-40, 1990.

21. Montalvo BM, Skaggs PH: The central canal of the spinal cord: ultrasonic identification (letter), *Radiology* May:536, 1985.

22. Naidich TP, Quencer RM, editors: *Clinical neurosonography: ultrasound of the Central Nervous System,* 1986, Springer-Verlag.

23. Nelson MD, Sedler JA, Gilles FH: Spinal cord central echo complex: histoanatomic correlation, *Radiology* 170:479-481, 1989.

24. Newton TH, Potts DG: *Computed tomography of the spine and spinal cord,* Modern Neuroradiology, volume 1, San Anselmo, CA, 1983, Clavadel Press.

25. Osborn AG: *Diagnostic neuroradiology,* St Louis, 1994, Mosby.

26. Platt JF, et al: Intraoperative sonographic characterization of a cystic intramedullary spinal cord lesion appearing as solid, *AJNR Am J Neuroradiol* 9:614, 1988.

27. Platt JF, et al: Intraoperative spinal sonography in the evaluation of intramedullary tumors, *J Ultrasound Med* 7:317-325, 1988.

28. Poser CM: The relationship between syringomyelia and neoplasm. In American Lecture Series No. 262: *American Lectures in Neurology,* Springfield, IL, Thomas, 1956.

29. Post MJD, et al: Intramedullary spinal cord metastases, mainly of nonneurogenic origin, *AJR Am J Roentgenol* 148:1015-1022, 1987.

30. Post MJD, et al: Spinal infection: evaluation with MR imaging and intraoperative US, *Radiology* 169:765-771, 1988.

31. Quencer RM, et al: Intraoperative spinal sonography: adjunct to metrizamide CT in the assessment and surgical decompression of post-traumatic spinal cord cysts, *AJR Am J Roentgenol* 142:593-601, 1984.

32. Quencer RM, et al: Intraoperative spinal sonography in thoracic and lumbar fractures: evaluation of Harrington Rod Instrumentation, *AJR Am J Roentgenol* 145:343-349, 1985.

33. Quencer RM, et al: Intraoperative spinal sonography of soft-tissue masses of the spinal cord and spinal canal, *AJR Am J Roentgenol* 143:1307-1315, 1984.

34. Quencer RM, Montalvo BM: Normal intraoperative spinal sonography, *AJNR Am J Neuroradiol* 5:501-505, 1984.

35. Quencer RM, Montalvo BM: Time requirements for intraoperative neurosonography, *AJNR Am J Neuroradiol* 7:155-158, 1986.

36. Rubin JM, Aisen AM, DiPietro MA: Ambiguities in MR imaging of tumoral cysts in the spinal cord, *JCAT* 10(3):395-398, 1986.

37. Rubin JM, Chandler WF: The use of ultrasound during spinal cord surgery, *World J Surg* 11:570-578, 1987.

38. Rubin JM, Chandler WF: *Ultrasound in Neurosurgery,* New York, 1990, Raven Press.

39. Rubin JM, Dohrmann GJ: Intraoperative sonography of the spine and spinal cord. In: *Seminars in Ultrasound CT and MR,* 6(1):48-67, 1985, Grune & Stratton.

40. Rubin JM, Dohrmann GJ: Intraoperative ultrasonography of the spine, *Radiology* 146:173, 1983.

41. Rubin JM, Dohrmann GJ: The spine and spinal cord during neurosurgical operations: real-time ultrasonography, *Radiology* 155:197-200, 1985.

42. Rubin JM, Knake JE: Intraoperative sonography of a spinal cord arteriovenous malformation, *AJNR Am J Neuroradiol* 8:730-731, 1987.

43. Sanders WP, et al: Ultrasonic features of two cases of spinal cord hemangioblastoma, *Surg Neurol* 26:453-456, 1986.

44. Sklar E, et al: Acquired spinal subarachnoid cysts: evaluation with MR, CT, myelography and intraoperative sonography, *AJNR Am J Neuroradiol* 10:1097-1104, 1989.

45. Smith SJ, et al: Brain edema: ultrasound examination, *Radiology* 155:379, 1985.

46. St Amour TE, Rubin JM, Dohrmann GJ: The central canal of the spinal cord: ultrasonic identification, *Radiology* 152:757-769, 1984.

47. Swany KS, et al: Intraspinal arachnoid cyst, *Clin Neurol Neurosurg* 86:145-148, 1984.

48. Vincent KA, Benson DR, McGahan JP: Intraoperative ultrasonography for reduction of thoracolumbar burst fractures, *Spine* 14(4):387-390, 1989.

49. Wilberger JE, Jr., et al: Magnetic resonance imaging and intraoperative neurosonography in syringomyelia, *Neurosurgery* 20(4):599-605, 1987.

38

Transcranial Doppler Monitoring of Carotid Endarterectomy

James H. Halsey, Jr.

Carotid endarterectomy represents an ideal procedure during which transcranial Doppler (TCD) can provide useful hemodynamic information. Monitoring of the middle cerebral artery (MCA) mean velocity (MV) can help detect serious cerebral ischemia when the carotid artery is clamped during endarterectomy, which occurs in approximately 25% of patients with contralateral carotid occlusion and in about 5% of those without it. Stroke occurs with relatively high frequency if the ischemia persists more than a few minutes. The risk is strongly diminished by shunting. In the absence of ischemia, however, the risks of shunting excede its potential benefit. Selective shunting can be based upon TCD monitoring, although it is technically difficult and cannot be done at all in some patients. The use of TCD monitoring during carotid endarterectomy, its technical problems, and partial solutions to these problems are discussed in this chapter.

MONITORING PROBLEMS

The principles of applying TCD monitoring to any clinical situation are beyond the scope of this discussion. The presentation is limited to the practical difficulties of using TCD to monitor carotid endarterectomy, as well as some of the solutions developed.

Failure to record

The temporal bone window deteriorates progressively with age, more severely in women than in men and more prominently in blacks. Calculations based on phantoms, measurements in cadaver skulls, and clinical research experience suggest that in order to maximize access through the temporal window, optimal power output for adult TCD practice should be about 1000 mW/cm^2. However, the current standard is 100 W, which is the approved power for fetal examination in utero. For each doubling of emitted power, the waveform intensity is increased by an average of 3 dB.[1] Instigated by these observations, one manufacturer has developed a prototype signal-averaging program. When the electrocardiogram (ECG) is simultaneously recorded and input into the instrument, a running average of 4 or 5 waveforms is displayed. This averaging procedure is widely used, for example, in the detection of cerebral cortical evoked potentials and reduces background noise while enhancing signal-to-noise ratio as the square root of the number

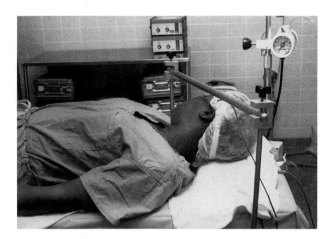

Fig. 38-1. The aluminum crossbar protects the transducer from the surgeon's assistant holding a retractor. The transducer is accessible to the sonographer from the head of the table.

of events averaged. The clinical experience with this program has been that, in fact, waveform intensity's enhancement is equivalent to the effect of approximately doubling the transducer power output. The use of signal averaging is ideally suited to the monitoring situation where the ECG is immediately available, the transducer position is stable, and the waveform is being continuously monitored. Averaging is less useful in initial window finding and handheld examination. It must be noted that it attenuates embolic signals, although the loudest ones can still be detected.

Loss of signal

The main problem, once a waveform has been obtained, is to maintain optimal insonation throughout the procedure. The surgeon's assistant, holding a retractor, rests a hand directly over the usual transducer position and often dislodges it. Some investigators simply hold the transducer manually in place, protecting it from the surgeon by hand. This practice can be fatiguing, may interfere with data recording, and may represent an inconvenience to the surgeon and anesthetist.

Some instruments have a "monitoring transducer," with detachable handles that reduce the transducer height to about 15 mm. It is held in place by a locking plate with an elastic Velcro strap, or the plate can be glued to the scalp with collodion. Even if the transducer is tightly attached to the scalp, any subsequent movement of the head during placement of electroencephalogram (EEG) electrodes, intubation, placement of surgical drapes, and surgery may disturb the point of insonation because of movement of the scalp in relation to the skull or because of asymmetric tension in the holding straps. Pressure on the transducer holder by the surgeon's hand may cause further disturbance.

The transducer can be protected from the surgeon by an aluminum crossbar held over the transducer, running in a line parallel with the jaw. It is held in place by two uprights attached to the operating table with obstetric stirrup clamps (Fig 38-1). In our procedures, following intubation, the patient's head is rotated to the opposite side and taped in place. This system does not disturb the surgeon who stands on the opposite side of the operating table from the assistant but is inconvenient if the surgeon stands at the head of the table. There may also be a problem in surgery performed under local anesthesia, when emergency intubation is required by severe ischemia complicated by unconsciousness or seizures. However, reliable TCD monitoring may make local anesthesia unnecessary because they both serve the same purpose: to monitor adequacy of cerebral blood flow.

INTERPRETATION OF THE TRANSCRANIAL DOPPLER WAVEFORM DURING MONITORING

Once the monitoring data are acquired, the next step is perhaps just as challenging: to interpret the significance of changes observed in the TCD Doppler waveform along the procedure.

Percent change at clamping

The magnitude of the MV varies along the course of the MCA. Proximally it is higher than distally. For this reason the most satisfactory index of ischemia is the MV during clamping expressed as a percent of the MV prior to clamping. The best definition of "MV prior to clamping" is the average of several measurements between the moment of first skin incision and clamping. This smooths the effects of incidental manual carotid compressions and random blood pressure changes.

Carotid siphon and anterior cerebral artery

If insonation is at 55 or 60 mm, part or all of the waveform may be from the carotid siphon. This waveform may disappear at clamping even if the MCA flow is adequate. Furthermore, at this depth, the insonation may also include the anterior cerebral artery (ACA). In this case, if the predominant collateral is via the anterior communicating artery, the MV of the reversed ACA flow may be higher than that of the siphon or proximal MCA recorded prior to clamping. This may rarely occur at 45 mm if a long sample volume is being used and the MCA and ACA insonation angles are the same. Often there is a harsh turbulent sound in this waveform, providing a clue to its identity. Although the appearance of the ACA signal is not a quantitatively accurate index of the change in MCA, MV, it does qualitatively indicate adequacy of the collateral as judged by EEG, stump pressure, and clinical outcome. In such cases, the waveform intensity is progressively stronger as depth of insonation is increased to 65 mm, confirming the ACA source and hiding the lower MCA waveform, which, coincidentally, has the same angle of insonation.

Lenticulostriate arteries

In some patients a narrow window may collimate the insonation angle above the main trunk of the MCA, revealing an inward-directed waveform. If this is in the depth range of 40 to 50 mm, the ACA is not a likely source (less than 1%). It is most often from inward-directed vectors of inward-directed branches of the MCA, the lenticulostriate arteries and within the sylvian fissure. Their MV is generally in the same range as that of the parent MCA. This waveform is a valid index to monitor for the assessment and detection of ischemia at clamping.

Posterior cerebral artery monitoring

Insonation of the posterior cerebral artery (PCA) does not yield a valid index of ischemia, except if the PCA arises from the carotid and there is no connection to the basilar artery. Under most conditions, however, the usual effect of carotid clamping is to increase the PCA MV. Although the PCA is not usually detected superficially to 50 mm, it has a branch supplying the inferior surface of the temporal lobe, which is detectable in about 5% of normal people and can often be followed out to 30 or 35 mm. This branch is more frequently detected in the presence of severe carotid stenosis or occlusion, when its MV may be increased. The most reliable way to be sure that monitoring is not being carried out from the PCA (including its inferior temporal branch) is to pay careful attention to the angle of insonation. Except in cases with extremely anterior window (mostly white men), the MCA is found 10 to 15° above the horizontal and anterior to the coronal planes, while the PCA is 10 to 15° below and posterior.

If MV is greater than 50 cm/s in the awake patient, MCA insonation is probable. During dissection, prior to clamping, the surgeon often compresses the carotid temporarily, at which time MV may decrease transiently, lending confidence in the insonation. The best way to be sure is to perform a test clamping combined with measurement of the stump pressure and EEG.

Simultaneous bilateral monitoring

Monitoring both MCAs simultaneously, using two transducers, is now technically feasible because of new software that alternates activation of each transducer sequentially many times per second while the waveforms are recorded on separate channels. This "beam splitting" eliminates the interference each transducer would have on the other if both were continuously activated. An incidental effect would be a 50% reduction of output power, unless instrument design compensated for it.

Although the electronic problem is thus solved, the practical difficulty of bilateral simultaneous monitoring remains significant. Beyond the increased difficulty of finding bilateral windows, the actual maintenance of the waveforms during surgery is also greater, especially in the opposite MCA. Because the head is ordinarily turned away from the side of surgery to facilitate exposure, the opposite transducer is likely to make contact with the table surface, resulting in its displacement, while the sonographer has greater difficulty reaching it to make position adjustments.

A major potential application of bilateral monitoring is when the contralateral carotid artery is occluded or severely narrowed. In the presence of a competent anterior communicating artery, ipsilateral clamping would cause contralateral ischemia. In a recent large study, severe (ipsilateral) ischemia occurred at clamping in 26% of cases with contralateral carotid occlusion, but in only 7% overall.[2] In my own experience of using ipsilateral TCD monitoring concurrently with bilateral EEG, the contralateral ischemia has been less severe than the ipsilateral, as judged by severity of EEG change. Because this is difficult to quantitate, a bilateral TCD study would be potentially interesting and useful.

MONITORING EXPERIENCES

Prior to the clamping of the internal carotid, MV is sometimes passively responsive to blood pressure changes. At clamping, MV falls immediately. The severity of the resulting ischemia is a function of the competence of the cerebral collateral circulation and an important determinant of this is the contribution of the contralateral carotid. In 40 patients with contralateral occlusion, MV fell to a mean of 39% of the preclamp value ($\pm 29\%$ = 1 standard deviation); in 209 without contralateral carotid stenosis, the mean was 68% ($\pm 30\%$). In the patients without contralateral occlusion, there was no relation between the severity of ischemia at clamping and the severity of contralateral stenosis.

Significance of the ischemia is suggested by concurrent EEG monitoring and by clinical outcome. If the MV falls to less than 15% of the preclamp level, ipsilateral EEG suppression occurs in about 50% of cases. If severe ischemia of this degree persists more than a few minutes, the risk of cerebral infarction is about 50%. Successful placement of a functioning shunt virtually always results in immediate correction of severe ischemia and protects against ischemia. If the MV remains above 15% but less than 40%, most such patients can tolerate clamping without shunting for up to 30 minutes; if the MV is above 40%, clamping times of up to an hour are well tolerated. Shunting is therefore beneficial in the presence of severe ischemia. In the absence of ischemia, it provides no benefit, and, in fact, its small risk constitutes a virtual contraindication (presuming reliability of the monitor-

Table 38-1. Effect of shunting on intraoperative ischemia

Severe ischemia (MV 0-15%)	Stroke	Total	
Shunt	0/74	0%**	
No shunt			p < 0.0001
Persisting ischemia (MV at 5 min <40%)	6*/13	46%	p < 0.01
Spontaneous recovery	0/13	0%	
Recovery unknown	0/7	0%	
Mild ischemia (MV = 16%-40%)			
Shunt	3/77	3.9%	0.10 > p > 0.05
No shunt	1/159	0.6%	
No ischemia (MV >40%)			
Shunt	6/136	4.4%**	
No shunt	7/1016	0.7%	
TOTAL	23/1495		

*One severely ischemic nonshunted case attributed to embolism.
**Difference between shunted severe ischemia and shunted no ischemia not significant (0.10 > p > 0.05).
MV, Mean velocity.

ing). One effective management scheme is to perform a test occlusion of 1 or 2 minutes, which provides assurance of correct MCA insonation and demonstrates the severity of ischemia. If the ischemia is mild or slight, endarterectomy can proceed directly without shunting. If ischemia is severe and does not begin to clear spontaneously or with induction of hypertension, the clamp can be released and final preparations for the shunt organized.

Complications of carotid endarterectomy are so infrequent that it would be difficult for one clinical center to collect sufficient cases to compare one treatment with another. For this reason, a cooperative study, comprising 1495 cases at 11 centers, was made.[2] It confirmed the high risk of hemodynamic infarction in the few cases of sustained severe ischemia, if not shunted, as well as the significant stroke risk that is due to shunting when ischemia was not present (Table 38-1). A policy of selective shunting of severe ischemia only, based on reliable monitoring, might result in a significant reduction of surgical morbidity.

REFERENCES
1. Halsey JH: Effect of emitted power on waveform intensity in transcranial Doppler, *Stroke* 21:1573-1578, 1990.
2. Halsey JH: The risks and benefits of shunting in carotid endarterectomy, *Stroke* 23:1583-1587, 1992.

Intraoperative Ultrasound during Carotid Endarterectomy

Gary J. Peterson
Cole A. Giller
Camilo R. Gomez

One important factor contributing to the success of carotid endarterectomy is the degree of technical precision that can be achieved by the surgeon, in that intimal defects, arterial narrowing, and thrombi can lead to devastating postoperative strokes. Technical imperfections have been reported with an incidence of as much as 25%, even in experienced hands.[6] This led to the utilization of a variety of methods to assess the results of the procedure intraoperatively, including palpation, angiography, and ultrasound. A combination of B-mode ultrasound imaging and Doppler techniques has emerged as a safe and reliable method of such assessment that rivals and in some cases surpasses the ability of angiography to detect surgical complications.[1-3] This chapter describes the technique of intraoperative ultrasonic assessment of carotid endarterectomy, including the interpretation of both the images and Doppler waveforms. It also provides a discussion of the efficacy of this technique.

TECHNIQUE

The purpose of intraoperative ultrasound is to image the cervical portion of the carotid system after endarterectomy in order to detect intimal flaps, thrombi, and stenoses. To provide optimal resolution, the frequency of the transducer should be between 7.5 and 10 MHz. Also, the probe needs to be either gas-sterilized or inserted inside a sterile plastic sleeve, which, in turn, should be filled with acoustic gel. Because insonation may involve gentle manipulation of the carotid vessels, some authors do not attempt it until after the wound is closed to avoid the risk of dislodging emboli.[1] A saline bath is also used for acoustic coupling, allowing the probe to be used without touching the carotid vessels and avoiding near-field artifact. The application of the saline bath can be facilitated by using retractors to lift the edges of the wound, providing a trough for the saline, and rotating the patient so that the saline bath is stable. Systematic scanning in the longitudinal, transverse, and oblique

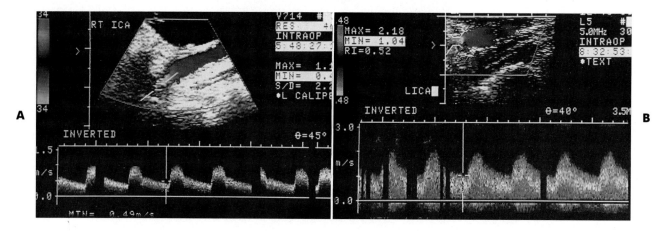

Fig. 39-1. A, Normal intraoperative color Doppler imaging and spectral analysis of a carotid endarterectomy site. Note peak velocity of 110 cm/s. **B,** Intraoperative color Doppler imaging and spectral analysis showing elevated peak velocities (218 cm/s) and spectral broadening. This is suggestive of residual stenosis, which eventually led to occlusion of the internal carotid artery.

planes is performed, with special attention to the end points of the endarterectomy, the points of shunt insertion, and the sites of clamping. From the practical point of view, the availability of the ultrasound instrument can be electively scheduled to coincide with the end of the procedure. Also, the presence of an ultrasound technologist greatly facilitates the study by freeing the surgeon to concentrate on scanning and viewing the images. Finally, the transducer can be angled under the mandible in order to insonate the distal portion of the internal carotid artery, even in the undissected field.

INTERPRETATION OF RESULTS

Although the images provided by B-mode are efficacious in detecting intimal flaps, stenoses, and thrombi, several authors also employ Doppler measurements to identify hemodynamic derangements (Fig. 39-1; see also Plates 109 and 110). Two major types of abnormalities must be sought when intraoperative carotid ultrasound is performed (see box): *Technical errors* directly result from the performance of the surgical procedure and include intimal flaps, ledges, dissections, suture strictures, and kinks. Intimal flaps appear as hyperechoic densities, sometimes mobile, within the vessel lumen. Step-offs, also known as *ledges,* are displayed as sudden changes in the vascular wall. *Intrinsic abnormalities* are pathologic conditions for which the procedure constitutes a risk factor, the most important of which is the formation of intravascular thrombi. An early thrombus may be difficult to detect with B-mode imaging because clots can be isointense with flowing blood. In these cases, the use of color Doppler imaging can call attention to areas devoid of flow, often equivalent to luminal defects caused by thrombi.

Regardless of the type of abnormality found, Dop-

Different types of abnormality that can be detected using intraoperative ultrasound	
Type of abnormality	**Examples**
Technical	Intimal flap
	Plaque dissection
	Suture stricture
	Kinking
	Step-offs
Intrinsic	Mural thrombus
	Platelet aggregate
	Obstructed flow

pler can be useful in assessing hemodynamic significance. Criteria for the classification of hemodynamic derangements, as measured by intraoperative Doppler, have been previously published (Table 39-1).[4,9] In general, these criteria rely upon flow acceleration at systole, as well as other secondary characteristics such as end-diastolic velocity, velocity ratios, and spectral broadening.

Although the detection of operative imperfections and other abnormalities using ultrasound is not difficult, the rules that govern surgical decisions based upon their discovery are less uniform. One problem is that, because ultrasound is extremely sensitive, many of the small defects detected may not lead to subsequent stenosis or require reexploration of the endarterectomy. Another is that a defect of the same magnitude may have different prognostic implications in different vessels. For example, Shawchuck and colleagues classified defects as small if the intimal flap was 1 mm or less in the internal carotid artery (ICA), if the intimal flap was 3 mm or less in the

Table 39-1. Previously published criteria used to characterize stenoses found intraoperatively

Stenosis category	Bandyk et al (1988)		Kinney et al	
	PSV (cm/s)	Vr	PSV (cm/s)	Spectral broadening
Normal	<125	1-1.4	<100	None
Mild	<125	1-1.4	100-125	Diastole
Moderate	125-180	1.5-2.4	125-150	Throughout
Severe	>180	2.5-4	>150	Throughout*

*And end diastolic velocity > 125 cm/s.
PSV, Peak systolic velocity; *Vr,* velocity ratio (PSV lesion/PSV proximal).

common (CCA) and external carotid arteries (ECA), or if the stenosis was less than 50% in diameter.[12] Although they noted that the vast majority of small lesions did not progress to cause either stenosis or flow disturbances, others have reported the opposite.[2] Therefore, the natural history of lesions that cause mild to moderate flow disturbances is unclear. However, the decision to reopen the endarterectomy because of a lesion that causes severe narrowing (as detected by ultrasonography) is on firmer ground.

COMPARISON WITH INTRAOPERATIVE ANGIOGRAPHY

Angiography has several disadvantages when it is used intraoperatively to assess carotid endarterectomy. The equipment is somewhat bulky, and its use in institutions where carotid endarterectomy is frequent poses a radiation load upon personnel. It also requires puncture of the carotid artery at a proximal point, potentially compromising the lumen of the vessel. In contrast, ultrasonography is simple, safe, and noninvasive. Careful comparisons of ultrasound (using B-mode only) and angiography in an animal model have shown that its accuracy surpasses that of angiography for intimal flaps and thrombi and that it is equal to angiography for the detection of stenoses.[7] This is supported by the fact that published rates of detection of flow disturbances of approximately 23% to 28%[1,8,12] are comparable to those of angiography.[6] These efficacy rates may be partly explained by the ability of the ultrasound beam to interrogate several planes cutting the carotid tree, whereas angiography can project to only one plane at a time. Furthermore, intraoperative ultrasound can be readily learned by the surgeon in just one or two sittings, even with no prior special training.[8]

EFFICACY OF INTRAOPERATIVE ULTRASOUND

Although the technique of intraoperative ultrasound is easily learned and the equipment is portable, it does represent added operative time, expense, and inconvenience. It is therefore proper to ask if this technique can detect technical imperfections and if such detection is relevant to the care of the patient.

There is ample evidence to suggest that carotid duplex ultrasound can detect surgical defects and that, in fact, it may be too sensitive. Several series have reported the overall detection of technical imperfections to be between 18% and 28%;[1-3,8,12] as noted, this compares well with the sensitivity of angiography.[6] The distribution of various types of defects, according to the literature, is 73% intimal flaps, 18% stenoses, and 9% a combination of thrombi, kinks, and residual plaques.[8,10] The incidence of technical imperfections felt to be severe has been consistent and ranges between 2% and 8%.[2,3,9,12] It therefore seems that the ultrasound technique is highly sensitive for the detection of technical imperfections following carotid endarterectomy and that it may be too sensitive, detecting mild defects not requiring surgical correction.

The clinical significance of these defects is difficult to assess because the severe ones should be surgically corrected. However, one series did show that even normal ultrasound findings were associated with an 8% risk of late ICA stenosis or occlusion after 4 years. Abnormal, severe defects detected with ultrasound were associated with a 20% risk.[3] Kinney and associates demonstrated an increased rate of restenosis if abnormal ultrasound findings were obtained and an increased risk of late ipsilateral stroke in the presence of recurrent stenosis.[9] They also noted that normal ultrasound findings produced a fivefold decrease in the incidence of late stroke. Defects detected by B-mode and in the Doppler measurements have been correlated to an increased risk of recurrent stenosis in other series.[4,9,11] Therefore, there seems to be an association between severe defects detected with ultrasound and subsequent clinical neurologic deterioration.

CONCLUSIONS

Intraoperative ultrasound during carotid endarterectomy is a safe, noninvasive method that surgeons can easily learn, and that has demonstrated efficacy in detecting surgical imperfections. Severe imperfections can lead to subsequent neurologic decline and should be repaired as soon as detected. Minor defects are frequently seen and may not be clinically significant. Their management may involve intraoperative angiography and will depend upon surgical judgment. Several authors have noted that the constant use of ultrasound in this setting has motivated improvements in surgical technique, which is an added benefit of this technology.[1,2] Intraoperative ultrasound has emerged as a convenient and useful tool in the intraoperative assessment of carotid endarterectomy.

REFERENCES

1. Ackroyd N, Lane R, Appleberg M: Intraoperative ultrasound during carotid artery surgery, *Aust N Z J Surg* 55:321-327, 1985.
2. Baker WH, Koustas G, Burke K, et al: Intraoperative duplex scanning and late carotid artery stenosis, *J Vasc Surg* 19:829-833, 1994.
3. Bandyk DF: *Intraoperative assessment of carotid endarterectomy.* In Bernstein EF, editor: *Vascular diagnosis,* ed 4, St Louis, 1993, Mosby–Year Book.
4. Bandyk DF, Mills JL, Gahtan V, Esses GE: Intraoperative duplex scanning of arterial reconstructions: fate of repaired and unrepaired defects, *J Vasc Surg* 20:426-433, 1994.
5. Bandyk DF, Moldenhauer P, Lipchik E, et al: Accuracy of duplex scanning in the detection of stenosis after carotid endarterectomy, *J Vasc Surg* 8:696-702, 1988.
6. Blaisdell FW, Lim R, Hall AD: Technical results of carotid endarterectomy, *Am J Surg* 114:239-245, 1967.
7. Coelho JCU, Sigel B, Flanigan DP, et al: An experimental evaluation of arteriography and imaging ultrasonography in detecting arterial defects at operation, *J Surg Res* 32:130-137, 1982.
8. Flanigan DP, Douglas DJ, Machi J, et al: Intraoperative ultrasonic imaging of the carotid artery during carotid endarterectomy, *Surgery* 11:893-899, 1986.
9. Kinney EV, Seabrook GR, Kinney LY, et al: The importance of intraoperative detection of residual flow abnormalities after carotid artery endarterectomy, *J Vasc Surg* 17:912-923, 1993.
10. Okuhn SP, Stoney RJ: Intraoperative use of ultrasound in arterial surgery, *Surg Clin North Am* 79:61-70, 1990.
11. Schwartz RA, Peterson GA, Noland KA, et al: Intraoperative duplex scanning after carotid artery reconstruction: a valuable tool, *J Vasc Surg* 7(5):620-624, 1988.
12. Shawchuck AP, Flanigan DP, Machi J, et al: The fate of unrepaired minor technical defects in intraoperative ultrasonography during carotid endarterectomy, *J Vasc Surg* 9:671-676, 1989.

40

Other Methods of Perioperative Ultrasonography

Cole A. Giller

Ultrasound equipment and expertise have become readily available to the clinician during the perioperative period and have led to the development of applications to a wide variety of specific clinical situations. This chapter is a discussion of a few of the most useful and interesting of these.

HYPERPERFUSION FOLLOWING CAROTID ENDARTERECTOMY

Cerebral autoregulation refers to the ability of the brain to maintain appropriate blood flow during changes in perfusion pressure or metabolic demand.[12] This ability is largely mediated by dilation or constriction of the small cerebral vessels (i.e., the pial vessels and arterioles) and can be evoked by the hemodynamic compromise arising from a severe carotid artery stenosis.[12,13,14] If this stenosis is long-standing, the cerebral bed may be chronically vasodilated and unable to vasoconstrict, should normal perfusion be suddenly restored by carotid endarterectomy. The result is an inappropriate cerebral hyperemia as normal pressure is introduced into the vasodilated tissue bed; it can lead to significant morbidity associated with edema, increased intracranial pressure, and hemorrhage.[17,20] This mecha-

nism has been described following the resection of arteriovenous malformations,[19] and the clinical syndrome includes unilateral headache or face pain, seizures, and delayed cerebral hemorrhage in the postoperative period, either immediately or after 24 to 48 hours.[1,10,13,15,20] Not surprisingly, this unusual increase in cerebral blood flow can be detected with ultrasound techniques, by the appearance of high-velocity, low-pulsatility signals in the cerebral vessels. Powers and Smith described two patients in whom middle cerebral artery (MCA) velocities measured with transcranial Doppler ultrasound (TCD) rose to 128 to 160 cm/s after carotid endarterectomy and were associated with headache.[13] Jorgensen and Schroeder have confirmed that a dramatic rise in MCA velocity after carotid endarterectomy is associated with the clinical syndrome of headaches and seizures and yields the diagnosis of postcarotid endarterectomy hyperemia.[10] Measured velocities were as much as 177% of preoperative values; the authors emphasized that the hyperemia may last 12 days and can be treated by carefully reducing systemic blood pressure until the MCA velocities on the affected side begin to normalize. Smith and Burt have also used MCA velocities to guide treatment by adjusting a special clamp

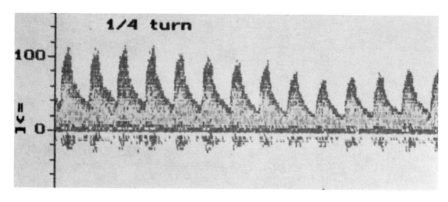

Fig. 40-1. Middle cerebral artery velocity in patient undergoing gradual ipsilateral carotid artery occlusion with a Selverstone clamp. The velocity is significantly affected by even a quarter-turn of the adjusting screw and can be used to guide the rate of occlusion.

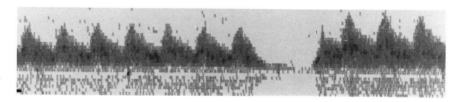

Fig. 40-2. Middle cerebral artery velocity falls to zero during ipsilateral carotid artery occlusion. This patient did not tolerate a trial of carotid occlusion with an angiographic balloon.

placed around the ipsilateral carotid artery until the MCA velocity is normalized.[18]

Although the incidence is low, cerebral hyperemia occurring after carotid endarterectomy can lead to serious neurologic complications. Transcranial Doppler studies can detect this hyperemia, are especially indicated in the presence of headaches or seizures, and can be used to guide subsequent therapy.

THERAPEUTIC CAROTID ARTERY OCCLUSION

Deliberate or anticipated carotid artery sacrifice has long been used for the treatment of surgically inaccessible aneurysms or vascular tumors.[16] Because sudden carotid occlusion may result in neurologic deficit, carotid occlusion is commonly performed gradually by means of an adjustable clamp placed surgically around the artery and that allows time for collateral flow and autoregulatory ability to develop. The precise amount by which to close the clamp at each setting can be difficult to determine, and many patients develop focal deficits when the clamp is even slightly tightened. This process can be guided, however, by monitoring the ipsilateral MCA velocity during clamp tightening,[5] continuing only until attenuation of the velocity waveform is first appreciated (Fig. 40-1). In this way, carotid occlusion may be safely achieved, even in brittle cerebral circulations.

With the advent of interventional angiographic techniques, tolerance to planned carotid artery occlusion can now be tested by temporarily inflating an angiographic balloon in the internal carotid artery for a short period of time while monitoring both the clinical exam and blood flow parameters. The effect upon MCA perfusion can also be evaluated by insonating the MCA during transient manual compression of the carotid artery, with a fall in velocity by more than 65% suggesting a significant impairment of perfusion[3,11] (Fig. 40-2). This manual TCD test has found to correlate well with the results of more formal balloon occlusion testing in a small series of patients.[3]

EXTRACRANIAL-INTRACRANIAL BYPASS

Vascular grafts between the extracranial and intracranial circulation are no longer commonly used in the treatment of chronic cerebral ischemia.[21] However, they are not infrequently placed when planning carotid sacrifice, and patients who have undergone these bypasses commonly require hemodynamic evaluation. Postoperative evaluation of the extracranial-intracranial (ECIC) graft's patency can be difficult because of local edema, and even the palpation of a pulse is no guarantee of unimpeded blood flow. Use of TCD ultrasound allows the insonation of the graft from its position in the superficial tissues to its insertion to the MCA circulation

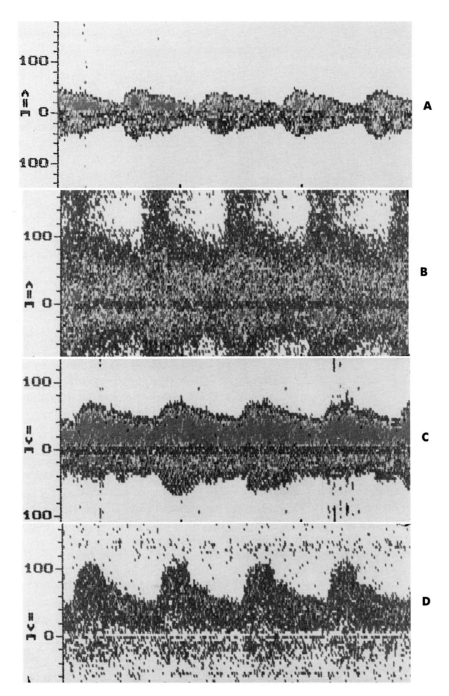

Fig. 40-3. A, Velocity obtained from external-internal carotid graft 30 mm deep to probe. Note the flow direction and low pulsatility, indicating connection to the cerebral circulation. **B,** Same patient at 51 mm, with velocity elevation suggesting mild stenosis at the anatomic site. **C,** Slightly deeper insonation that in **B,** Showing waveform of middle cerebral artery. **D,** Middle cerebral artery velocity from opposite side of same patient, shown for comparison. This has a more normal, less blunted appearance than the side dependent upon the graft.

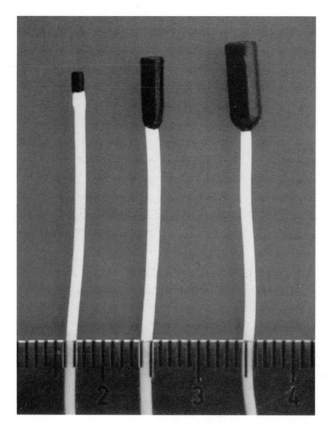

Fig. 40-4. Examples of microprobes available for intraoperative use.

(Fig. 40-3). This demands a shallow probe angle, with patency confirmed by the detection of velocity waveforms with a low pulsatility of intracranial characteristic, intracranial characteristic and with flow directed away from the insonating probe. Following the vessel to its junction with the MCA branch often reveals a focal area of high velocity representing an anastomotic stenosis, which is usually not hemodynamically significant unless markedly elevated. Flow direction in the MCA branches can be variable, depending upon whether flow through the graft is orthograde or retrograde in relation to the MCA vasculature. Because the diameter of the graft may enlarge with time, serial changes in velocity may represent changes in either caliber or flow and thus are difficult to interpret. Nevertheless, TCD evaluation provides an accurate assessment of graft patency and allows the graft flow to be assessed during provocative maneuvers such as vessel compression or administration of acetazolamide.[7]

MICROVASCULAR DOPPLER RECORDINGS

Small, sterilizable 20-MHz pulsed Doppler probes are available for use during surgery and have been extensively investigated by Gilsbach[6] and others (Fig. 40-4). The advantages include the ability to place the probe directly on an otherwise inaccessible arterial segment and to detect the hemodynamic effect of such operative maneuvers as clip placement as soon as they are performed. There are, however, significant limitations of this technology. The sample volume is small compared to the arterial lumen; thus, the Doppler waveform is exquisitely sensitive to the probe angle and the chosen depth of insonation within the blood column. Furthermore, velocity elevation may arise from several sources and can be difficult to interpret. Retraction at surgery can lead to local ischemia with velocity rising because of postischemic hyperemia after retraction release, the insonated vessel may have become stenotic, and, most unpredictably, vessels of smaller size may change diameter during even small changes in blood pressure or CO_2 to cause significant velocity elevations.[2]

Despite these difficulties, several useful applications have emerged. For example, effective placement of an aneurysm clip not only requires complete obliteration of the aneurysm neck but also must avoid stenosis of nearby vessels due to the clip itself or due to any subsequent crimping. Microprobe insonation of these vessels just before and after clip application can detect obstruction that may be difficult to appreciate by visual inspection alone, and the sudden appearance of a high-velocity signal is more likely due to stenosis than to hyperemia. Low velocities may indicate hypoperfusion even when intraoperative angiography shows vessel patency, as in one case in which slow filling of a superior cerebellar artery led to infarction in that distribution (Fig. 40-5). Absent or low velocities after clip placement can alert the neurosurgeon to the possibility of vessel compromise, allowing crucial clip readjustment.

Gilsbach[6] has used microprobe techniques to assess patency of ECIC bypass grafts and anastomotic stenoses. Surprisingly, the velocity waveform demonstrated vessel occlusion in 10% of grafts in which stenosis was not suspected. Signals from vessels feeding arteriovenous malformations (AVM) have also been studied,[9] revealing the expected high-velocity, low-pulsatility characteristics but also challenging the concept of normal perfusion breakthrough by indicating intact autoregulation. Detection of these distinctive signals can also be used to find small AVMs at operation.

Spinal vessels can also be insonated with this method, although the problem is that these arteries may change diameter unpredictably. However, one interesting application requires only the ability of the Doppler signal to indicate flow direction. By insonating the enlarged vessels exiting over a nerve root from a spinal AVM, a dural AVM that would require only vessel ligation can easily be distinguished from an intraparenchymal AVM (i.e., requiring extensive dissection) by its flow direction away from or toward the AVM, respectively.[4,8,9]

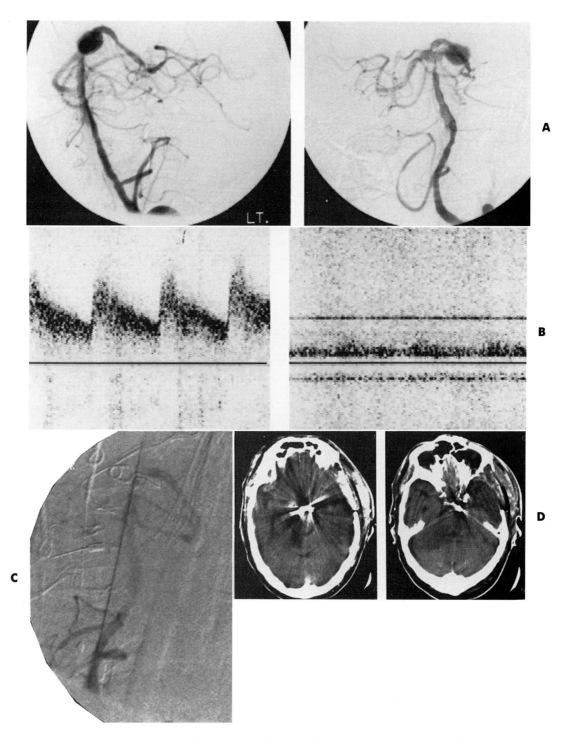

Fig. 40-5. A, Preoperative basilar artery angiogram of patient with superior cerebellar artery (SCA) aneurysm. **B,** Microprobe velocity recordings of the SCA contralateral *(left)* and ipsilateral *(right)* to clip placement, showing significant attenuation of ipsilateral SCA velocity. **C,** Intraoperative angiogram of same patient showing filling of ipsilateral SCA. The flow in this vessel was noted to be significantly slow. **D,** Postoperative computed tomographic scan showing SCA infarct ipsilateral to aneurysm. In this case, the Doppler changes were more predictive then angiography.

REFERENCES

1. Bernstein M, Flemming JFR, Deck JHN: Cerebral hyperperfusion after carotid endarterectomy: a cause of cerebral hemorrhage, *Neurosurgery* 15:50-56, 1984.
2. Giller CA, Bowman G, Dyer H, et al: Cerebral arterial diameters during changes in blood pressure and CO_2 during craniotomy, *Neurosurgery* 32:737-742, 1993.
3. Giller CA, Mathews D, Walter B, et al: Prediction of tolerance to carotid artery occlusion using transcranial Doppler ultrasound, *J Neurosurg* 81:15-19, 1994.
4. Giller CA, Meyer YJ, Batjer HH: Hemodynamic assessment of the spinal cord arteriovenous malformation with intraoperative microvascular Doppler ultrasound: case report, *Neurosurgery* 25:270-275, 1989.
5. Giller CA, Steig P, Batjer HH, et al: Transcranial Doppler ultrasound as a guide to graded therapeutic occlusion of the carotid artery, *Neurosurgery* 26:307-311, 1990.
6. Gilsbach JM: *Intraoperative Doppler sonography in neurosurgery,* New York, 1983, Springer-Verlag.
7. Harders A: *Neurosurgical application of transcranial Doppler sonography,* New York, 1986, Springer-Verlag.
8. Hassler W, Steinmetz H: Cerebral hemodynamics in angioma patients: an intraoperative study, *J Neurosurg* 67:822-831, 1987.
9. Hassler W, Thron A, Grote EH: Hemodynamics of spinal dural arteriovenous fistula, *J Neurosurg* 70:360-370, 1989.
10. Jorgensen LG, Schroeder TV: Defective cerebrovascular autoregulation after carotid endarterectomy, *Eur J Vasc Surg* 7:370-379, 1993.
11. Maurer J, Ungershock K, Amedee RG, et al: Transcranial Doppler ultrasound recording with compression test in patients with tumors involving the carotid arteries, *Skull Base Surg* 3:11-15, 1993.
12. Miller JD, Bell BA: *Cerebral blood flow variation with perfusion pressure and metabolism.* In Wood JH, editor: *Cerebral Blood Flow,* New York, 1987, McGraw-Hill.
13. Powers AD, Smith RR: Hyperperfusion syndrome after carotid endarterectomy: a transcranial Doppler evaluation, *Neurosurgery* 26:56-60, 1990.
14. Powers WJ: Cerebral hemodynamics in ischemic cerebrovascular disease, *Ann Neurol* 29:231-240, 1991.
15. Reigel MM, Hollier LH, Sundt TM, et al: Cerebral hyperperfusion syndrome: a cause of neurologic dysfunction after carotid endarterectomy, *J Vasc Surg* 5:628-634, 1987.
16. Roski RA, Spetzler RF: *Carotid ligation.* In Wilkins RH, Rengachary SS, editors: *Neurosurgery,* New York, 1985, McGraw-Hill.
17. Schroeder T, Sillesen H, Sorensen O, Engell HC: Cerebral hyperperfusion following carotid endarterectomy, *J Neurosurg* 66:824-829, 1987.
18. Smith RR, Burt T: Hyperperfusion after carotid endarterectomy managed by a removable clamp, *J Neuroimaging* 3:16-19, 1993.
19. Spetzler RF, Wilson CB, Weinstein P, et al: Normal perfusion pressure breakthrough theory, *Clin Neurosurg* 25:651-672, 1978.
20. Sundt TM, Sharbrough FW, Piepgras DG, Correlation of cerebral blood flow and electroencephalographic changes carotid endarterectomy, *Mayo Clin Proc* 56:533-543, 1981.
21. The EC/IC Bypass Study Group: Failure of extracranial-intracranial arterial bypass to reduce the risk of ischemic stroke: results of an international randomized trial, *N Engl J Med* 313:1191-1200, 1985.

Integrated Neurosonology in Clinical Practice

41

Imaging of the Nervous System: Ultrasound and Other Modalities

Roger E. Kelley

This chapter compares the information provided by carotid and/or vertebral ultrasonography and transcranial Doppler ultrasonography (TCD) with that provided by other modalities that have the potential to provide physiologic information. These modalities include magnetic resonance angiography (MRA), functional magnetic resonance imaging (FMRI), xenon-derived cerebral blood flow, single photon emission computed tomography (SPECT), and positron emission tomography (PET). These modalities should not be necessarily viewed as competitive. They provide complementary information, but it is important that the potential information provided by a particular study justifies the cost.

The basic principles of the imaging modalities to be discussed in this chapter are summarized in Table 41-1. There has recently been an effort to correlate information provided by duplex scanning and TCD with the results of other physiologic studies. In a dynamic process such as acute stroke, for example, there are a number of simultaneous physiologic alterations. A tracer modality such as PET or SPECT can capture only the evolving pathology at one point in time. This information can be interfaced with the results of serial TCD monitoring to follow the evolution of circulatory compromise or identify possible improvement in cerebral hemodynamics.

MAGNETIC RESONANCE ANGIOGRAPHY

Magnetic resonance angiography (MRA) is based on the finding that one can differentiate the spin-signal MR characteristics of flowing blood from static cerebral tissue with application of a 90° radio frequency (RF) pulse. Protons within the magnetic field, which orient along the longitudinal magnetic field lines in a parallel fashion, "flip" their orientation following the RF pulse so that the magnetization vector is in the transverse plane. As the protons "relax" back to their baseline magnetization vector, a signal is emitted. The signal intensity is a function of whether the protons of the cerebral tissue within the magnetic field have had recovery of their net longitudinal magnetization after the effect of the RF pulse has ceased. This is termed *relaxation.*

With repetitive RF pulsations, the protons cannot all return to their baseline magnetization in which the spins are termed *unsaturated.* The partial saturation of static cerebral tissue, secondary to failure of the net longitudinal magnetization vector to recover between repetitive

Table 41-1. Imaging modalities that provide physiologic information

Modality	Imaging principle	Utility
Carotid/vertebral pulsed wave and continuous-wave Doppler	The shift in Doppler frequency is reflective of the flow dynamics of the moving column of blood	Extracranial arterial stenosis and dissection
Transcranial Doppler ultrasonography (TCD)	Pulsed Doppler to derive flow velocity information that is reflective of intracranial vessel diameter	Intracranial stenosis, extracranial stenosis, and aneurysmal rupture-mediated vasospasm
Magnetic resonance angiography (MRA)	Use of time-of-flight and phase contrast MR technique to outline the cerebral vasculature	Evaluation of extracranial and intracranial stenosis as well as vascular anomalies
Functional magnetic resonance imaging (FMRI)	Use of ultrafast MR technique to detect changes in cerebral blood flow and metabolism; magnetic resonance spectroscopy (MRS) makes use of chemical shift characterization of normal versus abnormal tissue	Primarily a research tool; might allow better delineation of reversibly infarcted cerebral tissue, in the hyperacute time frame, and epileptic foci
Positron emission tomography (PET)	Ring system captures coincident events produced by a positron colliding with an electron; the information derived from appropriate tracer compounds includes cerebral blood flow, blood volume, metabolism, pH, and neurotransmission	Can provide quantitative physiologic information in a tomographic plane; allows determination of pharmakinetics of labeled drugs
Single photon emission computed tomography (SPECT)	Use of rotating gamma camera (multihead) or a ring system to detect emitted photons from radionuclide-labeled compound	Allows measurement of cerebral perfusion or metabolism in a semiquantitative fashion; can aid in the characterization of abnormal tissue, e.g., hyperacute stroke, epileptic foci
Xenon-derived cerebral blood flow	The derivation of the washout of administered xenon-133 or stable xenon from the cerebral circulation via either dynamic computed tomography scanning or scintillation detectors	Modeling of the xenon clearance curves allows determination of fast cerebral blood flow (gray matter) and slow cerebral blood flow (white matter)

RF pulses, contrasts with unsaturated blood entering the image slice. The signal intensity of moving columns of blood (i.e., cerebral vessels) can be enhanced by increasing the repetition rate of the RF pulses. The resultant increase in the degree of saturation of stationary brain tissue augments the signal intensity of the unsaturated blood entering the imaging slice.

The vascular signal component of MRI is related to several variables, including the pulse sequence, repetition time, slice orientation, and flip angle. These are termed *time-of-flight* (TOF) effects. They can either augment the vascular signal or diminish the signal. The latter is referred to as *flow void*. The vascular MRI signal is also influenced by the signal localization gradients. When blood flows into the imaging plane, low signal intensity is generated because the proton spins, which precess within the magnetic field gradient, rotate at a speed that is reflective of the gradient field strength they are exposed to. This activity results in a rotation that is either slower or faster than stationary tissue. The image

produced reflects an accumulation of the phase changes of the proton spins.

The contrast of the phase change of the stationary brain tissue versus the moving blood is termed *phase contrast*. The MRA represents the signal characteristics of the moving column of blood entering a static magnetic field (cerebral tissue). Information provided by MRA is primarily physiologic. Turbulence of flow by nonspecific eddying effects can alter the image produced and can result in false-positive evidence of stenosis.

Most commonly, MRA is performed with a TOF approach that can be obtained in either two dimensions (2D) or three dimensions (3D). Two-dimensional MRA tends to be more useful for evaluation of the extracranial vasculature, whereas 3D MRA tends to be favored for the intracranial vasculature (Fig. 41-1, *A*). Phase contrast MRA is generally less popular than TOF MRA as it is more time-consuming and does not provide as complete information (Fig. 41-1, *B*).

Duplex imaging of the carotid bifurcation and the

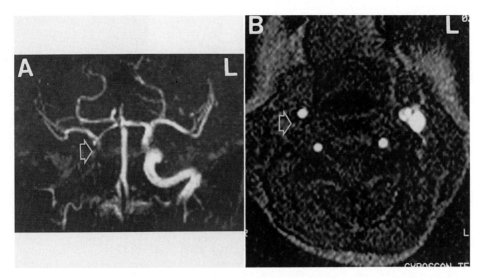

Fig. 41-1. Magnetic resonance angiogram of a 26-year-old woman with traumatic occlusion of the right internal carotid artery. **A,** The three-dimensional time-of-flight study, in anterior-posterior view, reveals an absent flow signal of the distal right internal carotid artery (*arrow*) with good cross-filling of the right middle cerebral artery via the anterior communicating artery. **B,** The phase contrast study, in transaxial plane, reveals a markedly attenuated flow signal of the distal right internal carotid artery (*arrow*).

proximal vertebral arteries has been compared to MRA and conventional cerebral arteriography. Kido and colleagues, in a comparison of MRA to cerebral angiography in the evaluation of stenosis of the carotid bifurcation, reported a sensitivity of 86% and a specificity of 92%.[24] Riles and associates, in their series published in 1992, reported a close correlation of MRA and contrast angiography in only 52% of cases, whereas duplex scanning correlated with contrast angiography in 65% of cases.

Mittl and co-workers compared 2D TOF MRA with duplex ultrasonography and arteriography in 73 carotid bifurcations to assess the determination of stenosis by the three techniques.[29] They found no significant difference between MRA and duplex ultrasonography in terms of both sensitivity and specificity. They concluded that neither technique was sufficiently accurate to preclude the need for routine angiography. In general, MRA tends to overestimate the actual degree of stenosis at the carotid bifurcation,[36] and neither MRA or duplex scanning can conclusively distinguish complete internal carotid artery (ICA) occlusion from very high-grade stenosis.

Röther and colleagues evaluated the combined use of MRA, duplex scanning, and TCD of the vertebrobasilar circulation in comparison to angiography in 41 subjects with symptoms of vertebrobasilar ischemia.[35] They reported that MRA had a sensitivity of 97% and a specificity of 98.9% in detecting obstructive lesions. The true degree of stenosis was difficult to assess accurately by MRA, however, and one case of vertebral artery

dissection was missed. Doppler ultrasonography was reported to provide complementary information.

In that MRA is capable of detecting cervicocranial dissection, it is quite possible that the combination of MRA and duplex ultrasonography will provide complementary information. Bui and associates found that MRA correlated with findings of conventional angiography in three of five patients.[6] They noted that MRA was associated with certain pitfalls. There can be a false appearance of vessel widening, presumably related to a combination of signal effects of the associated clot and the high-flow lumen. In addition, turbulence associated with the sharp turn of the carotids within the petrous canal can result in signal alteration that simulates vessel narrowing.

It is possible to calculate flow velocities of the intracranial arteries with MRA.[3] With application of an RF presaturation pulse, signal from cerebral tissue and intracranial vessels can be eliminated within a defined rectangular volume. Over a specific time interval (t), unsaturated spins flow into the volume of presaturation. The velocity (v), which reflects the fastest-flowing arterial spins, is then calculated as:

$$v = d/t$$

where d = maximal length of travel of the arterial inflowing spins over the time interval t. The arterial inflowing spins are of high signal intensity, and the information derived is correlated with phases of the cardiac cycle via electrocardiographic gating.

In a study of MRA-derived flow velocities compared

to TCD, Mattle and co-workers correlated velocity values at rest and during finger movement in six normal volunteers.[28] The authors reported an average velocity increase above baseline, during finger movement, of 11% for MRA and 11.3% for TCD. The correlation values for the two techniques were r = .86, p = 0.0001 during rest and r = 0.84, p = 0.0001 during finger movement.

This study serves as a further validation of TCD methodology in the assessment of cerebral activation. There has been increasing interest in the noninvasive evaluation of cortical function with stimulatory activity. This has involved the realms of PET[13,33] and functional MRI.[4,38] Transcranial Doppler is unique in this regard, however, in view of its ability to allow selective serial monitoring of cerebral vessels in a well-tolerated fashion.

Aaslid reported an average 16% increase in the flow velocity of the posterior cerebral arteries, with TCD, during visual stimulation.[1] Droste and colleagues reported that mental activity was associated with an increase of between 1.6% and 10.6% in middle cerebral artery flow velocity.[10] A selective circulatory correlate of mental activity can be detected with TCD. We observed a selective elevation of the flow velocity within both middle cerebral arteries and the left posterior cerebral artery while playing a commercial video game.[22] During a spatial task, we observed selective increase of the flow velocity within the right hemisphere.[23] As an example of a potential practical application of this methodology, Markus and Boland reported in right-handers a relative increase in left middle cerebral artery flow velocity during a word association task.[26] This could possibly serve as a tool for determining cerebral dominance.

FUNCTIONAL MAGNETIC RESONANCE IMAGING

Functional magnetic resonance imaging (FMRI) is based upon ultrafast scanning techniques that allow the sequential recording of perfusion or diffusion brain activity over split seconds. This is a rapidly evolving field, and a number of methodologies have been developed. Rapid sequential imaging with a gradient-echo echo-planar pulse sequence, for example, has been termed *echo-planar imaging* (EPI).[37] This technique can provide an entire image of the brain in less than a second with information extracted from one nuclear spin. Other modifications of the gradient-echo pulse sequence allow ultrafast scanning as well.[7]

Changes related to regional cerebral blood flow (rCBF)[32] and tissue oxygenation[12,30] can be detected by FMRI. This has allowed noninvasive assessment of cognitive stimulation with MR techniques. Signal intensity changes can be detected within specific regions of the brain during such maneuvers as visual stimulation, primary sensory stimulation and finger movements. Rao and colleagues, for example, reported an activation

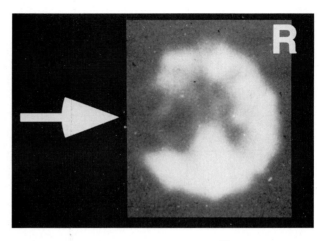

Fig. 41-2. Positron emission tomography ^{15}O cerebral blood flow scan. Note reduction of blood flow within the distribution of the left middle cerebral artery (*arrow*), which correlated with the area of infarction seen on computed tomographic brain scan.

pattern that correlated with the nature of the motor task.[32] With the use of refined diffusion-weighted imaging (DWI)[39] and perfusion imaging,[11] it may well be possible to quantitate CBF. Such information could be compared to patterns provided by TCD in an effort to noninvasively assess circulatory correlates of neurobehavior.

POSITRON EMISSION TOMOGRAPHY

Positron emission tomography (PET) is an imaging technique that uses radioactive molecules as tracers to assess brain chemistry and physiology.[8] This scanning provides cross-sectional images of positron-emitting radiopharmaceuticals (Fig. 41-2). The information provided by the coincident events, as a positron collides with an electron, can allow quantitative measurement of brain function through the use of sophisticated computer-based modeling. Oxygen metabolism, CBF, glucose metabolism, various neurotransmitter systems, and pharmacologic processes can be assessed.

Position emission tomography has provided interesting studies of human brain function in normals. The 2-[^{18}F]fluoro-2-deoxy-D-glucose technique, which quantitatively assesses regional cerebral metabolic rate of glucose, allows metabolic mapping of functional brain activity.[14] Visual stimulation, for example, is associated with an increase in glucose metabolism within the visual cortex, while the converse is seen with visual deprivation.[31]

Moreover, PET provides regional CBF in a quantitative fashion. The most common methodology makes use of the short-lived tracer oxygen-15 (^{15}O). This tracer can be administered either by continuous inhalation of $C^{15}O_2$[2] or by intravenous ^{15}O water bolus.[18] Theoretically, the information provided by TCD could be correlated with CBF data in the assessment of cerebral ischemia.

In a study of the blood flow velocity of the middle cerebral artery in acute hemispheric infarction, Kushner and co-workers reported that TCD provided pertinent prognostic information.[25] An unobtainable middle cerebral artery flow signal or a markedly reduced flow velocity was associated with proximal vessel occlusion by angiography and a poorer outcome. Hedera and colleagues, in a TCD study of the middle cerebral artery flow velocity in patients with internal carotid artery occlusion, noted a negative relationship between the blood flow velocity and the degree of acute neurologic dysfunction, as well as with the degree of neurologic recovery over the first 28 days.[17]

Despite these reports, a recent study did not find a correlation between middle cerebral artery blood velocity values and PET-derived CBF.[20] No relationship between TCD velocity and CBF measured by $^{15}O-H_2O$ was observed in 26 subjects with acute cerebral infarction, middle cerebral artery stenosis, or controls. The authors concluded that TCD could not be used as a reliable determinant of regional tissue perfusion. This study was limited by the fact that cerebral angiography was not obtained and in some subjects the two studies were performed up to 2 days apart. In addition, a somewhat heterogeneous group of subjects with cerebral ischemia was studied. This study underscores the challenges that are faced in comparing a relatively simple, noninvasive procedure like TCD to a powerful but highly sophisticated and complicated device such as PET. It is possible that changes in CBF are more reliably reflected by changes in velocity.

SINGLE PHOTON EMISSION COMPUTED TOMOGRAPHY

Single photon emission computed tomography (SPECT) provides a semiquantitative assessment of cerebral perfusion.[19] Like PET, this technique provides cross-sectional images of the distribution of a radiotracer. The agents used in imaging are designed to cross the blood-brain barrier and to follow a distribution in the brain that is proportional to the regional CBF. In addition, the radiopharmaceutical must remain within the brain substance for a time period sufficient to allow cross-sectional imaging. Imaging can be achieved with either a rotating gamma camera or, preferably, a ring system that allows more efficient capture of photon emissions.

Efforts have been made to correlate the findings of TCD and SPECT in pathologic conditions. Davis and associates reported that increasing TCD flow velocity values in aneurysmal subarachnoid hemorrhage, indicative of vasospasm, tended to predict ischemic changes

seen on SPECT.[9] Grosset and co-workers, in a similar study population, reported that abnormal perfusion patterns on SPECT correlated with sites of increased flow velocities by TCD.[15]

We have looked at the ability of TCD to detect acute changes in the cerebral and retinal circulation during cerebral angioplastic balloon occlusion of the internal carotid artery. This procedure is becoming increasingly popular for the management of vascular processes such as cavernous carotid fistula and for invasive lesions of the carotid artery. Plate 111, *A* shows the preocclusion SPECT study of a patient with a recent right middle cerebral artery distribution infarct and a right cavernous carotid fistula. Following occlusion, there is more prominent hypoperfusion of the right cerebral hemisphere (Plate 111, *B*). The correlative TCD study of the right middle cerebral artery before occlusion (Plate 112, *A*) and during occlusion (Plate 112, *B*) is also shown. Thus, the TCD study provides reliable information about the perfusion of the affected hemisphere.

Plate 113, *A* shows the right ophthalmic artery Doppler flow pattern before test occlusion of the right internal carotid artery in a patient with invasive squamous cell carcinoma. The flow pattern disappears during the test occlusion (Plate 113, *B*). The correlative SPECT scan is demonstrated in Plate 114, *A* (preocclusion) and Plate 114, *B* (during occlusion). Once again, hypoperfusion demonstrated by SPECT correlates with TCD findings and mitigates against a permanent procedure.

Plate 115 shows the SPECT study of a 52-year-old man who presented with an acute left hemiparesis and had a relatively small subcortical infarct by computed tomographic (CT) brain scan. He was found to have a positive serum fluorescent teponemal antibody, absorbed (FTA-ABS) test with cerebrospinal fluid (CSF) pleocytosis and a positive CSF Venereal Disease Research Laboratory (VDRL) syphilis test. His cerebral arteriogram was performed for possible vascular dissection, as he had suffered recent trauma. The arteriogram revealed prominent vasculitic changes with greatest involvement of the right middle cerebral artery, right anterior cerebral artery, right posterior cerebral artery, and the right carotid siphon. Figure 41-3 illustrates the serial TCD results after initiation of intravenous penicillin therapy, which was started on the day of the arteriogram. These studies reveal a trend toward lower flow velocities over time as well as detectable right posterior cerebral and right anterior cerebral artery Doppler signals over time. Thus, one can noninvasively monitor for response to therapy in such a process with TCD. Unfortunately, this patient never returned for a follow-up SPECT study.

XENON-DERIVED CEREBRAL BLOOD FLOW

Measurement of CBF by radioactive xenon-133 or stable xenon is based upon determination of xenon

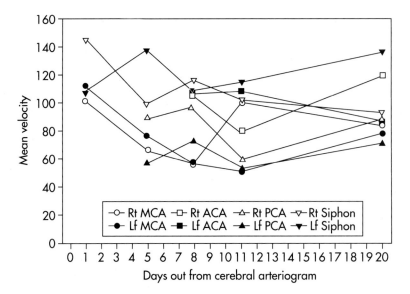

Fig. 41-3. Serial transcranial Doppler velocities of the middle cerebral artery (MCA), anterior cerebral artery (ACA), posterior cerebral artery (PCA), and the carotid siphon following the initiation of intravenous penicillin at the time of the cerebral arteriogram. Note that the PCAs could not be insonated initially but were insonated by Day 5 of therapy. In addition, the right ACA became detectable at Day 8 of therapy. By Day 11 of therapy, a Doppler signal could be detected in all 8 vessels of this patient with meningovascular syphilis.

clearance from brain tissue. The clearance curve is reconstructed by dynamic CT scanning in the first few minutes after xenon inhalation or by detection of gamma emission, with the use of crystal detectors, after injection or inhalation of xenon-133. Bishop and associates correlated flow velocity values of intracranial arteries, as measured by TCD, with CBF measurements obtained with the intravenously administered xenon-133 technique.[5] Measurements were made at rest and during hypercapnia in patients with symptoms of cerebrovascular disease. They found a poor correlation between the absolute MCA flow velocity and hemispheric CBF at rest. This was attributed to wide between-patient variations. A good correlation was observed, however, between blood velocity and blood flow response to hypercapnia.

In a study of posttraumatic cerebral arterial spasm, Martin and co-workers reported a statistically significant correlation between the highest middle cerebral artery flow velocity and the lowest CBF during vasospasm.[27] It is important to recognize the limitations of xenon-derived CBF in pathologic conditions as the two- and three-compartment models are based on the normal human condition with a known partition coefficient. In an acute brain insult, the scintillation detectors tend to "look through" the area of insult, and there is compartmental shifting of what constitutes gray and white matter flows.

The inhalation of nonradioactive (stable) xenon during CT brain scanning allows derivation of regional CBF and local partition coefficients. This technique has not achieved clinical utility, however, because of the expense, high-dose radiation exposure, and the anesthetic effect of inhaled xenon.

SUMMARY

From a practical and cost-effective standpoint, TCD appears to be the procedure of choice for noninvasive monitoring of cerebral hemodynamics. By contrast, MRA is a costly and time-consuming procedure. It does not hold a clear advantage over duplex ultrasonography in the evaluation of extracranial occlusive disease and may well be less accurate. Furthermore, MR techniques are limited in terms of patient tolerance, especially when there is alternation of consciousness.

None of the MR techniques are feasible for short-term monitoring when the pathophysiologic changes associated with acute cerebral ischemia are so dynamic and susceptible to sudden change. The same problems apply both to PET, which remains primarily in the research realm, although it is quite useful to attempt to correlate the quantitative changes it provides with serial TCD results, and to SPECT, a more readily available and practical procedure but one that, like PET, involves radiation exposure. Studies to date indicate that the perfusion information provided by SPECT correlates with that provided by TCD.

Transcranial Doppler can predict ischemic changes in aneurysmal subarachnoid hemorrhage and can provide prognostic information in acute intracerebral thromboembolic disease. It has the potential to allow noninvasive monitoring of interventional therapy in acute stroke. In the future, physiologic measures may help to supplement clinical assessment of neurologic status in acute therapeutic stroke trials.[16] As an example of this potential use for TCD, Karnik and associates reported on the ability of TCD to detect progressive recanalization of embolic occlusion of the middle cerebral artery during thrombolytic therapy.[21] It is hoped that convincing studies of large numbers of patients will be forthcoming to establish the reliability of TCD in such an important clinical realm.

REFERENCES

1. Aaslid R: Visual evoked response of the cerebral circulation, *Stroke* 18:771-775, 1987.
2. Ackerman RH, et al: Positron imaging in ischemic stroke disease using compounds labeled with oxygen 15: initial results of clinicophysiologic correlations. *Arch Neurol* 38:537-543, 1981.
3. Axel L, Shimakawa A, MacFall J: A time-of-flight method of measuring flow velocities by magnetic resonance imaging, *Magn Reson Imaging* 4:199-205, 1986.
4. Binder JR, et al: Functional magnetic resonance imaging of human auditory cortex, *Ann Neurol* 35:662-672, 1994.
5. Bishop CCR, et al: Transcranial Doppler measurement of middle cerebral artery blood flow velocity: a validation study, *Stroke* 17:913-915, 1986.
6. Bui LN, et al: Magnetic resonance angiography of cervicocranial dissection, *Stroke* 24:126-131, 1993.
7. Chien D, Edelman RR: Ultrafast imaging using gradient echoes, *Magn Reson Q* 7:35-56, 1991.
8. Council on Scientific Affairs: Report of the Positron Emission Tomography Panel: positron emission tomography, a new approach to brain chemistry, *JAMA* 260:2704-2710, 1988.
9. Davis SM, et al: Correlations between cerebral arterial velocities, blood flow, and delayed ischemia after subarachnoid hemorrhage, *Stroke* 23:494-497, 1992.
10. Droste DW, Harders AG, Rastogi E: A transcranial Doppler study of blood flow velocity in the middle cerebral arteries performed at rest and during mental activity, *Stroke* 20:1005-1011, 1989.
11. Fisher M, et al: New magnetic resonance techniques for evaluating cerebrovascular disease, *Ann Neurol* 32:115-122, 1992.
12. Frahm J, et al: Dynamic MR imaging of human brain oxygenation during rest and photic stimulation, *J Magn Reson Imag* 2:501-505, 1992.
13. Grafton ST: Cortical control of movement, *Ann Neurol* 36:19-26, 1994.
14. Greenberg JH, et al: Metabolic mapping of functional activity in human subjects with the [18F] fluoro-deoxyglucose technique, *Science* 212:678-680, 1981.
15. Grosset DG, et al: Prediction of symptomatic vasospasm after subarachnoid hemorrhage by rapidly increasing transcranial Doppler velocity and cerebral blood flow changes, *Stroke* 23:674-679, 1992.
16. Hanson SK, et al: Value of single-photon emission-computed tomography in acute stroke therapeutic trials, *Stroke* 24:1322-1329, 1993.
17. Hedera P, Traubrer P, Gujdková J: Short-term prognosis of stroke due to occlusion of internal carotid artery based on transcranial Doppler ultrasonography, *Stroke* 23:1069-1072, 1992.
18. Herholz K, et al: Regional cerebral blood flow measurement with intravenous 15O water bolus and 18F fluoromethane inhalation, *Stroke* 20:1174-1181, 1989.
19. Holman BL, Tumeh SS: Single-photon emission computed tomography (SPECT): applications and potentials, *JAMA* 263:561-564, 1990.
20. Huber M, et al: Transcranial Doppler and 15O-H2O-positron emission tomography findings in patients with acute brain infarction and middle cerebral artery stenosis, *J Stroke Cerebrovasc Dis* 4:23-29, 1994.
21. Karnik R, Stelzer P, Slany J: Transcranial Doppler sonography in monitoring local intra-arterial thrombolysis in acute occlusion of the middle cerebral artery, *Stroke* 23:284-287, 1992.
22. Kelley RE, et al: Transcranial Doppler assessment of cerebral flow velocity during cognitive tasks, *Stroke* 23:9-14, 1992.
23. Kelley RE, et al: Selective increase in the right hemisphere transcranial Doppler velocity during a spatial task, *Cortex* 29:45-52, 1993.
24. Kido DK, et al. Clinical evaluation of stenosis of the carotid bifurcation with magnetic resonance angiographic techniques, *Arch Neurol* 48:484-489, 1991.
25. Kushner MJ, et al: Transcranial Doppler in acute hemispheric brain infarction, *Neurology* 41:109-113, 1991.
26. Markus HS, Boland M: "Cognitive activity" monitored by noninvasive measurement of cerebral blood flow velocity and its application to the investigation of cerebral dominance, *Cortex* 28:575-581, 1992.
27. Martin NA, et al: Posttraumatic cerebral arterial spasm: transcranial Doppler ultrasound, cerebral blood flow, and angiographic findings, *J Neurosurg* 77:575-583, 1992.
28. Mattle H, et al: Middle cerebral artery: determination of flow velocities with MR angiography, *Radiology* 181:527-530, 1991.
29. Mittl RL, et al: Blinded-reader comparison of magnetic resonance angiography and duplex ultrasonography for carotid bifurcation stenosis, *Stroke* 25:4-10, 1994.
30. Ogawa S, et al: Oxygen sensitive contrast in magnetic resonance image of rodent brain at higher magnetic fields, *Magn Reson Med* 14:68-78, 1990.
31. Phelps ME, et al: Tomographic mapping of human cerebral metabolism: visual stimulation and deprivation, *Neurology* 31:517-529, 1981.
32. Rao SM, et al: Functional magnetic resonance imaging of complex human movements, *Neurology* 43:2311-2318, 1993.
33. Remy P, et al: Movement- and task-related activations of motor control areas: a positron emission tomographic study, *Ann Neurol* 36:19-26, 1994.
34. Riles TS, et al: Comparison of magnetic resonance angiography, conventional angiography and duplex scanning, *Stroke* 23:341-346, 1992.
35. Röther J, et al: Magnetic resonancy angiography in vertebrobasilar ischemia, *Stroke* 24:1310-1315, 1993.
36. Ruggieri PM, Masory KTJ, Ross JS: Magnetic resonance angiography: cerebrovascular applications, *Stroke* 23:774-780, 1992.
37. Stehling MK, Turner R, Mansfield P: Echo planar imaging: magnetic resonance imaging in a fraction of a second, *Science* 254:43-50, 1991.
38. Turner R: Magnetic resonance imaging of brain function, *Ann Neurol* 35:637-638, 1994.
39. Warach S, et al: Fast magnetic resonance diffusion-weighted imaging of acute human stroke, *Neurology* 42:1717-1723, 1992.

Neurosonology in the Evaluation of Ischemic Stroke and Transient Ischemic Attacks

Daryl R. Gress

Stroke remains a leading killer in this country. Although the mortality and morbidity are concentrated in late adulthood, the death and disability stretches through all age groups. Stroke occurs at an estimated rate of 400,000 to 500,000 per year in the United States and in clear relationship to the risk factors of smoking, hypertension, diabetes, and hyperlipidemia. The term usually includes sudden, focal neurologic deficits of a vascular etiology, including both hemorrhage and ischemia. Some 70% to 80% of stroke is ischemic in nature, and this group is the major focus of this discussion.

Efficient and effective care of the patient with stroke or stroke risk requires an understanding of the underlying vascular pathophysiology. Ultrasound, given its safety and high degree of accuracy, is an important tool for the clinician attempting to unravel the etiology of ischemia. The mechanisms underlying stroke are varied and must be kept in mind when planning the diagnostic evaluation.

Ischemia occurs when an area of brain tissue is deprived of its blood supply. Infarction occurs after prolonged ischemic injury, although tissue can recover if the blood supply is restored before irreversible cellular injury has taken place. The neurologic deficits caused by the ischemia are described as *stroke,* unless they resolve rapidly (standard convention is less than 24 hours), in which case the term *transient ischemic attack* (TIA) is used. Stroke and TIA are clinical terms and do not imply presence or absence of infarction.

STROKE MECHANISMS
Small vessel stroke

Small 100- to 200-micron vessels arise from the basal arteries and penetrate into the deep substance of the brain as end arterioles. These penetrating vessels provide irrigation of the deep nuclei and fiber tracts of the cerebrum as well as the deep tracts of the brainstem. Hypertension and diabetes are the major recognized risk factors for small vessel disease. Careful pathologic examination of these vessels has shown a scarring and occlusion termed *segmental arterial disorganization* or *lipohyalinosis.*[13] Small emboli are felt to be uncommon causes of small vessel occlusion. Infarction associated with small vessel occlusion commonly occurs in the striatum, thalamus, and deep white matter tracts and has been described as lacunar in pathologic studies. Stroke deficits are often characteristic, with pure motor hemiparesis, hemisensory loss, and ataxic hemiparesis most commonly seen. Small vessel stroke accounts for 15% to 20% of all ischemic stroke.

Large vessel stroke

The anterior, middle, and posterior cerebral arteries branch successively as they course over the cortical surface before penetrating in a radial fashion to irrigate cortex and underlying white matter. Blockage of these vessels is often by embolism and most commonly occurs in a division or branch with diameters of 1 to 2 mm. The resultant ischemia or infarction is characteristically a wedge-shaped area involving cortex and underlying white matter. Stroke deficits typically relate to the affected cortical function, with aphasia, anosognosia, hemianopia, and ipsilateral gaze preference providing the signature of cortical involvement.

Intracranial disease

Although atheromatous disease usually spares these intracranial vessels, it has been recognized more recently that cultural differences relate to the sites of atheromatous involvement, with intracranial disease seen more frequently in Asian and African-American populations. In the setting of stenosis of the proximal large intracranial vessels, local thrombosis leads to ischemia and infarction and can be associated with more distal embolization. Large vessel stroke related to local atheroma may account for 10% to 20% of all ischemic stroke.

Embolism—carotid source

Atherosclerotic disease at the carotid bifurcation is a common source of embolism leading to stroke. Atherosclerotic plaque is a common finding in the older age groups at higher risk for stroke, with a predilection for involvement at the distal common carotid, bifurcation, and proximal internal carotid artery. The plaque material consists of varying ratios of lipid and collagen with a complex surface topography. The plaque can have dystrophic calcification, intraplaque hemorrhage, and ulceration. Plaque can increase to compromise the vessel lumen, and progressive disease eventually results in vessel occlusion. Although the topography and ulceration may be related to platelet or thrombin emboli in some cases, the most significant correlate to stroke risk

is degree of stenosis. It is presumed that severe stenosis compromises distal flow with emboli formation in the slower moving blood just distal to the stenosis. Embolism related to carotid disease may account for some 20% of ischemic stroke.

Embolism—cardiac source

The mechanism of occlusion of the large vessels is most commonly thromboembolism related to a more proximal lesion. Cardiac embolism related to a defined pathology accounts for approximately 20% of all ischemic stroke. Atrial fibrillation increases stroke risk dramatically in the elderly. Mitral stenosis and other valvular lesions are known risks of embolism as well, as are most prosthetic valves. Low ejection fraction and severe regional wall motion abnormalities, particularly in the postmyocardial infarction period, have been associated with increased embolic risk. Septal defects and paradoxic emboli have been seen in stroke, especially in younger age groups.

Embolism—unknown source

A large proportion of embolic stroke occurs with no clearly demonstrable source of embolism. This category of "embolism of unknown origin" is applied to cases in which carotid and cardiac studies have not revealed an explanation; it accounts for up to 40% of ischemic stroke. Clearly, more careful evaluation with newer technology, such as transesophageal echo, can identify previously undetected aortic arch atheroma, patent foramina, and valvular lesions. It is likely the "unknown origin" category will become less frequently needed as other sources of embolism become understood.

Low flow

A final stroke mechanism to be considered here concerns circumstances where ischemia is related to low flow rather than embolism. Arterial stenosis commonly progresses to hemodynamic compromise without neurologic symptoms because of collateral flow either via the circle of Willis, retrograde ophthalmic flow, or pial surface collaterals. However, in some cases collateral flow is not possible because of the rather common developmental inadequacy of a communicating artery or vascular disease involving the collateral pathways. In this setting, as the arterial stenosis progresses, a critical point is reached when insufficient blood is delivered distally and ischemic symptoms appear. The ischemia usually appears most severely in the most distal territories of the stenosed vessel, described as *watershed zones.* These spells often coincide with transient decreases in blood pressure or cardiac output, and "low flow" TIAs often occur as multiple, similar spells with an associated hemodynamic fluctuation, such as orthostatic blood pressure changes or following cardiovascular medication doses. These arterial lesions are also risk factors for embolism, and associated strokes can occur from either mechanism. Low flow stroke is relatively uncommon outside the setting of profound hypotension surrounding hemodynamic collapse.

CLINICAL APPLICATIONS

Clinicians faced with patients with stroke symptoms or stroke risk must quickly and efficiently establish the underlying vascular pathology in each case. The clinical presentation and neurologic clues may provide direction, but vascular studies are necessary, and the options are extensive. For the clinician to accomplish this task requires tailoring the diagnostic studies to the individual case and keeping in mind the specific vascular question at each step.

Symptomatic carotid disease

The question of disease at the carotid bifurcation is often the starting point for the clinical investigation, in part because it is a common cause of stroke and also because it has specific treatment implications. The finding of no significant carotid disease is also clinically important in order to focus the investigation toward other possible causes of stroke. Carotid ultrasound provides an excellent means for the safe and reliable evaluation of the carotid bifurcation. Most patients require carotid testing as an early part of the evaluation.

The carotid bifurcation is a common source of embolism and has specific treatment. The preliminary results of the North American Symptomatic Carotid Endarterectomy Trial (NASCET) demonstrated that in patients presenting with TIA or mild stroke and severe carotid stenosis (greater than 70%), the risk of recurrent stroke was high and increased with increased stenosis.[24] The study clearly demonstrated the benefit of surgical endarterectomy compared to aspirin therapy. Ultrasound evaluation of the cervical carotid can provide safe and rapid evaluation of the bifurcation. The clinical question most often centers on severity of stenosis. In this setting, sensitivity of the technique is important, and with duplex evaluation alone, a sensitivity greater than 90% can be achieved while preserving specificity greater than 85%.[22] Degree of stenosis as determined by continuous-wave Doppler spectral analysis has been shown to correlate well with the residual lumen as measured from carotid endarterectomy specimens.[5]

Attempts have been made to correlate specific morphologic features of carotid plaque endarterectomy specimens, sonographic features, and neurologic symptoms. Atherosclerotic plaque at the carotid bifurcation is well visualized with B-mode ultrasound imaging. Low-echogenic plaque correlates with fibrofatty material with a high lipid content; increased collagen content is associated with an increase in echogenicity. Strongly echogenic material is associated with dystrophic calcifications. Most plaques are homogeneous unless intraplaque hemorrhage or lipid deposits create a complex heterogeneous appearance. An increased risk of symptoms has been associated with high lipid content[31] and intraplaque hemorrhage,[17,19] although the latter has been found in patients without symptoms.[2] An association between stroke and plaque ulcerations has also been reported,[35] and ultrasound has been used to quantify ulcer depth as a stroke risk factor.[18] A study of ultrasonographic plaque morphology in stenosis less than 60% found a significant correlation between neurologic events, radiographic strokes, and heterogeneous or complex, irregular plaques with calcification.[3] However, other studies have been less compelling, and current clinical evidence is strongest for the correlation of stroke risk and degree of stenosis.

Carotid ultrasound is of limited value in some settings. Carotid dissection can be detected, although usually only when significant stenosis occurs, and then the underlying mechanism cannot be reliably determined. Optimal studies can visualize an intimal flap or a duplicated lumen.[32] In the setting of suspected dissection, carotid duplex alone is not adequate evaluation to exclude the diagnosis. Standard carotid ultrasound studies also do not adequately assess the carotid siphon. However, the absence of severe stenosis at the bifurcation usually prompts the clinician to consider other sources of embolism, including the heart and intracranial arteries, and further studies may be necessary.

Hemodynamic information can also be important to the clinician. Assessment of downstream arteries can provide information about the severity of the proximal stenosis and the resultant consequences in perfusion. Transcranial Doppler (TCD) can assess the direction of flow as well as the flow velocity in the ophthalmic artery. With progressive stenosis of the internal carotid, flow in the ophthalmic artery can be seen to decrease in velocity and finally reverse in direction as collateral flow from the external carotid artery comes into play. Likewise, TCD can demonstrate reversal in flow direction in the proximal anterior cerebral artery distal to a severe carotid stenosis as evidence of collateral flow from the contralateral carotid. A decrease in velocity and pulsatility can be seen in the ipsilateral middle cerebral artery above severe carotid stenosis and suggests significant hemodynamic effect. These signs of hemodynamic compromise provide further evidence of the severity of the more proximal stenosis. Complete ultrasound evaluation of the carotid should include duplex, graphic Doppler spectral analysis, and some assessment of downstream hemodynamic effect.

Transcranial Doppler is also useful in the evaluation of distal internal carotid and intracranial disease. The siphonous portion of the internal carotid can be assessed via the transorbital approach. Middle cerebral artery stem stenoses are demonstrated by TCD, and lesions affecting the distal vertebral and basilar arteries can be detected. Findings of focal segments with abnormally high velocities are associated with intracranial stenoses. It has been possible to detect postural hemodynamic flow changes in the posterior circulation to further the understanding of the vascular mechanisms underlying ischemic symptoms.[33]

Transcranial Doppler then complements carotid duplex in the evaluation of cerebrovascular disease. The technique can be used as a screen for suspected intracranial disease, with either magnetic resonance angiography (MRA) or conventional angiography used as confirmatory studies. In cases where the clinical features and TCD findings are clear and in agreement, diagnostic certainty is such that therapeutic decisions can be made.

Because of relative cost, safety, and accuracy, carotid ultrasound is usually favored as the screening study. Now MRA can also provide noninvasive assessment of the carotid bifurcation. These imaging sequences most often utilize a two-dimensional or three-dimensional time-of-flight technique, and reliable studies can be achieved. Series comparing MRA to conventional angiography have demonstrated a sensitivity greater than 90% with specificity greater than 80% for the detection of severe stenoses.[16] Current MRA is limited by signal dropout in regions of severe stenosis, with a "skip sign" commonly seen associated with overestimation of the degree of stenoses. Little hemodynamic information is readily available from MRA evaluation. Comparison of MRA and carotid duplex studies have demonstrated comparable reliability in terms of sensitivity and specificity.[4,21]

Conventional contrast angiography remains the standard for evaluation of arterial disease. The costs and risks make conventional angiography a tool the clinician uses for a specific targeted question, not screening for severe disease. The risks of angiography relate to operator experience as well as the extent of vascular disease. The overall risks of angiography for permanent morbidity and mortality are as low as 0.5% to 1% or less, although in elderly patients with severe, diffuse atherosclerotic disease the risks may be several-fold higher.[9,14] Angiography also provides hemodynamic information and allows visualization of intracranial vessels as well. It is commonly done to confirm and visualize the stenosis at the bifurcation following detection of severe disease by ultrasound.

A 65-year-old man is seen following two 5-minute episodes of right face and arm weakness with loss of speech. He has a history of diabetes and hypertension. A left cervical bruit is heard.

The clinical question is focused on large vessel pathology because of the cortical deficits. The first urgent task is to identify the underlying vascular cause in an effort to most effectively reduce the risk of recurrent ischemia and stroke. The clinician must attempt to identify clinically relevant carotid disease. This task is not simple[1] and involves several issues. Carotid stenosis is often referred to as "mild," "moderate," or "severe." However, there are no consistent criteria for this division. Angiography has been taken as the standard, but some lesions are clearly not easily measured, even on cut film. The calculation of percent stenosis requires comparing the stenotic diameter to a reference with a segment of distal "normal" vessel chosen as that reference in NASCET. This distal segment may not be truly normal, and therefore the calculated percentage may not reflect the residual lumen. Other angiographic criteria compare the stenotic diameter to the estimated diameter were the vessel disease-free. This method was used in the European Carotid Surgery Trial (ECST)[11] and may give somewhat different results.

Vascular laboratories may also use different ultrasound and Doppler criteria for estimation of percent stenosis. Many use criteria based on comparison to angiography, in which stenotic diameter is compared to the estimated diameter were the vessel disease-free.[28] Clinicians need to understand the criteria of the local laboratory, and laboratories must strive for consistency in study quality. Additional ultrasound criteria have been proposed to improve the correspondence of carotid duplex results and NASCET angiographic criteria.[12,22]

Recognizing the technical limitations of quantifying the severity of stenosis, it remains reasonable to use carotid ultrasound or Doppler as the initial screening study in the evaluation of a patient with carotid territory TIA or stroke. A finding of "mild" stenosis (less than 50%) suggests a very low probability of a carotid source for the symptom, and the diagnostic attention should focus on cardiac issues or more distal intracranial disease. The finding of "severe" stenosis (greater than 70%) suggests a high probability of a carotid source, and surgical intervention should be considered. In centers where studies are reliable and of consistent high quality, it now seems possible to proceed, in selected cases, to surgical endarterectomy after careful noninvasive evaluation utilizing ultrasound and MRA. In routine cases with the ultrasound result in clear agreement with the findings on MRA, there can be adequate diagnostic certainty to defer conventional angiography. Magnetic resonance angiography can display the anatomic configuration of the bifurcation and help exclude other lesions, while ultrasound and Doppler confirm the degree of stenosis and provide hemodynamic data. In clinical situations with contradictory data or diagnostic uncertainty, conventional angiography remains the most definitive vascular study.

A carotid ultrasound or Doppler result of "moderate" stenosis (50% to 70%) is more problematic. The limitations of current technique and clinical knowledge overlap in that it is possible neither to distinguish a 60% stenosis from one of 70% nor to distinguish a difference in associated stroke risk. The clinician must make an individual decision in each case. Consideration must be given to the possibility of other embolic sources, including cardiac, and conventional angiography should be considered to provide additional anatomic detail. In a patient with a TIA, no cardiac source found on evaluation, and a 60%, heavily ulcerated, stenotic carotid lesion on both ultrasound and conventional angiography, the management decisions are not clear. Medical management with aspirin or warfarin should be considered. Surgical endarterectomy should also be considered, recognizing that no definitive data are yet available for this set of circumstances. It seems most reasonable to assess all risk factors carefully and thoroughly and make individualized management decisions until further information is available.

A particularly vexing problem for the clinician arises when the ultrasound study fails to detect flow in the internal carotid. The ultrasound criteria cannot distinguish complete occlusion from near occlusion with a trickle of slow flow. Particularly when the patient has had recent symptoms, there is an urgent need to distinguish these possibilities in order to choose appropriate treatment. Color flow imaging has not relieved this problem. Initially MRA had poor ability to resolve occlusion and slight flow, but current sequences can more reliably distinguish total and subtotal occlusion. However, conventional angiography again provides the standard for comparison, and the question of near occlusion often requires careful study, even with contrast angiography.

A 70-year-old woman is seen for evaluation of two episodes of left monocular blurring and several spells of speech difficulty, one with right arm weakness. Initial carotid duplex studies revealed mild to moderate disease bilaterally.

The clinician is faced with multiple spells in the left carotid territory despite no severe disease at the bifurcation. Based on duplex scanning, one can distinguish less than 50% stenosis from more serious disease with a positive predictive value of 97% and a negative predictive value of 96% as compared to conventional angiography.[28] A TCD evaluation may provide helpful information in this setting. It may reveal slow flow in the ophthalmic artery with reversal of flow in the anterior cerebral artery, and siphon disease would then be a likely explanation for the symptoms and findings. Carotid ultrasound does not adequately assess the carotid siphon, but TCD can provide indirect evidence of an

intervening stenosis. It is also often possible to evaluate flow directly in at least portions of the carotid siphon via the transorbital approach. It is then possible to demonstrate segments of increased velocity in the siphon corresponding to the stenosis.

Magnetic resonance angiography provides images of flow in the carotid siphon, although this region is particularly prone to imaging artifacts. For this reason it is difficult to rely on MRA for the diagnosis of siphon stenosis. Definitive diagnosis may require conventional contrast angiography.

A 58-year-old man with a history of heavy smoking is seen for evaluation of multiple episodes of left arm weakness. Initial carotid duplex and cardiac studies were unremarkable.

Here again the clinician is confronted with multiple events in a single arterial territory. A reasonable next step in the evaluation would be TCD, with intracranial disease a consideration. Middle cerebral artery stenosis can be detected by TCD and can be reliably diagnosed when the classic pattern of very high velocity flow in a proximal segment is associated with slow, dampened flow distally. In assessing distal arterial branches, TCD is of little value, but most clinically significant intracranial disease occurs in the more proximal segments.

Magnetic resonance angiography has provided a new level of noninvasive imaging of the intracranial vessels. A three-dimensional time-of-flight technique is most often used, and good visualization of flow is usually possible. Distal branches are again not assessed with this technique, although the proximal vessels out through the middle cerebral artery division are usually well seen. One of the major limitations of MRA is the lack of hemodynamic information. The pattern of collateral supply is not easily delineated, and the status of small communicator vessels is often beyond the resolution of the routine studies. Nonetheless, MRA can provide definitive diagnosis in many cases of middle cerebral stem stenosis, although the severity and extent are not readily discerned. The combined noninvasive evaluation with TCD and MRA can provide adequate diagnostic certainty to support treatment decisions such as long-term anticoagulation.

A 67-year-old man with a history of diabetes and neuropathy is seen for evaluation of multiple episodes of left arm and leg weakness. These have occurred with increasing frequency and have most often begun after standing.

Here the clinician is again faced with multiple events in a single arterial territory, but the postural nature of the presentation suggests inadequate flow rather than embolism as the underlying mechanism. The diagnostic effort should be directed to detection of severe, hemodynamically significant stenosis with compromised collateral. Carotid duplex examination is a practical starting point for the evaluation. Assessment of the carotid siphon may be necessary as well.

Evaluation of collateral flow is important in this setting. Transcranial Doppler is useful in determining flow velocities in the major vessels, comparing side to side as well as to absolute standards. Flow velocities may be very reduced in the middle cerebral artery above a carotid stenosis if communicating arteries are inadequate, or they can be normal above an occluded carotid with a widely patent anterior communicating artery. This hemodynamic information can be important in understanding the mechanism of ischemia.

Transcranial Doppler can also be used to assess the degree of relative compromise of cerebral perfusion. It is used to assess the cerebral circulation reserve, the ability of the vasculature to deliver more blood to the tissue. Autoregulation is felt to control cerebrovascular tone to optimize blood flow. As pressure drops or demand increases, vessels dilate to deliver more blood. As blood pressure increases, the vessels constrict to prevent excessive tissue perfusion. In the setting of low flow ischemia, the distal vasculature is thought to be chronically dilated to sustain flow. Then TCD is used to establish baseline velocities and to assess vasoreactivity. The latter can be tested after the administration of 3% to 5% CO_2. In the setting of relative ischemia, the vessels are already dilated and have a diminished ability for further dilatation. The TCD provocation study then documents an abnormal and diminished response to CO_2. An alternate method involves the administration of acetazolamide rather than the use of inspired CO_2. This technique can be used to detect relative ischemia and situations in which diminished reserve may help explain the etiology of symptoms.[27]

This concept of relative ischemia related to low flow and compromised collaterals has been evaluated with other modalities as well. Cerebral blood flow, blood volume, oxygen extraction fraction, and metabolism can be assessed by positron emission tomography (PET). Studies by PET have demonstrated that a decrease in cerebral perfusion pressure can be accommodated by vasodilatation, and it is only after maximal dilatation in the face of decreasing perfusion that ischemia develops.[26] Single photon emission computed tomography (SPECT) can also provide an assessment of cerebral blood flow, and the phenomenon of vasoreactivity has also been demonstrated.[8] A third technology utilizing radioactive xenon and computed tomography (CT) has been used to demonstrate the same vascular phenomenon. Recently, MRA has quantitatively evaluated acetazolamide-induced vasoreactivity.[20]

The clinical hypothesis put forth suggests that these technologies can identify populations of patients with severe occlusive disease who, by virtue of the loss of vasoreactivity, have a higher risk of subsequent stroke.

Initial applications were to identify those likely to benefit from extracranial-intracranial bypass procedures. However, since the publication of the international extracranial-intracranial (EC-IC) bypass study,[10] the procedure has essentially disappeared from clinical practice. Studies of this type are still important to further identify patients at risk for low flow ischemia. There may be a small population of patients who will benefit from the bypass procedure, and careful selection is appropriate.

In the setting of symptomatic carotid stenosis or occlusion, this loss of vasoreactivity as assessed by xenon CT was reported to be associated with a significantly higher incidence of subsequent stroke.[34] Similar reports have been made associated with TCD assessment of vasoreactivity in the setting of occlusive disease.[7] The results of recent endarterectomy trials have confirmed the clinical impression favoring surgical intervention in these cases.

Asymptomatic carotid disease

A 68-year-old woman with a history of stable angina is referred by her internist for evaluation of a left carotid bruit noted on a routine physical examination. She denies any neurologic symptoms.

A bruit heard over the cervical region may reflect underlying stenosis of the internal carotid artery, although it often reflects external carotid disease or transmission of cardiac murmurs. A focal ipsilateral bruit provides inadequate predictive power for detecting high-grade stenosis, with one study demonstrating a sensitivity of 63% and a specificity of 61%.[30] The absence of a bruit has little predictive power. Carotid ultrasound provides an excellent screening test in this situation. Even in asymptomatic patients, severe internal carotid artery stenosis represents a risk factor for stroke,[6] and a benefit from surgical endarterectomy has been suggested.[15,23]

The recent announcement of a definitive positive surgical benefit in the setting of asymptomatic severe stenosis will have great impact on clinical management.[25] The Asymptomatic Carotid Atherosclerosis Study (ACAS) enrolled 1662 patients with asymptomatic internal carotid stenosis greater than 60% as detected by carotid duplex or angiography who were randomized to medical management or surgical endarterectomy. The preliminary results revealed an absolute risk reduction of 5.8% over 5 years of primary end points. Routine screening of the asymptomatic population at risk for vascular disease and stroke is now important, but further details of the ACAS data will be helpful in developing a clinical strategy. Because the disease is progressive, effective management will require not only detection but also monitoring of progression.

Carotid ultrasound is also useful for monitoring the progression of disease safely and providing the clinician with information about both the progression and severity of the stenosis. A prospective study of the natural history of asymptomatic carotid stenosis in 167 patients revealed that 80% of the patients who developed symptoms also had ultrasound evidence of disease progression.[29] Carotid lesions were categorized as normal, 1% to 15%, 16% to 49%, 50% to 79%, 80% to 99%, or 100%, and progression of at least one category was observed in more than 35% of patients over 3 years. Given the rate of progression, 6- to 12-month follow-up intervals were recommended, and progression to more than 80% stenosis carried a 35% risk of ischemic symptoms or occlusion within 6 months. Agreement of duplex ultrasound and angiographic assessment of degree of stenosis exceeded 80%.

As the question of management for asymptomatic stenoses evolves, the possibility of selecting from the population a group at increased risk will remain critical. Further analysis of the ACAS data with respect to stroke risk stratified to degree of stenosis will help to focus clinical decisions. It has also been hypothesized that, in the setting of high-grade stenosis, loss of vasoreactivity may identify a group at particularly high risk for stroke. Clearly, TCD is a technique that can noninvasively assess vasoreactivity, and results of further studies will be important in clarifying this issue.

Vertebrobasilar disease

A 64-year-old man is seen for evaluation of episodes of unsteadiness and diplopia lasting minutes. The most severe spell involved several minutes of quadriplegia.

The clinician is faced with evaluation of recurrent spells referable to the posterior circulation. A single spell may result from an embolic event, but recurrent events suggest intrinsic vertebrobasilar disease. Atheromatous disease is most common at the vertebral origins and is also seen in the intracranial segment of the vertebral and basilar arteries. Duplex sonography has been utilized less in the posterior circulation than in the carotid system, in part because of technical difficulties. The course of the vessel is long, and it is frequently impossible to comment on presence or absence, size of vessel, flow velocity, spectral parameters, and flow direction as determined only at some point in the cervical portion. The sensitivity of duplex sonography as a screen for vertebral disease is therefore not as high as for carotid disease. The study can be done in conjunction with the carotid examination and in some clinical situations can provide adequate information. In addition to duplex scanning, TCD can be used to evaluate the intracranial vertebral and basilar arteries. The study can be technically challenging, and in some instances it is not possible to insonate along the entire course of the basilar artery. Direction of flow, flow velocity, and spectral parameters can be evaluated.

These studies together can be clinically useful when a definite and clinically consistent abnormality is identified. Antiplatelet or anticoagulant medication is the standard therapy for symptomatic posterior circulation ischemic events. Revascularization, either via surgery or angioplasty, is possible but is usually considered only after failure of medical management. In a patient with clear TCD evidence of vertebrobasilar stenosis and consistent clinical symptoms, it is reasonable to initiate medical therapy based upon the results. Usually MRI is necessary for adequate evaluation of the brain parenchyma in the posterior fossa in symptomatic patients, and MRA can be included to add diagnostic certainty. Magnetic resonance angiography of the posterior circulation can provide information of the cervical vertebral and intracranial vertebral and basilar arteries. Visualization of the vertebral origins is not consistently seen in sufficient detail to evaluate origin disease. In patients with symptoms that are less precise, such as isolated dizziness or presyncope, who are found to have normal or unremarkable TCD findings, it is reasonable to defer further evaluation of the posterior circulation. Likewise, in patients with medical illnesses that increase risks of angiography, such as renal insufficiency, TCD and MRA can provide safe, noninvasive evaluation. However, in the setting of threatening posterior circulation events and a normal TCD study, the diagnostic certainty of vertebral duplex and TCD is not adequate to exclude vascular pathology, and other evaluation is necessary. Conventional angiography may then be necessary for diagnostic clarity in the evaluation of threatening posterior circulation disease. The absolute diagnostic certainty of angiography may also be necessary when anticoagulant risks are higher than usual or when symptoms occur despite anticoagulation and invasive therapies are considered.

REFERENCES

1. Ackerman RH, Candia MR: Identifying clinically relevant carotid disease, *Stroke* 25:1-3, 1994.
2. Ammar AD, Wilson RL, Travers H, et al: Intraplaque hemorrhage: its significance in cerebrovascular disease, *Am J Surg* 148:840-843, 1984.
3. Belcaro G, Laurora G, Cesarone MR, et al: Ultrasonic classification of carotid plaques causing less than 60% stenosis according to ultrasound morphology and events, *J Cardiovasc Surg (Torino)* 34:287-294, 1993.
4. Buijs PC, Klop RB, Eikelboom BC, et al: Carotid bifurcation imaging: magnetic resonance angiography compared to conventional angiography and doppler ultrasound, *Eur J Vasc Surg* 7:245-251, 1993.
5. Call GK, Abbott WM, Macdonald NR, et al: Correlation of continuous-wave Doppler spectral flow analysis with gross pathology in carotid stenosis, *Stroke* 19:584-588, 1988.

6. Chambers BR, Norris JW: Outcome in patients with asymptomatic neck bruits, *N Engl J Med* 315:860-865, 1986.

7. Chimowitz MI, Furlan AJ, Jones SC, Transcranial doppler assessment of cerebral perfusion reserve in patients with carotid occlusive disease and no evidence of cerebral infarction, *Neurology* 43:353-357, 1993.

8. Chollet F, Celsis P, Clanet M, et al: SPECT study of cerebral blood flow reactivity after acetazolamide in patients with transient ischemic attacks, *Stroke* 20:458-464, 1989.

9. Davies KN, Humphrey RP: Complications of cerebral angiography in patients with symptomatic carotid territory ischaemia screened by carotid ultrasound, *J Neurol Neurosurg Psychiatry* 56:967-972, 1993.

10. EC/IC Bypass Study Group: Failure of extracranial-intracranial arterial bypass to reduce the risk of ischemic stroke, *N Engl J Med* 313:1191-1200, 1985.

11. ECST Collaborative Group: MRC European carotid surgery trial: interim results for symptomatic patients with severe (70-99%) or with mild (0-29%) carotid stenosis, *Lancet* 337:1235-1243, 1991.

12. Faught WE, Mattos MA, van Bemmelen PS, et al: Color-flow duplex scanning of carotid arteries: new velocity criteria based on receiver operator characteristic analysis for threshold stenoses used in the symptomatic and asymptomatic carotid trials, *J Vasc Surg* 19:818-827, 1994.

13. Fisher CM: The arterial lesions underlying lacunes, *Acta Neuropathol (Berl)* 12:1-15, 1969.

14. Hankey GJ, Warlow CP, Seller RJ: Cerebral angiographic risk in mild cerebrovascular disease, *Stroke* 21:209-222, 1990.

15. Hobson RW 2d, Weiss DG, Fields WS, et al: Efficacy of carotid endarterectomy for asymptomatic carotid stenosis. The Veterans Affairs Cooperative Study Group, *N Engl J Med* 328:221-227, 1993.

16. Huston J, Bradley LD, Wieberg DO, et al: Carotid artery prospective blinded comparison of two-dimensional time-of-flight MR angiography with conventional angiography and duplex US, *Radiology* 186:339-344, 1993.

17. Imparato AM, Riles TS, Mintzer R, Bauman FG: The importance of hemorrhage in the relationship between gross morphologic characteristics and cerebral symptoms in 376 carotid artery plaques, *Ann Surg* 197:195-203, 1983.

18. Johnson JM, Ansel AL, Morgan S, DeCesare D: Ultrasonographic screening for evaluation and follow-up of carotid artery ulceration: a new basis for assessing risk, *Am J Surg* 144:614-618, 1982.

19. Lusby RJ, Ferrell LD, Ehrenfeld WK, et al: Carotid plaque hemorrhage: its role in production of cerebral ischemia, *Arch Surg* 117:1479-1487, 1982.

20. Mandai K, Sueyoshi K, Fukunaga R, et al: Evaluation of cerebral vasoreactivity by three-dimensional time-of-flight magnetic resonance angiography, *Stroke* 25:1807-1811, 1994.

21. Mittl RL, Broderick M, Carpenter JP, et al: Blinded-reader comparison of magnetic resonance angiography and duplex ultrasonography for carotid artery bifurcation stenosis, *Stroke* 25:4-10, 1994.

22. Moneta GL, Edwards JM, Chitwood RW, et al: Correlation of NASCET angiographic definition of 70% to 99% internal carotid artery stenosis with duplex scanning, *J Vasc Surg* 17:152-159, 1993.

23. Moneta GL, Taylor DC, Nicholls SC, et al: Operative versus nonoperative management of asymptomatic high-grade internal carotid artery stenosis: improved results with endarterectomy, *Stroke* 18:1005-1010, 1987.

24. NASCET Collaborators: Beneficial effect of carotid endarterectomy in symptomatic patients with high-grade carotid stenosis, *N Engl J Med* 325:445-453, 1991.

25. National Institute of Neurological Disorders and Stroke: Carotid endarterectomy for patients with asymptomatic internal carotid artery stenosis. *Clinical Advisory;* September 28, 1994.

26. Powers WJ, Press GA, Grubb RL, et al: The effect of hemodynamically significant carotid artery disease on the hemodynamic status of the cerebral circulation, *Ann Intern Med* 106:27-35, 1987.

27. Ringelstein EB, Sievers C, Ecker S, et al: Noninvasive assessment of CO_2-induced cerebral vasomotor response in normal individuals and patients with internal carotid artery occlusions, *Stroke* 19:963-969, 1988.

28. Roederer GO, Langlois YE, Chan AW, et al: Ultrasonic duplex scanning of extracranial carotid arteries: improved accuracy using new features from the common carotid artery, *J Cardiovasc Ultrasonogr* 1:373-380, 1982.

29. Roederer GO, Langlois YE, Jager KA, et al: The natural history of carotid arterial disease in asymptomatic patients with cervical bruits, *Stroke* 15:605-613, 1984.

30. Sauve JS, Thorpe KE, Math M, et al: Can bruits distinguish high-grade from moderate symptomatic carotid stenosis? *Ann Intern Med* 120:633-637, 1994.

31. Seeger JM, Klingman N: The relationship between carotid plaque composition and neurologic symptoms, *J Surg Res* 43:78-85, 1987.

32. Sturzenegger M: Ultrasound findings in spontaneous carotid artery dissection: the value of duplex sonography, *Arch Neurol* 48:1057-1063, 1991.

33. Sturzenegger M, Newell DW, Douville C, et al: Dynamic transcranial doppler assessment of positional vertebrobasilar ischemia, *Stroke* 25:1776-1783, 1994.

34. Yonas H, Smith HA, Durham SR, et al: Increased stroke risk predicted by compromised cerebral blood flow reactivity, *J Neurosurg* 79:483-489, 1993.

35. Zukowski AJ, Nicolaides AN, Lewis RT, The correlation between carotid plaque ulceration and cerebral infarction seen on CT scan, *J Vasc Surg* 1:782-785, 1984.

43

Neurosonology in Critical Care

Lawrence R. Wechsler

Ultrasound has become an integral component of the diagnostic workup of many neurologic illnesses. These applications are well described in previous chapters of this book. In critically ill patients, ultrasound contributes to rapid diagnosis but also may be used in an additional capacity, to monitor essential cerebral parameters and guide management.

Not all critically ill patients with neurologic disease require ultrasound studies. Acute neuropathic processes, spinal cord disease, or myasthenic crisis would not likely involve ultrasound unless peripheral studies are needed to rule out deep vein thrombosis. Illnesses in which blood flow is critical or alters outcome are best suited to ultrasound monitoring. Most acute injuries to the central nervous system (CNS) are affected by blood flow changes either directly or because of the relationship between blood flow and intracranial pressure (ICP) and might benefit from application of ultrasound techniques.

Monitoring of neurologic status is central to the management of critically ill patients with neurologic disease. Aspects of the neurologic examination such as level of consciousness, orientation, focal neurologic abnormalities, and cranial nerve signs indicate improvement or deterioration and guide therapeutic interventions. Changes in status may occur rapidly; even when examinations are performed at frequent intervals, rapid

deterioration may be undetected. Monitoring allows continuous assessment of parameters that reflect immediate changes in cerebral function. In many conditions, sedation is necessary to control agitation or improve ventilation, rendering the neurologic examination less helpful. Alternative means of cerebral monitoring are essential in these situations, providing the only measure of neurologic function.

Several methods of monitoring the CNS are available. Each has strengths and weaknesses and may be best suited for a particular clinical situation. The choice of monitoring agents at an individual center also depends on available equipment, local interests, and experience with each technique. The clinician must be aware of the strengths and weaknesses of each monitoring technique and judge the value and reliability of information obtained in the clinical setting accordingly. This chapter contrasts available monitoring methods and reviews the role of ultrasound in the management of acutely ill patients with neurologic disease.

MONITORING TECHNIQUES
Electroencephalography

Electroencephalographic (EEG) monitoring is useful in identifying subclinical seizure activity and detecting changes in amplitude or focal slowing due to underlying brain injury. Derivations of EEG such as spectral edge (frequency which includes 90% of EEG power) and compressed spectral array (CSA) may be more sensitive than EEG and have been used to detect CNS changes, particularly ischemia. In patients comatose after head injury, CSA patterns correlate with prognosis[10,57] but have few implications for changes in therapy. Unfortunately, artifacts are difficult to distinguish from brain activity and frequently interfere with interpretation. The optimal parameter or derivation for monitoring remains uncertain,[38] and little information is available regarding sensitivity and specificity in specific clinical situations. Raw EEG data are probably not a particularly sensitive measure of small CNS changes, and difficulties with interpretation limit the usefulness of derivations such as CSA. An experienced examiner is necessary to properly interpret abnormalities and assure good technical quality of the traces.

Evoked potentials

Brainstem auditory evoked potentials (BAEPs) and somatosensory evoked potentials (SSEPs) have been used extensively to monitor CNS function. However, each test depends on conduction in specific pathways and can detect pathology only in those areas of the brain. Early negative and positive SSEP potentials recorded over the hemispheres correlate with activity in the cortex and thalamocortical projections.[4] Others correspond to conduction in the cervical and lumbar cord. Waves I through V of BAEPs are generated from specific sites along the auditory pathways from nerve VIII to the lateral lemniscus.[15] Abnormalities in BAEP and SSEP predict prognosis in comatose patients following head injury[32] and after global ischemia,[23] but, as is the case with EEG, typically no direct intervention results from these data. The SSEPs can be used to monitor hemispheric function in patients prone to ischemic injury such as following carotid endarterectomy; unless the somatosensory cortex is involved by the ischemic process, however, no changes will occur. Evoked potentials can be monitored noninvasively with standard equipment used for diagnostic studies. However, as in EEG, an experienced examiner is needed to properly interpret the significance of abnormalities appearing with serial or continuous recordings. Evoked potential monitoring is most easily accomplished in unresponsive patients because the stimulus may be uncomfortable over a prolonged time in an awake patient.

Cerebral blood flow techniques

Measurements of cerebral blood flow (CBF) are ideally suited to monitor patients with neurologic diseases that potentially reduce cerebral perfusion. Xenon-133, stable xenon computed tomography (CT), and single photon emission computed tomography (SPECT) assess CBF either qualitatively or quantita-

tively. SPECT depends on fixation of a tracer that distributes in proportion to blood flow. Imaging can be performed hours later, but the measurement reflects blood flow at the time of injection. However, values obtained are only relative to other areas of brain. Asymmetries may be due to an absolute increase on one side or a decrease on the other. Xenon-133 and stable Xenon CT provide quantitative measurement of blood flow. Xenon CT has the added advantage of imaging in the same plane as CT sections, allowing direct comparison of CBF values in CT-defined areas of the brain. Xenon, in concentrations used for xenon CT, increases CBF somewhat,[47] but this effect is minimal because most of the data used for calculation of CBF are obtained in the first few minutes of inhalation, before significant enhancement of CBF occurs. Radiation exposure limits the frequency with which xenon CT can be repeated, making it less useful in critically ill patients with rapidly changing physiology.

Positron emission tomography (PET) scanning provides additional information about cerebral metabolism, as well as CBF. In some cases, this information is invaluable because it demonstrates whether the level of blood flow is appropriate to the metabolic demands of the brain tissue. Low levels of CBF may occur in infarcted brain with little or no metabolism. Alternatively, metabolism may be normal or only slightly reduced with the same low level of CBF, indicating an ischemic area at risk for infarction.[3] Although such information is desirable, accurate measurements require a cooperative patient. A considerable support staff and a cyclotron are needed to maintain a PET scanner, which will likely be available only at selected institutions.

Although data obtained with these techniques are valuable in certain clinical settings, measurements are limited to infrequent intervals, and necessary equipment is large and not mobile. Usually the patient must be transported to another area of the hospital, often a difficult task for an unstable patient. The CBF studies may complement ultrasound, and using both together may provide a more complete assessment of the adequacy of the cerebral circulation. Ultrasound allows frequent or continuous monitoring of flow in large arteries, whereas CBF techniques, applied at intervals determined by changes in ultrasound parameters or clinical findings, indicate the status of hemispheric perfusion in brain territories supplied by the large arteries.

Ultrasound

Ultrasound provides a noninvasive means of monitoring the cerebral circulation at the bedside without many of the difficulties inherent in blood flow techniques. Blood flow in the extracranial cerebral arteries or the arteries of the circle of Willis are monitored by ultrasound techniques. Carotid duplex (CD) ultrasound allows evaluation of the internal carotid arteries, and transcranial Doppler (TCD) ultrasound assesses blood flow in the major intracranial arteries, including the middle, anterior, and posterior cerebral arteries; the vertebral arteries; and the basilar artery. Both techniques permit repeat testing at frequent intervals at the bedside without risk to the patient. Using special probes and appropriate software, TCD also permits continuous monitoring. Doppler shift frequency correlates with blood velocity,[60] and, assuming no change in vessel size, changes in velocity over time correspond to changes in CBF.[10] Xenon CBF studies, SPECT, and PET scans measure cerebral perfusion, whereas ultrasound of the large intracranial or extracranial arteries monitors bulk flow in specific arterial territories. In many circumstances, variations in the two parameters correlate well,[8,16] and blood flow velocity can be used as an indicator of CBF. When artery diameter changes (e.g., vasospasm) or arterial narrowing occurs distal to the basal cerebral arteries, velocity changes cannot be relied on to reflect CBF.

Experience and training are necessary to identify significant changes in ultrasound parameters during monitoring or on serial studies. However, this technique is more amenable to strict criteria (velocity changes of a certain amount or percent of baseline) than electrophysiologic methods. The TCD probes may become dislodged, particularly in agitated patients, causing velocity to decrease or pulsatility to increase. In most cases, an experienced examiner can distinguish such artifacts from physiologic changes. In addition, critically ill patients cannot always be adequately monitored with ultrasound techniques. Internal jugular catheters preclude placement of CD probes on the neck. Head bandages may limit access to the appropriate "windows" for monitoring intracerebral arteries by TCD. Nursing staff should be trained to adjust the continuous monitoring probe to obtain adequate signals when head movements or jarring causes displacement. Nurses or critical care staff must also be able to recognize significant abnormalities that require quick intervention or a change in therapy. Finally, brain injury can occur in the absence of blood flow changes in a particular monitored artery. Choice of monitoring technique depends on the function most frequently altered by the underlying disease process and the relative sensitivity of the technique to changes in brain function. Combinations of monitoring methods often prove useful when no one method is likely to detect all abnormalities.

ULTRASOUND IN SPECIFIC CLINICAL SETTINGS
Acute stroke

Until recently, therapy for stroke consisted primarily of supportive care and, for some patients, antiplatelet agents or anticoagulation to prevent recurrence. After failures in the 1960s, thrombolytic therapy was reintroduced initially with small groups of patients treated with intraarterial urokinase or streptokinase. Clinical improvement was demonstrated, with an acceptably low incidence of hemorrhage.[18,27] Subsequent trials also suggested the feasibility of intravenous therapy with tissue plasminogen activator (tPA) in the first few hours after stroke.[17,28] In one study, recanalization by angiography occurred in 30% of patients treated with intravenous tPA within 8 hours of stroke onset.[17] Greater recanalization rates were observed with branch occlusions than more proximal lesions such as middle cerebral artery (MCA) or internal carotid artery (ICA) occlusions.[63]

Angiographic studies are limited by the risk and impracticality of performing serial angiography to assess timing of recanalization. TCD ultrasound allows continuous monitoring of the MCA from the temporal window and can document the precise time of recanalization. During intravenous infusion of a thrombolytic agent, TCD ultrasound provides the only indication of arterial patency. Transcranial Doppler detection of flow in the occluded artery during constant intraarterial infusion determines the limits of the infusion and helps restrict the amount of thrombolytic agent to the minimum necessary to open the occluded artery.

Management of blood pressure, sedation, and anticoagulation is frequently changed when recanalization is achieved. Partial or complete large vessel occlusion may benefit from a somewhat higher than normal blood pressure to increase perfusion beyond the obstruction or by way of collateral pathways. Once blood flow has been reestablished, a decrease in blood pressure to nearnormal levels is advisable to minimize hyperemia that can predispose a patient to hemorrhage in previously ischemic brain. Anticoagulation may be instituted to help maintain patency of the previously occluded artery after recanalization. These measures help reduce complications and, it is hoped, improve overall outcome after thrombolytic therapy.

After thrombolysis, monitoring should be continued during transport and after arrival in the intensive care unit. The frequency of repeat occlusion after recanalization is unknown, but loss of TCD signals from a recently recanalized artery dictates reversal of blood pressure management and consideration of repeat efforts at thrombolysis. When recanalization does not occur immediately, intensive care unit (ICU) monitoring may reveal late recanalization, requiring appropriate adjustment in therapy.

Monitoring an occluded intracranial artery during thrombolysis is difficult because, initially, no signal is obtained. Only after partial flow is reestablished can the artery be identified with certainty. However, the probe position from the temporal window for detection of the

MCA stem is sufficiently predictable that a skilled examiner can properly place the probe and detect return of flow when it occurs. In patients with suspected MCA occlusion, finding an anterior cerebral artery (ACA) signal, typically at depths of 70 to 75 mm, then tracing backward to depth of 50 to 60 mm, should position the Doppler gate in the area of the MCA. The ACA velocity may be elevated ipsilateral to the occlusion as a result of collateral flow in leptomeningeal pathways.[9] Shifting the probe posteriorly to detect the signal from the posterior cerebral artery gives further credibility to the probe position. During thrombolysis, small adjustments should be made with the TCD probe to ensure that even a small amount of flow in the area is detected. Frequent, brief, high-amplitude signals suggesting emboli may occur early during recanalization, possibly signifying fragmentation of the thrombus. The character of the MCA signal also depends on the site of vascular occlusion. Occlusion of the MCA at its bifurcation into major divisions may result in a highly pulsatile velocity curve recorded from the proximal MCA stem; partial occlusion distal to the site of insonation causes a high resistance pattern. As clot is dissolved and the normal caliber of the artery is restored, pulsatility decreases. Multiple branch occlusions also produce a low velocity and highly pulsatile velocity curve in the proximal MCA, although in this situation some MCA flow is recorded even initially. Recanalization of most of the branches is signaled by increasing peak velocity and decreasing pulsatility (Fig. 43-1). Velocity may overshoot levels recorded from the contralateral, presumably normal MCA, and pulsatility may decrease because of hyperemia in the previously ischemic territory.[4]

Rapid diagnosis of stroke mechanism is also facilitated by ultrasound. When angiography in anticipation of intraarterial thrombolysis is not performed, CD and TCD ultrasound provide assessment of the extracranial and intracranial circulation that can be used to identify appropriate patients for thrombolytic therapy or anticoagulation. In patients with fluctuating neurologic deficits, knowledge of the site of vascular occlusion helps guide blood pressure management and select appropriate cases for further interventions such as thrombolysis or surgical revascularization, should the ischemic process progress. Although such interventions do not have proven benefits, they may be helpful in highly selected patients. In patients with transient ischemic attacks (TIAs) or minor stroke, carotid duplex may demonstrate carotid occlusion or intraluminal thrombus associated with stenosis. These patients are at risk for recurrent stroke, and anticoagulation with heparin is often recommended.[11,20] Although the value of heparin in preventing progression of stroke deficits is controversial, a subset of patients with high-grade carotid stenosis likely benefits from this therapy.[44] Similarly, patients with a crescendo pattern of TIAs and severe carotid stenosis should be considered for anticoagulation.[44] Carotid duplex identifies severe carotid stenosis and virtual or complete carotid occlusion with great reliability.[59] This test can be performed rapidly in the emergency room or at the bedside to facilitate decisions in the setting of recent or unstable neurologic events.

Magnetic resonance angiography (MRA), if available, also detects stenosis or occlusion of the extracranial and intracranial cerebral arteries, although the severity of stenosis is often overestimated.[45] Combining ultrasound and MRA provides a check on each technique and may be more accurate than either test alone. Measurements of CBF with xenon CT, xenon-133, or SPECT may add information about the adequacy of cerebral perfusion in the territory of stenotic or occluded arteries. In patients with multiple arterial lesions or puzzling symptoms, CBF data may clarify the site and extent of hemodynamic compromise.

Monitoring in an intensive care unit is necessary for most patients after carotid endarterectomy. Neurologic deterioration in the immediate postoperative period is rare but suggests reocclusion at the endarterectomy site due to thrombosis. Emergency ultrasound examination of the carotid bifurcation identified such patients quickly so that exploration and restoration of carotid patency can be rapidly accomplished. Rarely, postoperative deterioration is caused by intracranial hemorrhage. A few patients monitored postoperatively by TCD demonstrate increased MCA velocities due to hyperemia. These patients appear to be at particular risk for hemorrhage, and rapid control of blood pressure to the high normal range is advisable to minimize this risk (Fig. 43-2 on p. 476).[48]

Subarachnoid hemorrhage

Although early surgery and calcium channel blockers have improved outcome after subarachnoid hemorrhage (SAH), delayed ischemic deficit remains a significant cause of morbidity. Clinical deterioration frequently occurs 4 to 14 days after SAH, whether or not surgery has been performed. Rapid identification of the cause of deterioration is crucial because prompt therapy may prevent permanent neurologic injury. Repeat bleeding, vasospasm, hydrocephalus, and metabolic abnormalities are possible causes. Laboratory studies and CT scans rule out most possibilities. Vasospasm can be diagnosed by angiography, but this may be hazardous in an unstable patient. Increased velocities in the MCA, ACA, or both in a patient after SAH with focal neurologic deficits attribute to these vascular territories suggest vasospasm as the cause of the neurologic symptoms. Sensitivity and specificity for MCA vasospasm exceed 90%.[53,55] Detection of ACA vasospasm[24,39] and posterior vasospasm[56] is less accurate.

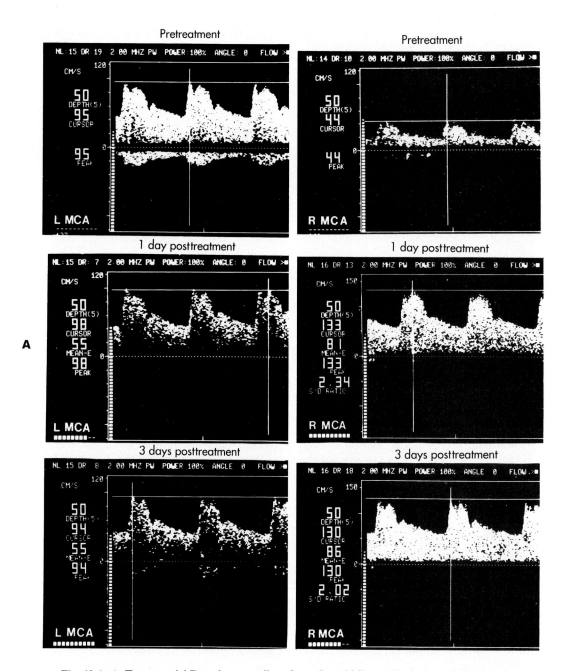

Fig. 43-1. A, Transcranial Doppler recordings from the middle cerebral artery (MCA) before treatment, 1 day, and 3 days after recanalization in a patient with multiple branch occlusions in the right MCA territory treated with tissue plasminogen activator (tPA). Recording from the right MCA *(left)* initially showed reduced peak velocity. After recanalization, velocities increased to levels greater than the contralateral MCA *(right)*. This increase persisted at 3 days. A repeat study at 14 days (not shown) demonstrated normal symmetric MCA velocities.

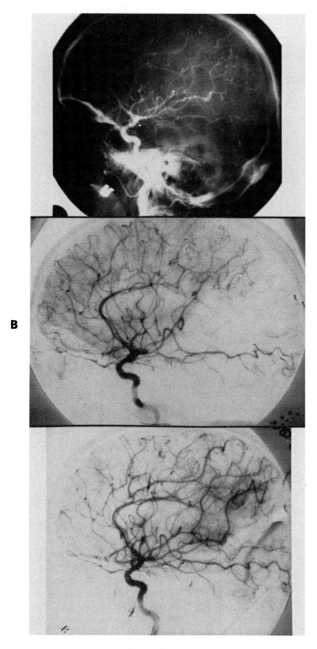

Fig. 43-1. B, Angiograms in the same patient before stroke *(top)*, immediately after stroke *(middle)* (angiographic complication), and after tPA treatment *(bottom)*. Multiple branches in the posterior parietal region, a few frontal branches, and branches of the anterior cerebral artery were occluded. Most of these were recanalized with engorged vessels in the posterior parietal region after thrombolytic therapy. (From Babikian VL: Transcranial Doppler ultrasonography in cerebrovascular disease. In Babikian VL, Wechsler LR, editors: *Transcranial Doppler ultrasonography,* St Louis, 1993, Mosby–Year Book.)

Ultrasound examinations can be performed at frequent intervals to follow the time course of velocity changes in the intracranial arteries. Rapidly rising velocities in the first few days identify patients with the severe spasm that is frequently associated with ischemic

symptoms.[26,52] Symptomatic vasospasm rarely occurs before day 3 or 4, but velocities may begin rising even before symptoms develop. Hypervolemic hemodilution or hypertensive therapy is often instituted to reverse ischemic deficits from vasospasm,[35] but whether these treatments should be started on the basis of increased velocities without neurologic symptoms is controversial. In some cases, increased perfusion pressure from induced hypertension or hypervolemia exacerbates edema or raises intracranial pressure, particularly when compliance is low. In patients with increased velocities, CBF studies detect those with hyperemia who may worsen with therapy aimed at increasing cerebral perfusion and select those likely to benefit from early aggressive treatment.

Because of the potential adverse effects, hypertensive and hypervolemic therapy should be discontinued as soon as vasospasm resolves. Follow-up angiography to assess resolution of vasospasm is usually avoided because of the risk of complications. Serial CBF studies demonstrate return of normal perfusion, but significant arterial narrowing may persist. Transcranial Doppler provides a noninvasive method of following not only the development of vasospasm but also the resolution phase (Fig. 43-3). When velocities return to near-normal values, therapy can be discontinued.[62]

Assessing the severity of vasospasm by TCD may be difficult. For any given velocity, the range of stenosis is broad in an individual patient. Mean velocity greater than 120 cm/s correlates with narrowing of the MCA, with a sensitivity of 84% and specificity of 89%;[55] when mean velocity exceeds 200 cm/s, vasospasm is generally considered severe.[52] In interpretation of TCD results, using ranges for stenosis based on velocity elevation is advisable; many factors influence absolute velocity. Fluctuations in Pco_2, hematocrit, cardiac output, and blood pressure all result in variations in velocity without any real change in arterial diameter. A pattern of steadily rising velocities is more valuable in clinical decision making than is attempting to estimate the residual lumen diameter based on a particular velocity reading. Once vasospasm becomes advanced, the hemodynamic consequences are the critical consideration. They are best assessed with CBF studies or, if the latter are not available, tests of reactivity such as changes in velocity in response to CO_2 or Diamox. Hypercarbia and acetazolamide (Diamox) cause cerebral vasodilation under normal circumstances, increasing velocity in the MCA as a result of increased volume flow. When vasospasm is sufficiently severe to cause ischemia, maximal vasodilation of the cerebral arterial bed occurs. No further vasodilation occurs in response to hypercarbia or acetazolamide. Similar information can be obtained with xenon-133 or stable xenon.

Raised ICP alters TCD velocity waveforms in a

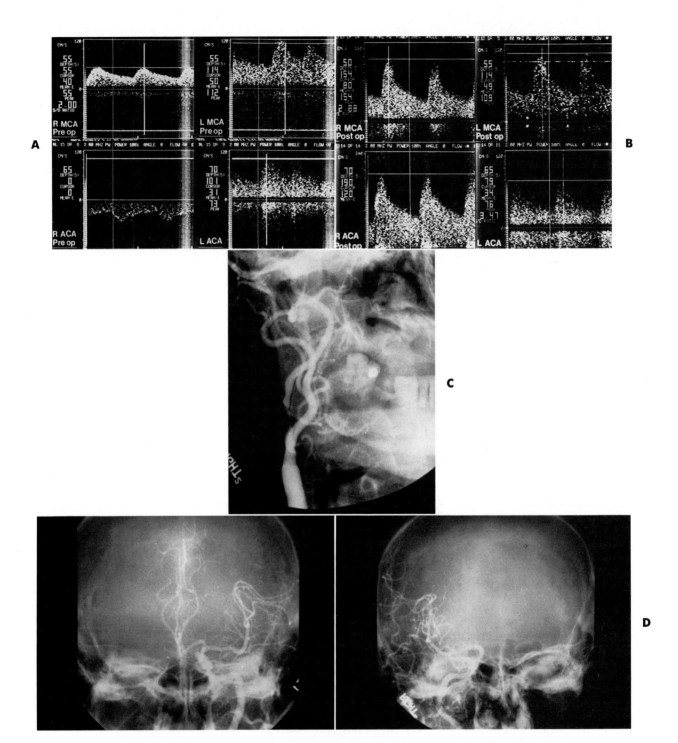

Fig. 43-2. Transcranial Doppler recording (**A**) before and (**B**) after carotid endarterectomy in a patient with severe right internal carotid stenosis. Before endarterectomy, right middle cerebral artery (MCA) velocity is decreased and pulsatility is diminished in comparison to the left MCA. Direction of flow is reversed in the anterior cerebral artery (ACA). Velocities in the right MCA and ACA are increased relative to the left after endarterectomy, indicating hyperemia. **C,** Preoperative angiogram showing severe stenosis of the right internal carotid artery. **D,** Intracranial views demonstrating both ACAs fill from the left carotid injection *(left)*. The right A1 segment is not visualized from the right carotid injection *(right)*.

Left MCA

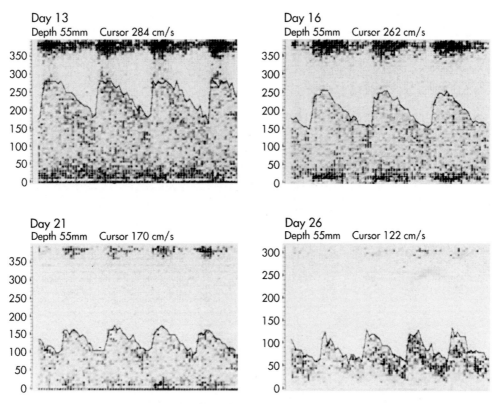

Fig. 43-3. Transcranial Doppler (TCD) studies in a patient with symptomatic vasospasm appearing 13 days after subarachnoid hemorrhage (SAH). Initial TCD showed high velocity in the left middle cerebral artery consistent with vasospasm. The symptoms resolved with vasopressors but recurred on day 16, when treatment was tapered. There was evidence of persistent vasospasm on TCD. On day 21, velocities were lower, indicating partial resolution of vasospasm, and hypertensive therapy was successfully tapered. The TCD recordings returned to normal by day 26. (From Wechsler LR, Ropper AH, Kistler JP: Transcranial Doppler in cerebrovascular disease, *Stroke* 17:906, 1986.)

predictable manner.[37] As ICP rises, diastolic velocity decreases, resulting in increased pulsatility and lower mean velocity.[37] Diagnosis of vasospasm becomes less reliable when ICP is increased. An increase in pulsatility across all arteries suggests raised ICP and limits the ability to monitor changes in vasospasm by means of comparison of serial TCD studies.

Detection of vasospasm in the ACA and posterior circulation is less accurate than MCA vasospasm.[24,39] This is likely due at least in part to the greater variability in the angle of insonation of these arteries. Assuming the same window is used for serial TCD studies, changes in velocities should correspond to changes in vasospasm more accurately than absolute velocities correlate with residual lumen diameter. Monitoring changes in ACA or basilar artery velocity, may provide clinically useful information about the course of vasospasm in arteries other than the MCA. Combining these data with CBF studies identifies decreased perfusion in the territory of arteries

narrowed by vasospasm, even when the extent of narrowing cannot be precisely predicted on the basis of velocity.

Increased velocities are not always due to vasospasm. Hyperemia can also cause elevated velocities, and in some cases mild vasospasm and hyperemia coexist. Cerebral blood flow studies with xenon, SPECT, or PET help distinguish hyperemia from vasospasm; blood flow is increased in the former and decreased in the latter.[33] When CBF studies are not available, pulsatility may be used as a crude index of hyperemia; pulsatility decreases with vasodilation and reduced cerebral vascular resistance. A single measurement of pulsatility may be difficult to interpret, but a decrease in pulsatility from a previous baseline associated with an increase in mean velocity suggests hyperemia.[21] This should be confirmed with a blood flow study because severe vasospasm may also cause vasodilation of distal arterioles and result in reduced pulsatility, mimicking the pattern seen with hyperemia.[30] The frequency of velocity increases due to

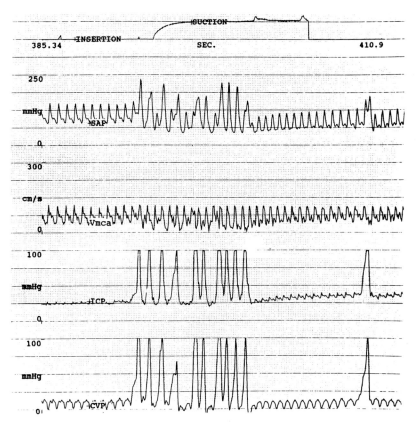

Fig. 43-4. Simultaneous recording of systemic arterial pressure (SAP), middle cerebral artery (MCA) velocity (V$_{MCA}$), intracranial pressure (ICP), and central venous pressure (CPV) during suctioning in a patient with cerebral edema due to head injury. Sudden increases in ICP are associated with increased pulsatility in the MCA and decreased diastolic velocity. (Courtesy of Dr. Mary Kerr.)

hyperemia is unknown. However, the excellent correlation between abnormal velocities and angiographic evidence of vasospasm in most studies[1,25,29,37] suggests that it is infrequent.

Another method for differentiating hyperemia from vasospasm by ultrasound compares the ICA velocity recorded from a submandibular approach to that in the MCA.[2,26,40] Hyperemia results from increased volume flow, which is associated with velocity increases of similar magnitude in both the ICA and the MCA. An MCA-ICA ratio less than 3 suggests hyperemia, and one greater than 3 indicates vasospasm.[40] Although small studies have shown a good correlation between this index and CBF evidence of hyperemia, large-scale comparisons are lacking. The variability of the insonation angle to the ICA from the submandibular approach reduces the reliability of the ratio. Consistent examination technique is essential to minimize misinterpretations due to inaccurate ICA velocity measurements. Only those practitioners with considerable experience and proven reliability should depend on this index for routine diagnosis.

Intracranial pressure

Measurement of ICP is valuable in managing patients with brain injury, although whether treatment of increased ICP alters outcome remains uncertain. Cerebral perfusion pressure (CPP = mean arterial pressure − ICP) must be maintained above 60 mm Hg to prevent ischemia.[34] Because blood pressure (BP) often fluctuates in patients with acute brain injury and pharmacologic agents to control blood pressure often become necessary, knowledge of ICP is critical to assuring adequate CPP.

Intracranial pressure can be measured with intraventricular or epidural catheters. Both techniques have advantages and disadvantages, particularly with focal mass lesions that may cause tissue shifts and uneven distribution of ICP in various brain compartments.[6] These techniques are invasive and are limited by the possibility of infection and intraparenchymal bleeding. In many situations, the risks of ICP monitoring outweigh the potential benefits, and ICP therapy is administered empirically, without specific knowledge of the response. A noninvasive method of measuring or following ICP changes would be desirable in such situations. Evoked potentials or EEG changes provide a crude tool because they enable detection of ischemic change caused by marked reductions in CPP. Typically, ICP is quite high when such changes occur. Loss of cortically generated waves on SSEPs and loss of waves II to V with preservation of wave I on BAEPs indicate severe cortical and brainstem injury associated with brain death.[23] Treatment must be instituted earlier, before ischemic levels of CPP are reached.

Transcranial Doppler has been proposed as a noninvasive index of ICP (Fig. 43-4). Several studies suggest a correlation between aspects of the TCD velocity curve and ICP.[22,31,36] As ICP increases, mean and diastolic velocities recorded from the MCA decrease and pulsatility increases. It is difficult to predict absolute ICP on the basis of a single recording of pulsatility, but changes in ICP correlate with changes in pulsatility, assuming other factors such as Pco_2 and arterial diameter remain constant.[31] In experimental models of increased ICP, pulsatility changes correlated with CPP;[46] this has also been demonstrated in clinical studies of patients with severe brain injury.[12,14] When CPP remains above 70 mm Hg, no change in pulsatility occurs, presumably as a result of the effects of autoregulation. As CPP falls below 70 mm Hg, autoregulation is lost and pulsatility increases. At CPP values of 20 mm Hg or less, there is a striking increase in pulsatility with small CPP changes.[12]

In patients with severe brain injury and no contraindication to invasive ICP monitoring, epidural or intraventricular catheters are the preferred method of monitoring. However, in individuals with bleeding diathesis, stroke with brain swelling, or other situations in which the benefits of invasive ICP monitoring are less certain, TCD monitoring provides an index of ICP that may be used to guide therapy. Continuous readout of velocity can be obtained with a monitoring probe fixed to the area of the temporal window. Software on some TCD instruments allows long-term trend monitoring of Doppler indices. Other factors that can affect pulsatility and mean velocity, particularly Pco_2, must also be monitored for proper identification of changes that correlate with CPP. Response to infusion of mannitol or diuretics can be assessed on the basis of changes in TCD pulsatility. Lowering BP even from high levels may reduce CPP below a critical threshold when ICP is elevated, and this should be reflected in increased pulsatility of the MCA velocity curve. Intracranial pressure increases in patients with edema after stroke can be identified, allowing initiation of treatment before clinical signs due to tissue shift and herniation occur.

Head injury

Severe head trauma results in focal or diffuse brain injury (or both), impairing consciousness or causing focal neurologic deficits. Patients are usually monitored in an intensive care unit and followed for evidence of clinical deterioration. Cerebral edema increases over the first few days after head injury, potentially leading to herniation and brain death. Hyperemia, probably due to loss of autoregulation, occurs in some cases and exacerbates edema if unchecked. Although less frequent than in aneurysmal SAH, vasospasm and ischemic infarction also are found in patients with head injury.[41]

The time course of velocity increases in the basal cerebral arteries of patients with traumatic SAH is quite similar to those with SAH from a ruptured aneurysm.[41] Transcranial Doppler abnormalities suggesting vasospasm have been found in up to 40% of patients with severe head injury.[61] Severe vasospasm and infarction occur less frequently but, when present, merit the same aggressive therapy as vasospasm due to aneurysmal SAH. Daily monitoring of velocity allows detection of those at risk for infarction due to vasospasm. Patients with mean velocity increases on serial studies to levels above 120 cm/s should be considered candidates for therapy aimed at reducing the hemodynamic effects of vasospasm. When velocities reach abnormal levels, CBF studies permit determination of whether stenosis is sufficiently severe to impair perfusion. If so, specific measures such as hypertensive therapy or hemodilution become more urgent. Cerebral blood flow studies also identify hyperemia, which can increase TCD velocities to the same levels as vasospasm.[13,51] This differentiation is critical; therapies for vasospasm are hazardous in patients with hyperemia.[54] Daily TCD monitoring with selected CBF studies minimizes the use of potentially harmful therapy by limiting its use to the minority of patients who have hemodynamically significant vasospasm.

After severe head injury, intubation and sedation are often necessary to induce hyperventilation and control agitation. Because these interventions may limit the neurologic examination, monitoring techniques become important in detecting evidence of tissue shifts and increased ICP. Clinical signs of herniation do not occur until ICP reaches a very high level[6,42] and cannot be relied on to guide therapy. Improved outcome after head injury has been demonstrated in patients with lower ICP;[7,43] however, whether ICP treatment alters outcome remains controversial.[50,58] If aggressive ICP therapy is planned, direct measurement of ICP with an epidural or intraventricular catheter is necessary. Transcranial Doppler monitoring of MCA velocity can be useful as a noninvasive index of ICP, in addition to conventional ICP monitoring or alone. As mentioned in previous sections, changes in the velocity and pulsatility provide a crude index of ICP but should not be relied upon without direct ICP monitoring unless invasive monitoring is contraindicated. Bedside monitors in the ICU usually display BP and ICP but not a continuous readout of CPP. Transcranial Doppler evidence of increased pulsatility may provide the first indication of reduced perfusion. Continuous TCD recording serves as a backup method of ICP monitoring in case an epidural or intraventricular catheter becomes plugged and no longer accurately reflects ICP.

Brain death

Extreme elevations in ICP result in irreversible ischemia and brain death. Confirmatory studies are often not necessary because the reason for increased ICP is known, and clinical criteria alone are sufficient to establish brain death. However, in children or patients treated with barbiturate coma, confirmation of brain death is necessary, and TCD offers a rapid, easily available diagnostic test.

A distinctive TCD pattern occurs in brain death, characterized by brief systolic spikes or a reverberating pattern, with brief forward flow during systole and reversed flow during diastole.[49] This pattern must be found in multiple arteries recorded from at least two windows because occlusion of a single intracranial artery can produce the same TCD pattern. In some patients, no TCD signals can be obtained from the intracranial circulation. Other tests such as xenon CBF, SPECT, and angiography may be used as a confirmatory test instead of TCD.

Other uses of ultrasound

The availability of ultrasound in the intensive care unit aids management of systemic problems in critically ill patients with neurologic illness. Deep vein thrombosis is a constant threat in bedridden patients, and duplex examination of the lower extremities should be performed whenever thrombosis is suspected. Ultrasound helps guide placement of catheters into the jugular vein for measurement of AVo_2 differences or the pulmonary artery for monitoring of pulmonary capillary wedge pressure. Color Doppler imaging of the intracranial arteries identifies arteries more accurately and provides more reliable velocity measurements than conventional TCD.[5] This may be helpful in patients with distorted intracranial anatomy due to mass lesions[19] and avoids errors due to monitoring of velocity in the wrong artery. Once the correct position of the artery has been identified on color Doppler imaging, the TCD probe can be quickly positioned for continuous monitoring.

SUMMARY

Ultrasound techniques are applicable to many critically ill patients with neurologic disease. Repeatability of ultrasound studies without risk to the patient, ease of use, and reliability of results make ultrasound an excellent choice for monitoring in a variety of settings.

The number of applications of TCD continues to expand. As more information is gathered about correlations between TCD velocity and blood flow or ICP, the role of TCD monitoring and its clinical value will be clarified. Although CD ultrasound has limited applications, in postoperative patients after endarterectomy or patients with acute stroke, the obtained information may be invaluable.

Further comparisons between TCD and other monitoring techniques would be helpful in defining the optimal method of approaching specific clinical problems. It should be emphasized that ultrasound measures velocity of flow in large arteries rather than brain perfusion. In many situations, ultrasound may be most reliable when combined with other tests such as CBF studies to examine not only flow in proximal arteries but tissue perfusion as well.

REFERENCES

1. Aaslid R, Huber P, Nornes H: Evaluation of cerebrovascular spasm with transcranial Doppler ultrasound, *J Neurosurg* 60:37-41, 1984.
2. Aaslid R, Huber P, Nornes H: A transcranial Doppler method in the evaluation of cerebrovascular spasm, *Neuroradiology* 28:11-16, 1986.
3. Ackerman RH, et al: Positron imaging in ischemic stroke disease using compounds labeled with oxygen 15, *Arch Neurol* 38:537-543, 1981.
4. Babikian VL: *Transcranial Doppler ultrasonography in cerebrovascular disease.* In Babikian VL, Wechsler LR, editors: *Transcranial Doppler ultrasonography,* St Louis, 1993, Mosby–Year Book.
5. Babikian V, Wechsler L: Recent developments in transcranial Doppler sonography, *J Neuroimaging* 4:159-163, 1994.
6. Barnett GH: *Intracranial pressure monitoring devices: principles, insertion and care.* In Ropper AH, editor: *Neurological and neurosurgical intensive care,* New York, 1993, Raven Press.
7. Becker D, et al: The outcome from severe head injury with early diagnosis and intensive management, *J Neurosurg* 47:491-502, 1977.
8. Bishop CCR, et al: Transcranial Doppler measurement of middle cerebral artery blood flow velocity: a validation study, *Stroke* 17:913-915, 1986.
9. Brass L, Duterte DL, Mohr JP: Anterior cerebral artery velocity changes in disease of the middle cerebral artery stem, *Stroke* 20:1737-1740, 1989.
10. Bricolo A, et al: Clinical application of compressed spectral array in long-term EEG monitoring of comatose patients, *Electroencephalogr Clin Neurophysiol* 45:211-225, 1978.
11. Buchan A, et al: Intraluminal thrombus in the cerebral circulation: implications for surgical management, *Stroke* 19:681-687, 1988.
12. Chan K-H, et al: The effect of changes in cerebral perfusion pressure upon middle cerebral artery blood flow velocity and jugular bulb venous oxygen saturation after severe brain injury, *J Neurosurg* 77:55-61, 1992.
13. Chan K-H, et al: Transcranial Doppler waveform differences in hyperemic and nonhyperemic patients after severe head injury, *Surg Neurol* 38:433-436, 1992.
14. Chan K-H, et al: Multimodality monitoring as a guide to treatment of intracranial hypertension after severe brain injury, *Neurosurgery* 32:547-553, 1993.
15. Chiappa KH: *Evoked potentials in clinical medicine,* New York, 1983, Raven Press.
16. Dahl A, et al: Local intra-arterial fibrinolytic therapy in acute carotid territory stroke: pilot study, *Stroke* 23:15-19, 1992.

17. del Zoppo G, et al: Recombinant tissue plasminogen activator in acute thrombotic and embolic stroke, *Ann Neurol* 32:78-86, 1992.

18. del Zoppo G, et al: Local intra-arterial fibrinolytic therapy in acute carotid territory stroke: pilot study, *Stroke* 19:307-313, 1988.

19. Finn JP, Quinn MW, Hall-Craggs MA, Kendall BE: Impact of vessel distortion on transcranial Doppler velocity measurements: correlation with magnetic resonance imaging, *J Neurosurg* 73:572-575, 1990.

20. Fisher CM: *Principles of diagnosis and management of occlusive cerebrovascular disease.* In Ropper AH, editor: *Neurological and neurosurgical intensive care,* New York, 1993, Raven Press.

21. Giller CA, Hodges K, Batjer HH: Transcranial Doppler pulsatility in vasodilation and stenosis, *J Neurosurg* 72:901-906, 1990.

22. Giulioni M, Ursino M, Alvisi C: Correlations among intracranial pulsatility, intracranial hemodynamics, and transcranial Doppler wave form: literature review and hypothesis for future studies, *Neurosurgery* 22:807-812, 1988.

23. Goldie WD, et al: Brainstem auditory and short latency somatosensory evoked responses in brain death, *Neurology* 31:248-256, 1981.

24. Grolimund P, et al: Evaluation of cerebrovascular disease by combined extracranial and transcranial Doppler sonography: experience in 1,039 patients, *Stroke* 18:1018-1024, 1987.

25. Grosset DG, et al: Angiographic and Doppler diagnosis of cerebral artery vasospasm following subarachnoid hemorrhage, *Br J Neurosurg* 7:291-298, 1993.

26. Grosset DG, et al: Use of transcranial Doppler sonography to predict development of a delayed ischemic deficit after subarachnoid hemorrhage, *J Neurosurg* 78:183-187, 1993.

27. Hacke W, et al: Intra-arterial thrombolytic therapy improves outcome in patients with acute vertebrobasilar occlusive disease, *Stroke* 19:1216-1222, 1988.

28. Haley EC, et al: Urgent therapy for stroke II: pilot study of tissue plasminogen activator administered 91-180 minutes from onset, *Stroke* 23:641-645, 1992.

29. Harders AG, Gilsbach JM: Time course of blood velocity changes related to vasospasm in the circle of Willis measured by transcranial Doppler ultrasound, *J Neurosurg* 66:718-728, 1987.

30. Hassler W, Chioffi F: CO_2 reactivity of cerebral vasospasm after aneurysmal subarachnoid hemorrhage, *Acta Neurochir (Wien)* 98:167-175, 1989.

31. Homburg AM, Jakobsen M, Enevoldsen E: Transcranial Doppler recordings in raised intracranial pressure, *Acta Neurol Scand* 87:488-493, 1993.

32. Hume AL, Cant BR: Central somatosensory conduction time after head injury, *Ann Neurol* 10:411-419, 1981.

33. Jakobson M, Enevoldsen E, Dalager T: Spasm index in subarachnoid haemorrhage: consequences of vasospasm upon cerebral blood flow and oxygen extraction, *Acta Neurol Scand* 82:311-320, 1990.

34. Jennet WB, et al: Relation between cerebral blood flow and cerebral perfusion pressure, *Br J Surg* 57:390-397, 1970.

35. Kassell NF, et al: Treatment of ischemic deficits from vasospasm with intravascular volume expansion and induced arterial hypertension, *Neurosurgery* 11:337-343, 1982.

36. Klingelhofer J, et al: Evaluation of intracranial pressure from transcranial Doppler studies in cerebral disease, *J Neurol* 235:159-162, 1988.

37. Klingelhofer J, et al: Cerebral vasospasm evaluated by transcranial Doppler ultrasonography at different intracranial pressures, *J Neurosurg* 75:752-758, 1991.

38. Labar DR, et al: Quantitative EEG monitoring for patients with subarachnoid hemorrhage, *Electroencephalogr Clin Neurophysiol* 78:325-332, 1991.

39. Lennihan L, et al: Transcranial Doppler detection of anterior cerebral artery vasospasm, *Stroke* 20:151, 1989 (abstract).

40. Lindegaard K-F, et al: Cerebral vasospasm after subarachnoid hemorrhage investigated by means of transcranial Doppler ultrasound, *Acta Neurochir Suppl (Wien)* 42:81-84, 1988.

41. Martin NA, et al: Posttraumatic cerebral arterial spasm: transcranial Doppler ultrasound, cerebral blood flow, and angiographic findings, *J Neurosurg* 77:575-583, 1992.

42. McDowall DG: Monitoring the brain, *Anesthesiology* 45:117-134, 1976.

43. Miller JD, et al: Significance of intracranial hypertension in severe head injury, *J Neurosurg* 47:503-515, 1977.

44. Miller VT, Hart RG: Heparin anticoagulation in acute brain ischemia, *Stroke* 19:403-406, 1988.

45. Mittl RL, et al: Blinded-reader comparison of magnetic resonance angiography and duplex ultrasonography for carotid artery bifurcation stenosis, *Stroke* 25:4-10, 1994.

46. Nelson RJ, et al: Experimental aspects of cerebrospinal hemodynamics: the relationship between blood flow velocity waveform and cerebral autoregulation, *Neurosurgery* 31:705-710, 1992.

47. Obrist WD, et al: Effect of stable xenon inhalation on human CBF, *J Cereb Blood Flow Metab* 5:557-558, 1985.

48. Powers AD, Smith RR: Hyperperfusion syndrome after carotid endarterectomy: a transcranial Doppler evaluation, *Neurosurgery* 26:56-60, 1990.

49. Ropper AH, Kehne SM, Wechsler L: Transcranial Doppler in brain death, *Neurology* 37:1733-1735, 1987.

50. Saul T, Ducker T: Effect of intracranial pressure monitoring and aggressive therapy on mortality in severe head injury, *J Neurosurg* 56:498-503, 1982.

51. Saunders FW, Cledgett P: Intracranial blood velocity in head injury: a transcranial ultrasound Doppler study, *Surg Neurol* 29:401-409, 1988.

52. Seiler RW, et al: Cerebral vasospasm evaluated by transcranial ultrasound correlated with clinical grade and CT-visualized subarachnoid hemorrhage, *J Neurosurg* 64:594-600, 1986.

53. Sekhar LN, et al: Value of transcranial Doppler examination in the diagnosis of cerebral vasospasm after subarachnoid hemorrhage, *Neurosurgery* 22:813-821, 1988.

54. Shigemori M, et al: Intracranial haemodynamics in diffuse and focal brain injuries: evaluation with transcranial Doppler (TCD) ultrasound, *Acta Neurochir (Wien)* 107:5-10, 1990.

55. Sloan MA, et al: Sensitivity and specificity of transcranial Doppler ultrasonography in the diagnosis of vasospasm following subarachnoid hemorrhage, *Neurology* 39:1514-1518, 1989.

56. Sloan MA, et al: Sensitivity and specificity of transcranial Doppler for detecting vertebral artery vasospasm, *Stroke* 23:469, 1992 (abstract).

57. Steudel WE, Druger J: Using the spectral analysis of the EEG for prognosis of severe brain injuries in the first post-traumatic week, *Acta Neurochir suppl (Wien)* 28:40-42, 1979.

58. Stuart G, et al: Severe head injury managed without intracranial pressure monitoring, *J Neurosurg* 59:601-605, 1983.

59. Taylor DC, Strandness DE Jr: Carotid artery duplex scanning, *J Clin Ultrasound* 15:635-644, 1987.

60. Tegeler CH, Eicke M: *Physics and principles of transcranial Doppler ultrasonography.* In Babikian VL, Wechsler LR, editors: *Transcranial Doppler ultrasonography,* St Louis, 1993, Mosby–Year Book.

61. Weber M, Grolimund P, Seiler RW: Evaluation of posttraumatic cerebral blood flow velocities by transcranial Doppler ultrasonography, *Neurosurgery* 27:106-112, 1990.

62. Wechsler LR, Ropper AH, Kistler JP: Transcranial Doppler in cerebrovascular disease, *Stroke* 17:905-912, 1986.

63. Wolpert SM, et al: Neuroradiologic evaluation of patients with acute stroke treated with recombinant tissue plasminogen activator, *AJNR Am J Neuroradiol* 14:3013, 1993.

Appendix I

GUIDELINES FOR PROFESSIONAL TRAINING AND CERTIFICATION IN NEUROSONOLOGY

Charles H. Tegeler

As seen in the preceding pages of this text, the scope, complexity, and clinical importance of neurosonology mandate extensive training to ensure that these services are provided in a safe, accurate, and appropriate way. This is true for the technical performance as well as the clinical interpretation and reporting of these studies. Documentation of training, qualifications, performance, and credentialing for all aspects of ultrasound testing is assuming ever greater importance and may ultimately be required for reimbursement. Voluntary accreditation of neurosonology laboratories is now available and discussed in detail in Appendix 2. The vital role for ongoing quality assurance programs is presented in Appendix 3. This Appendix addresses training and credentials for the medical staff, who interpret studies and may also perform neurosonographic exams.

In the past, specific guidelines for the training of physicians in neurosonology have been lacking. This is, in part, due to the diversity of the backgrounds and specialties represented by the physicians involved in such testing. However, as with other diagnostic procedures, the guidelines of the American Medical Association (AMA) state that physicians should be allowed access to the performance and interpretation of diagnostic procedures based on adequate training in that specific modality, irrespective of specialty or type of practice.[4]

Guidelines for training in ultrasound have now been established by several organizations. The American Institute of Ultrasound in Medicine (AIUM) has published training guidelines for those preparing to be able to interpret the entire gamut of ultrasound procedures.[2] To prepare for the interpretation of studies in a general ultrasound laboratory, the AIUM recommends completion of an approved residency program, fellowship, or postgraduate training program, which includes the equivalent of at least 3 months of diagnostic ultrasound training under supervision of a qualified physician, with documentation of the evaluation and interpretation of at least 500 studies. Without such formal experience in residency, fellowship, or postgraduate training, the AIUM recommends at least 100 hours of AMA Category I CME activity devoted to ultrasound and documentation of the evaluation and interpretation of at least 500 studies within a 3-year period. The American College of Cardiology has outlined the training needed to become certified for the interpretation of echocardiographic studies,[6] and guidelines are available for training in radiology residency.[3]

Guidelines specific to neurosonology have been in place for a number of years. The American Academy of Neurology (AAN) and the American Society of Neuroimaging (ASN) provided guidelines on the minimum training for those wishing to interpret neurosonographic studies.[1] The ASN has offered a certification examination in neurosonology for physicians since 1980. This examination has specific criteria for eligibility, including documentation of training in residency or CME experience, as well as the documentation of the interpretation and/or performance of at least 100 neurosonographic studies, under supervision. An outline of what is felt to constitute the core curriculum of knowledge in the field (physics, instrumentation, anatomy, pathology, pathophysiology, technique, indications, alternatives, interpretation, biologic effects, and quality control) and what candidates for the certification examination are responsible for is also available. Maintenance of certification both for the ASN and for the accreditation of the laboratory also require ongoing participation in CME programs relevant to neurosonology: at least 15 hours of AMA category I CME dedicated to neurosonology, every 3 years.

Similar guidelines are being created worldwide. Germany has very specific and quite complex guidelines for training required before a physician can bill for such studies.[5] These requirements may be met during residency training (18 months of training) or through a course system combined with documented case performance and/or interpretation. Pertinent ultrasound procedures are divided into extracranial Doppler, extracranial duplex (including color flow), and transcranial Doppler. Performance and interpretation of 200 cases is required for each category. On average, about 50 hours of CME is required as coursework for those not receiving documented training during residency.

Thus, while the specifics may vary, there are common threads to all of the available guidelines for training in ultrasound and neurosonology. Virtually all include 3 months of focused experience during residency, fellowship, or postgraduate training, with documentation of the performance and/or interpretation of a number of cases (from 100 to 500), a valid medical license, and often the necessity for board eligibility or certification. For those receiving such training outside a residency, fellowship, or a postgraduate training program, the common threads are extensive participation in approved CME (40 to 100 hours), with similar documentation of the performance and/or interpretation of cases under supervision, as well as a valid medical license, and often board eligibility or certification. In addition, physicians who wish to perform, evaluate, or interpret neurosonographic studies must have a broad knowledge of neuroanatomy, neuropathology, pathophysiology, and clinical aspects of neurologic and cerebrovascular disease. This also includes knowledge of the effects of disease on the neurosonographic examination, the indications, and the limitations of the procedures. The physician must have knowledge of alternative and complementary diagnostic procedures and should be capable of correlating the neurosonographic results with such results of other procedures.

The process of credentialing for hospital privileges is usually built on similar requirements and often includes a requirement for the performance and/or interpretation of a standard panel of example or test cases. The use of standardized, practical assessment of skills has long been used to evaluate internal medicine residents.[7]

Those wishing to direct laboratories, carry out academic ultrasound research activities, or be course directors are held to more rigorous standards. In Germany, this means that course directors must demonstrate a tenfold increase in the number of documented cases, twice the amount of time in training (36 months), and 400 cases per year of ongoing activity. In the United States, this often means at least a 1 year postresidency fellowship in neurosonology.

As the need for credentialing and certification becomes more acute, everyone wishing to pursue this exciting field is encouraged to obtain at least 3 months of specific training during residency, with documentation from the training director, or plan to attend extensive amounts of AMA Category I–accredited CME activities specific to neurosonology. In either case, all must maintain records of all cases performed and interpreted under supervision. For those physicians who are eligible, participation in the neurosonology certification examination from the American Society of Neuroimaging is recommended.

REFERENCES

1. American Academy of Neurology: Guidelines for training of the performance/interpretation of neurosonographic studies, *American Society of Neuroimaging Newsletter 1:* January 1992.
2. American Institute of Ultrasound in Medicine: Training guidelines for physicians who evaluate and interpret diagnostic ultrasound examinations, *AIUM Reporter* May 1993.
3. Filly RA: Radiology residency training in diagnostic sonography, *J Ultrasound Med* 8:475, 1989 (letter).
4. McKinney WM: AMA practice guidelines for members seeking to obtain hospital privileges for the performance and interpretation of neuroimaging studies, *J Neuroimaging* 2:46, 1992 (letter).
5. Niederkorn K: Training and qualification regulations for neurosonology in Germany, 1994 (personal communication).
6. Popp RL, Winters WL, et al: Clinical competence in adult echocardiography: a statement for physicians from the ACP/ACC/AHA Task Force on Clinical Privileges in Cardiology, *J Am Coll Cardiol* 15:1465-1468, 1990.
7. Stillman P, Swanson D, Regan MB, et al: Assessment of clinical skills of residents utilizing standardized patients: a follow-up study and recommendation for application, *Ann Intern Med* 114:393-401, 1991.

Appendix II

ACCREDITATION OF VASCULAR ULTRASOUND LABORATORIES

Sandra L. Katanick

The Intersocietal Commission for the Accreditation of Vascular Laboratories (ICAVL) is a nonprofit organization that provides a mechanism for voluntary accreditation of facilities performing noninvasive vascular diagnostic testing. It was established with the initial support of eight sponsoring organizations representing the full range of clinical specialties involved in noninvasive vascular testing. In April of 1989, at a meeting of the American Institute of Ultrasound in Medicine, several key individuals active in the practice of noninvasive vascular testing met to discuss the concept of forming an independent organization devoted to the mission of providing a process of recognition for facilities performing noninvasive testing for the diagnosis of vascular disease. The commission's primary objective in recognizing these facilities is to ensure high-quality patient care through a process of voluntary accreditation. The initial sponsoring organizations were the American Academy of Neurology (AAN), American College of Radiology (ACR), American Institute of Ultrasound in Medicine (AIUM), North American Chapter for International Society for Cardiovascular Surgery (ISCVS), Society of Vascular Medicine and Biology, Society for Vascular Surgery (SVS), Society of Diagnostic Medical Sonographers (SDMS), and the Society of Vascular Technology (SVT). In January 1993, the ICAVL expanded its board of directors by adding six new members representing three new sponsoring organizations. These newly added organizations are the American Association of Neurosurgeons/Joint Council on Cerebrovascular Surgery, the American College of Cardiology (ACC), and the Society of Cardiovascular and Interventional Radiology (SCVIR). All of these organizations have a significant percentage of their membership involved in noninvasive vascular diagnostic testing. Each organization provides two representatives to the ICAVL Board of Directors. Sponsoring organizations also participate in the development and review of the ICAVL standards and nominate candidates to be considered for vacant positions on the ICAVL Board of Directors.

The first assignment that the Board of Directors completed was to develop and publish the essentials and standards for noninvasive vascular testing in the areas of cerebrovascular, peripheral arterial, peripheral venous, and visceral vascular testing, as well as laboratory organization. These are the generalized guidelines for testing and are discussed later in the chapter. Following the development of the standards, a self-study mechanism for review of a laboratory was developed based on the standards. The self-studies are a series of detailed questions designed to enable an outside peer reviewer to determine if there is compliance to the published standards and that the facility is performing high-quality noninvasive vascular testing. If substantial compliance is demonstrated, accreditation is granted for a period of 3 years. If a determination of compliance is uncertain, a site visit may be necessary or the laboratory may be denied accreditation.

ESSENTIALS AND STANDARDS

The essentials and standards are the guidelines developed for the performance and interpretation of noninvasive vascular testing. They are written for the areas of cerebrovascular (both extracranial and intracranial), peripheral arterial, peripheral venous, and visceral vascular testing, as well as for the organization of a vascular laboratory. The organization standard begins by addressing the operational structure of the laboratory by defining the duties, responsibilities, and qualifications necessary for the medical director, technical director, and the medical and technical staff. All members of the medical staff, including the medical director, must be legally qualified physicians and have appropriate experience, evidenced by graduate or postgraduate education, a residency or fellowship with vascular laboratory rotations, or a number of years in the field combined with continuing medical education (CME) relevant to noninvasive vascular diagnosis. It is necessary to maintain adequate, ongoing continuing education specific to the field. The technical staff, including the technical director, should also possess appropriate training and experience suitable for the services provided. They are encouraged to obtain the registered vascular technologist (RVT) certification as evidence of a high level of commitment. The commission's recommendation for CME for all staff personnel is a minimum of 15 hours every 3 years relevant to the services provided. Section 2 of organization outlines the recommended laboratory support services. It is necessary to provide appropriate administration, clerical, nursing, and any other support services necessary to maintain adequate support for safe and efficient patient care. These services must be supervised. Section 3 requires that the physical facilities for testing be of adequate size and cleanliness to conduct testing and that they ensure patient comfort and privacy. It is also necessary to have adequate interpretation and storage space. Reports and record keeping are the topic of Section 4. The standard requires that all studies be interpreted and the final report verified by a qualified physician in a timely fashion. Permanent records must be made and retained, using the legal guidelines of the state in which the laboratory practices. If preliminary reports are issued, they must be clearly identified as preliminary, and a policy must be in place to address how any discrepancies between the preliminary and final report, should they occur, are resolved. Patient safety is addressed in Section 5 of the standard and requires that policies be in place for the reporting of patient or staff incidents, infection control, and transducer cleaning,

and that appropriate equipment and personnel are present to handle any medical emergencies. The final section of this standard addresses continuing education requirements. It specifies that personnel participate in current, relevant continuing education and that adequate reference textbooks and journals are available.

The essentials and standards for cerebrovascular, peripheral arterial, peripheral venous, and visceral vascular testing have identical sections. Because of the specific audience of this text, the Cerebrovascular Testing Standard is used as the example. Section 1 addresses the instrumentation necessary for testing and is separated into primary and secondary instrumentation. In order to be compliant, primary instrumentation must be used for testing patients. For extracranial cerebrovascular testing, duplex scanning is the only primary instrument. The standard outlines the requirements for transducer frequency for both imaging and Doppler, the importance of angle correction, and the ability to adjust the size and location of the sample volume. Other instruments such as continuous-wave Doppler and oculoplethysmography are considered secondary and should not be used alone for the diagnosis of cerebrovascular disease. Indications for testing are the focus of Section 2. All patients being tested should be referred for appropriate indications for testing. These indications vary, depending on clinical conditions. The application for accreditation requires listing the indications by percent. Section 2 also outlines the techniques necessary to complete an examination. In general terms, the standard describes imaging, hemodynamics, and views appropriate for testing. Section 3 describes the diagnostic criteria to be used for reporting. It requires reporting both image and Doppler information, as well as adherence to the stated criteria in the final report. It allows for the use of published or internally generated criteria. Procedure volumes is the topic of Section 4. For all four areas of testing, it is necessary to perform and interpret a minimum number of procedures annually to remain competent. The commission has determined that a laboratory must perform at least 100 carotid duplex examinations annually in order to maintain proficiency. The final section in each standard addresses quality assurance. This section is divided into two areas: instrument maintenance and correlation and confirmation of results. Instrument maintenance requires that all instrumentation used in the laboratory is maintained in good operating condition and undergoes periodic calibration. Each piece of equipment should have regular, documented inspections for electrical safety, and it is recommended that tissue-equivalent phantom testing be done on all imaging systems on a regular basis either by laboratory personnel or as part of a manufacturer's maintenance agreement. For correlation and confirmation of test results, the standard requires ongoing

Table 1. Sample of accuracy determination

		Carotid angiogram categories[1]						
		Norm	1-19%	20-39%	40-59%	60-79%	80-99%	Occl
Carotid	Norm	6	4	1				
Duplex	1-19%	2	7	1	3			
Scan	20-39%		3	4	2	1		
Categories	40-59%		1	1	10	1	2	
	60-79%				2	8	3	1
	80-99%				2	1	12	3
	Occl						2	5
		Exact correlation = 52		Total exams = 88		Percent agreement = 52/88 = 59%		

[1]The above chart is only a suggestion and is not required for accreditation. Laboratory personnel may submit documentation of alternate methods or techniques for quality assurance.

comparison with a reference standard. For carotid duplex scanning, this standard is generally arteriography. The commission suggests that a table be utilized to determine the overall accuracy of carotid duplex scanning (Sample: Table 1). The table should be edited to use the laboratory's specific criteria for categories of stenosis. In addition to completing the table, laboratories applying for accreditation must support these figures with logs, records, arteriogram reports, and any other materials used to compile the statistical analysis.

SELF-STUDIES

The self-study documents are detailed questionnaires that, once completed by the laboratory, become the application for accreditation. The organization self-study requires documentation of education, experience, background, and relevant continuing medical education for the past 3 years for the medical and technical directors and all members of the medical and technical staff. It requires each member to list the number of procedures they perform or interpret in an average week. It requires a listing of the support services available and a schematic drawing of the physical facility. It asks specific questions regarding record retention, report generation and physician reading policies. The organization self-study also requires submission of a laboratory-specific policy for reading privileges as well as policies for infection control, patient safety, incident reporting, and emergency medical procedures. The final section requires detailed information about each piece of equipment used in the laboratory and the maintenance procedures for each piece. Like the standards, the self-study documents are divided into sections. Each specific area of testing has its own self-study to be completed, and all are organized in similar fashion. Section 1 requires the laboratory to identify which pieces of equipment are used for specific areas of testing. It is

necessary to list all indications for each area of testing by percent in Section 2. There are also questions asked about referral patterns in this section. Section 2 also requires a technical protocol for each procedure performed in the laboratory. The protocols should be laboratory-specific and not a copy of a manual or textbook. They should provide sufficient detail to allow the reviewer a clear picture of how a test is completed, such as patient position, image and Doppler acquisition information including frequency of image and Doppler sampling information, angle correction details, worksheet information, and reporting routines. Section 3 requires a listing and referencing of the diagnostic criteria used for reporting, which may include a chart or graph of the criteria used and proof of validation of the criteria in the quality assurance section. Section 4, procedure volumes, requires specific statistics for a 1-year period that list the volume of procedures performed. It also asks what percentage are performed on a bedside and portable basis. In addition, this section requires submission of a specific number of completed case studies. Each case must have enough hard copy to support both the technique and the diagnosis. The case studies should also contain any worksheets used and any reports of correlation that may have been obtained. The final section of the self-study asks specific questions regarding correlation policies. It requires documentation of responsibility for obtaining the correlation results and comparing them to the noninvasive studies, how frequently these procedures are carried out, and how the resulting information regarding accuracy is disseminated to the staff.

COST OF ACCREDITATION

A laboratory may apply for accreditation in a single area of testing or all areas of testing that are currently offered, provided the volume requirements are met. The fees for accreditation are $1000 for one area of testing and $1500 for two or more areas applied for at the same time. Accreditation fees are the primary source of revenue for the commission. Accreditation is valid for a period of 3 years.

DECISIONS

Once an application has been reviewed, it is either granted accreditation, required a site visit, or is denied. Occasionally the decision will be deferred because additional information is required before a decision can be made.

APPLICATION INFORMATION

Completed applications for accreditation are accepted at any time in the ICAVL office; however, quarterly deadlines have been established that allow for a schedule of review activities. Deadlines generally occur on March 1, June 1, September 1, and November 1 of each year. Once an application is received in the office, it is processed and reviewed for completeness and assigned to two reviewers. It is then sent to the reviewers, whose findings are discussed at a scheduled meeting of the board of directors, usually 2 months following a deadline. The board decides whether substantial compliance to the standards has been demonstrated and agrees to either accredit, deny, or visit the laboratory. Occasionally the decision may be deferred for additional information. If a laboratory is accredited, the reviewer's findings are compiled into a critique letter and sent to the laboratory approximately 6 to 8 weeks following the review meeting. If a laboratory is denied, it also takes approximately 6 to 8 weeks for that decision as well. In the case of denial, a laboratory has the right to appeal the decision if they feel it has been made in error. If a site visit is necessary, notification is sent within 1 week of the meeting, and arrangements are made for the site visit to be completed prior to the next scheduled board meeting.

STATISTICS

The first orders for standards and self-studies were processed in May of 1991. Since that time, more than 2000 orders for accreditation materials have been processed. As of November 1994, there are more than 500 accredited laboratories in Canada and the United States, including Puerto Rico. Of the laboratories applying for accreditation, 63% are hospital based and 37% are private office, mobile, or clinic-based practices. The medical director is a vascular or general surgeon in 67% of the accredited laboratories; a neurologist is the medical director in 4% of the laboratories applying for accreditation.

BENEFITS OF ACCREDITATION

Through accreditation, peer recognition of the high-quality noninvasive vascular testing is granted. This permits the accredited laboratory to distinguish itself

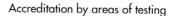

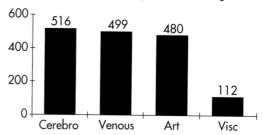

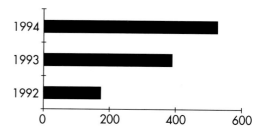

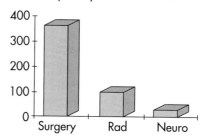

through its commitment to providing high-quality patient care. When a laboratory is granted accreditation, a detailed letter outlining the strengths and weaknesses, as identified through the review process, is sent to the medical director of the laboratory along with a certificate of accreditation for each area of testing that has been granted accreditation. In addition to this letter and the certificates, a press release that details the prevalence of vascular disease and the importance of accurate noninvasive diagnosis is also sent. An accredited laboratory may use this press release, in whole or part, in their marketing efforts and, in addition, may also submit the names and addresses of local newspapers, radio stations, and television stations for the ICAVL to send this release on official letterhead. A camera-ready logo, identifying the laboratory as accredited by the ICAVL, is also sent to the laboratory and may be used on letterhead, report forms, or other printed material as chosen by the laboratory.

EFFECTS OF ACCREDITATION

Since the inception of vascular laboratory accreditation, many positive results have been reported as a result of completing the process. Almost all laboratories that have completed the process report improved organization. The area most often improved appears to be that of quality assurance. Although most laboratories previously had some degree of correlation efforts, many were informal with little documentation. As a result of completing the accreditation process, those efforts are now more formalized and well documented. It also has necessitated the review and update of all policies and testing procedures. The need for more relevant continuing education is usually identified, and policies are initiated that ensure ongoing relevant education for all members of the laboratory staff. There is also an increase in the number of technologists and physicians applying to take the RVT (Registered Vascular Technologist) examination through the American Registry of Diagnostic Medical Sonographers. This increase in formal qualifications of laboratory staff is felt to be directly related to the requirements for accreditation.

FOR MORE INFORMATION

The office of the ICAVL is staffed to answer any questions regarding the accreditation process. The commission's office is located at 14750 Sweitzer Lane, Suite 102, Laurel, MD 20707. The telephone number is (301)317-1700; fax (301)317-0256.

Appendix III

QUALITY ASSURANCE IN THE VASCULAR LABORATORY

Anne M. Jones

The purpose of a noninvasive neurovascular laboratory is to indentify, localize, and quantify the severity of extracranial and intracranial stenoses and to assess the contribution of the collateral network to brain perfusion. According to Sumner,[8] measurements completed in the vascular laboratory should be simple, accurate, and reproducible, providing unique information pertinent to the clinical evaluation; they should also be cost-effective, not duplicating information already available to the clinician. In most clinical settings, noninvasive anatomic and physiologic studies are the test of choice for the initial assessment of patients with suspected cerebrovascular disease.

ESTABLISHING THE NONINVASIVE VASCULAR LABORATORY

The growing interest in standardization, quality assurance, and appropriate utilization of noninvasive testing creates an environment requiring accountability, commitment, and expertise. Noninvasive laboratories must be able to support their findings with statistics and demonstrate compliance with nationally recognized standards.[6,10] Prior to opening a neurosonology laboratory, considerable thought must be given to the purpose and scope of the lab. Which studies should be completed? Which measurements should be made? The choices of how and what to measure are important for a number of reasons. First, the methods help to define standards used to separate normals from abnormals. By defining specific, objective, measurable parameters, the severity of disease or degree of physiologic impairment can be defined. In addition, serial examinations can recognize, document, and quantify changes since the previous noninvasive examination.

Measurements are important for another reason – to convey information from one laboratory to another. All too often, duplicate studies must be done because one laboratory did not complete the examination or report results according to a standard format. In order to report objective findings to the academic or clinical community, specific guidelines for measurement and interpretation must be defined and followed. In doing so, the added benefit of objectively assessing the incidence prevalence and natural history of cerebrovascular disease can be accomplished.

LABORATORY STAFF: PREREQUISITES

Often, the decision to establish a noninvasive neurovascular laboratory is made by planners or administrators, who pay little attention to the scope and purpose of the laboratory or to the choice of medical director. These decisions are crucial to the ultimate success of the laboratory. Even a medical director who does not define the purpose of the lab should agree with the scope of the lab and define all aspects of laboratory operations. The choice of medical director is not a popularity contest; the person with the busiest clinical practice is not necessarily the person for the job. The medical director should be a physician with a keen understanding of cerebrovascular disease who has experience or training in noninvasive testing. Prior experience, acquired during a residency or fellowship, should be a prerequisite, as it adds stability and credibility to the laboratory. In the absence of these credentials, the medical director should have a working knowledge of noninvasive techniques and an appreciation of the capabilities and limitations of each procedure. This knowledge base will help the medical director make informed decisions about instrumentation, medical and technical staff, and the choice of procedures provided by the lab. The medical director is ultimately responsible for clinical and administrative duties; a long-term commitment is required to develop and manage a noninvasive neurovascular lab.

The choice of a qualified medical director is important; the choice of a qualified technical director is vital. The technical director is responsible for the day-to-day operation of the laboratory. This individual must be extremely knowledgeable about vascular disease, noninvasive testing modalities, and the strengths and limitations of each procedure offered by the lab. The technical director should have at least 5 years of clinical experience and be capable of evaluating data, modifying procedures, and working closely with the medical staff to maximize laboratory productivity. Although a certification examination designed for neurovascular technologists is not currently available, the vascular technology examinations offered by the American Registry of Diagnostic Medical Sonographers (ARDMS) include noninvasive evaluation of cerebrovascular disease.[1] The vascular technologist is encouraged to sit for this exam and acquire the Registered Vascular Technology (RVT) credential as proof of competence in the field.[2,3,5]

SUPPORT STAFF

The medical director and technical director should collaborate to define the job descriptions and prerequisites for potential members of the medical, technical, and ancillary staff. Although experienced individuals are occasionally available, most laboratories must provide educational support and "on-the-job" training for support staff. In the most recent survey of the responsibilities of vascular technologists performed by the American Registry of Diagnostic Medical Sonographers (ARDMS), 73% of the respondents stated that they were trained on the job, and only 13% had completed some type of allied health program.[9] Therefore, it is essential that the medical and technical directors design an educational program for technologists in training, as well as for physicians seeking reading privileges in the lab. The educational program can include reading assignments, didactic and technical components, as well as supervision by experienced members of the staff. Well-defined guidelines can define short-term and long-term objectives for technologists and physicians

and provide a basis for objective performance appraisals. The technologists should be provided an extensive period of supervised patient testing so that they are adequately exposed to all required techniques. The training period for technologists can vary but is usually 6 months.[4]

Members of the medical staff may be required to work closely with the medical director, completing a type of "apprenticeship." This apprenticeship allows the medical director to share expertise, define interpretive protocols, and confirm that all members of the medical staff are interpreting studies according to the protocols established by the laboratory. Upon completion of the training period, the medical director should routinely review studies interpreted by the medical staff members for 3 to 6 months and then randomly review studies as a part of an ongoing quality control program. All members of the medical and technical staff should understand the technical and diagnostic protocols of the laboratory.

As previously mentioned, a major component of the technical director's job is education and instruction of the technical staff. The laboratory's educational program must be clearly defined. The training may include short-term, educational programs specifically tailored to meet the needs of the neurovascular technologist. Before attending such a program, the technologist should review the course objectives and content and be assured that the faculty members have adequate clinical expertise. The program should provide a focused, comprehensive introduction to the fundamentals of noninvasive cerebrovascular testing and include hands-on training. After attending the program, the technologist should return to the clinical setting and have adequate time and supervision to develop the necessary technical skills. To familiarize the new technologist with instrumentation, examination techniques, and normal anatomy, it is helpful to provide scanning of "normal volunteers"—individuals who do not have disease but are willing to have a study completed by the novice technologist. After completing a series of normals, the technologist is allowed to complete studies on patients with known pathology, to familiarize them with the anatomic changes and flow characteristics associated with disease. Finally, the technologist is prepared to perform clinical examinations on patients, under the supervision of the technical director. The technical director should perform at least a limited examination on all of these patients during the initial training period and, for at least 6 months, review all studies on patients before they are allowed to leave the laboratory. Although every technologist develops expertise at a different rate, in a high-volume laboratory (100 exams/week), the technologist should be prepared to work independently within 3 to 6 months.

INSTRUMENTATION

Second only to the choice of medical and technical staff is the choice of instrumentation. For extracranial cerebrovascular evaluation, the primary instrumentation includes either a duplex or color flow duplex system. These systems are the backbone of the laboratory, providing anatomic and physiologic evaluation of extracranial and, in some cases, intracranial vasculature. Because most of the commercially available duplex systems provide similar features, it is important to define the specific needs of the laboratory before considering a purchase. A list of required components is defined; it should include the required transducer(s) and frequencies, image quality, Doppler quality, hard-copy capabilities, software needs, and cost. If money is not an issue, color flow Doppler and a selection of transducers should be considered. Other parameters to consider may include size, portability, noise and heat output, ease of operation, educational and technical support, and cost of service contracts after the initial warranty has expired. In addition, it is important to explore the geographic location, availability, and experience of technical support personnel as well as the availability of loaner systems, should your system experience extended down time. If the laboratory only performs transcranial Doppler examinations (TCD), the same considerations apply.

During the evaluation period, request that the imaging systems being seriously considered for purchase remain in the laboratory for a short period; despite the staff's lack of familiarity with the system, a clinical trial period can be very useful and may have an impact on the purchase decision. It is also useful to request a reference list so that current users can be contacted.

Secondary instrumentation may also be purchased for the vascular laboratory. These studies provide additional physiologic data and are performed as an adjunct to the primary duplex evaluation; they may include oculopneumoplethysmography (OPG), TCD, and periorbital Doppler. Although the "secondary" instruments are much less costly than the duplex systems, accurate performance requires considerable expertise, and adequate educational support should be provided by the manufacturer.

PROTOCOLS AND VALIDATION STUDIES

Because the results of noninvasive neurovascular studies have an impact on the clinical management of the patient, the results must be validated prospectively against an established standard. To do this, technical protocols defining data acquisition and diagnostic protocols for data interpretation must be developed. Although these protocols may be based on published scientific data, they should be laboratory-specific. The data acquired in each laboratory may vary slightly because of the instrumentation, technique, patient population, or the gold standard available for correlation. Therefore, the diagnostic criteria for a specific laboratory will be accurate only if validated internally, using published data as a foundation or starting point; a new laboratory will complete prospective validation of data, while an established laboratory may review data retrospectively to assess the strengths and limitations of the lab. If sources of error are defined by the retrospective review, an improved plan for data acquisition can be defined and areas of concern corrected. Once the guidelines and protocols have been adopted, it is imperative that they be consistently applied by all members of the technical and medical staff.

STATISTICAL ANALYSIS OF DATA

Methods of analysis of scientific data can be highly variable, often providing vague and ambiguous results. It is important to decide in advance which information will be most useful to the clinician, the patient, and the laboratory. It is advisable to calculate overall accuracy, sensitivity, and specificity as well as positive and negative predictive values.[7] Although other parameters can also be reviewed, this information is useful to the clinician who is managing the patient and to the laboratory performing noninvasive studies. To calculate these statistics, laboratory test results must be compared to the established gold standard, usually cerebral angiography or surgery. It is advisable to utilize a double-blind method, so that the individual reading the noninvasive results is unaware of the results of the gold standard and vice versa.

The simplest statistic compares the outcome of each test as either positive or negative. A true-positive result indicates that both tests are positive. A true-negative result indicates that both tests are negative. A false-positive result means that the gold standard is negative, indicating the absence of disease, while the noninvasive study was positive, indicating the presence of disease. A false-negative result occurs when the noninvasive test indicates the absence of disease but the gold standard is positive.

True-positive and true-negative results can be used to calculate sensitivity and specificity. *Sensitivity* is the ability of a test to recognize disease. It can be calculated by dividing the number of true-positive tests by the total number of positive results obtained by the gold standard.

Specificity is the ability to recognize the absence of disease and is calculated by dividing the true negatives by the total number of negative results obtained by the gold standard.

The clinician ordering the noninvasive test is eager to know the predictive value of the test. In other words, what is the likelihood that a positive result actually proves that disease is present and that a negative result

$$\text{Sensitivity} = \frac{\text{True positives}}{\text{True positives} + \text{false negatives}}$$

$$\text{Specificity} = \frac{\text{True negatives}}{\text{True negatives} + \text{false positives}}$$

$$\text{Positive predictive value (PPV)} = \frac{\text{True positives}}{\text{True positives} + \text{false positives}}$$

$$\text{Negative predictive value (NPV)} = \frac{\text{True negatives}}{\text{True negatives} + \text{false negatives}}$$

proves the absence of disease? These results can be obtained by calculating the positive predictive value (PPV), or likelihood that disease is present, and the negative predictive value (NPV), the likelihood that disease is not present. The calculations are described in the accompanying figures. Overall accuracy can be calculated by dividing the number of true negatives and true positives by the total number of tests performed. These results are not very specific and can be highly variable, based on the incidence of disease in the patient population.

It is often difficult to know the best type of noninvasive test to use for a given disease process or patient population. Sumner states that the role of the test in clinical practice should be kept in mind.[8] If the goal of the test is to rule out the presence of disease, then a sensitive test should be used. If the goal of the noninvasive test is to confirm the presence of disease, then a specific test should be used. Because the patient population referred to the noninvasive lab is diverse, high levels of sensitivity and specificity help to make the level of diagnostic confidence optimal.

CONTINUING MEDICAL EDUCATION

Although the initial education of the medical and technical staff may be adequate, it must be continually updated and reinforced through continuing medical education. If the cost of attending a national symposium is prohibitive, alternative methods of continuing medical education can be developed. These methods may include grand rounds, journal clubs, laboratory staff meetings for correlation data reviews, or invited lectures by members of the medical and technical staff. Many of these activities qualify for CME recognition by the Continuing Medical Education Department of a medical center or the professional ultrasound or vascular technology associations. Because CME is required to maintain the ARDMS credential and receive vascular lab accreditation, it is important to explore all possible avenues for continuing medical education and to establish policies and funding to support these efforts.

LABORATORY ACCREDITATION

The collaborative effort among specialists in noninvasive vascular testing has resulted in the creation of standards for cerebrovascular, peripheral arterial, peripheral venous, and visceral vascular testing. At this

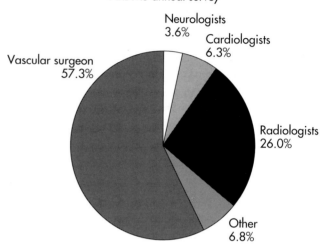

Who read the studies of RVT's
ARDMS annual survey

Neurologists 3.6%
Cardiologists 6.3%
Vascular surgeon 57.3%
Radiologists 26.0%
Other 6.8%

time, standards for transcranial Doppler are being tested in pilot laboratories. The standards were developed as a guideline for vascular laboratory accreditation by the Intersocietal Commission for the Accreditation of Vascular Laboratories (ICAVL). The accreditation process, outlined in another appendix, has been endorsed by most of the professional organizations involved in noninvasive peripheral vascular and cerebrovascular testing. The accreditation process is designed to improve patient care and establish guidelines for appropriate utilization of noninvasive techniques. It is in the best interest of the profession to endorse the process of accreditation and to support voluntary certification of personnel as the gold standard of quality control. Imposing voluntary standards on our profession may be the best way to assure competence.

CONCLUSION

Establishing a neurovascular laboratory requires more than space and instrumentation; it requires carefully planned goals and objectives, committed medical and technical directors, and well-trained and competent medical and technical staff. The clinical neurologist is in the minority in this area of vascular testing and may therefore be held to a higher standard of accountability. Appropriate studies must be performed and interpreted according to well-defined, statistically validated protocols. Results must show acceptable sensitivity, specificity, and accuracy. Continuing medical education must be provided for all members of the medical and technical staff; certification should be encouraged, if not required. The ultimate reward will be a financially self-supporting, high-volume laboratory that provides appropriate care to patients and accurate results to the referring physician.

REFERENCES

1. ARDMS examination and information booklet, Cincinnati, 1994, American Registry of Diagnostic Medical Sonographers.
2. Burnham CB, Nix ML: *Establishing technical competence in the vascular laboratory.* In Bernstein EF, editor: *Vascular diagnosis,* St Louis, 1993, Mosby–Year Book.
3. Cardullo PA: Support the RVT credential, *J Vasc Technol* 11:164, 1987 (editorial).
4. Jones AM: *Education and training of the vascular technologist.* In Bernstein EF, editor: *Vascular diagnosis,* St Louis, 1993, Mosby–Year Book.
5. Jones AM: Is the RVT credential necessary? In support of the RVT credential, *J Vasc Technol* 17:99-100, 1993.
6. Kempczinski RF: *Quality control in the vascular laboratory.* In Bernstein EF, editor: *Vascular diagnosis,* St Louis, 1993, Mosby–Year Book.
7. Sumner DS: *Evaluation of noninvasive testing procedures: data analysis and interpretation.* In Bernstein EF, editor: *Vascular diagnosis,* St Louis, 1993, Mosby–Year Book.
8. Sumner DS: *What should we measure?* In Bernstein EF, editor: *Vascular diagnosis,* St Louis, 1993, Mosby–Year Book.
9. *Survey of the responsibilities of vascular technologists,* Cincinnati, 1994, American Registry of Diagnostic Medical Sonographers.
10. Thiele BL: *Accreditation of vascular laboratories.* In Bernstein EF, editor: *Vascular diagnosis,* St Louis, 1993, Mosby–Year Book.